I0072030

Drug Safety and Pharmacoepidemiology

Drug Safety and Pharmacoepidemiology

Editor: Avianna Stokes

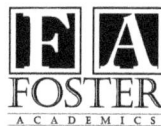

FA
FOSTER
ACADEMICS

www.fosteracademics.com

www.fosteracademics.com

FA FOSTER
ACADEMICS

Cataloging-in-Publication Data

Drug safety and pharmacoepidemiology / edited by Avianna Stokes.
    p. cm.
Includes bibliographical references and index.
ISBN 978-1-63242-578-2
1. Drugs--Side effects. 2. Drugs--Safety measures. 3. Pharmacoepidemiology.
4. Drugs--Safety regulations. I. Stokes, Avianna.
RM302.5 .D78 2019
615.704 2--dc23

© Foster Academics, 2019

Foster Academics,
118-35 Queens Blvd., Suite 400,
Forest Hills, NY 11375, USA

ISBN 978-1-63242-578-2 (Hardback)

This book contains information obtained from authentic and highly regarded sources. Copyright for all individual chapters remain with the respective authors as indicated. All chapters are published with permission under the Creative Commons Attribution License or equivalent. A wide variety of references are listed. Permission and sources are indicated; for detailed attributions, please refer to the permissions page and list of contributors. Reasonable efforts have been made to publish reliable data and information, but the authors, editors and publisher cannot assume any responsibility for the validity of all materials or the consequences of their use.

Trademark Notice: Registered trademark of products or corporate names are used only for explanation and identification without intent to infringe.

Contents

Preface

Pharmacoepidemiology is concerned with the study of the uses of drugs and their effects in specific populations. It builds on the principles of pharmacology and epidemiology. Drug safety is a significant area of pharmacoepidemiology. It studies the adverse effects of drugs. It is concerned with the assessment, detection, monitoring and prevention of adverse drug reactions. Overdose, misuse and abuse of drugs as well as drug exposure during critical stages of human life such as pregnancy and breastfeeding, are also studied in this field. This book aims to shed light on some of the unexplored aspects of drug safety and pharmacoepidemiology. It strives to provide a fair idea about these disciplines and to help develop a better understanding of the latest advances within these fields. Students, researchers, experts, pharmacologists and all associated with these fields will benefit alike from this book.

After months of intensive research and writing, this book is the end result of all who devoted their time and efforts in the initiation and progress of this book. It will surely be a source of reference in enhancing the required knowledge of the new developments in the area. During the course of developing this book, certain measures such as accuracy, authenticity and research focused analytical studies were given preference in order to produce a comprehensive book in the area of study.

This book would not have been possible without the efforts of the authors and the publisher. I extend my sincere thanks to them. Secondly, I express my gratitude to my family and well-wishers. And most importantly, I thank my students for constantly expressing their willingness and curiosity in enhancing their knowledge in the field, which encourages me to take up further research projects for the advancement of the area.

Editor

Adverse Drug Events Related to Canagliflozin: A Meta-Analysis of Randomized, Placebo-Controlled Trials

Shawaqfeh MS*, Bhinder MT, Halum AS, Harrington C, Muflih S and Do T
Nova Southeastern University, Palm Beach Gardens, Florida, United States

Abstract

Canagliflozin, a sodium-glucose co-transporter 2 (SGLT2) inhibitor, was recently approved in United States for the treatment of type 2 diabetes mellitus in combination with diet and exercise. Two strengths were approved, 100 mg and 300 mg. The US label warns of a dose-dependent increase in volume depletion-related adverse reactions on the 300 mg dose. The purpose of this meta-analysis was to assess the dose response of canaglifozin on safety and tolerability outcomes.

A search was performed through MEDLINE, EMBASE, and Cochrane Library for clinical trials comparing canagliflozin with placebo or active controls. Keywords include canagliflozin, and meta-analysis. Reference lists of relevant articles were also used as sources. Two reviewers extracted data and evaluated pertinent studies. Study characteristics, safety outcomes of interest, and risk of bias were collected, verified and further analyzed. Canagliflozin was studied as monotherapy in 2 trials (n=270) and as an add-on therapy in 10 studies (n=2525). Ten of the studies were included in the analysis of selected safety outcomes. Length of intervention ranged from 12 to 52 weeks. All studies were randomized, comparative to either placebo or active controls. Canagliflozin treatment, , increased the risk of vulvovaginal mycotic infection (RR 4.11; CI 3.01-5.60; P<0.01), pollakiuria (RR 2.89, CI 1.84-4.53), polyuria (RR 3.87; CI 1.66-9.05), hypoglycemia (RR 1.22; CI 1.10-1.35) and hypovolemia (RR 2.04; CI 1.13-3.68). There were no significant dose responses among observed safety outcomes with the exception of genital infections (RR 4.12; CI 2.47-6.87). Additionally, the canagliflozin treatment group experienced a 24% reduction in serious adverse events when compared to controls (RR 0.76; 0.62-0.93; P<0.01).

This meta-analysis did not show a dose response effect of canaglifozin on treatment emergent adverse events in type 2 diabetics.

Keywords: Canagliflozin; Meta-analysis; Diabetes; Adverse events

Introduction

Diabetes Mellitus is fast becoming one of the most prevalent chronic diseases in the United States, with 14.3% of the population over 20 years of age suffering from this malady [1]. Patients are educated about the importance of having a multi-pronged approach in management of their disease, where one combines diet and exercise regimens with medications. Due to the constant advancement in medical research and innovation, new treatment regimens are constantly being invented to keep pace with the demand for better antidiabetic medications. As with any drug therapy regimen, there has to be a balance between its effectiveness and tolerability, and this is no different for new antidiabetic medications such as canagliflozin; a sodium-glucose co-transporter 2 (SGLT2) inhibitor. The drug, was the first of its kind (SGLT2s) to be approved for treatment of Type 2 Diabetes Mellitus in the United States [2,3]. These questions were answered in several clinical studies variably; this analysis will compile all these reports together in one report that will strengthen the evidence of adverse events reporting.

The drug is to be used as an adjunct with diet, exercise, and other antidiabetic drug classes. There are 100 mg and 300 mg strengths dosage approved, with the former being the starting dosage, incremented to the latter in patients who have normal renal function. Drug label warns of a dose-dependent increase in volume depletion-related adverse reactions on the 300 mg dose [4] the purpose of this meta-analysis is to assess the occurrence of drug-related adverse events associated with the use of canagliflozin at varying doses. The meta-analysis will have all randomized controlled trials that reported adverse events in a systematic way combined in one report that will verify the significance of dose related adverse events. This type of information will help the clinicians to decide safely about the appropriateness of their selection of canagliflozin.

Method

A systematic review was performed from September 2013–July 2015 using the EMBASE and MEDLINE databases, identifying Cochrane reviews, controlled clinical trials, randomized control trials, meta-analyses and systematic reviews, using search terms canagliflozin, placebo, adverse events, and humans. The studies were limited to those published in the English language, and conducted on humans. The Trial Registry website ClinicalTrials.gov was also searched for studies relating to canagliflozin.

The pertinent data describing adverse events was extracted from the safety results sections of the articles, including relevant text and tables. This data was then subsequently entered into Review Manager Software, Version 5.3 (The Nordic Cochrane Centre, The Cochrane Collaboration, and Copenhagen, Denmark) for analysis [5]. The

*Corresponding author: Shawaqfeh MS, Nova Southeastern University, Palm Beach Gardens, Florida, United States, E-mail: mshawaqfeh@nova.edu

aforementioned software has been made available by the Cochrane Collaboration to facilitate meta-analyses.

The data was combined for meta-analysis employing the Mantel-Haenszel method, random effects model at 95% confidence for the RR. Study characteristics and safety outcomes of interest were collected, verified and further analyzed, focusing on the frequencies of dose dependent adverse events for both the canagliflozin group and the placebo populations.

Results

Description of the included studies

In the initial stages of the study, there were 678 citations which were subjected to elemental review (Figure 1). Of those studies, randomized, placebo-controlled trials which described data on dose-related adverse events in adult patients taking canagliflozin were sent for further analysis while the others, which did not contain relevant information on adverse reactions, or did not have a placebo control were not included. Following this elemental review, there were 49 articles which were used for adverse event data extraction. Of those articles, 19 were included in the final analysis [6-24]. All of the studies were randomized, placebo controlled trials and one was the US label for brand name canagliflozin (Invokana; Janssen Pharmaceuticals, Inc., Titusville, NJ) [4].

All studies were conducted in adults, from varying centers in over 22 different countries around the world. The studies varied in length from 4 weeks up to 104 weeks. The trials included a total of 8932 patients, with population sizes ranging from 10-1452 patients in each trial. Canagliflozin doses ranged from 10 mg-800 mg/day.

Any adverse event

The overall rate of adverse events (Tables 1 and 2) in both the canagliflozin group and the placebo group were similar with the exception of a few adverse events. Furthermore, there was no dose-

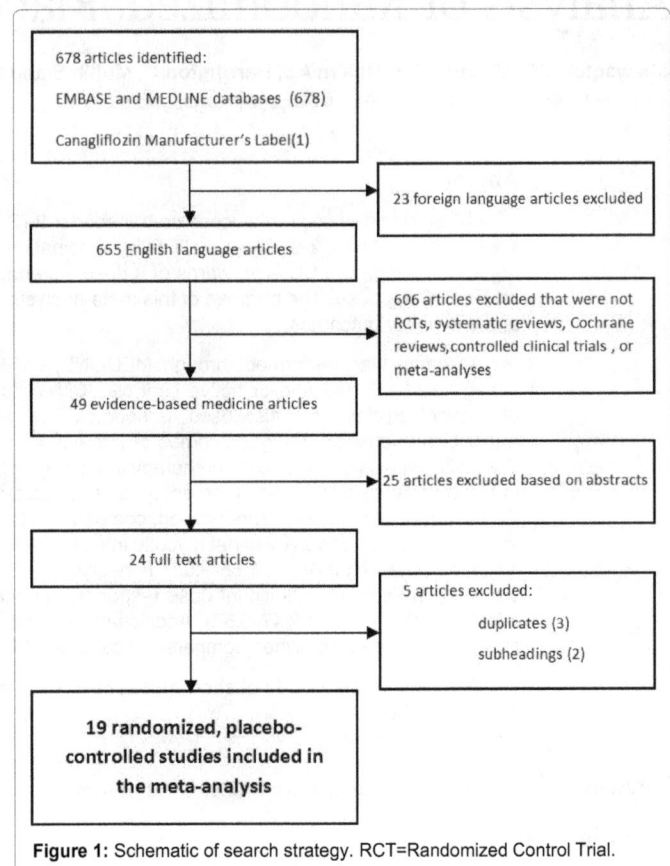

Figure 1: Schematic of search strategy. RCT=Randomized Control Trial.

Table 1: Treatment-emergent adverse events of canagliflozin 100 mg vs. control.

Adverse Event	No. of Studies	No. of Patients		Adverse Event Rate (%)		Risk Ratio
		Drug	Control	Drug	Control	M-H, Random, 95%
Any Adverse Event	16	2521	2512	65	64	1.02 [0.98, 1.06]
Serious Adverse Event	15	2737	2725	6.2	7.2	0.86 [0.71, 1.04]
AEs Leading to Discontinuation	14	2496	2488	4	3.9	1.01 [0.74, 1.39]
Postural Dizziness	8	1495	1480	0.87	0.675	1.20 [0.54, 2.68]
Hypovolamia	7	1505	1497	1.32	0.46	2.52 [1.10, 5.78]
Polyuria	5	1377	1367	0.726	0.14	3.22 [0.86, 12.02]
Pollakiuria	7	1505	1497	3.5	0.868	3.30 [1.48, 7.37]
Hypoglycaemia	11	1446	1435	15.97	11.2	1.40 [1.18, 1.66]
Vulvovaginal Mycotic Infection	9	781	741	12.03	2.56	4.24 [2.65, 6.78]
Genital Mycotic Infections	13	1678	1709	7.15	1.87	3.57 [2.40, 5.32]
Nasopharyngitis	4	295	294	3.72	6.12	0.69 [0.31, 1.52]
Nausea	4	231	228	4.32	2.19	1.68 [0.61, 4.66]
Headache	4	231	228	10.3	5.26	1.82 [0.94, 3.54]
Diarrhea	4	231	228	2.16	4.38	0.51 [0.19, 1.41]
Urinary Tract Infection	13	2422	2413	6.85	5.71	1.20 [0.96, 1.49]
Urinary Tract AEs	2	128	130	9.375	6.92	1.35 [0.59, 3.10]
Postural Hypotension	6	1441	1432	0.55	0.13	2.94 [0.81, 10.75]
Osmotic Diuresis-Related AEs	5	827	823	5.68	2.67	1.98 [1.02, 3.84]
Volume-Related AEs	5	824	827	3.03	1.45	2.09 [1.03, 4.23]

I^2 Index (%) =<50%

Table 2: Treatment-emergent adverse events of canagliflozin 300 mg vs. control.

| Adverse Event | No. of Studies | No. of Patients | | Adverse Event Rate (%) | | Risk Ratio |
		Drug	Control	Drug	Control	M-H, Random, 95%
Any Adverse Event	18	2836	2835	67	65	1.02 [0.99, 1.06]
Serious Adverse Event	15	3019	3010	6.29	7.17	0.89 [0.74, 1.07]
AEs Leading to Discontinuation	14	2783	2773	5.19	3.85	1.32 [1.03, 1.69]
Postural Dizziness	8	1857	1843	0.8	0.67	1.31 [0.58, 2.98]
Hypovolemia	8	1879	1875	0.9	0.54	1.63 [0.70, 3.79]
Polyuria	6	1751	1745	1.08	0.11	4.41 [1.45, 13.40]
Pollakiuria	8	1879	1875	2.92	0.96	2.64 [1.52, 4.61]
Hypoglycaemia	10	1721	1713	22.3	17.5	1.32 [1.08, 1.62]
Vulvovaginal Mycotic Infection	10	966	907	11.4	2.86	3.69 [2.45, 5.57]
Genital Mycotic Infections	13	1780	1830	8.53	1.47	4.88 [3.27, 7.28]
Nasopharyngitis	5	317	312	4.73	6.41	0.78 [0.41, 1.51]
Nausea	5	244	238	5.32	2.94	1.50 [0.62, 3.61]
Headache	4	234	228	6.83	5.26	1.37 [0.57, 3.30]
Diarrhea	5	252	246	5.15	4.47	1.13 [0.48, 2.66]
Urinary Tract Infection	13	2708	2698	6.61	5.85	1.14 [0.92, 1.40]
Urinary Tract AEs	2	128	130	9.37	6.92	1.35 [0.59, 3.10]
Postural Hypotension	7	1815	1810	0.49	0.16	1.99 [0.70, 5.62]
Osmotic Diuresis-Related AEs	5	829	823	6.87	2.67	2.42 [1.31, 4.48]
Volume-Related AEs	4	733	734	3.41	1.49	2.20 [1.08, 4.50]

I^2 Index (%) =<50%

dependent response associated with the development of any particular adverse event, generally being equally present in both cohorts. Additionally, the rate of inconsistency or heterogeneity, measured by I^2 was low, with many of the analyses presenting with no inconsistencies at all. The overall rate of any adverse event in the 100 mg Canagliflozin group was 65% and the 100 mg placebo group was 64%, with a risk ratio of 1.02 [0.98, 1.06]. In the 300 mg canagliflozin group, the rate of any adverse event was once again comparable to the placebo at 67% for the canagliflozin group and 65% for the placebo group. The risk ratio was 1.02 [0.99, 1.06].

Vulvovaginal mycotic infections/genital mycotic infections

The adverse events with the highest risk were the vulvovaginal mycotic infections and the genital mycotic infections, which showed a significant difference between the canagliflozin group and the placebo group. The adverse event rate of vulvovaginal mycotic infections (Figure 2) in the 100 mg canagliflozin group was 12% versus 2.56% in the placebo group, with a risk ratio of 4.24 [2.65, 6.78]. In the 300 mg canagliflozin group, the rate of vulvovaginal mycotic infections was 11.4% and the placebo group had 2.86%, with a RR of 3.69 [2.45, 5.57]. In the 100 mg canagliflozin group, the rate of genital mycotic infections was 7% versus 1.8% in the placebo group, RR 3.57 [2.40, 5.32]. In the 300 mg canagliflozin cohort, the rate of genital mycotic infection was 8.53% versus 1.47% in the placebo group with a RR of 4.88 [3.27, 7.28].

Osmotic diuresis-related adverse events

The adverse event rate of osmotic-diuresis related adverse events in the 100 mg group was 5.68% and 2.67% for the drug and placebo respectively, RR 1.98 [1.02, 3.84]. In the 300mg canagliflozin group, the rate of osmotic-diuresis related adverse events was 6.87% and the placebo group had 2.67%, with a RR of 2.42 [1.31, 4.48].

Volume-related adverse events

In the 100mg canagliflozin group, the rate of volume-related adverse events was 3.03% versus 1.45% in the placebo group, RR 2.09

[1.03, 4.23] (Figure 3). In the 300mg canagliflozin cohort, the rate of volume-related adverse events was 3.41% versus 1.49% in the placebo group with a RR of 2.20 [1.08, 4.50].

Hypoglycaemia

The adverse event rate of hypoglycaemia (Figure 4) in the 100 mg canagliflozin group was 15.97% versus 11.2% in the placebo group, with a risk ratio of 1.40 [1.18, 1.66]. In the 300 mg canagliflozin group, the rate of hypoglycaemia was 22.3% and the placebo group had 17.5%, with a RR of 1.32 [1.08, 1.62].

Other adverse events

Urinary tract adverse events had an adverse event rate of 9.375% in the canagliflozin group and 6.92% in the placebo group, RR 1.35 [0.59, 3.10]. The adverse event rate of pollakiuria in the 100 mg cohort was 3.5% for canagliflozin and 0.868% for the placebo, RR 3.30 [1.48, 7.37].

Discussion

There were 16 different types of adverse events associated with the use of canagliflozin. Overall, use of canagliflozin did not increase the incidence of any adverse event or serious adverse events. At the higher dose (300 mg), there was an increased risk of discontinuation of the drug due to adverse events RR 1.32 [1.03, 1.69]. Both the 100 mg and 300 mg dose of canagliflozin increased the risk of genital mycotic/vulvovaginal mycotic infections. To a lesser degree was the incidence of urinary tract adverse events. As is common knowledge, patients suffering from Type 2 Diabetes Mellitus are more prone to both urinary tract infections and genital mycotic infections due to a number of different rationale, such as decreased humoral immunity, increased urination, and possible urinary retention/ incontinence due to diabetic neuropathies.

However, when looking at canagliflozin and all SGLT2's role in the development of genital mycotic infections, one must look at its mechanism which facilitates glycosuria, likely a causative factor. It is

Study or Subgroup	Experimental Events	Total	Control Events	Total	Weight	Risk Ratio M-H, Random, 95% CI
1.9.1 100mg dose						
Bode 2013 PBO + AAD	18	117	2	94	4.7%	7.23 [1.72, 30.38]
Cefalu 2012 v GLIM + Met	26	231	5	219	10.9%	4.93 [1.93, 12.61]
Chen, 2015	2	15	0	15	1.1%	5.00 [0.26, 96.13]
Inagaki 2013 PBO Mono	1	22	0	21	1.0%	2.87 [0.12, 66.75]
Lavalle-G 2013 Sita + Met	22	194	5	194	10.6%	4.40 [1.70, 11.38]
Rosenstock 2012 PBO + Met	7	28	1	34	2.3%	8.50 [1.11, 65.03]
Rosenstock 2012 Sita Met	7	28	2	27	4.4%	3.38 [0.77, 14.82]
Stenlof 2013 PBO Mono	10	114	4	104	7.5%	2.28 [0.74, 7.05]
Yale 2013 PBO + OAD	1	32	0	33	1.0%	3.09 [0.13, 73.19]
Subtotal (95% CI)		781		741	43.4%	4.24 [2.65, 6.78]
Total events	94		19			

Heterogeneity: Tau² = 0.00; Chi² = 2.48, df = 8 (P = 0.96); I² = 0%
Test for overall effect: Z = 6.02 (P < 0.00001)

Study or Subgroup	Experimental Events	Total	Control Events	Total	Weight	Risk Ratio M-H, Random, 95% CI
1.9.2 300mg dose						
Bode 2013 PBO + AAD	12	107	2	94	4.4%	5.27 [1.21, 22.95]
Cefalu 2012 v GLIM + Met	34	244	5	219	11.3%	6.10 [2.43, 15.33]
Inagaki 2013 PBO Mono	1	20	0	21	1.0%	3.14 [0.14, 72.92]
Lavalle-G 2013 Sita + Met	20	202	5	194	10.4%	3.84 [1.47, 10.03]
Rosenstock 2012 PBO + Met	4	28	1	34	2.1%	4.86 [0.58, 41.01]
Rosenstock 2012 Sita Met	4	28	2	27	3.7%	1.93 [0.38, 9.68]
Schernthaner Sit + OAD	26	170	7	163	14.7%	3.56 [1.59, 7.98]
Sha, 2014	1	18	0	18	1.0%	3.00 [0.13, 69.09]
Stenlof 2013 PBO Mono	8	108	4	104	7.0%	1.93 [0.60, 6.20]
Yale 2013 PBO + OAD	1	41	0	33	1.0%	2.43 [0.10, 57.73]
Subtotal (95% CI)		966		907	56.6%	3.69 [2.45, 5.57]
Total events	111		26			

Heterogeneity: Tau² = 0.00; Chi² = 3.40, df = 9 (P = 0.95); I² = 0%
Test for overall effect: Z = 6.22 (P < 0.00001)

Total (95% CI)		1747		1648	100.0%	3.92 [2.88, 5.34]
Total events	205		45			

Heterogeneity: Tau² = 0.00; Chi² = 6.07, df = 18 (P = 1.00); I² = 0%
Test for overall effect: Z = 8.64 (P < 0.00001)
Test for subgroup differences: Chi² = 0.19, df = 1 (P = 0.67), I² = 0%

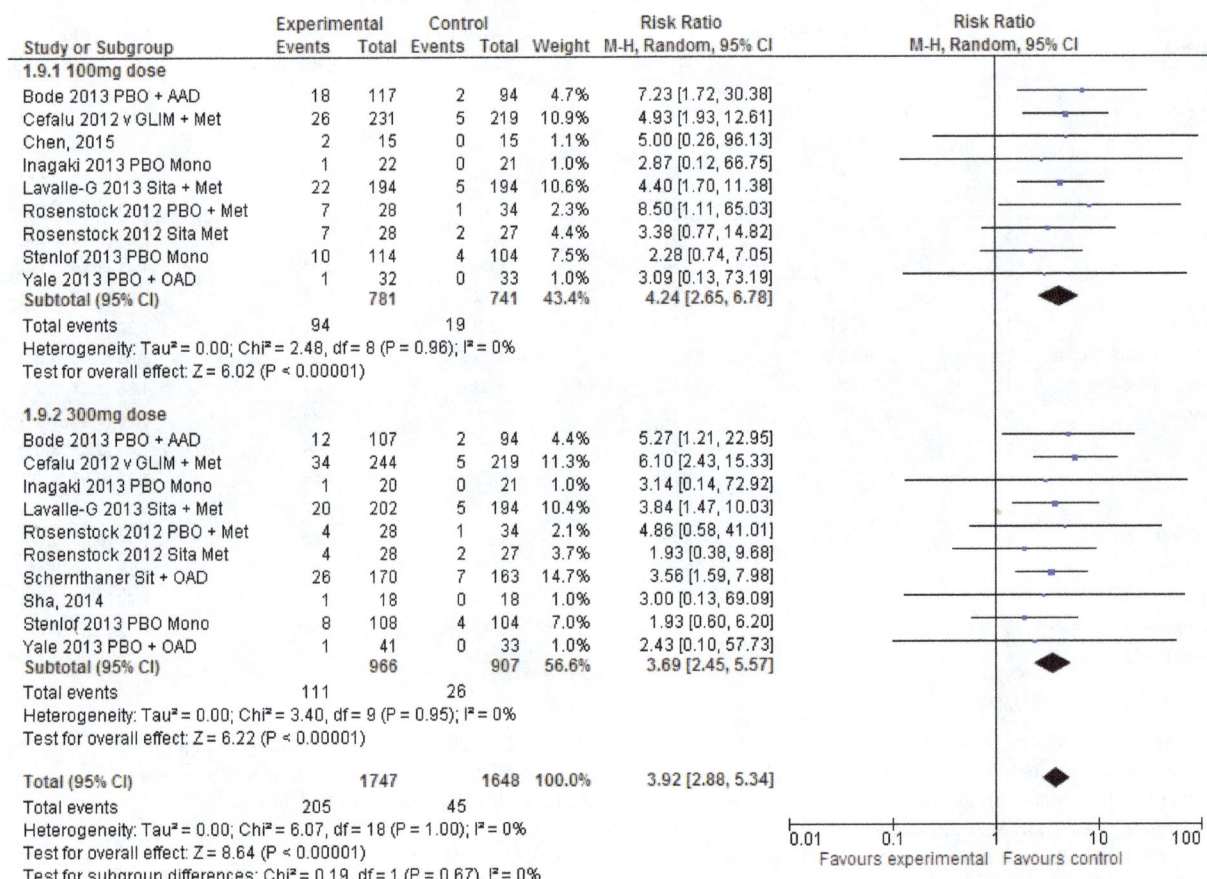

Figure 2: Forest plot of comparison of treatment-emergent vulvovaginal mycotic infection with canagliflozin 100 mg and 300 mg.

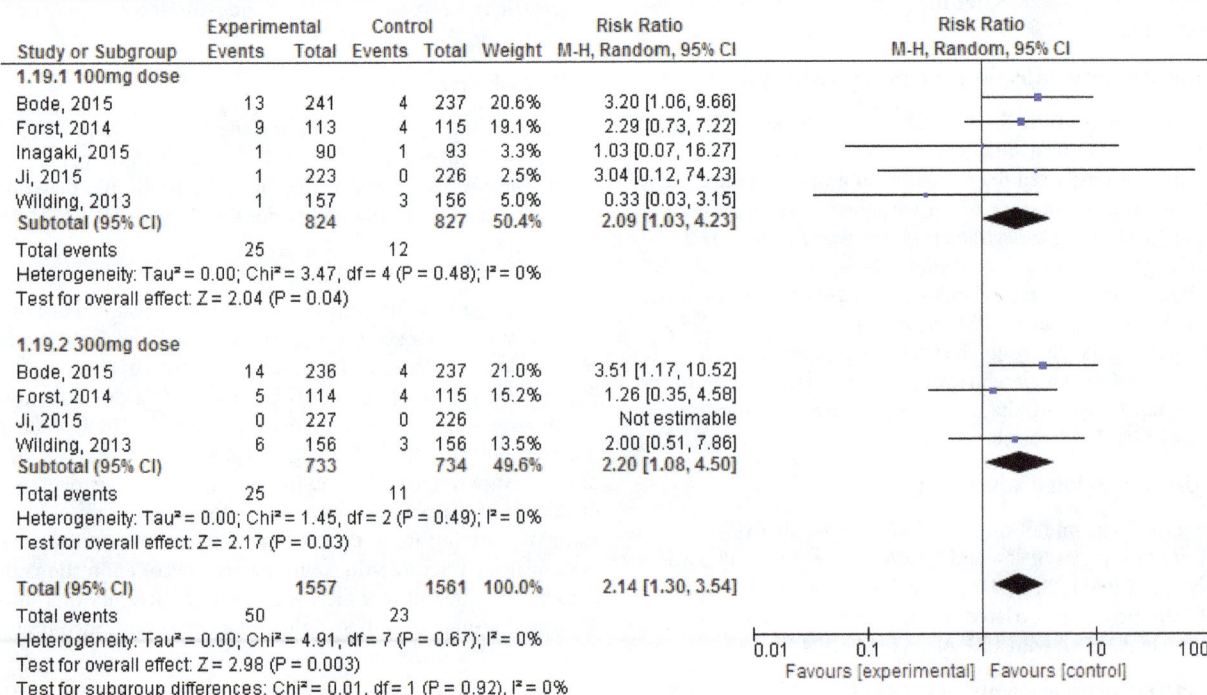

Study or Subgroup	Experimental Events	Total	Control Events	Total	Weight	Risk Ratio M-H, Random, 95% CI
1.19.1 100mg dose						
Bode, 2015	13	241	4	237	20.6%	3.20 [1.06, 9.66]
Forst, 2014	9	113	4	115	19.1%	2.29 [0.73, 7.22]
Inagaki, 2015	1	90	1	93	3.3%	1.03 [0.07, 16.27]
Ji, 2015	1	223	0	226	2.5%	3.04 [0.12, 74.23]
Wilding, 2013	1	157	3	156	5.0%	0.33 [0.03, 3.15]
Subtotal (95% CI)		824		827	50.4%	2.09 [1.03, 4.23]
Total events	25		12			

Heterogeneity: Tau² = 0.00; Chi² = 3.47, df = 4 (P = 0.48); I² = 0%
Test for overall effect: Z = 2.04 (P = 0.04)

Study or Subgroup	Experimental Events	Total	Control Events	Total	Weight	Risk Ratio M-H, Random, 95% CI
1.19.2 300mg dose						
Bode, 2015	14	236	4	237	21.0%	3.51 [1.17, 10.52]
Forst, 2014	5	114	4	115	15.2%	1.26 [0.35, 4.58]
Ji, 2015	0	227	0	226		Not estimable
Wilding, 2013	6	156	3	156	13.5%	2.00 [0.51, 7.86]
Subtotal (95% CI)		733		734	49.6%	2.20 [1.08, 4.50]
Total events	25		11			

Heterogeneity: Tau² = 0.00; Chi² = 1.45, df = 2 (P = 0.49); I² = 0%
Test for overall effect: Z = 2.17 (P = 0.03)

Total (95% CI)		1557		1561	100.0%	2.14 [1.30, 3.54]
Total events	50		23			

Heterogeneity: Tau² = 0.00; Chi² = 4.91, df = 7 (P = 0.67); I² = 0%
Test for overall effect: Z = 2.98 (P = 0.003)
Test for subgroup differences: Chi² = 0.01, df = 1 (P = 0.92), I² = 0%

Figure 3: Forest plot of comparison of treatment-emergent volume-related adverse events with canagliflozin 100 mg and 300 mg.

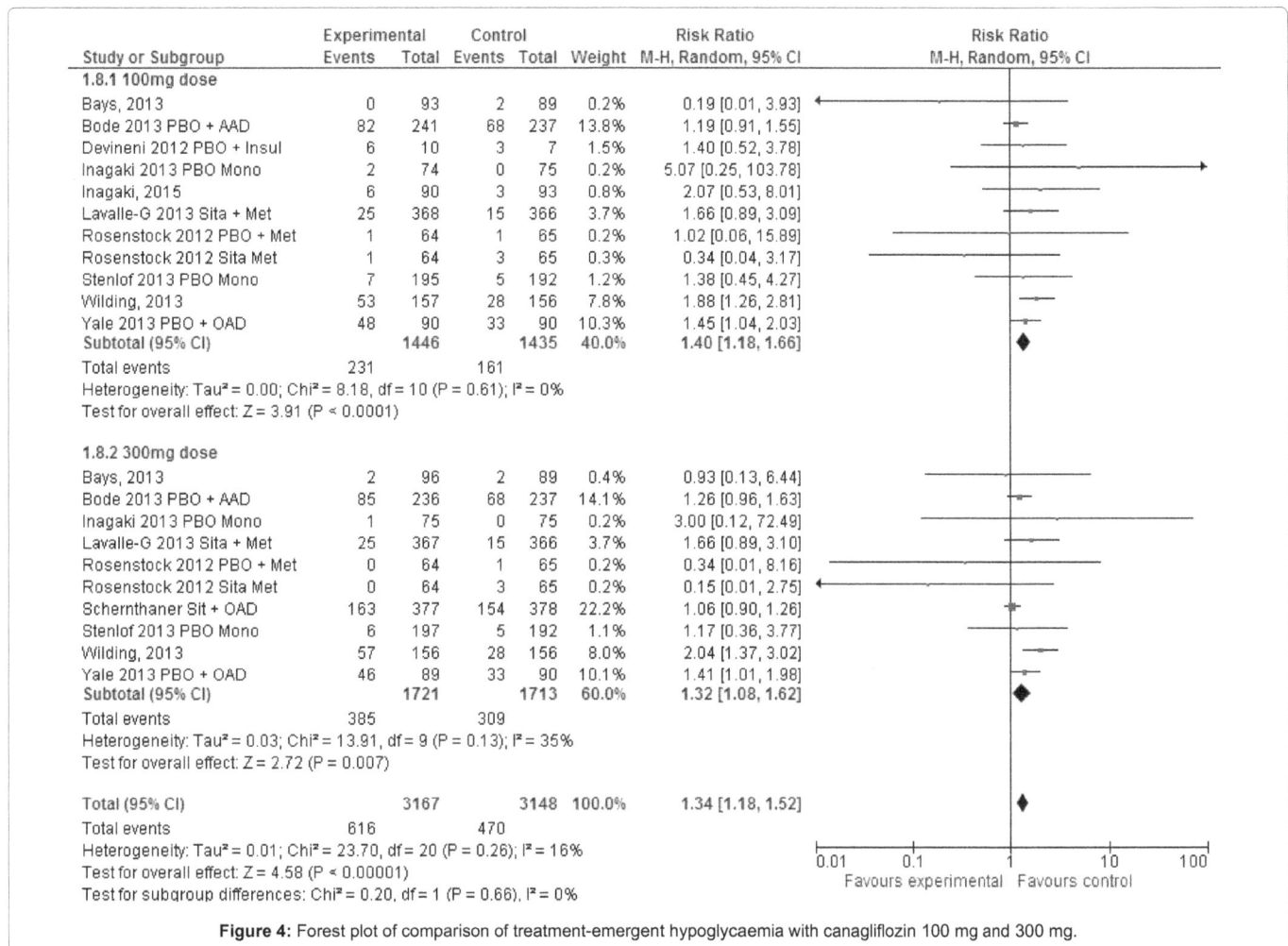

Figure 4: Forest plot of comparison of treatment-emergent hypoglycaemia with canagliflozin 100 mg and 300 mg.

purported that glycosuria maintains a welcoming environment for the major hyphal cell wall protein 1 of the fungi to attach to the uro-epithelium, grow and multiply. The philosophy behind this is that as the major hyphal wall protein 1 (hwp1) plays an integral role in mating, normal hyphal development, cell-to-cell adhesive functions necessary for biofilm integrity, attachment to host, and virulence, it must be involved in the overall mechanism advanced to describe the phenomenon in question [25]. Furthermore, its properties promote the effective interaction between both fungal and host molecules, which leads to effective colonization, especially when humoral immunity is decreased [25].

It is possible that, due to the widely acknowledged association of increased urinary tract infections and genital mycotic infections associated with diabetes, that there is increased surveillance leading to increased diagnosis of infections [26]. However, as SGLT2s are associated with an increase in osmotic-diuresis related adverse events such as polyuria and pollakiuria, there could be an increased tendency to report infections in those patients [26].

As with any antidiabetic agent, there is always the possibility of patients experiencing hypoglycaemic attacks. As a result of this, patients should exercise caution whenever taking any hypoglycemic agent, being cognizant of the associated clinical manifestations related to the adverse event, in order to prevent development of serious complications. The FDA approval promotes canagliflozin as an adjunct

with other antidiabetics. This might add up some concern about the added risks and safety issues in elderly.

It has been reported by the FDA that canagliflozin is associated with an increased risk for bone fractures, thus causing the mentioned organisation to strengthen its warning for the drug [20]. This information is based on new confirmatory information from nine clinical trials [20]. The logic behind the development of these fractures stems from the fact that SGLT2 inhibitors increase serum concentrations of phosphate through increased tubular resorption, which has the potential to adversely affect bone. These inhibitors also increase the concentration of parathyroid hormone, which enhances bone resorption, thus increasing the risk of pathologic fractures [20]. In the included studies of this meta-analysis, there was no reported data relating to the association of canagliflozin with bone fractures. This could be due to the fact that the number of cases is not significant, and, therefore, the results were not included in the studies.

Canagliflozin showed in various studies almost an increasing number of adverse events that was not clearly stating whether these events are dose related or not. But this analysis compiled all reported data from all strictly randomized controlled studies to verify the strength of evidence that the adverse events are dose related or not.

Limitations

The results in this study are limited to the data that is currently available. A limitation of this study could stem from limited sample sizes and treatment durations in some of the included studies, which could affect conclusions pertaining to the safety and efficacy of canagliflozin. Furthermore, the patient populations reflect the strength of the study. In order to represent a true diabetic population, patients from a broad age group and varying ethnicities, especially black or African-American and Hispanic populations where diabetes is highly prevalent coupled with overweight and obese patients should have been included in the studies to ensure that the data found can be generalized to the diabetic population as a whole. Also, these trials did not report data for subgroups of high risk patients with low renal function, advanced age, or those taking loop diuretics.

Conclusion

Canagliflozin has been associated with an increased incidence of genital mycotic infections and vulvovaginal mycotic infections, and to a lesser degree urinary tract infections. While the exact mechanism is not known, it is believed that there could be an interaction between the glycosuria effect of the SGLT2 and the hwp1 which is allowing fungus to grow and flourish in those regions. No dose dependent adverse events were noted, as they were equally prevalent in both dosing cohorts. The risk of hypoglycaemia is increased, as is the case with most of the antidiabetic agents. The risk of volume depletion is significant, and high-risk patients such as the elderly, those with chronic renal failure, or those taking diuretics should be monitored closely if prescribed canagliflozin.

References

1. Tucker M (2015) Diabetes Prevalence in the US May Have Plateaued. Medscape.

2. http://www.reuters.com/article/johnsonjohnson-diabetes-idusl3n0cl1fv20130329

3. American Diabetes Association (2013) Economic Costs of Diabetes in the US in 2012. Diabetes Care. 36: 1033-1046.

4. https://www.invokana.com/about-invokana/what-is-invokana?

5. http://tech.cochrane.org/revman/about-revman-5

6. Bays HE, Weinstein R, Law G, Canovatchel W (2014) Canagliflozin: Effects in overweight and obese subjects without diabetes mellitus. Obesity 22:1042-1049.

7. Bode B, Stenlöf K, Harris S, Sullivan D, Fung A, et al. (2015) Long-term efficacy and safety of canagliflozin over 104 weeks in patients aged 55-80 years with type 2 diabetes. Diabetes Obes Metab 17:294-303.

8. Bode B, Stenlöf K, Sullivan D, Fung A, Usiskin K (2013) Efficacy and Safety of Canagliflozin Treatment in Older Subjects With Type 2 Diabetes Mellitus: A Randomized Trial. Hosp Pract 41:72-84.

9. Cefalu WT, Leiter LA, Yoon K-H, Arias P, Niskanen L, et al. (2013) Efficacy and safety of canagliflozin versus glimepiride in patients with type 2 diabetes inadequately controlled with metformin (CANTATA-SU): 52 week results from a randomized, double-blind, phase 3 non-inferiority trial. Lancet 382:941-950.

10. Chen X, Hu P, Vaccaro N, Polidori D, Curtin CR, et al. (2015) Pharmacokinetics, Pharmacodynamics, and Safety of Single-Dose Canagliflozin in Healthy Chinese Subjects. Clin Ther 37:1483-1492.

11. Devineni D, Morrow L, Hompesch M, Skee D, Vandebosch A, Murphy J, et al. (2012) Canagliflozin improves glycemic control over 28 days in subjects with type 2 diabetes not optimally controlled on insulin. Diabetes Obes Metab. 14:539-545.

12. Forst T, Guthrie R, Goldenberg R, Yee J, Vijapurkar U et al. (2014) Efficacy and safety of canagliflozin over 52 weeks in patients with type 2 diabetes on background metformin and pioglitazone. Diabetes Obes Metab. 16:467-477.

13. Inagaki N, Kondo K, Yoshinari T, Takahashi N, Susuta Y, et al. (2015) Efficacy and safety of canagliflozin monotherapy in Japanese patients with type 2 diabetes inadequately controlled with diet and exercise: a 24-week,

14. Inagaki N, Kondo K, Yoshinari T, Maruyama N, Susuta Y, et al. (2013) Efficacy and safety of canagliflozin in Japanese patients with type 2 diabetes: a randomized, double-blind, placebo-controlled, 12-week study. Diabetes Obes Metab. 15:1136-1145.

15. https://www.invokana.com/about-invokana/what-is-invokana?

16. Ji L, Han P, Liu Y, Yang G, Van NKD, et al. (2015) Canagliflozin in Asian patients with type 2 diabetes on metformin alone or metformin in combination with sulphonylurea. Diabetes Obes Metab Diabetes Obes Metab. 17:23-31.

17. Lavalle-González FJ, Januszewicz A, Davidson J, Tong C, Qiu R, et al. (2013) Efficacy and safety of canagliflozin compared with placebo and sitagliptin in patients with type 2 diabetes on background metformin monotherapy: a randomized trial. Diabetologia. 56:2582-2592.

18. Polidori D, Sha S, Heise T, Natarajan J, Artis E, et al. (2015) Effect of canagliflozin, a sodium glucose co-transporter 2 inhibitor, on C-peptide kinetics. Clin Pharmacol Drug Dev 4:12-27.

19. Rosenstock J, Aggarwal N, Polidori D, Zhao Y, Arbit D, et al. (2012) Dose-Ranging Effects of Canagliflozin, a Sodium-Glucose Cotransporter 2 Inhibitor, as Add-On to Metformin in Subjects With Type 2 Diabetes. Diabetes Care 35:1232-1238.

20. Schernthaner G, Gross J, Rosenstock J, Guarisco M, Fu M, et al. (2013) Canagliflozin compared with sitagliptin for patients with type 2 diabetes who do not have adequate glycemic control with metformin plus sulfonylurea: a 52-week randomized trial. Diabetes Care 36:2508-2515.

21. Sha S, Polidori D, Heise T, Natarajan J, Farrell K, et al. (2014) Effect of the sodium glucose co-transporter 2 inhibitor canagliflozin on plasma volume in patients with type 2 diabetes mellitus. Diabetes Obes Metab 16:1087-1095.

22. Stenlöf K, Cefalu WT, Kim K-A, Alba M, Usiskin K, et al. (2013) Efficacy and safety of canagliflozin monotherapy in subjects with type 2 diabetes mellitus inadequately controlled with diet and exercise. Diabetes Obes Metab. 15:372-382.

23. Wilding JPH, Charpentier G, Hollander P, González-Gálvez G, Mathieu C, et al. (2013) Efficacy and safety of canagliflozin in patients with type 2 diabetes mellitus inadequately controlled with metformin and sulphonylurea: a randomized trial. Int J Clin Pract 67:1267-1282. Yale J-F, Bakris G, Cariou B, Yue D, David-Neto E, et al. (2013) Efficacy and safety of canagliflozin in subjects with type 2 diabetes and chronic kidney disease. Diabetes Obes Metab. 15:463-473.

24. Tucker M (2015) FDA Strengthens Fracture Warning for Canagliflozin. Medscape.

25. Staab JF (1999) Adhesive and Mammalian Transglutaminase Substrate Properties of Candida albicans Hwp1. Science. 5407:1535-1538.

26. Geerlings S, Fonseca V, Castro-Diaz D, List J, Parikh S (2014) Genital and urinary tract infections in diabetes: Impact of pharmacologically-induced glycosuria. Diabetes Res Clin Pract 103:373-381.

Cholesterol Drugs Improve Breast Cancer Prognosis in Women with Diabetes Mellitus

Chi-Chen Hong[1], Anand B Shah[2], Caitlin M Jackowiak[2], Ellen Kossoff[3], Hsin-Wei Fu[2], George K Nimako[2], Dimitra Bitikofer[2], Stephen B Edge[4] and Alice C Ceacareanu[2]*

[1]Department of Cancer Prevention and Control, Roswell Park Cancer Institute, Buffalo NY, USA
[2]Department of Pharmacy Practice, School of Pharmacy and Pharmacy and Pharmaceutical Sciences, State University of New York at Buffalo, Buffalo NY, USA
[3]Department of Pharmacy, Roswell Park Cancer Institute, Buffalo NY, USA
[4]Department of Surgical Oncology, Roswell Park Cancer Institute, Buffalo NY, USA

Abstract

Study objective: To evaluate the impact of Cholesterol management on breast cancer recurrence and survival (CHOLBRES) in diabetic women with breast cancer.

Design: Cholbres study included all incident breast cancer cases with pre-existing diabetes mellitus diagnosed with cancer between 01/01/2003-12/31/2007. Clinical characteristics, outcomes, and pharmacotherapy were abstracted from medical records or hospital-developed databases. The follow-up, with a median of 31 months, began at breast cancer diagnosis and ended at first recurrence, death, or date of last contact.

Patients: All diabetes mellitus women with incident breast cancer were identified (n=269); of these 208 met the inclusion criteria and were used for analysis.

Methods: The association between self-reported cholesterol-lowering medications and breast cancer outcomes was evaluated with multivariate Cox proportional hazards models.

Main results: Women taking cholesterol-lowering drugs were found to have fewer recurrences (HR=0.54, 95% CI: 0.24 to 1.18, p=0.12), improved overall survival (HR=0.48, 95% CI: 0.27 to 0.86, p=0.01), and better disease-free survival (HR=0.65, 95% CI: 0.35 to 1.21, p=0.17) than women who did not take any cholesterol-lowering medication. Cholesterol management employing statins as a mono-therapy was associated with better overall survival (HR=0.42, 95% CI: 0.21 to 0.84, p=0.08) and slightly improved disease-free survival (HR=0.49, 95% CI: 0.23 to 1.04, p=0.24).

Conclusion: Our findings demonstrate that cholesterol-lowering therapy significantly improves breast cancer prognosis in women with diabetes mellitus. Though larger studies are needed to confirm this potential added benefit, efforts to ensure that women with breast cancer and diabetes receive guideline-appropriate cholesterol-lowering medications should have significant impact on breast cancer outcomes.

Keywords: Cholesterol; Statins; Breast cancer; Prognosis; Diabetes

Introduction

Diabetes mellitus's hallmarks, insulin resistance, dyslipidemia and inflammation, are all associated with increased breast cancer risk and poorer prognosis in diabetic women [1-11]. According to American Diabetes Association guidelines, statins (3-hydroxy-3-methylglutaryl Coenzyme A reductase inhibitors) should be initiated regardless of lipid levels in 98.5% of diabetes mellitus patients, however, over one-third of eligible patients do not receive a prescription for statins in US clinical practices [12]. Statins exhibit pleiotropic effects that can affect carcinogenesis and cancer outcomes through several pathways, including inflammation, immune response, cell migration, and apoptosis [13-17]. While dyslipidemia management recommended by the American Diabetes Association targets prevention of cardiovascular disease events [18], addition of statins may also improve cancer outcomes in diabetic women with breast cancer. Currently, the association between statin use and breast cancer risk is unclear, with some data suggesting that statin use may reduce the risk of breast cancer recurrence [19-21]. Since statin therapy can positively influence several key risk factors related to breast cancer prognosis that are more prevalent among women with diabetes mellitus, we hypothesize that diabetic women will derive greater breast cancer-outcome related benefits from statin therapy compared to the general population of breast cancer patients [20,22-24]. This study examined whether cholesterol-lowering therapy improves breast cancer outcomes in a hospital-based retrospective cohort of women with pre-existing diabetes mellitus.

Methods

Patient population and data collection

This study was approved by the Institutional Review Board of Roswell Park Cancer Institute and State University of New York at Buffalo. All women with incident breast cancer treated at RPCI with a diagnosis date from 01/01/2003-12/31/2007 were reviewed (n=2,149). Eligible cases were those >18 years of age with pre-existing diabetes and no previous history of cancer. Presence of diabetes was determined by cancer-center coding of the International Classification of Diseases, Ninth Revision (ICD-9), and by self-reported pharmacotherapy and/

*Corresponding author: Alice C Ceacareanu, New York State Center of Excellence in Bioinformatics and Life Sciences, 701 Ellicott Street, Buffalo NY 14203, USA, E-mail: acc36@buffalo.edu

or medical history. Based on the ICD-9 codes, 170 cases with diabetes were identified. Of the remaining 1,979 cases, chart review identified 99 additional diabetes mellitus patients, for a total of 269 cases. Of these, 61 were excluded due to: male gender (n=3), unknown or type 1 diabetes (n=19), gestational diabetes or diabetes mellitus diagnosed post- breast cancer diagnosis (n=9), unclear date of breast cancer diagnosis (n=5), personal history of prior breast cancer (n=8), and incomplete data (n=16). A total of 208 individuals were included in the final analyses.

Date of breast cancer diagnosis, age, race, body mass index (BMI), patient- and tumor-related clinical parameters were obtained from a hospital-developed prospective database of the Roswell Park Cancer Institute Breast Program; medical history and pharmacotherapy at diagnosis were documented by individual chart review. Data collection accuracy was ensured by comparison of at least two independent review reports for each patient. Any discrepancies were resolved on a case-by-case basis by a third reviewer in consultation with ACC. The

Variable	Non-Users No.	%	Users No.	%	P^1	Non-statin Only No.	%	Statin Only No.	%	Non-statin + Statin No.	%	P^2
All Patients	69 (33.2)		139 (66.8)			26	18.7	75	54.0	38	27.3	
Age, years												
<50	14	20.3	13	9.4	0.09	3	23.1	7	53.9	3	23.1	0.97
50 to 59	21	30.4	37	26.6		5	13.5	20	54.1	12	32.4	
60 to 69	19	27.5	44	31.7		9	20.5	23	52.3	12	27.3	
≥ 70	15	21.7	45	32.4		9	20.0	25	55.6	11	24.4	
Race/ethnicity												
White	49	71.0	103	74.1	0.78	23	22.3	50	48.5	30	29.1	0.20
African American	18	26.1	33	23.7		3	9.1	23	69.7	7	21.2	
Other	2	2.9	3	2.2		0	0	2	66.7	1	33.3	
Menopausal Status												
Premenopausal	14	20.3	12	8.6	0.04	2	16.7	7	58.3	3	25.0	0.02
Postmenopausal	53	76.8	125	89.9		23	18.4	67	53.6	35	28.0	
Unknown	2	2.9	2	1.4		1	50.0	1	50.0	0	0	
BMI, Kg/m²												
<25	7	10.1	6	4.3	0.39	1	16.7	4	66.7	1	16.7	0.90
25 to <30	13	18.8	26	18.7		2	7.7	16	61.5	8	30.8	
30 to <40	23	33.3	61	43.9		12	19.7	32	52.5	17	27.9	
40+	16	23.2	28	20.1		7	25.0	13	46.4	8	28.6	
Unknown	10	14.5	18	13.0		4	22.2	10	55.6	4	22.2	
Tumor Stage												
0	3	4.4	19	13.7	0.08	0	0.0	13	68.4	6	31.6	0.21
I	27	39.1	54	38.9		12	22.2	25	46.3	17	31.5	
II	22	31.9	33	23.7		6	18.2	19	57.6	8	24.2	
III	13	18.8	20	14.4		3	15.0	13	65.0	4	20.0	
IV	2	2.9	12	8.6		4	33.3	5	41.7	3	25.0	
X (Unknown)	2	2.9	1	0.7		1	100.0	0	0	0	0	
Tumor Grade												
1	10	14.5	12	8.6	0.61	0	0	6	50.0	6	50.0	0.19
2	29	42.0	59	42.5		14	23.7	27	45.8	18	30.5	
3	21	30.4	46	33.1		7	15.2	29	63.0	10	21.7	
Unknown	9	13.0	22	15.8		5	22.7	13	59.1	4	18.2	
Tumor Size, cm												
0–2.0	37	53.6	81	58.3	0.79	19	23.5	40	49.4	22	27.2	0.38
>2.0 to 5.0	14	20.3	24	17.3		1	4.2	16	66.7	7	29.2	
> 5	4	5.8	5	3.6		1	20.0	2	40.0	2	40.0	
Unknown	14	20.3	29	20.9		5	17.2	17	58.6	7	24.1	
ER Status												
ER+	51	73.9	90	64.8	0.12	23	25.6	46	51.1	21	23.3	0.03
ER-	15	21.7	30	21.6		3	10.0	16	53.3	11	36.7	
Unknown	3	4.4	19	13.7		0	0.0	13	68.4	6	31.6	
ACE-27 Comorbidity Scores												
Mild	10	14.5	11	7.9	0.23	2	18.2	5	45.5	4	36.4	0.57
Moderate	13	18.8	36	25.9		4	11.1	23	63.9	9	25.0	
Severe	46	66.7	92	66.2		20	21.7	47	51.1	25	27.2	

Columns grouped under **Type of Cholesterol-lowering Medication**.

Abbreviations: BMI, body mass index. [1]P-value associated with Fisher's exact test comparing women taking any cholesterol management medication versus women who do not take any. [2]P-value associated with Fisher's exact test comparing 3 groups of medication users: non-statin only, statin only, and both statins and non-statins.

Table 1: Use of cholesterol therapy according to patient- and tumor-related variables (n=208).

Cholesterol Management	Breast Cancer Recurrence[1]						Overall Mortality						Disease Free Survival					
			Age-adjusted		Multivariate[2]				Age-adjusted		Multivariate[2]				Age-adjusted		Multivariate[2]	
	No.	No of Events	HR	95% CI	HR	95% CI	No	No of Events	HR	95% CI	HR	95% CI	No	No of Events	HR	95% CI	HR	95% CI
No Medication (group 1)	64	13	Ref	-	Ref		69	22	Ref	-	Ref		64	19	Ref		Ref	
Non-statin only (group 2)	26	5	1.29	0.44 to 3.78	0.71	0.24 to 2.12	26	8	0.50	0.21 to 1.18	0.50	0.21 to 1.18	26	11	1.48	0.67 to 3.24	0.96	0.43 to 2.16
Statin only (group 3)	71	8	0.66	0.27 to 1.63	0.51	0.20 to 1.32	75	17	0.42	0.21 to 0.84	0.42	0.21 to 0.84	71	14	0.59	0.29 to 1.22	0.49	0.23 to 1.04
Both Non-statin & Statin (group 4)	36	2	0.33	0.07 to 1.47	0.38	0.08 to 1.81	38	7	0.61	0.26 to 1.45	0.61	0.26 to 1.45	36	6	0.59	0.23 to 1.49	0.73	0.28 to 1.88
P			0.31		0.43				0.08		0.08				0.09		0.24	
Any cholesterol medication (groups 2+3+4 vs. 1)	133	15	0.67	0.31 to 1.45	0.54	0.24 to 1.18	139	32	0.59	0.34 to 1.03	0.48	0.27 to 0.86	133	31	0.74	0.40 to 1.34	0.65	0.35 to 1.21
P			0.30		0.12				0.06		0.01				0.32		0.17	

Abbreviations: HR, hazard ratio; 95% CI, 95% confidence interval.[1]Disease recurrence and disease free survival analysis limited to N=197 women, excluding 11 women who were never disease free. [2]All multivariate analyses are adjusted for cancer stage (0, 1 to IIIa, IIIB+, unknown), ER status (positive, negative, unknown), age at breast cancer diagnosis (continuous variable), race (Caucasian, African American, other), and ACE-27 comorbidity score (1-2, 3).

Table 2: Associations of Cholesterol Medicatiom with Breast Cancer Outcomes: Proportional Hazards model.

grade of cogent comorbid ailments at diagnosis was estimated using the Adult Comorbidity Evaluation 27 (ACE-27) score (http://oto2.wustl.edu/clinepi/calc.html) [25].

Ascertainment of vital status and cancer outcome variables

Information on vital status and breast cancer recurrences were obtained from the National Comprehensive Cancer Network (NCCN) Breast Cancer Outcomes Database at Roswell Park Cancer Institute, with ≥ 92% complete follow-up. NCCN-coordinated linking with the National Death Index for all patients who were defined as "lost to follow-up" was completed 12/08/2011. Outcomes of interest were breast cancer recurrence, disease free survival, and overall mortality. Disease-free survival was defined as the time from initial diagnosis to breast cancer recurrence, death from any cause, or end of follow-up. If alive, individuals were followed through their last day of contact or vital status update, whichever was more recent. Follow-up began at diagnosis and ended at first confirmed recurrence and/or death depending on the analysis. Women lost to follow-up were censored at the date of last contact. Events documentation was limited to data collected through to 02/14/2012.

Statistical analysis

Baseline cohort characteristics in cholesterol therapy users versus non-users and, respectively, users of statins, non-statins, and statin-nonstatin combined regimens were compared using Fisher's exact tests. Kaplan-Meier (KM) log-rank tests were used to evaluate differences in breast cancer outcomes by type of cholesterol medications used. Two sets of analyses were performed for each outcome: 1) comparison of non-users versus users of any cholesterol-lowering pharmacotherapy; and 2) comparison of non-users, non-statin users, statin users, and users of combined statin and nonstatin regimens. Cox proportional hazard models were used to calculate hazard ratios (HR) and 95% confidence intervals (95% CI) for univariate and multivariate analyses examining associations between a defined event and use of statins and/or non-statins. Multivariate models were adjusted for cancer stage, ER status, age-at-diagnosis, race, BMI, and ACE-27 score as *a priori* adjustment factors (Table 1). SAS for Windows, version 9.2 or 9.3 were used for all statistical analyses.

Results

The mean age at breast cancer diagnosis was 63.0 ± 11.3 years, with 86% of women being postmenopausal; mean BMI was 35.3 ± 8.3 Kg/m². Unknown ER status was noted in approximately 10% of women and this was attributed to the information not being required to guide treatment. Two-thirds (66.8%) of the study population received cholesterol-lowering medications, with 54.3% receiving statin therapy. Older and postmenopausal women were more likely to receive cholesterol-lowering drugs, although only menopausal status was statistically significant, p=0.04. Cases with unknown ER status (86% stage 0) were more likely to have received a statin alone or in combination, p=0.03 (Table 1). Type of cholesterol-lowering medication did not vary with ACE-27 scores or with any other variable analyzed.

After a median follow-up of 59.7 months (ranging from 3 to 105 months), fewer recurrences (15/133 versus 13/64), overall deaths (32/139 versus 22/69) and disease-free survival events (31/133 versus 19/64) were reported in cholesterol-lowering medication users versus non-users, with a trend towards higher 5-year recurrence-free (0.89 versus 0.78), overall (0.82 versus 0.75), and disease-free survival (0.81 versus 0.71) (Figure 1). In fully adjusted multivariate Cox proportional hazards models, cholesterol-lowering medications were associated with approximately 2-fold reduced mortality (HR=0.48, 95% CI, 0.27 to 0.86, p=0.01) and recurrences (HR=0.54, 95% CI, 0.24 to1.18, p=0.12), and approximately 50% longer disease-free survival (HR=0.65, 95% CI, 0.35 to 1.21, p=0.17) as compared to non-users (Table 2). Statin mono-therapy had the most beneficial effect on overall mortality (HR=0.42, 95% CI,0.21 to 0.84, p=0.01) and disease-free survival (HR=0.49, 95% CI,0.23 to 1.04, p=0.06), while addition of non-statins to statin regimens attenuated the benefit of statins alone increasing HR for overall mortality and disease-free survival to HR=0.61 (95% CI, 0.26 to 1.45, p=0.26) and HR=0.73 (95% CI,0.28 to 1.88, p=0.51), respectively.

Discussion

Our data demonstrates a strong association between use of cholesterol-lowering drugs and improved breast cancer prognosis in type 2 diabetic women, resulting in approximately 2-fold reduced mortality and breast cancer recurrences, and 54% improved disease-free survival. The benefit appeared to be stronger among women

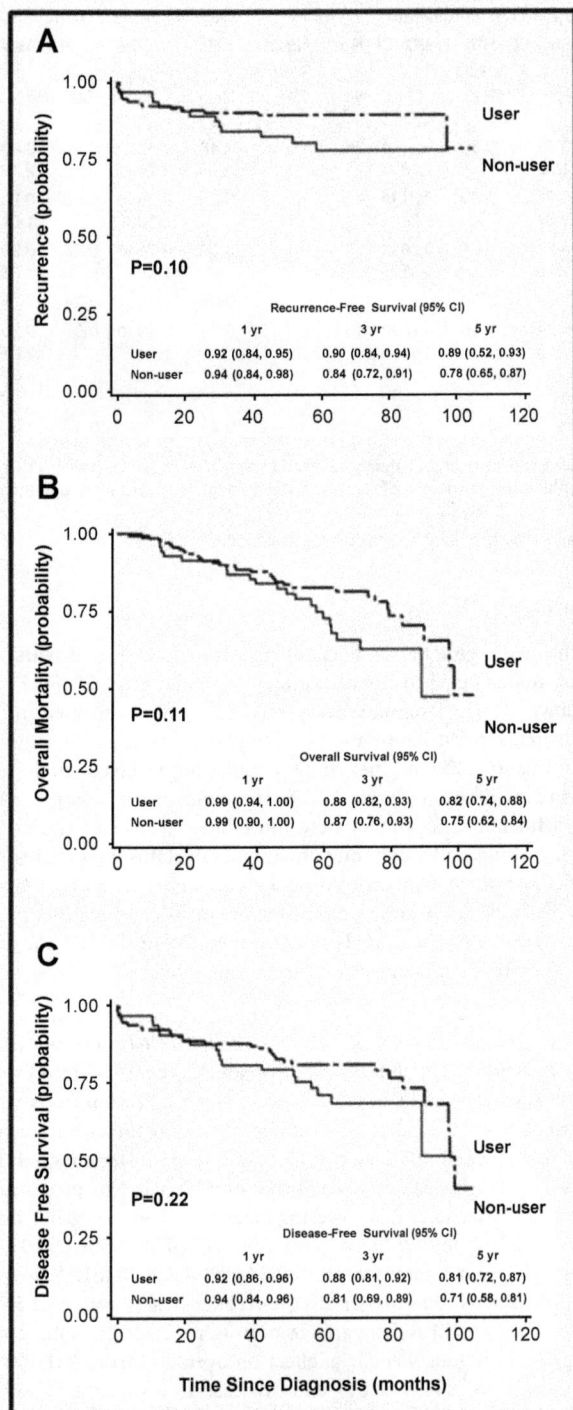

Figure 1: Kaplan-Meier plots indicating a trend towards fewer breast cancer recurrences (A), lower overall mortality (B), and better disease free survival (C) in cholesterol-lowering drug users as compared to non-users. Disease recurrence and disease free survival analysis limited to N=197 women, excluding 11 women who were never disease free.

To date, only a few studies examined the prognostic significance of cholesterol-lowering medications with most providing some evidence for improved breast cancer outcomes [17-19]. The largest population-based study thus far (18,800 women) reported HR estimates similar to those reported in smaller studies [19-21] and found lipophilic statins to be associated with 43% lower 5-year breast cancer recurrence rates (HR= 0.70, 95% CI, 0.53 to 0.92)[17]. Given that cholesterol-lowering drugs users may have more cogent ailments than non-users, the magnitude of protective effects observed among users may be underestimated [25]. Such considerations merit attention as recent studies have associated statin use with increased risk for diabetes mellitus [26-28] and could contribute to underutilization of statins in specific patient populations who are most likely to benefit from statin therapy.

From a mechanistic stand-point, diabetes mellitus hallmarks are also risk factors for breast cancer and are positively impacted by statin pharmacotherapy [9]. Potentially, mevalonate pathway inhibition [29,30], down-regulation of proteins responsible for breast cancer invasiveness [29-32], or prevention of insulin receptor inactivation may each reduce breast cancer recurrence [33,34]. Further evidence is, however, needed to verify whether observed statins benefits occur through any of these mechanisms.

The primary limitation of our study was small sample size, which prevented us from exploring subclasses of cholesterol-lowering medication in relationship with breast cancer outcomes and also precluded us from exploring associations stratified by tumor stage. Larger studies may clarify whether the statin benefits identified by us are a class effect or could potentially differ between lipophilic and hydrophilic members [19,35]. Unfortunately, no studies evaluating statin use and breast cancer prognosis have been able to address this question due to limited sample size [20,21]. Another limitation was that our study could not account for new prescriptions or drug changes occurring post-diagnosis. Such misclassifications are expected to underestimate the magnitude of protective effects.

In summary, this study shows that cholesterol-lowering medications, particularly statins, are significantly associated with improved breast cancer prognosis in women with diabetes mellitus. Although larger prospective studies are needed to confirm this benefit, efforts to assure that women with breast cancer and diabetes mellitus receive guideline-appropriate dyslipidemia management should have a significant positive impact on breast cancer outcomes.

Acknowledgements

Authors are grateful to Linda Hauck and Nancy Watroba (Roswell Park Cancer Institute) for providing patient follow-up data from tumor registry and breast surgery databases. Thanks are due to Kevin Patel, PharmD, Christopher Martens, PharmD and David Yeow, PharmD (University at Buffalo) for identifying cases eligible for study inclusion. We acknowledge here the invaluable help received from Sharon Kiley (Roswell Park Cancer Institute), CHOLBRES study Clinical Research Associate, and Diane Fisher (University at Buffalo), CHOLBRES study administrator, throughout the duration of this study. Last, not least, we thank Drs. Christine Ambrosone, PhD (Roswell Park Cancer Institute), and Alan Forrest, PharmD (University at Buffalo) for constructive discussions related to this research. CH and ACC had full access to all the data in the study and takes responsibility for the integrity of the data and the accuracy of the data analysis.

References

1. Coughlin SS, Calle EE, Teras LR, Petrelli J, Thun MJ (2004) Diabetes mellitus as a predictor of cancer mortality in a large cohort of US adults. Am J Epidemiol 159: 1160-1167.

2. Verlato G, Zoppini G, Bonora E, Muggeo M (2003) Mortality from site-specific malignancies in type 2 diabetic patients from Verona. Diabetes Care 26: 1047-1051.

3. Lipscombe LL, Goodwin PJ, Zinman B, McLaughlin JR, Hux JE (2008) The

receiving statins alone and support recent findings that statin use may be linked to better breast cancer prognosis [19-21]. Similar to previous observations [23], one-third of our eligible patients were not receiving any form of cholesterol-lowering medication at the time of breast cancer diagnosis.

impact of diabetes on survival following breast cancer. Breast Cancer Res Treat 109: 389-395.

4. Lipscombe LL, Goodwin PJ, Zinman B, McLaughlin JR, Hux JE (2006) Diabetes mellitus and breast cancer: a retrospective population-based cohort study. Breast Cancer Res Treat 98: 349-356.

5. Wolf I, Sadetzki S, Gluck I, Oberman B, Ben-David M, et al. (2006) Association between diabetes mellitus and adverse characteristics of breast cancer at presentation. Eur J Cancer 42: 1077-1082.

6. Kaplan MA, Pekkolay Z, Kucukoner M, İnal A, Urakci Z, et al. (2011) Type 2 diabetes mellitus and prognosis in early stage breast cancer women. Med Oncol 29: 1576-1580.

7. Schrauder MG, Fasching PA, HÃberle L, Lux MP, Rauh C, et al. (2011) Diabetes and prognosis in a breast cancer cohort. J Cancer Res Clin Oncol 137: 975-983.

8. Shoelson SE, Lee J, Goldfine AB (2006) Inflammation and insulin resistance. J Clin Invest 116: 1793-1801.

9. Pierce BL, Ballard-Barbash R, Bernstein L, Baumgartner RN, Neuhouser ML, et al. (2009) Elevated biomarkers of inflammation are associated with reduced survival among breast cancer patients. J Clin Oncol 27: 3437-3444.

10. Goodwin PJ (2008) Insulin in the adjuvant breast cancer setting: a novel therapeutic target for lifestyle and pharmacologic interventions? J Clin Oncol 26: 833-834.

11. Tsugane S, Inoue M (2010) Insulin resistance and cancer: epidemiological evidence. Cancer Sci 101: 1073-1079.

12. Fu AZ, Zhang Q, Davies MJ, Pentakota SR, Radican L, et al. (2011) Underutilization of statins in patients with type 2 diabetes in US clinical practice: a retrospective cohort study. Curr Med Res Opin 27: 1035-1040.

13. Lopez-Pedrera C, Ruiz-Limon P, Valverde-Estepa A, Barbarroja N, Rodriguez-Ariza A (2012) To cardiovascular disease and beyond: new therapeutic perspectives of statins in autoimmune diseases and cancer. Curr Drug Targets 13: 829-841.

14. Fritz G (2005) HMG-CoA reductase inhibitors (statins) as anticancer drugs (review). Int J Oncol 27: 1401-1409.

15. Bellosta S, Ferri N, Bernini F, Paoletti R, Corsini A (2000) Non-lipid-related effects of statins. Ann Med 32: 164-176.

16. Demierre MF, Higgins PD, Gruber SB, Hawk E, Lippman SM (2005) Statins and cancer prevention. Nat Rev Cancer 5: 930-942.

17. Xiao H, Yang CS (2008) Combination regimen with statins and NSAIDs: a promising strategy for cancer chemoprevention. Int J Cancer 123: 983-990.

18. American Diabetes Association (2011) Standards of medical care in diabetes--2011. Diabetes Care Suppl 1: S11-61.

19. Ahern TP, Pedersen L, Tarp M, Cronin-Fenton DP, Garne JP, et al. (2011) Statin prescriptions and breast cancer recurrence risk: a Danish nationwide prospective cohort study. J Natl Cancer Inst 103: 1461-1468.

20. Kwan ML, Habel LA, Flick ED, Quesenberry CP, Caan B (2008) Post-diagnosis statin use and breast cancer recurrence in a prospective cohort study of early stage breast cancer survivors. Breast Cancer Res Treat 109: 573-579.

21. Chae YK, Valsecchi ME, Kim J, Bianchi AL, Khemasuwan D, et al. (2011) Reduced risk of breast cancer recurrence in patients using ACE inhibitors, ARBs, and/or statins. Cancer Invest 29: 585-593.

22. Meex RC, Phielix E, Schrauwen-Hinderling VB, Moonen-Kornips E, Schaart G, et al. (2010) The use of statins potentiates the insulin-sensitizing effect of exercise training in obese males with and without Type 2 diabetes. Clin Sci (Lond) 119: 293-301.

23. Hoenig MR, Sellke FW (2010) Insulin resistance is associated with increased cholesterol synthesis, decreased cholesterol absorption and enhanced lipid response to statin therapy. Atherosclerosis 211: 260-265.

24. Haukka J, Sankila R, Klaukka T, Lonnqvist J, Niskanen L, et al. (2010) Incidence of cancer and statin usage--record linkage study. Int J Cancer 126: 279-284.

25. Piccirillo JF, Tierney RM, Costas I, Grove L, Spitznagel EL Jr (2004) Prognostic importance of comorbidity in a hospital-based cancer registry. JAMA 291: 2441-2447.

26. Culver AL, Ockene IS, Balasubramanian R, Olendzki BC, Sepavich M, et al. (2012) Statin Use and Risk of Diabetes Mellitus in Postmenopausal Women in the Women's Health Initiative. Arch Intern Med 172: 144-152.

27. Preiss D, Seshasai SR, Welsh P, Murphy SA, Ho JE, et al. (2011) Risk of incident diabetes with intensive-dose compared with moderate-dose statin therapy: a meta-analysis. JAMA 305: 2556-2564.

28. Sattar N, Preiss D, Murray HM, Welsh P, Buckley BM, et al. (2010) Statins and risk of incident diabetes: a collaborative meta-analysis of randomised statin trials. Lancet 375: 735-742.

29. Denoyelle C, Vasse M, KÃ¶rner M, Mishal Z, GannÃ© F, et al. (2001) Cerivastatin, an inhibitor of HMG-CoA reductase, inhibits the signaling pathways involved in the invasiveness and metastatic properties of highly invasive breast cancer cell lines: an in vitro study. Carcinogenesis 22: 1139-1148.

30. Kusama T, Mukai M, Tatsuta M, Nakamura H, Inoue M (2006) Inhibition of transendothelial migration and invasion of human breast cancer cells by preventing geranylgeranylation of Rho. Int J Oncol 29: 217-223.

31. Berndt N, Hamilton AD, Sebti SM (2011) Targeting protein prenylation for cancer therapy. Nat Rev Cancer 11: 775-791.

32. Shimoyama S (2011) Statins are logical candidates for overcoming limitations of targeting therapies on malignancy: their potential application to gastrointestinal cancers. Cancer Chemother Pharmacol 67: 729-739.

33. McFarlane SI, Muniyappa R, Francisco R, Sowers JR (2002) Clinical review 145: Pleiotropic effects of statins: lipid reduction and beyond. J Clin Endocrinol Metab 87: 1451-1458.

34. Oh SW, Park CY, Lee ES, Yoon YS, Lee ES, et al. (2011) Adipokines, insulin resistance, metabolic syndrome, and breast cancer recurrence: a cohort study. Breast Cancer Res 13: R34.

35. Hamelin BA, Turgeon J (1998) Hydrophilicity/lipophilicity: relevance for the pharmacology and clinical effects of HMG-CoA reductase inhibitors. Trends Pharmacol Sci 19: 26-37.

3

Clinical Characteristics of Systemic Lupus Erythematosus Patients with Coronary Artery Disease

Guo Y, Li Y and Jia Y*

Scientific Research Building, Fuwai Hospital, No 167 Beilishi Road, West District, Beijing, People's Republic of China

Abstract

Purpose: The aim of this study was to analyze the clinical characteristics of Systemic Lupus Erythematosus (SLE) patients with Coronary Artery Disease (CAD).

Methods: This study used data from electronic medical records system from Fuwai Hospital. Subjects included SLE patients with CAD and gender-and, age-matched CAD patients without autoimmune connective tissue diseases in a ratio of 1:4. All CAD patients were confirmed by Coronary Angiography (CAG). Data from all subjects was abstracted for Cardiovascular Disease (CVD) risk factors, laboratory test results, echocardiography and CAG.

Results: The proportion of old myocardial infarction (OMI) (p=0.000), myocardial infarction (MI) (p=0.001), family history of premature CAD (p=0.023), hypercholesterolemia (p=0.005), menopause (p=0.015), renal disease manifestation (p=0.000), and higher CRP (p=0.000) in SLE patients with CAD (n=22) were significantly higher than in CAD patients (n=88). CAG showed more multi-vessel lesions (p=0.015) and vascular occlusion lesions (p=0.006) in SLE patients with CAD. Total cholesterol (TC), serum creatinine, urine protein and B-type natriuretic peptide precursor (pro-BNP) were significantly higher in SLE patients with CAD (p=0.000). SLE patients with CAD had higher mortality than CAD patients (p=0.029).

Conclusions: These results indicate that SLE patients with CAD have more renal insufficiency, hypercholesterolemia, and family history of premature CAD than matched patients. In addition, SLE patients with CAD have more extensive and severe coronary artery lesions, and are easily combined with cardiac dysfunction.

Keywords: Systemic Lupus Erythematosus (SLE); Coronary Artery Disease (CAD); Clinical characteristics

Introduction

With the advance of diagnostic and treatment technologies, the prognosis for patients with Systemic Lupus Erythematosus (SLE) has been greatly improved. However, long-term survival remains poor, most likely due to late disease complications. In 1976 Urowitz et al. identified the bimodal mortality pattern, with early deaths due to active disease and infections, and late deaths due to Cardiovascular Disease (CVD) [1]. SLE patients have an increased risk for CVD. The risk of Myocardial Infarction (MI) is increased 50-fold in women with SLE aged 35-44 years old than in women of similar ages without SLE [2].

The increased risk of CVD in SLE patients is under debate. The reason for the increased risk of CVD is likely to be multifactorial. Traditional CVD risk factors include gender, age, obesity, dyslipidemia, hypertension, smoking, family history of premature Coronary Artery Disease (CAD), diabetes mellitus, and menopause. Traditional CVD risk factors are important, but do not, however, fully explain the increased risk of CVD in SLE patients. SLE patients have a 10- to 17-fold higher risk related to CAD than expected taking into account the traditional risk factors [3]. The non-traditional factors are associated with SLE itself like renal disease manifestation, pro-inflammatory cytokines, inflammatory mediators, anti-oxLDL antibodies, antiphospholipid antibodies, and corticosteroid use. CAD is one of the cardiovascular manifestations observed in SLE patients. Although it has been reported that CAD is clinically identifiable in 6.1%-8.9% SLE patients, the occurrence of subclinical CAD is more frequent. Because the clinical manifestations of CAD are more subtle and complex in SLE patients, more attention should be paid to SLE patients

with CAD. To understand and manage risk factors for CAD in SLE patients, diagnostic tools such as laboratory tests, echocardiography and Coronary Angiography (CAG) are important.

The aims of this matched study were to investigate CVD risk factors to help us understand clinical characteristics and to analyze clinical characteristics such as demographics, medical history, medication, test results, and motality in SLE patients with CAD.

Methods

Data source

Data for this study were collected through electronic medical records system from Fuwai Hospital, Beijing, China. The electronic medical records system is a database that covers 100% of inpatients since 2002 in Fuwai Hospital. The electronic medical records system has a range of data, including demographics, personal statistics like age and weight, vital signs, medical history, medication, allergies, laboratory test results, radiology images, and billing information. Outpatient visits including return visits are also well recorded in this system.

*Corresponding author: Jia Y, Scientific Research Building, Fuwai Hospital, No 167 Beilishi Road, West District, Beijing, People's Republic of China, E-mail: yhjia2002@yeah.net

Study population

From 2002 to 2014, in the electronic database of 103,136 CAD patients from Fuwai Hospital which is a national center specialized in cardiovascular diseases, there were 22 SLE patients with CAD confirmed by CAG (0.21‰ of inpatients in the electronic database). Group 1 consisted of 22 SLE patients with CAD. Group 2 was 88 gender-, and age-matched CAD patients who were randomly selected from the same time of initial hospital admission.

The inclusion criteria were: The diagnosis of SLE was earlier than CAD. Group 1 was in the hospital at the same time of initial hospital admission in group 2. All CAD patients had undergone CAG. Exclusion criteria were: Matched CAD patients with autoimmune connective tissue diseases such as SLE, rheumatoid arthritis, scleroderma, and mixed connective tissue disease.

All SLE patients fulfilled the revised American College of Rheumatology criteria for SLE and had been confirmed by specialists [4]. The CAD diagnosis was confirmed by clinical manifestations, Electrocardiogram (ECG), myocardial enzymes, echocardiography, and CAG. CAD patients were defined as those who had a stenosis ≥ 50% of the time and in at least one of major coronary arteries or their main branches on cardiac catheterization. MI was defined on the basis of definite ECG abnormalities or manifestations of chest pain with probable ECG abnormalities and abnormal myocardial enzymes. Patients who experienced more than one cardiac event were only counted once. The event date for each case was defined as the hospital admission date.

In this study, patients were followed-up through telephone interviews and asked about cardiovascular and SLE outcomes in 2014. They were also asked about past and present medication use in detail. Through electronic medical records and telephone follow-ups we collected information for group 1 including SLE duration, medications, cardiovascular events, and other chronic organ damage. Medications included aspirin, statins, anticoagulants, current and past use of corticosteroid, immunosuppressive drugs (azathioprine and cyclophosphamide), and antimalarial drugs (hydroxychloroquine).

Risk factors for CVD

CVD risk factors included traditional CVD risk factors and non-traditional disease-specific factors. Gender, age, obesity (body mass index ≥ 28.0 kg/m², using the 'China' cut-points) [5], dyslipidemia (determined by ESC/EAS Guidelines for the management of dyslipidemia) [6], hypercholesterolemia (defined as cholesterol>5.2 mmol/L), hypertension (defined as a systolic blood pressure ≥ 140 mmHg and/or a diastolic blood pressure ≥ 90 mmHg on 2 or more occasions and/or patient self-reported intake of antihypertensive medications) [7], smoking ('ever' or 'never', 'ever' defined as having smoked more than 1 cigarette per day for more than 1 year), family history of premature CAD (defined as MI or sudden death in a first-degree relative: male, age<55 years or female, age<65 years), diabetes mellitus (fasting plasma glucose>7.0 mmol/L, or current diabetic therapy) [8], menopause, renal disease manifestation (serum creatinine>1.4 mg/dl, or significant proteinuria (>1+ on dipstick analysis or >500 mg/day)), C-reactive protein (CRP) (0-8 mg/L), lipoprotein(a) (Lpa) (10-300 mg/L), and corticosteroid use were collected for all the subjects from the electronic medical records [5-8]. Moreover, blood lipids, B-type natriuretic peptide precursor (pro-BNP), serum creatinine, blood urea nitrogen, urine protein, coagulation, chest radiography, echocardiography, and CAG (recorded locations of stenosis, stenosis (with stenosis ≥ 50% is significant stenosis), two and more vessels involved is defined as multi-vessel lesion, stenosis=100% is occlusion) results were collected.

Statistical analysis

Statistical analyses were performed using the SPSS statistical package (SPSS version 21.0). Data presented are the mean ± SD for continuous variables as well as percentages for categorical variables. Qualitative variables were compared using chi- square test and quantitative variables were compared using independent samples t test. As a descriptive measure of association, $p<0.05$ is considered to be statistically significant. Finally, multiple logistic regression models were performed to define the possible role of factors associated with CAD.

Results

In this study, 22 SLE patients with CAD were included in group 1 and 88 gender-, and age-matched CAD patients were included in group 2. Group 1 had 4 patients with stable angina pectoris, 5 patients with unstable angina pectoris, 4 patients with acute myocardial infarction (AMI), 9 patients with old myocardial infarction (OMI), and 13 patients with MI. Group 2 had 33 patients with stable angina pectoris, 36 patients with unstable angina pectoris, 13 patients with AMI, 6 patients with OMI, and 19 patients with MI. There was a significant trend towards OMI ($p=0.000$) and MI ($p=0.001$) in group 1 than in group 2.

CVD risk factors between the 2 groups

There were no differences in hypertension, dyslipidemia, obesity, smoking, diabetes, and Lpa (Table 1). Group 1 was significantly more likely to have family history of premature CAD ($p=0.023$), hypercholesterolemia ($p=0.005$), menopause ($p=0.015$), renal disease manifestation ($p=0.000$), and higher CRP ($p=0.000$) compared to group 2. The average number of risk factors per person was 3.32 ± 1.70.

Tests and mortality between the 2 groups

Table 2 showed clinical data from the two groups. Both groups had similar triglycerides, low-density lipoprotein cholesterol, and high-density lipoprotein cholesterol. SLE patients with CAD had higher values of total cholesterol (TC) ($p=0.013$), serum creatinine ($p=0.000$), blood urea nitrogen ($p=0.000$), urine protein ($p=0.000$), and pro-BNP ($p=0.000$) when compared to CAD patients. Group 1 patients had lower echocardiography ejection fraction (EF) than their matched peers ($p=0.000$). CAG showed single coronary vessel lesions were significantly less ($p=0.015$) in SLE patients with CAD. However, there were more multi-vessel ($p=0.015$) and vascular occlusion lesions ($p=0.006$) in group 1 compared with group 2. No difference was found in the proportion of Coronary Artery Bypass Grafting (CABG) surgery between the two groups.

The telephone follow-up data demonstrated that 4 patients had died, of which 2 patients died due to lupus nephritis and others died of MI. The average survival time for the 4 patients was 13.87 ± 9.31 years old after SLE diagnosis. There were 3 patients who had died in group 2, of which 2 patients died of MI and 1 patient died of heart failure. SLE patients with CAD had higher mortality compared to CAD patients ($p=0.029$).

Clinical characteristics of SLE patients with CAD:

There were 22 SLE patients with CAD; with a male to female ratio was 3:19. In group 1, the average age of SLE at diagnosis was 36.54 ± 8.54 years old. The average age of when cardiac events first occurred was 53.27 ± 8.75 years old. The SLE patients developed CAD in 16.29 ± 8.70 years after the diagnosis of SLE. CAG showed multi-vessel lesions in 18 patients (81.82%) and vascular occlusion lesions in 9 patients (40.91%). As for chronic organ damage, 4 patients had musculoskeletal damage, 4 patients had renal damage, 3 patients had neuropsychiatric damage, 2 patients had skin damage, and 2 patients had pulmonary damage (Table 3).

Table 3 shows all patients used corticosteroid, with 9 patients that discontinued corticosteroid and 12 patients that were taking corticosteroid during study timeframe. The average dose of corticosteroid (prednisone equivalent) was 8.46 ± 7.32 mg and the cumulative lifetime dose (prednisone equivalent) was 13.33 ± 5.63 g. Among these 22 SLE patients with CAD, there was 1 patient taking antimalarial drugs, 2 patients taking tripterygium wilfordii and 3 patient taking immunosuppressive drugs. 20 patients used statins including atorvastatin (accounting for 90%), simvastatin and pravastatin. Apart

from a patient with upper gastrointestinal bleeding, 21 patients were taking aspirin and 6 of these patients were taking clopidogrel at the same time. Moreover, 4 patients were taking low molecular weight heparin (ranging from enoxaparin to fondaparinux) in addition to aspirin and clopidogrel.

Discussion

SLE is an inflammatory rheumatic disease of immunologic origin. The overall age-adjusted incidence and prevalence (ACR definition) per 100,000 persons is 5.5 and 72.8, respectively. SLE patients have an increased risk for CVD. More than 50% of SLE patients have cardiac involvement [9]. Risk of SLE patients developing CAD is 4-8 times higher than in healthy controls. CAD has been confirmed as a major cause of mortality in SLE patients. The clinical manifestations of CAD in SLE can result from several pathophysiologic mechanisms, including atherosclerosis, arteritis, thrombosis, embolization, spasm, and abnormal coronary flow. Clinically, non-atherosclerotic factors will be considered, if CAD patients are younger than 30 years old

Cardiovascular risk factors	SLE with CAD (n=22)	CAD (n=88)	P
Age (years)	57.41 ± 10.19	57.50 ± 9.65	NS
Gender (female/male)	3/19	3/19	NS
Family history of premature CAD n (%)	9 (40.91)	16 (18.18)	0.023
Hypertension n (%)	11 (50.00)	58 (65.91)	NS
Obesity n (%)	6(27.27)	32(36.36)	NS
Dyslipidemia n (%)	14 (63.64)	37 (42.05)	NS
Hypercholesterolemia n (%)	11 (50.00)	17 (19.32)	0.005
Diabetes mellitus n (%)	5 (22.73)	29 (32.95)	NS
Smoking n (%)	4 (18.18)	21 (23.86)	NS
Menopause (years)	48.42 ± 3.99	50.13 ± 2.26	0.015
Renal disease manifestation n (%)	8(36.36)	4(4.55)	0.000
CRP (mg/L)	9.59 ± 10.79	3.18 ± 4.80	0.000
Lpa (mg/L)	320.68 ± 303.31	289.94 ± 276.92	NS

˙Data are expressed as mean ± SD, n (%) Abbreviations: CAD= coronary artery disease, CRP= C-reactive protein, Lpa= Lipoprotein(a); NS = non-significant.
Table 1: Prevalence of CVD risk factors between the 2 groups

Variable	SLE with CAD(n=22)	CAD(n=88)	P
Triglycerides (mmol/L)	1.43 ± 0.52	1.76 ± 1.36	NS
Total cholesterol (mmol/L)	5.22 ± 0.63	4.31 ± 1.06	0.000
LDL-C (mmol/L)	2.53 ± 1.01	2.39 ± 0.99	NS
HDL-C (mmol/L)	1.27 ± 0.43	1.38 ± 0.33	NS
Serum creatinine (mmol/L)	73.37 ± 20.14	60.89 ± 11.84	0.000
Blood urea nitrogen (mmol/L)	8.47 ± 7.32	4.94 ± 1.45	0.000
Urine protein n (%)	8(36.36)	4(4.55)	0.000
Pro-BNP (pmol/L)	1200.84 ± 1316.48	626.95 ± 317.61	0.000
EF (%)	55.18 ± 12.26	65.11 ± 5.65	0.000
Coronary angiography			
Single vessel n (%)	4 (18.18)	41 (46.59)[b]	0.015
Two vessels n (%)	8 (36.36)	24 (27.27)	NS
Three vessels n (%)	10 (45.45)	23 (26.14)	NS
Multi-vessel n (%)	18 (81.82)	47 (53.41)	0.015
Vascular occlusion n (%)	9 (40.91)	13 (14.77)	0.006
CABG surgery n (%)	3 (13.64)	5 (5.68)	NS
Mortality n (%)	4(18.18)	3(3.41)	0.029
Lupus nephritis n (%)	2(9.09)	0(0)	
MI n (%)	2(9.09)	2(2.27)	
Heart failure n (%)	0(0)	1(1.14)	

˙Data are expressed as mean ± SD, n (%) Abbreviations: LDL-C= Low-density lipoprotein cholesterol, HDL-C= High-density lipoprotein cholesterol, pro-BNP: B-type natriuretic peptide precursor, EF=Ejection fraction (From echocardiography), CABG: Coronary artery bypass grafting, MI: myocardial infarction.
Table 2: Tests and mortality between the 2 groups

Variable	SLE with CAD (n=22)
Corticosteroid n (%)	22 (100.00)
average dose (prednisone equivalent) at study (mg/d)	8.46 ± 7.32
cumulative lifetime dose (prednisone equivalent) (gm)	5.35 ± 2.72
Antimalarial drugs n (%)	1 (4.55)
Tripterygium wilfordii n (%)	2 (9.09)
Immunosuppressive drugs n (%)	3 (13.64)
Aspirin	21 (95.45)
Statins n (%)	20 (90.91)
Chronic damage	1.68 ± 0.78
Musculoskeletal n (%)	4 (18.18)
Renal damage n (%)	4 (18.18)
Malignancy n (%)	0 (0.00)
Neuropsychiatric n (%)	3 (13.64)
Skin damage n (%)	2 (9.09)
Pulmonary n (%)	2 (9.09)

without CVD risk factors. In our study, as for when cardiac events first occurred, the minimum age was 34 years old and the average age of was 53.27 ± 8.75 years old. The average number of risk factors per person was 3.32 ± 1.70. CAG has a certain role in identification of arteritis. In the CAG results of SLE patients, there were no vasculitis typical changes like cystic change and aneurysm. In the occurrence of MI, coronary thrombosis has an important position. The occurrence of thrombosis is related to endothelial injury mediated by immune complex and anti-phospholipid antibodies. Almost all thrombosis occurs on the basis of atherosclerosis. Although there is an increased relative risk for CAD in SLE patients, the risk factors that may contribute to this increased risk is unclear.

In this retrospective study, we focused on the clinical characteristics of SLE patients with CAD by checking related risk factors, laboratory data and myocardial perfusion abnormalities. Features of this study are that all CAD patients had undergone CAG and SLE patients with CAD were compared with CAD patients. Univariate analyses demonstrate that, SLE patients with CAD were more likely to have risk factors for atherosclerotic disease than their matched peers. Our study found family history of premature CAD, hypercholesterolemia, renal disease manifestation, earlier menopause, and higher CRP were more common in SLE patients with CAD. The study showed hypercholesterolemia to be a significant CVD risk factor in SLE patients. In many studies, hypercholesterolemia has been proven to be associated with the increased risk of CVD events in SLE patients [10]. Many studies have demonstrated that SLE is a multi-gene related disease. Urowitz et al. found that SLE patients with CAD are more likely to have a family history of premature CAD [11]. Our study demonstrated family history of premature CAD was significantly associated with the increased risk of CAD in SLE patients. Renal disease manifestation is known to be one of the important factors for accelerated atherosclerosis in SLE [12]. Renal impairment and proteinuria are likely to have an adverse effect on CVD risk [13]. Our results about renal disease manifestation are similar to the studies above. SLE patients with CAD had their menopause an average of 2 years earlier than did the CAD patients (at a mean age of 48.4 years versus 50.1 years). Premature menopause was more prevalent in SLE patients with CAD than in CAD patients in our study. SLE patients have menopause on average 3-4 year earlier than healthy people in previous studies [14]. This is associated with the SLE itself and usage of corticosteroid, antimalarial drugs, and immunosuppressive drugs in these patients. Group1 had significantly higher CRP compared to group 2. Inflammatory mediators and endothelial activation are associated to atherosclerosis. Elevated high sensitivity CRP (hsCRP) is

considered a powerful independent predictor of vascular events in the LUMINA study [15]. Genetic variations in the CRP gene(s) and disease activity may account for elevated CRP levels in SLE patients.

Although no statistically significant correlation was found between the presence CAD in SLE patients and a number of risk factors, this does not mean those factors are irrelevant. Among the risk factors, hypertension, dyslipidemia and hypercholesterolemia are more common in SLE patients [16]. Some studies have identified hypertension as the modifiable risk factor which is most closely linked to the onset of SLE patients with CAD [14-17]. However, in our study, there was no difference in hypertension between the two groups. This is most likely due to the limited number of studied SLE patients with CAD. Almost all SLE patients with CAD had been treated with corticosteroid and 36.36% of patients had renal disease manifestation. Although dyslipidemia is a feature of patients with steroid-treated SLE and patients with renal disease manifestation, no difference was found in dyslipidemia between the two groups. There were 78.57% of dyslipidemia patients with hypercholesterolemia in group 1 and 45.94% in group 2. Whether dyslipidemia is associated with the increased risk of CVD in SLE patients need further evidence. No differences were found in obesity and diabetes mellitus between the two groups. High prevalence of metabolic syndrome in patients with SLE has been repeatedly established in previous studies. However, most controls of previous studies are general population. Our control group consisted of CAD patients who also had a lot of atherosclerotic risk factors.

The average age of first cardiac event in SLE patients was 53.27 ± 8.75 years old. This age is 10.5 years earlier than the age of non-SLE patients, which suggests SLE is an independent risk factor which increases the risk of CAD in SLE patients [18]. The SLE patients developed CAD in 16.29 ± 8.70 years after the diagnosis of SLE. Patients with SLE have cardiovascular events at a much younger age compared with the general population. Having a cardiovascular event in 9-18years after the diagnosis of SLE has been demonstrated in some studies.[2] Fuwai Hospital is a center specialized in cardiovascular diseases. This hospital does not have autoimmune related texts. In group 1, there was a lack of sufficient clinical immunology data. Therefore, this study is not a comprehensive evaluation of risk factors which should account for the increased risk of CAD in SLE patients, and the role of other variables, such as hypertension, stroke, and smoking needs further investigation.

CAG is regarded as the gold standard for CAD diagnosis. SLE patients with CAD had more MI, multi-vessel lesions and vascular occlusion lesions compared with the matched patients. The multi-vessel lesions proportion reached as high as 81.8% and nearly half of the SLE with CAD patients had vascular occlusion lesions. Our data suggests that patients in group 1 have more extensive coronary artery lesions, vascular occlusion lesions, and are easily combined with cardiac dysfunction. There were 13.64% SLE with CAD patients and 5.68% matched patients that had CABG surgery. No difference was found in the proportion of CABG surgery between the two groups. For SLE patients with CAD, there might have been some operation contraindications, including multi-systems involvement and concomitant likelihood of postoperative complications, such as poor healing due to steroid use.

Data from ultrasound and pro-BNP demonstrated that SLE patients with CAD had poorer cardiac pump function, and were more easily combined with cardiac dysfunction. Karadag et al. have found that SLE patients without clinical signs of ischemic heart disease have increased levels of BNP [19]. Increased BNP levels in SLE patients may reflect myocardial damage. Results of serum creatinine, blood urea nitrogen, and urine protein suggest that renal disease manifestation is a CVD risk factor in SLE patients. Studies have shown that increasing level of serum creatinine and the presence of proteinuria are associated with SLE patients with CAD [20]. In addition, kidney damage and use of glucocorticoid (>30 mg/d) can induce dyslipidemia in SLE patients [21]. In group 1, there were 8 patients with kidney disease (36.36%), 2 patients with pulmonary involvement (9.09%), and 2 patients with strokes (9.09%). All of these results suggest that SLE has multi-systems involvement. Data suggests that high cholesterol levels, increased serum creatinine levels, and the presence of urine protein are most likely to be CVD predictive factors in SLE patients.

The average survival time was 13.87 ± 9.31 years in the 4 dead patients from group 1after SLE diagnosis. Kaditanon et al. have reported the overall cumulative probability of survival after SLE diagnosis at 5, 10, 15, and 20 years is 95%, 91%, 85%, and 78%, respectively [22]. Our data showed SLE patients with CAD had higher mortality than CAD patients. This is most likely due to SLE patients with CAD have more severe coronary lesions, worse cardiac function and more serious complications. SLE itself may directly responsible for increased mortality. Renal involvement is also associated with significantly increased mortality in SLE patients [23]. In our study, musculoskeletal damage and renal damage were more common in SLE patients with CAD. An observation of 232 SLE patients reveals that musculoskeletal, cardiovascular and renal damage are the most common on the SLE chronic organ damage list [24]. The average dose (prednisone equivalent) during the study was 8.46 ± 7.32 mg and the cumulative lifetime dose (prednisone equivalent) was 13.33 ± 5.63 g. Compared with other studies, our SLE patients with CAD had higher cumulative lifetime dose, which may partly explain the increased CVD risk. In group 1, there were 95.45% patients taking aspirin and 90.91% patients taking statins. Some studies have reported the beneficial effect of aspirin in SLE patients [25]. Statins not only exert favorable effects on lipoprotein metabolism, but may also have an increasingly recognized immunomodulatory role. Some studies propose that (like diabetes mellitus) SLE should be considered a 'CAD-equivalent' condition for baseline risk. The increased use of aspirin, statins, needs to be more-widely investigated.

In conclusion, several CVD risk factors may account for the development of CAD in SLE patients. The approach to the prevention of cardiovascular events in SLE should include the control of risk factors to substantially reduce or delay the occurrence of these potentially fatal events. SLE patients with CAD have more extensive coronary artery lesions, vascular occlusion lesions, and are easily combined with MI, cardiac dysfunction and multi-systems involvement. SLE patients with CAD have more severe CAD clinical manifestations and poor prognosis. Most early CAD clinical manifestations of SLE patients are complicated and atypical. Coronary assessment and early screening should be strengthened in SLE patients with CAD with clinical manifestations or not. Early intervention of CVD risk factors should not be ignored. We ought to assess SLE activity and involvement of other systems, thereby delaying or preventing the progression of CAD.

References

1. Urowitz MB, Bookman AA, Koehler BE, Gordon DA, Smythe HA, et al. (1976) The bimodal mortality pattern of systemic lupus erythematosus. Am J Med 60: 221-225.

2. Manzi S, Meilahn EN, Rairie JE, Conte CG, Medsger TA Jr, et al. (1997) Age-specific incidence rates of myocardial infarction and angina in women with systemic lupus erythematosus: Comparison with the Framingham study. Am J Epidemiol 145: 408-415.

3. Esdaile JM, Abrahamowicz M, Grodzicky T, Li Y, Panaritis C, et al. (2001) Traditional Framingham risk factors fail to fully account for accelerated atherosclerosis in systemic lupus erythematosus. Arthritis Rheum 44: 2331-2337.

4. Hochberg MC (1997) Updating the American College of Rheumatology revised criteria for the classification of systemic lupus erythematosus. Arthritis Rheum 40:1725.

5. Zhou BF(2002) Cooperative Meta-analysis Group of the Working Group on Obesity in China: Predictive values of body mass index and waist circumference for risk factors of certain related diseases in Chinese adults-study on optimal cutoff points of body mass index and waist circumference in Chinese adults. Biomed Environ Sci 15: 83-95.

6. Reiner Z, Catapano AL, De Backer G, Graham I, Taskinen MR et al. (2011) ESC/EAS Guidelines for the management of dyslipidemia: The task force for the management of dyslipidemia of the European Society of Cardiology (ESC) and the European Atherosclerosis Society (EAS). Eur Heart J 32: 1769-1818.

7. Mancia G, De Backer G, Dominiczak A, Cifkova R, Fagard R et al. (2007) 2007 ESH-ESC practice guidelines for the management of arterial hypertension: ESH-ESC task force on the management of arterial hypertension. J hypertens 25: 1751-1762.

8. Expert Committee on the Diagnosis and Classification of Diabetes Mellitus (2003) Report of the expert committee on the diagnosis and classification of diabetes mellitus. Diabetes Care 26 Suppl 1: S5-20.

9. Nikpour M, Urowitz M B, Ibanez D, Harvey PJ, Gladman DD (2011) Importance of cumulative exposure to elevated cholesterol and blood pressure in development of atherosclerotic coronary artery disease in systemic lupus erythematosus: a prospective proof-of-concept cohort study. Arthritis Res Ther13: R156.

10. Urowitz MB, Gladman D, Ibañez D, Bae SC, Sanchez-Guerrero J, et al. (2010) Atherosclerotic vascular events in a multinational inception cohort of systemic lupus erythematosus. Arthritis Care Res (Hoboken) 62: 881-887.

11. Serikova Slu, Kozlovskaia NL, Shilov EM (2008) Lupus nephritis as a factor of atherosclerosis risk in patients with systemic lupus erythematosus. Ter Arkh 80: 52-58.

12. Bruce IN, Gladman DD, Urowitz MB (2000) Premature atherosclerosis in systemic lupus erythematosus. See comment in PubMed Commons below Rheum Dis Clin North Am 26: 257-278.

13. Bruce IN, Urowitz MB, Gladman DD, Ibañez D, Steiner G (2003) Risk factors for coronary heart disease in women with systemic lupus erythematosus: the Toronto Risk Factor Study. Arthritis Rheum 48: 3159-3167.

14. Szalai AJ, Alarcón GS, Calvo-Alén J, Toloza SM, McCrory MA, et al. (2005) Systemic lupus erythematosus in a multiethnic US Cohort (LUMINA). XXX: association between C-reactive protein (CRP) gene polymorphisms and vascular events.Rheumatology (Oxford) 44: 864-868.

15. Bessant R, Duncan R, Ambler G, Swanton J, Isenberg DA, et al. (2006) Prevalence of conventional and lupus-specific risk factors for cardiovascular disease in patients with systemic lupus erythematosus: A case-control study. Arthritis Rheum 55: 892-899.

16. Nuttall SL, Heaton S, Piper MK, Martin U, Gordon C (2003) Cardiovascular risk in systemic lupus erythematosus--evidence of increased oxidative stress and dyslipidaemia.Rheumatology (Oxford) 42: 758-762.

17. Scalzi LV, Hollenbeak CS, Wang L (2010) Racial disparities in age at time of cardiovascular events and cardiovascular-related death in patients with systemic lupus erythematosus.Arthritis Rheum 62: 2767-2775.

18. Scalzi LV, Hollenbeak CS, Wang L (2010) Racial disparities in age at time of cardiovascular events and cardiovascular-related death in patients with systemic lupus erythematosus.Arthritis Rheum 62: 2767-2775.

19. Karadag O, Calguneri M, Yavuz B, Atalar E, Akdogan A, et al. (2007) B-type natriuretic peptide (BNP) levels in female systemic lupus erythematosus patients: what is the clinical significance?Clin Rheumatol 26: 1701-1704.

20. Selzer F, Sutton-Tyrrell K, Fitzgerald SG, Pratt JE, Tracy RP, et al. (2004) Comparison of risk factors for vascular disease in the carotid artery and aorta in women with systemic lupus erythematosus. Arthritis Rheum 50: 151-159.

21. Urquizu-Padilla M, Balada E, Chacon P, Pérez EH, Vilardell-Tarrés M, et al. (2009) Changes in lipid profile between flare and remission of patients with systemic lupus erythematosus: a prospective study. J Rheumatol 36: 1639-1645.

22. Kasitanon N, Magder LS, Petri M (2006) Predictors of survival in systemic lupus erythematosus. Medicine (Baltimore) 85: 147-156.

23. Chambers SA, Allen E, Rahman A, Isenberg D (2009) Damage and mortality in a group of British patients with systemic lupus erythematosus followed up for over 10 years. Rheumatology (Oxford) 48: 673-675.

24. Wahl DG, Bounameaux H, de Moerloose P, Sarasin FP (2000) Prophylactic antithrombotic therapy for patients with systemic lupus erythematosus with or without antiphospholipid antibodies: do the benefits outweigh the risks? A decision analysis.Arch Intern Med 160: 2042-2048.

25. Haque S, Bruce IN (2005) Therapy insight: systemic lupus erythematosus as a risk factor for cardiovascular disease.Nat Clin Pract Cardiovasc Med 2: 423-430.

Co-prescribing of Warfarin with Statins and Proton Pump Inhibitors in Elderly Australians

Gadzhanova S* and Roughead E

Division of Health Sciences, School of Pharmacy and Medical Sciences, University of SouthAustralia, City East Campus-R3-17B,Australia

Abstract

Background: Comorbidity is common in individuals with atrial fibrillation (AF). The predominant treatment for AF is warfarin and medicine interactions with warfarin represent a challenge for optimising treatment of AF in older people with comorbidities. Statins and Proton Pump Inhibitors are commonly prescribed therapies and in both classes, there are medicines with greater or lesser potential to interact with warfarin.

Objective: The aim of this study was to examine use of antithrombotic treatment in elderly Australians, and the extent of concurrent use of interacting statins and proton pump inhibitors (PPIs) with warfarin.

Methods: A retrospective cohort study was conducted using data from the Australian Government Department of Veterans' Affairs. The cohort included all patients who had at least one hospitalisation with a primary diagnosis for AF between 2007 and 2011. Individuals contributed person-months from the date of first AF hospitalisation to death or end of study (December 2011). Monthly utilisation of antithrombotics was assessed. A sub-cohort of warfarin users was defined as those with AF who received warfarin as monotherapy and the proportions of those co-dispensed statins or PPIs were established.

Results: Around 70% of patients with AF were receiving antithrombotic treatment, with 35% dispensed warfarin, 17% aspirin, and 7% clopidogrel as monotherapy. In December 2011, 54% of patients with AF on warfarin monotherapy were co-dispensed a statin, with the statins with potential for interaction dispensed at highest rates; atorvastatin followed by simvastatin and rosuvastatin. At study end, 43% of the warfarin cohort were also dispensed PPIs, with one-third using esomeprazole, followed by pantoprazole, both of which have the potential to interact with warfarin.

Conclusion: 30% of patients with AF were not receiving antithrombotic treatment. In those receiving an antithrombotic agent, warfarin was the most commonly dispensed (35%). The most common statin and PPI co-prescribed with warfarin were agents with the potential to interact with warfarin, despite alternative agents being available. Raising awareness of the safer alternative for people with comorbidities may improve warfarin management.

Keywords: Atrial fibrillation; Statins; Proton pump inhibitors; Warfarin; Comorbidity

Introduction

Atrial Fibrillation (AF) is a common form of irregular heart rhythm increasing a person's risk for ischaemic stroke by about five-fold [1]. The condition affects around 1.1% of Australians [2] and the prevalence increases with age, more than half of all atrial fibrillation patients are aged over 75 years [2]. Antithrombotic (anticoagulation or antiplatelet) therapy is recommended to reduce the risk of stroke, with warfarin being the most commonly used oral anticoagulant in Australia [3]. Dose-adjusted-warfarin reduces stroke risk by 64%, while antiplatelet agents reduce risk by 22% [4].

Bleeding is the most common complication of warfarin therapy and the risk is related to factors such as advanced age, prior bleeding or stroke, and specific comorbidities [3,5]. Treatment for comorbid conditions may require medications which increase the probability of interactions with warfarin. Some drugs alter the pharmacokinetics or pharmacodynamics of warfarin which impacts on the bleeding risk; these include concomitant antiplatelet therapy [3,5], statins for lowering of high cholesterol [3,6], and Proton Pump Inhibitors (PPI) for reducing gastric acid production [7,8].

Warfarin is metabolised by liver enzymes from the Cytochrome P450 (CYP) family. S-warfarin is a CYP2C9 substrate, for which fluvastatin and rosuvastatin are also substrates [9,10]. R-warfarin is a substrate of CYP3A4, for which atorvastatin and simvastatin are also

substrates [9,10]. Only pravastatin is excreted predominantly by renal mechanisms and does not undergo significant metabolism via the CYP system [9,10]. The administration of statins (except pravastatin) to patients receiving warfarin could competitively inhibit warfarin metabolism causing potentiation of the anticoagulant effect [6], requiring a dosage adjustment.

PPI medications undergo considerable biotransformation in the liver before elimination [11]. Omeprazole, esomeprazole, pantoprazole and lansoprazole are extensively metabolised by CYP2C19 and CYP3A4 and as a consequence they also might interact with warfarin as it is also metabolised by the same hepatic CYP enzymes [8,11]. Only rabeprazole has primary nonenzymatic metabolism with an insignificant percent metabolised by CYP system [11]. Both statins and PPIs are among the

*Corresponding author: Svetla Gadzhanova, Research Fellow, Division of Health Sciences, School of Pharmacy and Medical Sciences, University of South Australia, City East Campus-R3-17B, Australia, E-mail: Svetla.Gadzhanova@unisa.edu.au

most prescribed medicines in Australia [12] with significant potential to interact with warfarin. The extent to which prescribers are aware of these interactions and preferentially prescribe the medicines in the class least likely to interact with warfarin is unknown.

Aim of the study

The aim of this study was to examine use of antithrombotic treatments to manage atrial fibrillation, and the extent of concurrent use of interacting statins and proton pump inhibitors with warfarin.

Methods

Data sources

Data for this study were sourced from the Australian Government Department of Veterans' Affairs (DVA) administrative claims database [13]. The DVA administrative claims database contains details of all prescription medicines, medical and allied health services and hospitalisations provided to veterans, their spouses and dependants, as well as details on patient gender, date of birth and date of death. At study entry (2007), the data covered approximately 293,000 members of the veteran community, who had a mean age of 76 years [14]. Medicines are coded in the dataset according to the World Health Organization (WHO) Anatomical Therapeutic Chemical (ATC) classification system [15] and the Schedule of Pharmaceutical Benefits item codes [16]. Hospitalisations are coded according to the WHO International Classification of Diseases (ICD) [17].

Study population and statistical analysis

The study period was 1 January 2007 to 31 December 2011. The study cohort included all patients who have had at least one hospitalisation with a primary diagnosis for AF (identified by ICD code I48) during the study period. These patients contributed person-months from the date of their first (earliest) hospitalisation until death or end of study (Dec 2011). Overall monthly utilisation of antithrombotics was reported as the proportion of people dispensed the medicine(s) of interest in each month among the AF population in that month. Results were stratified by those using monotherapy or combination therapies. Medicine utilisation in a given month was determined using the dispensing date and the estimated prescription duration. The estimated prescription duration was calculated from the data for each medicine and was defined as the time period in which 75% of prescriptions for that medicine were refilled. It was assumed that a person continued to use the medicine from the dispensing date for the prescription duration.

A sub-cohort of warfarin users was defined as those with AF who received warfarin as monotherapy. The age-standardised monthly proportions of those co-dispensed Proton Pump Inhibitors (PPI), or statins were established.

Participants were censored at the time of death or end of study. Medicine utilisation rates were age-standardised using the veteran population in January 2007 as the standard population in five-year categories. Poisson regression models were used to calculate age-Standardised Rate Ratios (SRR) comparing the rate in one year to the previous year to test for linear trend over time in 2007-2011. Analyses were performed using a SAS 9.4 statistical package (SAS Institute, Cary NC, USA).

Definition of medicines included in the analyses

The medicines and ATC codes included in this study:

Antithrombotics

-   Oral anticoagulants: warfarin (B01AA03). Note: the newer oral anticoagulants dabigatran and rivaroxaban for AF were subsidised after the end of study and were not analysed;

-   Antiplatelets: clopidogrel (B01AC05), aspirin (B01AC06), dipyridamole (B01AC07), ticlopidine (B01AC05), aspirin plus dipyridamole (B01AC30–PBS code 8382E), aspirin plus clopidogrel (B01AC30 - PBS code 9296G);

Proton pump inhibitors: esomeprazole (A02BC05), lansoprazole (A02BC03), omeprazole (A02BC01), pantoprazole (A02BC02), rabeprazole (N02BC04).

Statins: simvastatin (C10AA01 and in fixed-dose combination (FDC)->C10BA02), atorvastatin (C10AA05 and in FDC-> C10BX03), pravastatin (C10AA03), fluvastatin (C10AA04), rosuvastatin (C10AA07).

Results

The AF cohort included 15,375 unique patients. Around 70% of the patients (Figure 1) were receiving antithrombotic treatment and the rate was stable over the years (SRR=0.998, 95% CI: 0.994-1.002, p=0.30). Stratification by the type of therapy (Figure 1) showed that the majority of patients were dispensed warfarin monotherapy (35%, SRR=1.002, 95% CI: 0.996-1.004, p=0.99), followed by aspirin monotherapy (17%, SRR=0.995, CI: 0.992-0.999, p=0.07) and clopidogrel monotherapy (7%, SRR=0.997, CI: 0.989-1.006, p=0.52). Dipyridamole and ticlopidine monotherapy had very limited use (below 0.1%). Nine percent of patients were managed on dual therapies (SRR=1.006, CI: 0.994, 1.016, p=0.37) and a further 2% on triple therapies (SRR=0.950, CI: 0.938-0.964, p=0.10). Of the patients with AF receiving dual therapy with antithrombotics, warfarin plus aspirin was the most commonly used (stable rate of 4.5%), followed by aspirin plus clopidogrel (around 3%), and aspirin plus dipyridamole (1.5%). Triple therapy of warfarin plus aspirin plus clopidogrel was dispensed for 0.5% of AF patients, while warfarin plus aspirin plus dipyridamole- for 0.1%.

Figure 2 presents concurrent use of statins and PPIs in patients with AF who were dispensed warfarin monotherapy. Overall statin use increased significantly from 41.6% in Jan 2007 to 54.2% in Dec 2011 (SRR=1.037, 95% CI: 1.031-1.042, p<0.0001) (Figure 2). Stratification by the type of statin (Figure 3) showed that atorvastatin was the most commonly dispensed in around half of the patients on any statin. Simvastatin use decreased over the study period (from 36% to 26%). Pravastatin use fell from 15% to 7%, while rosuvastatin increased from

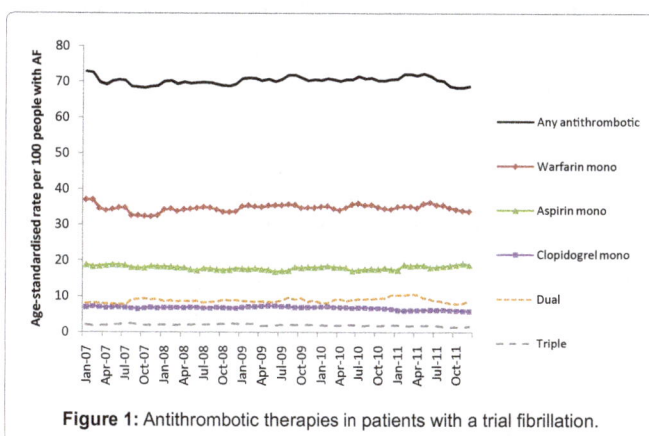

Figure 1: Antithrombotic therapies in patients with a trial fibrillation.

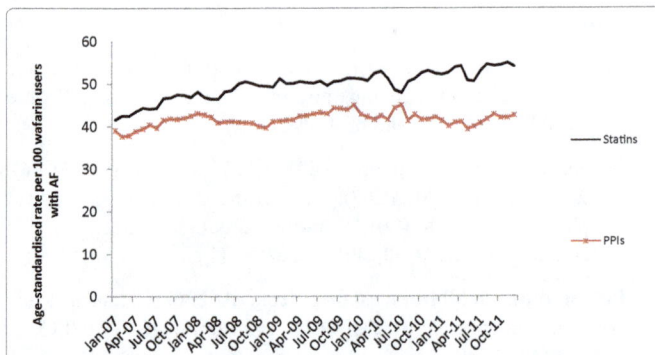

Figure 2: Dispensing of statins and PPIs in patients with AF on warfarin monotherapy.

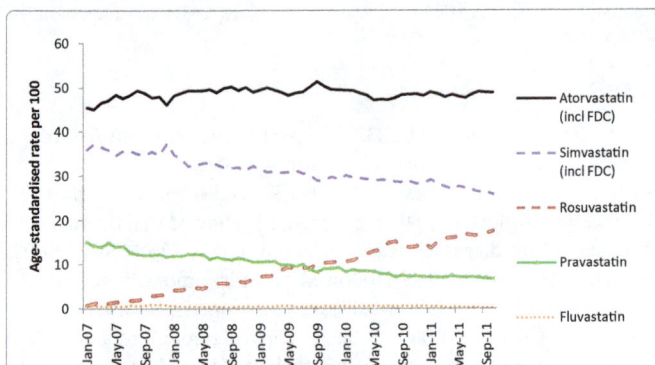

Figure 3: Statins by type in patients with AF dispensed warfarin monotherapy and any statin.

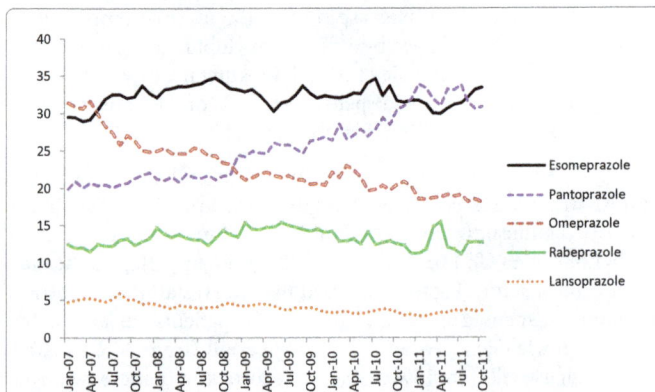

Figure 4: PPIs by type in patients with AF dispensed warfarin monotherapy and any PPI.

1% to 18%. Fluvastatin had very limited use, below 1%.

Overall PPI use also increased from 39.3% to 42.7% (SRR=1.024, CI: 1.020-1.028, p<0.0001) (Figure 2). Stratification by the type of PPI (Figure 4) revealed that esomeprazole contributed for around one-third of all PPI use, pantoprazole use increased from 20% in January 2007 to 31% in Dec 2011, omeprazole use decreased from 31% to 18% in the same period, rabeprazole use was around 13%, and lansoprazole was used in less than 4% of patients on PPIs at the end of the study period.

Discussion

Antithrombotic treatment is recommended to reduce the risk of

stroke in people with AF [3], with warfarin recommended in those who are at moderate to high risk of stroke, and aspirin when the risk is low [18,19], as warfarin has been shown to be significantly more effective than aspirin for stroke reduction [3]. Our results demonstrate that antithrombotics were dispensed in approximately 70% of patients with AF. Around 35% of patients received warfarin as sole treatment for atrial fibrillation, and another 17% received aspirin as monotherapy. The warfarin results are comparable with a US study reporting utilisation of warfarin by 42% of patients with high level of stroke, and by 44% with moderate stroke risk [20]. We did not measure individual stroke risk, however, our population may represent more severe disease as, by definition, all patients had had a prior hospitalisation for AF.

The combination of warfarin and aspirin is associated with increased incidence of major bleeding [21] and should be used with caution in elderly patients [22]. Our results showed that 4.5% of patients with AF were receiving aspirin concurrently with warfarin.

Comprehensive management of AF requires identification and treatment of predisposing factors and concomitant disorders (e.g. hypercholesterolemia) that increase the risk of stroke and other cardiovascular conditions [23]. In managing comorbid conditions, such as oesophageal reflux, practitioners also need to avoid therapies that may reduce the effectiveness of medicines for AF. Knowledge of the pharmacokinetic-pharmacodynamic properties of medicines that are prescribed for common comorbid conditions enables avoidance of drug interactions when concurrent therapy is necessary. However, our results suggest prescribers are not aware of some of these interactions and appropriate alternative therapies.

The administration of statins (except pravastatin) to patients receiving warfarin could competitively inhibit warfarin metabolism. We found that in Dec 2011 more than half the patients (54%) with AF dispensed warfarin as a monotherapy were also dispensed a statin, with atorvastatin dispensed at highest rates, followed by simvastatin and rosuvastatin. Case reports have shown a potentiation of the anticoagulant effect of warfarin when administered with fluvastatin [6] and that warfarin is a commonly co-administered medicine in cases of statin induced rhabdomyolysis [24]. A nested case-control study found no difference in risk of bleeding in warfarin users with recent statin use [25]. Conflicting results were found over the longer term use, however a healthy user effect may have confounded the longer term results [25]. Pravastatin, which is not metabolised by the CYP system and is not expected to interact with warfarin [6], was not widely prescribed with its use decreasing from 15% to 7% during the study; implying that prescribers might not be recognising the potential interactions between warfarin and statins.

Certain PPIs have been shown to reduce warfarin metabolism and clearance leading to increased warfarin concentration as they are metabolised by competing pathways [7]. Clinical evidence suggest significant hazard of over-anticoagulation for esomeprazole (HR 1.99, 95% CI 1.55-2.55) and lansoprazole (HR 1.49, 95% CI 1.05-2.10) when used concurrently with anticoagulant treatment [26]. A lower and non-significant risk increase was found for the other PPIs [26]. Patients on anticoagulants and PPIs should be monitored cautiously [7]. An Italian study on simultaneous use of warfarin and PPIs, found that 62% were using omeprazole, around 10% pantoprazole, and very few, rabeprazole [27]. Our data showed that overall 43% of patients with AF receiving warfarin as sole treatment were also dispensed a PPI in Dec 2011. The majority of those using PPIs (one-third) received esomeprazole followed by increasing use of pantoprazole. Rabeprazole, which has primarily nonenzymatic metabolism, had stable use in around 13%

of people on warfarin and PPIs, suggesting low awareness of potential differences in interactions in this class.

Our study had a number of limitations associated with use of administrative claims data. We used dispensing data as a surrogate for patient's use, however, we were unable to determine whether dispensed medicines were actually taken by the study participants. Also, as dose of prescribed medicines was not available in the data, dosage adjustment (e.g. warfarin dosage reduction) could not be established. We did not assess the length of co-dispensing and harm associated with those potentially interacting medicines. We could not account for other risk factors such as body weight, diet and genetics which may have had an impact on warfarin efficacy.

All subjects in this study receive subsidised medicines from the Department of Veterans' Affairs. Patient co-payments are $6.00 for all medicines and there is no price differential between the medicines for veterans, so pricing factors will not have influenced our results. Additionally, age is unlikely to have influenced our results as the veteran cohort is elderly, with a mean age of 76 years. The older age may make them even more vulnerable to interactions, as a result of age-related changes in kidney and liver function. This further highlights the need to encourage prescribers to be aware of potential pharmacokinetic interactions and consider alternative therapies for elderly people.

We analysed data from a national dataset of around 300,000 predominantly older Australian. The results are likely to reflect the general elderly Australian population, but may slightly over-estimate the utilisation rates as similar numbers of prescriptions per general practitioner visit are observed between the veteran population and the Australian population; however, because of the higher rate of GP visits, veterans receive slightly more prescriptions annually than other Australians (rate ratio 1.13; p<0.05) [13]. Veterans with no service related disability have similar levels of use to other Australians [13].

Conclusion

This study has identified that 30% of patients with AF were not receiving antithrombotic treatment. In those receiving an antithrombotic agent, warfarin was the most commonly dispensed (35%). In December 2011, above half of those with AF who were managed on warfarin as a sole therapy were co-dispensed statins, and around 43% were co-dispensed PPIs. The most common statin and PPI co-prescribed with warfarin were agents with the potential to interact with warfarin, despite alternative agents being available. Raising awareness of the safer alternative for people with comorbidities may improve warfarin management.

References

1. Wolf PA, Abbott RD, Kannel WB (1991) Atrial fibrillation as an independent risk factor for stroke: the Framingham Study. Stroke 22: 983-988.

2. Atrial Fibrillation Association (2010) The economic cost of atrial fibrillation, Australia.

3. Hart RG, Benavente O, McBride R, Pearce LA (1999) Antithrombotic therapy to prevent stroke in patients with atrial fibrillation: a meta-analysis. Ann Intern Med 131: 492-501.

4. Tran HA, Chunilal SD, Harper PL, Tran H, Wood EM, et al. (2013) An update of consensus guidelines for warfarin reversal. Med J Aust 198: 198-199.

5. Department of Health, Western Australia. Quick reference guide: atrial fibrillation information for the health practitioners. Perth: Health networks branch, Department of Health, Western Australia; (2011)

6. Andrus MR (2004) Oral anticoagulant drug interactions with statins: case report of fluvastatin and review of the literature. Pharmacotherapy 24: 285-290.

7. Agewall S, Cattaneo M, Collet JP, Andreotti F, Lip GY, et al. (2013) Expert position paper on the use of proton pump inhibitors in patients with cardiovascular disease and antithrombotic therapy. Eur Heart J 34: 1708-1713, 1713a-1713b.

8. Sansom L (2012) Australian pharmaceutical formulary and handbook. (22nd edition), Pharmaceutical Society of Australia.

9. Corsini A, Bellosta S, Baetta R, Fumagalli R, Paoletti R, et al. (1999) New insights into the pharmacodynamic and pharmacokinetic properties of statins. Pharmacol Ther 84: 413-428.

10. Williams D, Feely J (2002) Pharmacokinetic-pharmacodynamic drug interactions with HMG-CoA reductase inhibitors. Clin Pharmacokinet 41: 343-370.

11. Hagymási K, Müllner K, Herszényi L, Tulassay Z (2011) Update on the pharmacogenomics of proton pump inhibitors. Pharmacogenomics 12: 873-888.

12. Top 10 drugs in Australia (2013) Aust Prescr 36: 211.

13. Lloyd J, Anderson P (2008) Veterans' use of health services. Australian Institute of Health and Welfare, Australia.

14. http://www.dva.gov.au/Pages/home.aspx

15. World Health Organization Collaborating Centre for Drug Statistics Methodology. Anatomical Therapeutic Chemical Code Classification index with Defined Daily Doses.

16. Australian Government. The Schedule of Pharmaceutical Benefits. Department of Health and ageing.

17. World Health Organization (2007) International Statistical Classification of Diseases and Related Health Problems.

18. National Prescribing Service Limited (2009) Antiplatelet and anticoagulant therapy in stroke prevention. Prescribing Practice Review 44.

19. Amerena JV, Walters TE, Mirzaee S, Kalman JM (2013) Update on the management of atrial fibrillation. Med J Aust 199: 592-597.

20. Zimetbaum PJ, Thosani A, Yu HT, Xiong Y, Lin J, et al. (2010) Are atrial fibrillation patients receiving warfarin in accordance with stroke risk? Am J Med 123: 446-453.

21. Dentali F, Douketis JD, Lim W, Crowther M (2007) Combined aspirin–oral anticoagulant therapy compared with oral anticoagulant therapy alone among patients at risk for cardiovascular disease: a meta-analysis of randomized trials. Arch Intern Med 167: 117-24.

22. Hart RG (2000) What causes intracerebral hemorrhage during warfarin therapy? Neurology 55: 907-908.

23. Lip GY, Tse HF, Lane DA (2012) Atrial fibrillation. Lancet 379: 648-661.

24. Omar MA, Wilson JP (2002) FDA adverse event reports on statin-associated rhabdomyolysis. Ann Pharmacother 36: 288-295.

25. Douketis JD, Melo M, Bell CM, Mamdani MM (2007) Does statin therapy decrease the risk for bleeding in patients who are receiving warfarin? Am J Med 120: 369.

26. Teichert M, van Noord C, Uitterlinden AG, Hofman A, Buhre PN, et al. (2011) Proton pump inhibitors and the risk of overanticoagulation during acenocoumarol maintenance treatment. Br J Haematol 153: 379-385.

27. Trifirò G, Corrao S, Alacqua M, Moretti S, Tari M, et al. (2006) Interaction risk with proton pump inhibitors in general practice: significant disagreement between different drug-related information sources. Br J Clin Pharmacol 62: 582-590.

5

Development of Psychiatric Symptoms during Antiviral Therapy for Chronic Hepatitis C

Vitale G[1], Simonetti G[1], Conti F[1]*, Taruschio G[2], Cursaro C[1], Scuteri A[1], Brodosi L[1], Vukotic R[1], Loggi E[1], Gamal N[1], Pirillo L[1], Cicero AF[1], Boncompagni G[2] and Andreone P[1]

[1]Department of Medical and Surgical Sciences, University of Bologna, Bologna, Italy
[2]Servizio Psichiatrico di Diagnosi e Cura, Azienda USL, Bologna, Italy

Abstract

Pegylated-interferon-α (Peg-IFN) are part of chronic hepatitis C (CHC) treatment. Among several side effects, it can induce psychiatric symptoms (PS) which could require discontinuation. The aim of this study was to evaluate the incidence, onset and risk factors of PS and antiviral treatment adherence in CHC patients treated with Peg-IFN plus ribavirin (RBV). All consecutive patients who received antiviral therapy between 2005 and 2011 were subjected to a psychiatric assessment before and during treatment. Of them, 49.2% reported PS especially during the first 4 weeks. Irritability was the predominant symptom recorded. The baseline factors associated with a higher risk of developing PS were: age ≤ 50 years (OR=1.67, 95% CI=1.15-2.43), living in Northern Italy (OR=1.88, 95% CI=1.31-2.70), genotype 1 (OR=1.82, 95% CI=1.28-2.60), previous antiviral treatment (OR=1.53, 95% CI=1.07-2.19) and history of mental disorders (MD) (OR=2.32, 95%CI=1.50-3.58). There was no difference in terms of sustained virologic response (SVR) between patients with and those without a history of MD (p=0.129). On the contrary, SVR was lower in patients who developed PS compared to other ones (p<0.001) due to the higher prevalence of difficult-to-treat patients. Only 1.7% of patients dropped-out for PS. In conclusion, most of patients receiving Peg-IFN develop PS, in particular irritability, especially during the first 4 weeks. Age ≤ 50, living in Northern Italy, genotype 1 infection, previous antiviral treatment and history of MD are associated with a higher chance of developing PS.

Keywords: Interferon; Adherence; Antiviral treatment; Hepatic disease; Mental disorders

Abbreviations

HCV: Hepatitis C Virus; Peg-IFN: Pegylated-Interferon-α; RBV: Ribavirin; DAAs: Direct Antiviral Agents; MD: Mental Disorders; PS: Psychiatric Symptoms; CHC: Chronic Hepatitis C; OR: Odds Ratios; CI: Confidence Intervals; SVR: Sustained Virologic Response

Introduction

Approximately 170 million people are infected with the hepatitis C virus (HCV) worldwide [1]. HCV infection is the most frequent cause of chronic hepatitis and an important risk factor for liver cirrhosis, end stage liver disease and hepatocellular carcinoma [2]. Treatment with Pegylated-interferon-α (Peg-IFN) and Ribavirin (RBV) associated or not with direct antiviral agents (DAAs), can lead to persistent eradication of HCV reducing rate of progression to end-stage liver disease and its complications [3]. An increased prevalence of mental disorders (MD) has been reported in HCV infection [4,5] and has been associated with the infection itself, possibly mediated by an effect on the central nervous system [2]. In addition, due to interaction of interferon and central nervous system [6-8], antiviral treatment is often associated with significant psychiatric symptoms (PS), such as depression, insomnia, anxiety, cognitive disturbances or suicide attempts [9,10]. In particular, depression rates during antiviral therapy range from 30 to 70% of cases [2,11-13]. The onset of PS during antiviral treatment has a strong impact on the quality of life and may affect treatment compliance leading to drug dose reduction or treatment discontinuation [11-13]. In order to avoid this even in patients with pre-existing MD and/or developing PS an adequate psychological and psychiatry counseling has been recommended [14]. Due to the scarcity of studies assessing the incidence of MD and PS during antiviral treatment in large cohorts of patients, we conducted this retrospective study to evaluate the incidence of psychiatric manifestations, their onset modalities, their impact on the adherence to and drop-out from antiviral treatment and the risk factors associated with development of PS in a large cohort of almost six-hundred patients with chronic hepatitis C (CHC) receiving Peg-IFN and RBV therapy at a single centre.

Methods and Patients

Selection of patient and data collection

All consecutive patients with CHC receiving Peg-IFN plus RBV treatment at our tertiary outpatient clinic for liver diseases at the Azienda Ospedaliero-Universitaria, Policlinico Sant'Orsola-Malpighi, Bologna, Italy between 2005 and 2011 were retrospectively enrolled in this study. The medical team consisted of both hepatologists and dedicated psychiatrists and psychologists experienced in the treatment of drug-induced psychiatric disorders. Each patient was evaluated by the same hepatologist for the entire duration of therapy. A telephone network was available for the management of patient's questions related to antiviral treatment. In that period, the standard of care was a combination of weekly subcutaneous Peg-IFN injections and daily weight-based oral RBV for genotypes 1 and 4 and fixed 800 mg RBV dose for genotypes 2 and 3 [15]. Two types of Peg-IFN were used: Peg-IFN 2a at dose of 180 mg/week (Pegasys, Hoffman-LaRoche, Nutley, NJ)

*Corresponding author: Fabio C, Department of Medical and Surgical Sciences, University of Bologna, Via Massarenti 9, 40138- Bologna, Italy,
E-mail: fabio.conti2@studio.unibo.it

and Peg-IFN 2b at dose of 1.5 mg/Kg/week (PegIntron, Merck/Schering Plough Corp., Whitehouse Station, NJ) [16]. The treatment duration was decided according to the standard clinical practice. Treatment stopping rules, in case of non-response, were applied following the international guidelines available in those years [17]. Patients were examined and monitored closely at the beginning of therapy, at weeks 4, 12, 24 (and also at weeks 36, 48 and 72 in patients treated for more than 24 weeks) and then followed for additional 24 weeks from the end of treatment. During the periodic visits, side effects were assessed and managed. Additional visits were scheduled to manage adverse events as needed. Data employed to perform this study were retrieved from an electronic data-base. Baseline data collected on each patient included: demographic characteristics, HCV genotype, presence of cirrhosis, type and duration of antiviral treatment, documented history of MD, PS arising during the treatment, date of symptoms onset. The presence of MD before treatment was defined according to patient's medical record and attending physician evaluation, while a history of MD leads to pre-treatment psychiatric consultation. The diagnosis of MD was made according to the criteria of the Diagnostic and Statistical Manual of Mental Disorders (DSM-IV TR) [18].

Statistical analysis

Continuous data were expressed as mean ± standard deviation, while categorical variables were summarized as absolute and relative frequencies. Non-parametric procedures were used to compare the characteristics of the patients, including Pearson chi-square test and Mann-Whitney U test. A p-value <0.05 was considered as statistically significant. Logistic regression models were used to evaluate possible predictors of development of PS and results were reported as odds ratios (OR) and their 95% confidence intervals (CI). All baseline characteristics were included in the univariate analysis. Covariates with a 2-sided P value <0.10 at univariate analysis were included for multivariate analysis. Backward stepwise elimination was used to remove non-significant factors from the model. All statistical analyses were performed using the SPSS software package (version 17.0 for Windows, SPSS Inc., Chicago, IL, USA).

Results

Characteristics of patients

Five hundred and ninety consecutive patients were included in this analysis. Baseline characteristics are summarized in Table 1. The mean age was 54 ± 13 years (range: 19-77) and most were males and came from Southern Italy. When the study population was subdivided in deciles, a higher prevalence of patients aged 51-60 years (27.6%) and 61-70 (26.6%) was observed. Data about employment status was available in 481 patients: more than half reported a stable employment status (39.5% employees and 18.5% freelancers) while the remaining (42%) were unemployed. Most patients were non-cirrhotic (77.8%) and treatment naive (59.3%). HCV genotype 1 was predominant (52.9%). Determination of interleukin-28B polymorphism was available in 76 (12.9%) patients: CC 25%, CT 56.6%, TT 18.4%. Peg-IFN 2a and 2b were equally prescribed. The duration of treatment was >48 weeks in 29% of patients. A history of MD was present in 130 (22%) patients. The types of MD are reported in Table 1. Among patients with a positive psychiatric history, 57 (43.8%) had already been treated with interferon-based antiviral therapy.

Development of psychiatric symptoms during treatment

During the antiviral treatment 290 patients (49.2%) developed the following PS: Irritability (54.1%), sleep disorders (38.6%), depressed mood (35.8%), anxiety (22.8%), neurocognitive dysfunctions (12.4%), confusion (5.5%), psychotic manifestations (2.1%) and behavioral disorders (1%). Gender distribution, presence of cirrhosis and type of Peg-IFN used were similar between subjects who developed PS and those who did not develop PS. Mean age was lower in patients with PS, among whom the rate of patients aged ≤ 50 years was significantly higher compared to those without PS (44.8% vs. 29.3%, respectively; p<0.001). The two groups also differed in term of history of MD, genotype distribution and treatment-experience. The development of PS was less frequent in patients who came from the southern Italy compared to those coming from the center or northern Italy; the incidence of PS was higher during the first 4 weeks of treatment (24.9%) and decreased progressively in the following weeks (Figure 1). The risk to develop PS was greater in patients with genotype 1 and 4 (Figure 1) and, as expected, in those with a history of MD (Figure 2). Irritability was the predominant symptom ranging from 40.8% to 54.3% of cases between week 4 and week 24 (Figure 3). Five baseline factors were associated with a higher chance of developing PS both at univariate and multivariate analysis: age ≤ 50 years, living in Northern Italy, genotype 1, previous antiviral treatment and history of MD (Table 2).

Treatment outcomes

Treatment was discontinued in 32/590 patients (5.4%): 22 patients (3.7%) for medical reasons and 10 (1.7%) for psychiatric complications, including also a case of completed suicide (0.2%) occurred in week 16. The rates of drop-out for psychiatric complications were higher in patients with than in those without MD history (4.6% vs. 0.9%, respectively; p=0.010). None of the patients with a history of psychiatric disorder induced by previous antiviral therapy dropped out during the new treatment course. Only eight subjects (1.4%) were lost during the follow-up. A sustained virologic response (SVR), defined as persistently negative HCV-RNA 24 weeks after end of treatment, was obtained in 353 patients (59.8%) while 95 (17.3%) did not respond to therapy and 102 (16.1%) had a viral relapse after treatment discontinuation. There was no SVR difference between patients with and those without a history of MD (53.8% vs. 61.5%, respectively; p=0.129).

Age	54 ± 13
Male gender	316 (53.6)
Area of recruitment: • Northern Italy • Central Italy • Southern Italy	 230 (39) 51 (8.6) 309 (52.4)
Genotype: • 1 • 2 • 3 • 4 • 5 • Mixed	 312 (52.9) 193 (32.7) 57 (9.7) 22 (3.7) 1 (0.2) 5 (0.8)
Cirrhosis	131 (22.2)
Previuos antiviral treatment	240 (40.7)
History of MD	130 (22)
Type of previous MD: • Substance abuse • Depression • Anxiety • Anxiety and depression • Psychiatric disorder interferon-induced • Bipolar disorder	 68 (52.3) 20 (15.4) 17 (13.1) 13 (10) 8 (6.2) 4 (3.1)
Type of Peg-IFN: • 2a • 2b	 305 (51.7) 285 (48.3)

Table 1: Baseline characteristics of the study population.

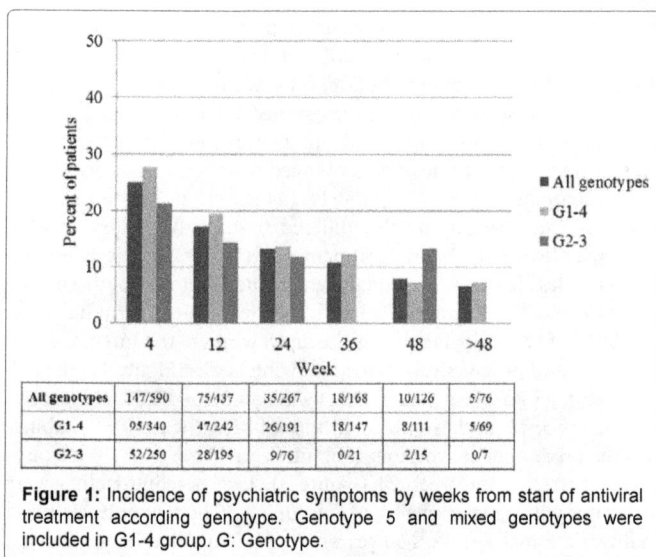

Figure 1: Incidence of psychiatric symptoms by weeks from start of antiviral treatment according genotype. Genotype 5 and mixed genotypes were included in G1-4 group. G: Genotype.

All genotypes	147/590	75/437	35/267	18/168	10/126	5/76
G1-4	95/340	47/242	26/191	18/147	8/111	5/69
G2-3	52/250	28/195	9/76	0/21	2/15	0/7

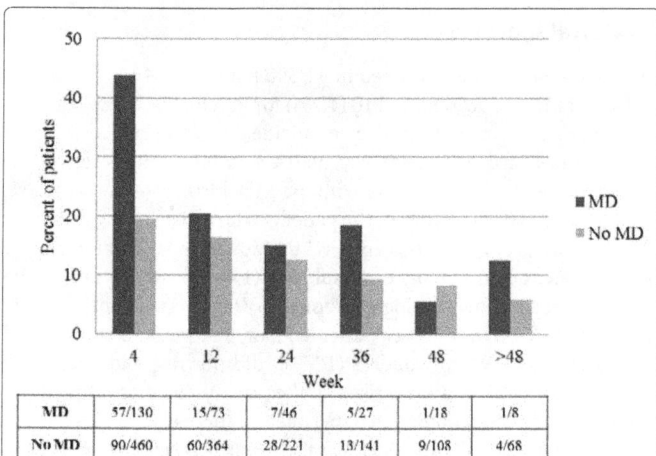

Figure 2: Incidence of psychiatric symptoms by weeks from start of antiviral treatment according presence or absence of mental disorders. MD: Mental Disorders.

MD	57/130	15/73	7/46	5/27	1/18	1/8
No MD	90/460	60/364	28/221	13/141	9/108	4/68

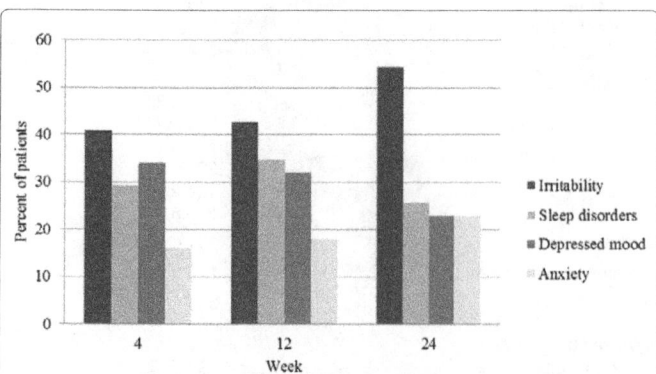

Figure 3: The most common psychiatric symptoms developed during the first 24 weeks of treatment with Pegylated-interferon-α and Ribavirin.

Conversely, the probability to achieve a SVR was significantly lower in patients who developed PS compared to those who did not (52.4% vs. 67%, respectively; p<0.001). However, this difference was related to the higher prevalence of most difficult-to-treat patients (genotype 1, cirrhosis and previous treatment failure) in PS group. Indeed, by

selecting only patients with genotype 1, or with cirrhosis, or previously treated, the response rates were not statistically different (p=0.138, p=0.170, p=0.117, respectively) between the two groups.

Discussion

This retrospective analysis of a large cohort of Italian patients with CHC treated with Peg-IFN and RBV provides comprehensive information on the prevalence and course of PS occurring during antiviral therapy, which could be relevant for the management of this complication. However, we have to recognize that this study has limitations due to its retrospective nature. Moreover, the definition of MD was not based on structured interviews or screening instruments collected prospectively, but derived from the clinical judgment of attending physicians and patients self-reports. A high prevalence of MD history (although it may be underestimated) was found in our patients confirming the reports from previous studies that pointed out that the prevalence of psychiatric disorders in patients with hepatitis C was higher than in the general population [19,20]. Interferon-based antiviral treatments, by acting on this background, further enhance these abnormalities, so that up to 70% of HCV-infected patients treated with interferon have been reported to have mild to moderate depressive syndromes [2,21-23] and 20% to 40% have major depression [2,23]. Our report fully confirms these data.

As in previous studies [24] irritability was the symptom that more frequently occurred in our patients. As it is often under-appreciated and under-recognized [25], irritability needs to be carefully assessed and managed, since it correction would likely improve the quality of life of patient and adherence to antiviral therapy.

Based on the current literature, the most interferon-inducted adverse psychiatric effects occur during the first 3 months of therapy [26,27]. Our data confirm these observations as 50.7% of PS occurred during the first 4 weeks of treatment and more than 75% during the first 12 weeks. During this period patients with unfavorable genotype (1 or 4) and a history of MD are most at risk. For this reason it would be advisable to intensifying patient surveillance in the first 12 weeks of treatment in order to recognize and treat PS as early as possible, thus reducing drop-out risk. Our study also showed that the incidence of PS generally deemed to be more serious, such as confusion and psychotic symptoms, is low. This finding should encourage clinicians not to stop treatment when PS arise, even though close monitoring and caring by a multidisciplinary is warranted [14,28]. It should not be disregarded, however, that suicidal ideation and attempts, even if rare [29], remains a relevant risk in these patients as also shown by our study.

	Development of PS			
	Univariate		Multivariate	
	OR	95% CI	OR	95%CI
Age ≤ 50 years	1.96	1.39-2.75	1.67	1.15-2.43
Male gender	1.17	0.86-1.61		
Northern Italy	2.05	1.47-2.87	1.88	1.31-2.70
Genotype 1	1.76	1.27-2.44	1.82	1.28-2.60
Cirrhosis	1.46	0.99-2.16		
Previous antiviral treatment	1.57	1.129-2.19	1.53	1.07-2.19
History of MD	2.80	1.85-4.23	2.32	1.50-3.58
Peg-IFN 2a	1.11	0.81-1.54		

PS: Psychiatric Symptoms, OR: Odds Ratio, CI: Confidence Interval, MD: Mental Disorders, Peg-IFN: Pegylated-Interferon-α

Table 2: Univariate and multivariate analyses of factors associated with the development of psychiatric symptoms during antiviral therapy with Pegylated-interferon-α and Ribavirin.

Several risk factors for developing PS during Peg-IFN plus RBV treatment were identified in this study. Contrary to what has been described for depression [30,31], age has not emerged as a consistent risk factor in our study. However, by stratifying our population using 50 years as a cut-off, younger patients have a greater risk. Northern Italians have an almost 2-fold chance of developing PS with respect to subjects from Central and Southern Italy, probably due to different life-style and social relationships and/or a different support received by the family during treatment. In our study, genotype 1 is another significant predictive factor to develop PS, as reported in a previous study [32]. This is likely due to the need of higher doses of drugs, longer treatment duration and higher rates of previous interferon-based treatment. In fact, we found a higher risk for psychiatric disorders in previously-treated patients, suggesting that a further interferon treatment could favor an exacerbation of PS in patients with an increased vulnerability to psychiatric manifestations due to a previous interferon treatment. Conversely, the type of Peg-IFN did not influence the occurrence of PS. It should also be noted that PS occurred in half of our patients, with a greater frequency in those with a positive history of MD. Therefore, a history of MD and of PS development during previous interferon-based treatment should alert the clinician to institute a careful longitudinal evaluation of mood status. It has to be underlined, however, that, despite the development of PS, patients with history of MD are still able to complete their programmed treatment course as those with no history of MD. This result was likely achieved thanks to the multidisciplinary approach employed in this study, which involved dedicated physicians, psychiatrists, psychologists and nurses. Although the evaluation of the virologic response to treatment was not the main objective of this study, it is interesting to note that SVR did not differ between patients with and without a history of MD.

Therefore, also patients with psychiatric comorbidity, if highly motivated, might be included in an intensive psychiatric care program to prepare them for the antiviral treatment and should not be excluded a priori from HCV therapy.

On the contrary, patients who developed PS showed a lower rate of SVR. However, this was mostly due to the higher prevalence of difficult-to-treat patients in this group, rather than to a higher drop-out rate considering that only 1.7% of patients discontinued therapy because of psychiatric adverse effects (all within the first 24 weeks of treatment). A large number of new antiviral drugs have now been investigated and treatment regimens in the near future will not require the use of interferon thus a reduced incidence of treatment-induced PS can be expected. Nonetheless, these drugs will have very high costs and will not be available for all patients. Therefore, especially in developing countries, the replacement of interferon therapy by all-oral regimens will probably take time. In addition, the most recently approved DAAs will still be used in combination with Peg-IFN (e.g., in genotype 1) [33] suggesting that the interferon era is not yet over and that the psychiatric and psychological counseling will be still necessary.

In conclusion, patients with CHC, aged $\leq$ 50 years, living in Northern Italy, previously treated with antiviral therapy, with genotype 1 infection and/or history of MD have high risk of developing PS during Peg-IFN plus RBV treatment. Although irritability is often disregarded by physicians, this symptom occurs more frequently than depression in the first three months of treatment. A main message that can be derived from this study is that patients with a clinical history of MD should not be excluded from antiviral treatment and that a multidisciplinary approach to interferon-induced PS can avoid premature treatment discontinuation, thus offering to patient full chance to achieve a SVR to therapy.

References

1. Wasley A, Alter MJ (2000) Epidemiology of hepatitis C: Geographic differences and temporal trends. Semin Liver Dis 20: 1-16.

2. Schaefer M, Capuron L, Friebe A, Diez-Quevedo C, Robaeys G, et al. (2012) Hepatitis C infection, antiviral treatment and mental health: A European expert consensus statement. J Hepatol 57: 1379-1390.

3. Singal AG, Volk ML, Jensen D, Di Bisceglie AM, Schoenfeld PS (2010) A sustained viral response is associated with reduced liver-related morbidity and mortality in patients with hepatitis C virus. Clin Gastroenterol Hepatol 8: 280-288, 288.

4. Dinwiddie SH, Shicker L, Newman T (2003) Prevalence of hepatitis C among psychiatric patients in the public sector. Am J Psychiatry 160: 172-174.

5. Batista-Neves SC, Quarantini LC, de Almeida AG, Bressan RA, Lacerda AL, et al. (2008) High frequency of unrecognized mental disorders in HCV-infected patients. Gen Hosp Psychiatry 30: 80-82.

6. Raison CL, Borisov AS, Majer M, Drake DF, Pagnoni G, et al. (2009) Activation of central nervous system inflammatory pathways by interferon-alpha: Relationship to monoamines and depression. Biol Psychiatry 65: 296-303.

7. Capuron L, Pagnoni G, Demetrashvili M, Woolwine BJ, Nemeroff CB, et al. (2005) Anterior cingulate activation and error processing during interferon-alpha treatment. Biol Psychiatry 58: 190-196.

8. Shuto H, Kataoka Y, Horikawa T, Fujihara N, Oishi R (1997) Repeated interferon-alpha administration inhibits dopaminergic neural activity in the mouse brain. Brain Res 747: 348-351.

9. Taruschio G, Santarini F, Sica G, Dragoni C, Migliorini S, et al. (1996) Psychiatric disorders in hepatitis C virus related chronic liver disease. Gastroenterology 110: 1342A.

10. Dieperink E, Willenbring M, Ho SB (2000) Neuropsychiatric symptoms associated with hepatitis C and interferon alpha: A review. Am J Psychiatry 157: 867-876.

11. Schaefer M, Engelbrecht MA, Gut O, Fiebich BL, Bauer J, et al. (2002) Interferon alpha (IFNalpha) and psychiatric syndromes: A review. Prog Neuropsychopharmacol Biol Psychiatry 26: 731-746.

12. Leutscher PD, Lagging M, Buhl MR, Pedersen C, Norkrans G, et al. (2010) Evaluation of depression as a risk factor for treatment failure in chronic hepatitis C. Hepatology 52: 430-435.

13. Raison CL, Borisov AS, Broadwell SD, Capuron L, Woolwine BJ, et al. (2005) Depression during pegylated interferon-alpha plus ribavirin therapy: prevalence and prediction. J Clin Psychiatry 66: 41-48.

14. Neri S, Bertino G, Petralia A, Giancarlo C, Rizzotto A, et al. (2010) A multidisciplinary therapeutic approach for reducing the risk of psychiatric side effects in patients with chronic hepatitis C treated with pegylated interferon I± and ribavirin. J Clin Gastroenterol 44: e210-217.

15. Hadziyannis SJ, Sette H Jr, Morgan TR, Balan V, Diago M, et al. (2004) Peginterferon-alpha2a and ribavirin combination therapy in chronic hepatitis C: A randomized study of treatment duration and ribavirin dose. Ann Intern Med 140: 346-355.

16. Zeuzem S, Welsch C, Herrmann E (2003) Pharmacokinetics of peginterferons. Semin Liver Dis 23 Suppl 1: 23-28.

17. Ghany MG, Strader DB, Thomas DL, Seeff LB; American Association for the Study of Liver Diseases (2009) Diagnosis, management, and treatment of hepatitis C: An update. Hepatology 49: 1335-1374.

18. American Psychological Association (2000) Diagnostic and statistical manual of mental disorders: DSM-IV-TR. (4th eds): American Psychiatric Pub.

19. Butt AA, Khan UA, McGinnis KA, Skanderson M, Kent Kwoh C (2007) Co-morbid medical and psychiatric illness and substance abuse in HCV-infected and uninfected veterans. J Viral Hepat 14: 890-896.

20. Yovtcheva SP, Rifai MA, Moles JK, Van der Linden BJ (2001) Psychiatric comorbidity among hepatitis C-positive patients. Psychosomatics 42: 411-415.

21. Reichenberg A, Gorman JM, Dieterich DT (2005) Interferon-induced depression and cognitive impairment in hepatitis C virus patients: A 72 week prospective study. AIDS 19 Suppl 3: S174-178.

22. Schaefer M, Schwaiger M, Garkisch AS, Pich M, Hinzpeter A, et al. (2005) Prevention of interferon-alpha associated depression in psychiatric risk patients with chronic hepatitis C. J Hepatol 42: 793-798.

23. Schäfer A, Wittchen HU, Seufert J, Kraus MR (2007) Methodological approaches in the assessment of interferon-alfa-induced depression in patients with chronic hepatitis C - a critical review. Int J Methods Psychiatr Res 16: 186-201.

24. Schaefer M, Schmidt F, Folwaczny C, Lorenz R, Martin G, et al. (2003) Adherence and mental side effects during hepatitis C treatment with interferon alfa and ribavirin in psychiatric risk groups. Hepatology 37: 443-451.

25. Blacklaws H, Gardner A, Usher K (2011) Irritability: An underappreciated side effect of interferon treatment for chronic hepatitis C? J Clin Nurs 20: 1215-1224.

26. Loftis JM, Hauser P (2004) The phenomenology and treatment of interferon-induced depression. J Affect Disord 82: 175-190.

27. Hauser P, Khosla J, Aurora H, Laurin J, Kling MA, et al. (2002) A prospective study of the incidence and open-label treatment of interferon-induced major depressive disorder in patients with hepatitis C. Mol Psychiatry 7: 942-947.

28. Schäfer A, Scheurlen M, Kraus MR (2012) Managing psychiatric side effects of antiviral therapy in chronic hepatitis C. Z Gastroenterol 50: 1108-1113.

29. Fattovich G, Giustina G, Favarato S, Ruol A (1996) A survey of adverse events in 1,241 patients with chronic viral hepatitis treated with alfa interferon. J Hepatol 24: 38-47.

30. Miyaoka H, Otsubo T, Kamijima K, Ishii M, Onuki M, et al. (1999) Depression from interferon therapy in patients with hepatitis C. Am J Psychiatry 156: 1120.

31. Kraus MR, Schäfer A, Faller H, Csef H, Scheurlen M (2003) Psychiatric symptoms in patients with chronic hepatitis C receiving interferon alfa-2b therapy. J Clin Psychiatry 64: 708-714.

32. Martín-Santos R, Díez-Quevedo C, Castellví P, Navinés R, Miquel M, et al. (2008) De novo depression and anxiety disorders and influence on adherence during peginterferon-alpha-2a and ribavirin treatment in patients with hepatitis C. Aliment Pharmacol Ther 27: 257-265.

33. Kim do Y, Ahn SH, Han KH (2014) Emerging therapies for hepatitis C. Gut Liver 8: 471-479.

6

Development of Opthalmic Formulation for Dry Eye Syndrome

Datar P*

Sinhgad Institute of Pharmacy, Narhe, Pune, Maharashtra, India

Abstract

Opthalmic formulation was prepared considering the essential requirements for the healthy eye. Acacia gum was used along with zinc sulphate as essential nutrients. The pH was adjusted to make the solution isotonic by using NaCl and other buffer solutions. The formulation was evaluated for viscosity and eye irritation test. The formulation was made in concerned with dry eye syndrome and associated disease due to old age. Formulation was observed for particle size and sterility test and finally stability test.

Keywords: Acacia; Ophthalmic drops; Dry eye syndrome; Keratoconjunctivitis sicca

Introduction

In today's scenario, working overtime on computers or watching television has been increased leading to early age dry eye syndrome. The stress can lead to adverse ocular conditions such as those associated with oxidative and/or free radical damage within the eye. These conditions can evolve a condition, disease, or disorder of the cornea, retina, lens, sclera, anterior segment, or posterior segment of the eye.

In dry eye, the eye becomes dry either because there is abnormally high rate of evaporation of tears or because there is not enough tears being produced. Individuals with dry eye experience heaviness of the eyelids or blurred or decreased vision referred to as keratoconjunctivitis sicca.

Healthy tears contain a complex mixture of proteins such as antimicrobial proteins such as lysozyme, lactoferrin, growth factors, inflammation suppressors and mucin which provides viscosity and stability of the tear and electrolytes for proper osmolarity. The contents of the tear in an eye suffering from dry eye are altered with lesser concentrations of proteins such as cytokine which promotes inflammation. Additionally, soluble mucin is greatly decreased due to loss of goblet cells which impacts viscosity of the tear film.

Mucus is a viscous, lubricating material that recruits and maintains moisture to the surfaces it coats. Mucus is actively secreted with salt and water onto surfaces that require these hydrating and lubricating properties for normal functioning. Mucus is particularly important in the normal functioning of the ocular surface [1].

The first line of treatment is usually eye drops, preferably preservative free, that act as artificial tears. Most artificial tears are hydrogels that increase the moisture content on the eye surface and give some temporary relief. These solutions and ointments give some temporary relief, but do little to arrest or reverse any damaging conditions.

Oral medicine for dry eye is also available. For example, pilocarpine, the active ingredient in Salagen TM or cevimeline, the active ingredient in Evoxac TM, is known to stimulate specific receptors in lacrimal gland and cause increased secretion of tears.

Currently, the pharmaceutical treatment of dry eye disease is mostly limited to administration of artificial tears (saline solution) to temporarily rehydrate the eyes. However, relief is short-lived and frequent dosing is necessary. In addition, artificial tears often have contra-indications and incompatibility with soft contact lenses [2].

Stimulation of tear secretion by topical application of melanocyte stimulating hormones is described [3].

Current medications that are used, including cyclosporine A, corticosteroids, tacrolimus, tetracycline derivatives and autologous serum, have been effective for management of dry eye. In addition, a topical ophthalmic formulation of cyclosporine (Restasis) has been investigated as a treatment of immune-based dry eye disease [4]. Stimulation of ocular mucin secretion has also been demonstrated with hydroxyeicosatetraenoic acid derivatives [5]. Nichols et al. [6] disclosed a method of stimulating tear secretion from lacrimal tissue by administering to the eyes an effective amount of purinergic receptor agonists such as uridine 5'-triphosphate, cytidine 5'-triphosphate, adenosine 5'-triphosphate, dinucleotides, and their analogs. Jumblatt and Jumblatt [7] demonstrated the effects of adenine analogues on secretion of high molecular weight, mucin-like glycoprotein by conjunctival goblet cells.

Acacia contains mucilage and chemical constituents such as quercetin, catechol, gallic acid, (+) catechin, (–) epicatechin, (–) epigallocatechin –5, 7–digallate and tannins [8,9]. Acacia has been used in pharmaceuticals as excipient for tablets, emulsifier and thickener. The decoction of bark yields spongy gum which is useful in sore throat, for washing ulcers, to stop bleeding from wounds, skin diseases, as an astringent for diarrhoea and leucorrhoea. Powdered gum is also given in dysentery and diabetes [10]. Gum Acacia consists principally of Arabin, a compound of Arabic acid with calcium, varying amounts of the magnesium and potassium salts of the same acid being present. Acacia is a demulcent and antioxidant [11]. It is also administered intravenously in haemolysis. Acacia is also known to have antibacterial and anti-inflammatory activities [12]. In the form of mucilage, it is used as a suspending agent. Acacia is a good emulsifying agent for fixed oils, volatile oils and also for liquid paraffin. The fried gum is considered a nutritive tonic, particularly in sexual debility. It also soothes inflamed membranes of the pharynx, alimentary canal and genito-urinary organs.

*Corresponding author: Datar P, Sinhgad Institute of Pharmacy, Narhe, Pune, Maharashtra, India, E-mail: d_pras_anna@rediffmail.com

Eye drops are sterile, aqueous or oily solutions or oil solutions or suspensions of one or more medicaments intended for instillation into the conjunctival sac. They may contain suitable auxiliary substances such as buffers, stabilizing agents, solubilizing agents and agents to adjust the tonicity or viscosity of the preparation. Unlike creams and ointments, these systems have obvious advantages such as ease of administration, ease of mixing with tear fluid and ability to spread over the corneal surface. Increased viscosity of the instilled drops improves contact time of drug with the site of application and can provide better therapeutic efficacy unlike eye solutions, which drain out rapidly from the eyes. In present study, the objective was to prepare ophthalmic drops using suitable concentration of acacia gum that enhances the contact time and also leaves a thin film of drug over the eye surface. Various concentrations of acacia were analyzed to find the suitable concentration for stability of formulation. Viscosity increases the contact time of the formulation. An ophthalmic formulation is provided for the prevention and treatment of adverse ocular conditions, including presbyopia, arcus senilis, age-related macular degeneration, and other conditions associated with aging.

In present study, the objective was to prepare ophthalmic drops using suitable concentration of acacia gum that enhances the contact time and also leaves a thin film of drug over the eye surface. Various concentrations of acacia were analyzed to find the suitable concentration for stability of formulation. Viscosity increases the contact time of the formulation. An ophthalmic formulation is provided for the prevention and treatment of adverse ocular conditions, including presbyopia, arcus senilis, age-related macular degeneration, and other conditions associated with aging.

Too much viscosity produces irritation in eye, hence optimal viscosity was achieved. Viscosity measurements were done using Oswald viscometer and Brookfield viscometer. Apart from providing viscosity to the ophthalmic solutions acacia is also a natural source of calcium and magnesium. These are essential nutrients to eye.

Isotonicity was adjusted and appropriate pH was set. Formulation was observed for particle size and sterility test. Formulation was kept for standing for 3 months any conglomeration was observed. Assay of drug $ZnSO_4$ was performed intermittently for stability studies. Formulations were instilled in to rabbit eye and were observed for any inflammatory response.

Experimental Methods

Materials

Acacia, Whatmann filter paper, autoclave, filter, Brookfield viscometer, Ostwald's viscometer.

Hydration of acacia gum was achieved as dispersion of gum in deionised water by heating while stirring at about 80°C, autoclaving at 121°C, 15 PSI and adding 0.2% sodium citrate and stirring. Solutions of gum were prepared in concentration of 0.3%, 0.6%, 0.9% and 1.2%,

1.5%, 1.8%, 2.0% w/v. The solutions were allowed to cool to room temperature.

Zinc sulphate is the optimum source of zinc. It gives symptomatic relief to tearing, photophobia, redness, swelling, blepharospasm and itching due to allergies. Also, it may be used to control hyperemia of the palpebral and bulbar conjunctiva resulting from bacterial, allergic and vernal conjunctivitis.

Stabilizing agent

Stabilizing agent is used to reduce degradation of drug during sterilization and storage. Sodium citrate is used as stabilizing agent and it prevents the sticking together of acacia gum and zinc sulphate. Since it is an anti-coagulant and as a buffering agent, sodium citrate helps maintain pH levels. Sodium citrate also acts as a sequestering agent, attaches to calcium ions in water.

Isotonicity adjustment

Sodium chloride equivalent method [13] for isotonicity was used. The "tonic equivalent" of a drug is the amount of sodium chloride that is equivalent to 1 gram, or other weight unit, of the drug.

Formulations were filtered to remove undispersed fibers before and after sterilization. They were observed for agglomerate formation and clarity. Table 1 gives the composition of formulations F1-F7.

Evaluation of formulation

1) pH: Formulation pH was determined using a digital pH meter. pH was set to 7.4.

2) Viscosity:

i) Oswald viscometer (Ubbelohde viscometer): Basically consist of a glass tube in the shape of a U held vertically in a controlled temperature bath. In one arm of the U is a vertical section of precise narrow bore (the capillary). Above this is a bulb, there is another bulb lower down in the other arm. In use, liquid is drawn into the upper bulb by suction, then allowed to flow down through the capillary into the lower bulb. Two marks (one above and one below the upper bulb) indicate a known volume. The time taken for the level of the liquid to pass between these marks is proportional to the kinematic viscosity.

ii) Brookfield Viscometer:

The instrument measures the shearing stress on a spindle rotating at a definite, constant speed while immersed in the sample. The degree of spindle lag is indicated on a rotating dial. This reading multiplied by a conversion factor based on spindle size and rotational speed, gives a value for viscosity in centipoise. By taking measurements at different rotational speeds, an indication of the degree of thixotropy of the sample is obtained.

3) Particle size: Injections must be examined for freedom from

Formulation	F1	F2	F3	F4	F5	F6	F7
Acacia gum	0.3 g	0.6 g	0.9 g	1.2 g	1.5 g	1.8 g	2.0 g
Boric acid	0.5 g	0.5 g	0.5 g	0.5 g	0.5 g	0.5 g	0.5 g
NaCl	0.896 g	0.896 g	0.896 g	0.896 g	0.896 g	0.896 g	0.896 g
ZnSO$_4$	0.22 g	0.22 g	0.22 g	0.22 g	0.22 g	0.22 g	0.22 g
Benzethonium chloride	0.01 g	0.01 g	0.01 g	0.01 g	0.01 g	0.01 g	0.01 g
Sodium citrate	0.2 g	0.2 g	0.2 g	0.2 g	0.2 g	0.2 g	0.2 g
Water for injection (q.s.)	100 ml	100 ml	100 ml	100 ml	100 ml	100 ml	100 ml

Table 1: Composition of Formulation.

foreign particles, before and after sterilization. The earlier inspection makes possible the re-filtration of unsatisfactory solutions, which may not be permissible after sterilization.

A convenient arrangement is a box with a shielded lamp at the top. To reduce refection it should be painted black inside, except for half the back. The container is held horizontally and rotated immediately under the lamp and then inverted once or to find heavy particles, such as glass. Movement must not be sufficiently vigorous to fill the solution with confusing air bubbles.

Human eye cannot detect particles smaller than about 50 µM. Hence samples were tested for microscopic evaluation for presence of agglomerates or particles smaller than 50 µM.

4) Assay of zinc sulphate- To 5.0 ml add 50 ml of water and 5 ml of ammonia buffer pH 10.9 and titrate with 0.1M disodium edentate using mordant black II solution as indicator each ml of 0.1M disodium edetate is equivalent to 0.002875 g of $ZnSO_4, 7H_2O$.

5) Sterility test: As per I.P. specifications.

6) Acute eye irritation test:

Six healthy young albino rabbits were used for the study with prior examination of both eyes of each experimental animal 24 hours before starting the experiment, to avoid any animals showing ocular defects or preexisting corneal injury. Animals should be individually housed. The temperature of the experimental animal room was kept at 20°C (± 3°C) for rabbits. The relative humidity was maintained at 50-60% and not exceeding 70%. Lighting was artificial and the sequence of light hours and dark hours being was maintained at 12 hrs each alternatively. Feeding was conventional laboratory diet with an unrestricted supply of drinking water. The test is carried out by applying 0.1 mL of each formulation was instilled in the conjunctival sac of one eye of rabbits after gently pulling the lower lid away from the eyeball. The lids are then gently held together for about one second in order to prevent loss of the material. The other eye, which remains untreated, served as a control. The eyes were examined at every one hour and continued for 72 hours after application. The grades of ocular reaction, in terms of redness to the conjunctivae and cornea were recorded at each examination as per OECD TG405 [14]. The cornea is visually observed and assessed for inflammation, tear production, reaction to light, hemorrhage and gross destruction. The conjunctiva is evaluated for the degree of redness, swelling and discharge.

Results and Discussions

Ophthalmic drop evaluation

pH was set to 7.4 for all formulations. pH did not changed even after standing for 3 months.

Particle size

Microscopic examination of formulations did not show not more than 20 particles that have maximum dimension greater than 25 µM, not more than 10 particles have a maximum dimension greater than 50 µM and none has a maximum dimension greater than 100 µM. Samples of formulation were tested. No particles were found in any of the formulations on standing for three months.

Sterility test

The test showed no growth of microorganisms even after keeping for incubation at 37°C for 7 days. The ophthalmic drop was found sterile.

Conc. % w/v	Brookfield Viscometer (Shearing stress in centipoises) for spindles 3,4,5,6,7 at 2,4,10 and 20 revolutions.	Ostwald's Viscometer (viscosity in poise)
0.3 (F1)	No Shearing stress	0.076
0.6 (F2)	No Shearing stress	0.081
0.9 (F3)	No Shearing stress	0.084
1.2 (F4)	No Shearing stress	0.089
1.5 (F5)	No Shearing stress	0.094
1.8 (F6)	No Shearing stress	0.099
2.0 (F7)	No Shearing stress	0.101

Table 2: Viscosity measurements for formulations F1-F7.

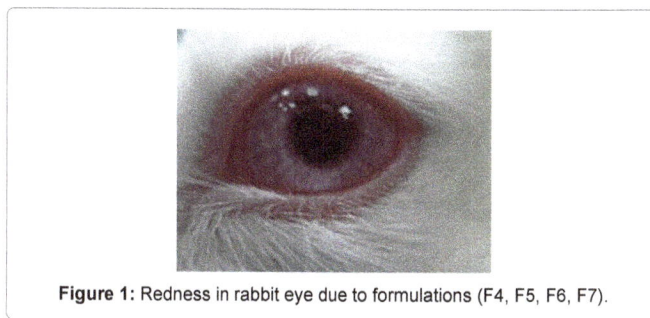

Figure 1: Redness in rabbit eye due to formulations (F4, F5, F6, F7).

Rheological studies of the gum formulation [15,16]

Rheological behavior of the formulations were performed by subjecting the formulation to various rates of shear using suitable spindle of Brookfield viscometer by using spindle no.'s 3, 4, 5, 6, 7 were utilized at revolutions 2, 4, 10 and 20. Formulation is expected to show no shearing stress in this study as too much viscosity may cause uneasiness for the patient. Ostwald's viscometer shows the viscosity in poise where all the formulations show viscosity below or equal to 0.1 poise. Limits of viscosity upto 0.1 poise was considered for easy instillation of drops.

Table 2 gives the viscosity measurements for formulations F1-F7.

Biological evaluation was carried out on rabbit eye which did not showed redness or inflammation for formulations (F1) 0.3, (F2) 0.6, (F3) 0.9% w/v concentrations of acacia gum formulations. Remaining higher concentrations in formulations F4 to F7 showed redness (Figure 1) but no inflammation.

Assay was carried out as per I.P. for all the formulation and it was observed that all contain not less than 95.0% and not more than 105.0% of Zinc sulfate.

Stability studies

Formulations were kept in a desicator at 27°C for 3 months in a sealed bottle. Formulations F3, F4, F5, F6 and F7 showed agglomeration after standing for two weeks. Formulations F1 and F2 did not showed agglomeration even after standing for 3 months.

Conclusion

Our studies have found that 0.6% w/v of acacia solution produce sufficient viscosity in ophthalmic eye drop formulation to serve the purpose of maximum contact of drop. We have further seen that 0.6% w/v acacia is also better stabilized formulation. The formulation was clear and did not showed agglomeration. The drug content of formulations shows no degradation of $ZnSO_4$ due to acacia gum interaction.

References

1. Forstner G, Wesley A, Forstner J (1982) Clinical aspects of gastrointestinal mucus. Adv Exp Med Biol 144:199-224.

2. Lemp MA (1990) Is the dry eye contact lens wearer at risk? Yes. Cornea 9:S48-S50.

3. Sulliva DA, Block L, Pena JD (1996) Influence of androgens and pituitary hormones on the structural   profile and secretory activity of the lacrimal gland. Acta Ophthalmol Scand 74:421-435.

4. Stern ME, Beuerman RW, Fox RI, Gao J, Mircheff AK, et al. (1998) A unified theory of the role of the ocular surface in dry eye. Adv Exp Med Biol 438: 643-651.

5. Gamache DA, Wei ZY, Weimer LK, Spellman JM, Yanni JM (2002) Preservation of corneal integrity by the mucin secretagogue 15(S)-HETE in a rabbit model of desiccation-induced dry eye. Adv Exp Med Biol 506: 335-340.

6. Nichols KK, Yerxa B, Kellerman DJ (2004) Diquafosol tetrasodium: a novel dry eye therapy. Expert Opin Investig Drugs 13: 47-54.

7. Jumblatt JE, Jumblatt MM (1998) Regulation of ocular mucin secretion by P2Y2 nucleotide receptors in rabbit and human conjunctiva. Exp Eye Res 67: 341-346.

8. Jahan N, Afaque SH, Khan NA, Ahmad G, Ansari AA (2008) Physico-chemical studies of the gum acacia, Natural product radiance 7: 335-337.

9. Montgomery R (1959) The Chemistry of plant Gum and Mucilage. Reinhold Publishers New York.

10. Duke JA (1985) Handbook of Medicinal Herbs. CRC Press Boca Raton, USA.

11. Abd-Allah AR, Al-Majed AA, Mostafa AM, Al-Shabanah OA, Din AG, et al. (2002) Protective effect of arabic gum against cardiotoxicity induced by doxorubicin in mice: a possible mechanism of protection. J Biochem Mol Toxicol 16: 254-259.

12. Adedapo AA, Sofidiya MO, Masika PJ, Afolayan AJ (2008) Anti-inflammatory and analgesic activities of the aqueous extract of Acacia karroo stem bark in experimental animals. Basic Clin Pharmacol Toxicol 103: 397-400.

13. Mellen M, Seltzer LA (1936) J Am Pharm Assoc Sci Ed 25:759.

14. Guideline OECD Draft 405 (2012) Organization For Economic Co-Operation And Development. Acute eye irritation and corrosion.

15. Sklubalová Z (2005) In situ gelling polymers for ophthalmic drops. Ceska Slov Farm 54: 4-10.

16. Ugriné-Hunyadvári E, Kissné-Koczka C (1995) Polymer-containing eye drops. I. Rheological characteristics of polymer solutions. Acta Pharm Hung 65: 9-13.

7

Evaluating Educational Intervention to Improve Drug Administration Practice in Out-Patient Children in Northwestern Nigeria

Chedi BAZ[1]*, Abdu-Aguye I[2] and Kwanashie HO[2]

[1]Department of Pharmacology, Bayero University Kano, Nigeria
[2]Department of Pharmacology and Therapeutics, Ahmadu Bello University, Zaria, Nigeria

Abstract

Drug administration practice of mothers from 20 facilities (12 primary and 8 secondary) in northwestern Nigeria were assessed prospectively with the aim of identifying the type, frequency and potential clinical significance of drug administration errors in paediatric outpatients. The data was analyzed and errors classified according to National Coordinating Council for Medication Error Reporting and Prevention taxonomy. Educational interventions were designed and administered to mothers of 10 (6 primary and 4 secondary) least performing facilities, while the remaining 10 facilities acted as control. The percentage of the parents that claimed to knew the correct dosage were relatively high (78% to 93%) and differ significantly between the secondary and primary facilities. Further assessment shows that the dose of the drugs dispensed, the time/frequency of administration, and the duration of use were not known by 68.2% (330/484), 63.0% (305/484), and 12.0% (58/484) of the mothers respectively. The overall total possibility of the drug administration errors significantly reduced in the right direction (p<0.0005; d=4.27) after the intervention.

Keywords: Drug administration errors; Paediatric; Outpatient; Health facilities; Nigeria

Introduction

A drug administration error was defined as any discrepancy between printed or handwritten prescribers' orders and drug delivery to the patient, or deviation from a prescriber's valid prescription, official pharmacopeia or manufacturer's literature. Administration errors were classified into wrong timing; that is greater than one hour difference compared with the ordered time [1], wrong dose (quantity), wrong drug, wrong frequency, wrong duration and wrong route. Many drugs used in paediatric units are either unlicensed or used off-label [2]. The need to prepare dilutions or to open capsules may increase the risk of drug administration errors [3]. When computing drug doses, health care personnel may make mistakes, which may be life threatening [4]. In paediatric units, the physiological immaturity and widely variable body weight of the patients may increase the risk and impact of errors. The incidence of medication errors and the risk of serious errors occurring in children are significantly greater than in adults. In USA alone, it was estimated that 100-150 deaths occur annually in children due to medication errors [5]. Studies by Freyn [6], King [7] and Miller [8] showed the rate of medication errors in paediatric practice as follows: 3-37% prescribing, 5-58% dispensing and 72-75% administration errors. The household administration of liquid dosage form has been identified as one of the important factors contributing to medication error in paediatric patients [9]. Teaspoons used at home vary greatly in size, causing many children to be under-dosed [10]. Since about 72% of the drugs were prescribed as syrups, this is an area of major public health concern [11].

Despite the awareness that paediatric patients are at increased risk for medication errors [12], little is known about their drug utilization and epidemiology of these errors. Much of the studies on drug utilization focused on general outpatient, few have been conducted in the paediatric setting and even fewer have concentrated on medication errors [13]. With our understanding of the problems and solutions of patient safety growing daily, it has become clear that the prescription, dispensing and administration of medication represent a substantial portion of preventable medical errors that occur in paediatric. The objective of this study was to identify the type, frequency and potential clinical significance of drug administration errors in paediatric outpatients with a view to intervening.

Materials and Method

Study design

The study was a cross sectional prospective survey involving twenty public health care institutions selected from Kano State by stratified random sampling using senatorial district as stratum. In each senatorial district, two secondary and four primary public health facilities were selected by simple random sampling using balloting system. Also the only available paediatric specialist and teaching hospitals were added to make-up the twenty facilities. After sampling, ten (four secondary and six primary) facilities were purposely selected to receive the intervention while the remaining acted as control.

Inclusion and exclusion criteria

The subjects included in this study were mothers that brought patients of either sex, aged 11 years or below with general illness. Mothers that present patients to the health care facilities for follow-up of chronic diseases or to receive services such as vaccination, and other specialized care services were excluded from the study sample.

Data collection

Consents of mothers that brought children to the selected facilities

---

*Corresponding author: Chedi BAZ, Department of Pharmacology, Bayero University Kano, Nigeria E-mail: b2chedi@yahoo.com

were sought at the point of exit. Those that accepted were recruited into the study and were asked whether they knew how to administer the drugs dispensed to their wards or not, the ones that claimed to know the correct dose were enlisted while the remaining were excluded. The data was collected in two waves:

(a) Pre-intervention (Baseline): Each mother was requested to (1) identify the drugs dispensed to her child from mix of other drugs, (2) state the route administration of each drug, (3) mentioned the times and number of days that each drug will be given and (4) mothers were provided with paracetamol syrup and all other requirements including a medium-sized teaspoon, at no cost. They were requested to measure one dose (5ml) three times the way they would normally do at home. After each pour, the quantity was withdrawn and measured using a syringe, the average was recorded. For the purpose of this study, failure to identify the right drugs, state right route, right duration, right time (schedule time ± one hour) and measure right q Nigeria uantity 4.75ml to 5.25ml (5 ml ± 5%) were considered as potential administration errors. The errors were calculated as percentages and classified according to standardized taxonomy of classifying errors [14].

For the purpose of this study, request for clarification or expression of doubt before any aspect of the drug administration practice was considered as category A error, while an error that was intercepted during the administration practice was categorized as B error. Errors that involved non-antimicrobial drugs and/or drugs with wide therapeutic range were considered as category C error and where an antimicrobial drug or drug with narrow therapeutic index was involved it was categorized as D error. When several errors were made during the same administration were counted as one and the highest level of severity that applies during the course of the event was selected as the outcome category.

(b) Post-intervention: mothers were allowed to rest for 30 minutes during which the pre-intervention (baseline) data was analyzed; areas that need intervention identified and appropriate interventions administered. The baseline procedure was repeated prior to the intervention in the control facilities and 15 minutes after the intervention in the intervention facilities.

(c) Intervention Description: Mothers were trained on good drug administration skills and enlightened about consequences of medication errors and importance of adhering to dosage regimens. They were showed what a 5 mL dose looked like and the meanings of twice daily, thrice daily etc in terms of hours.

(iv) Statistical Analysis

The percentage error (pE) was calculated as the number of administrations with one or more errors (nE) divided by the total number of observed drug administration (nA) times 100. Data collected was entered into HP laptop and coded. Analysis was carried out using Microsoft excel 2007 and SPSS version 15; values were express as mean ± SEM. Drug administration errors were computed and compared

between the primary and secondary facilities by Student's t-test. To evaluated the impact of the intervention, the difference (net gain scores) was computed by subtracting the mean difference (gain scores) of the control group (post minus pre) from mean difference (gain scores) of the intervention group as suggested by Tumwikirize et al. [15]. Plus sign (+) indicates increase and negative sign (-) signifies decrease. Secondly, mean differences of control and intervention groups were compared using unpaired Student's t-test [16,17] and values of $p<0.05$ were considered statistically significant. Thirdly, to know if an observed difference is not only statistically significant but also important or meaningful, effect size [18] was calculated for each indicator. Cohen's effect size (d) was determined by mean difference of intervention group (m1) minus mean difference of control (m2)/pooled standard deviation. By convention the subtraction (m1-m2), was done so that the difference is positive if it is in the direction of improvement or in the predicted direction and negative if in the direction of deterioration or opposite to the predicted direction. Cohen's d<0.2=trivial effect; 0.2-0.4=small effect; 0.5-0.8=moderate effect; >0.8=large difference effect.

Result

During the study, 484 drug administration practices by 242 mothers were assessed. The percentage of the mothers that claimed to knew the correct dosage were relatively high (78% to 93%) and differ significantly between the secondary and primary facilities (Table 1), but this does not necessarily reflect reality because the response "Yes or I know the dose" was accepted as positive answer.

Further assessment of knowledge of those mothers that claimed to know the dose of drugs dispensed in relation to the quantity to administer, the time/frequency of administration, and the duration of use were not known by 68.2% (330/484), 63.0% (305/484), and 12.0% (58/484) of the mothers respectively (Table 2).

These errors occurred for more than 90% pre-intervention ally but significantly reduced in the right direction (p<0.0005; d=4.27) after the intervention (Table 3).

Discussions

About 90% and 80% of parents in the secondary and primary health care facilities respectively claimed to know the correct dosage schedule, and significant (p<0.05; d=1.22) increase was recorded in secondary facilities after the intervention. These figures, though higher than 55% to 68.3% reported in Bangladesh [19], Burkina Faso [20], Cambodia [21] and Indian [22], did not necessarily reflect reality since the response "Yes, I know the dose" was accepted as positive answer. The claim was proved wrong after the drug administration error analysis.

Assessment of possibilities of drug administration errors proved most parents that claimed to have adequate knowledge on dosage schedule wrong. This was evidenced by the high value of 88.5-100% total errors obtained in the both secondary and primary facilities before

Table 1: Percentage of parents who claimed to have adequate knowledge.

	Control group		Intervention group		Group comparison		
	Pre	Post	Pre	Post	Diff	P Value	Effect Size
Sec. (n=4)	93.18 ± 2.80	92.65 ± 2.70	85.35 ± 1.46	89.75 ± 1.11	4.93	0.03a	2.46***
Pri. (n=6)	78.12 ± 1.183	80.85 ± 1.842	79.95 ± 2.750	84.48 ± 1.721	1.80	0.44ns	1.02***
Overall (n=10)	84.14 ± 2.75	85.57 ± 2.41	82.11 ± 1.89	86.59 ± 1.37	1.43	0.04a	1.76***

Group comparison: Difference (-)=decrease and (+)=increase; P value–ns–not significant; a=<0.05; b=< 0.005; c=< 0.0005; Effect size (Cohen's d)-* =0.2-0.4 (small); **=0.5-0.8 (medium); ***=>0.8 (strong); (+)=improvement, (-)=deterioration;

Facilities comparison P value–0=not significant; 1=<0.05; 2=<0.005; 3=< 0.0005.

Table 2: Rates of Administration Error.

Error Category	Type of Error	Frequency of Errors (n)	Percentage (%)	Pre-intervention (n=242)	Post-intervention (n=242)
				Rate per 100 Parents	Rate per 100 Parents
A (Circumstances or events that have the capacity to cause error)	TOTAL	63	100.0	14.8	22.4
	Look Alike	23	36.5	5.1	4.4
	Inadequate Information	45	71.4	9.8	8.8
C (An error occurred that reached the patient, but may not cause patient harm)	TOTAL	226	100.0	50.0	43.0
	Wrong Quantity	214	94.7	48.8	39.6
	Wrong Time	197	87.2	40.8	40.6
	Wrong Duration	31	13.7	7.0	5.8
D (An error occurred that required monitoring or intervention to preclude harm)	TOTAL	128	100.0	25.8	27.2
	Wrong Quantity	116	90.6	24.2	23.7
	Wrong Time	108	84.4	22.8	21.9
	Wrong Duration	27	21.1	6.3	4.8

Table 3: Percentages of Administration Error.

		Control group		Intervention group		Group comparison		
		Pre	Post	Pre	Post	Diff	P Value	Effect Size
Category A (Circumstances or events that have the capacity to cause error).	Sec (n=4)	11.28 ± 4.13	3.85 ± 3.85	13.80 ± 0.23	1.68 ± 1.68	-4.70	0.08ns	3.54***
	Pri (n=6)	21.83 ± 1.30^1	18.13 ± 2.58^1	21.13 ± 1.52^2	2.78 ± 2.59ns	-11.65	0.02a	6.17***
	Overall (n=10)	17.61 ± 2.41	12.42 ± 3.10	18.20 ± 1.49	4.14 ± 1.75	-8.87	0.0005c	4.07***
Category C (An error occurred that reached the patient, but may not cause patient harm).	Sec (n=4)	53.63 ± 5.13	54.55 ± 3.36	51.80 ± 1.04	34.60 ± 0.64	-18.13	0.001b	10.78***
	Pri (n=6)	49.52 ± 2.08^0	45.77 ± 3.06^0	47.42 ± 2.63^0	37.58 ± 3.26^0	-6.08	0.07ns	2.32***
	Overall (n=10)	51.16 ± 2.32	49.28 ± 2.58	36.39 ± 1.96	36.39 ± 1.96	-10.90	0.002b	4.20***
Category D (An error occurred that reached the patient and required monitoring or intervention to preclude harm).	Sec (n=4)	23.63 ± 5.05	23.88 ± 5.56	34.35 ± 0.78	22.23 ± 2.98	-12.30	0.02a	5.51***
	Pri (n=6)	28.60 ± 1.68^0	25.55 ± 2.77^0	31.45 ± 1.90^0	21.62 ± 4.73^0	-6.78	0.03a	2.71***
	Overall (n=10)	26.61 ± 2.24	24.88 ± 2.60	32.61 ± 1.23	21.89 ± 2.94	-8.99	0.005b	3.63***
Total	Sec (n=4)	88.53 ± 4.37	82.28 ± 6.69	99.95 ± 0.03	58.58 ± 3.55	-35.13	<0.0005c	15.46***
	Pri (n=6)	99.95 ± 0.02^1	89.45 ± 2.64^0	100.00 ± 0.04^0	64.95 ± 2.83^0	-24.55	<0.0005c	16.92***
	Overall (n=10)	95.38 ± 2.46	86.58 ± 3.11	99.98 ± 0.02	62.40 2.33	-28.78	<0.0005c	11.17***

Group comparison: Difference (-)=decrease and (+)=increase; P value-ns–not significant; a=<0.05; b=<0.005; c=<0.0005; Effect size (Cohen's d)- *=0.2-0.4 (small); **=0.5-0.8 (medium); ***=>0.8 (strong);

(+)=improvement, (-)=deterioration;

Facilities comparison P value–0=not significant; 1=<0.05; 2=<0.005; 3=<0.0005.

the intervention; however significant (p<0.0005; d=4.27) improvement was observed after the intervention. Previous studies reported 67% [23] and 72-75% [8].

More than 60% of the parents could not measure 5 ml correctly; about 47% overdosed while the remaining under-dosed. The consequences of a single dosing error may be minimal. But these types of overdosing and under-dosing errors are likely to accumulate especially in children that were administered drug(s) every four to eight hours for several days and accounted for some of the C and D errors recorded in this study. Other causes of C and D errors observed were the inability of parents to state the administration time precisely i.e. every 6, 8 or 12 hours for qds, tid and bd) and the number of days the drugs should be given accurately. Most parents (>60%) would have given the drugs within 12 hours irrespective of the frequency of dosing interval (8 am to 8 pm); this could lead to development of resistance and treatment failures. Look-alike, anxiety and inadequate information from the health care providers could be the cause of the errors recorded. With proper training, parents can dose liquid medication accurately, understand and adhere to correct dosing timing and duration as evidenced in the result obtained after the intervention.

Conclusion

This study provides insights into the drug administration practice in paediatric outpatient departments in Kano, Nigeria. Though drug administration errors were extremely frequent in this study, and many had more than one error, the intervention resulted to significant decrease the possibilities of drug administration error.

References

1. American Society of Hospital Pharmacists (1982) ASHP Standard definition of a medication error. Am J Hosp Pharm 39: 321.

2. Avenel S, Bomkratz A, Dassieu G, Janaud JC, Danan C (2000) The incidence of prescriptions without marketing product license in a neonatal intensive care unit. Arch Pediatr 7: 143-147.

3. Roberts R, Rodriguez W, Murphy D, Crescenzi T (2003) Pediatric drug labeling: improving the safety and efficacy of pediatric therapies. JAMA 290: 905-911.

4. Rowe C, Koren T, Koren G (1998) Errors by paediatric residents in calculating drug doses. Arch Dis Child 79: 56-58.

5. McIntyre J, Conroy S, Avery A, Corns H, Choonara I (2000) Unlicensed and off label prescribing of drugs in general practice. Arch Dis Child 83: 498-501.

6. Frey B, Buettiker V, Hug MI, Waldvogel K, Gessler P, et al. (2002) Does critical

incident reporting contribute to medication error prevention? Eur J Pediatr 161: 594-599.

7. King WJ, Paice N, Rangrej J, Forestell GJ, Swartz R (2003) The effect of computerized physician order entry on medication errors and adverse drug events in pediatric inpatients. Pediatrics 112: 506-509.

8. Miller MR, Robinson KA, Lubomski LH, Rinke ML, Pronovost PJ (2007) Medication errors in paediatric care: a systematic review of epidemiology and an evaluation of evidence supporting reduction strategy recommendations. Qual Saf Health Care 16: 116-126.

9. Nsimba SE (2006) Assessing prescribing and patient care indicators for children under five years old with malaria and other disease conditions in public primary health care facilities. Southeast Asian J Trop Med Public Health 37: 206-214.

10. Hyam E, Brawer M, Herman J, Zvieli S (1989) What's in a teaspoon? Underdosing with acetaminophen in family practice. Fam Pract 6: 221-223.

11. Kohn LT, Corrigan JM and Donaldson MS (2000) Committee on quality of health care in America. In: To Err Is Human: Building a Safer Health System. Washington, DC: National Academy Press, 1-287.

12. Kaushal R, Jaggi T, Shojania KG, Bates DW and Walsh K (2004) Pediatric medication errors: what do we know? What gaps remain? Ambulatory Pediatrics 4:73-81.

13. Grasso BC, Rothschild JM and Genest R (2003) What do we know about medication errors in inpatient psychiatry? Joint Commission Journal on Quality and Safety, 29:391-400.

14. http://www.nccmerp.org/pdf/taxo2001-07-31.pdf

15. Tumwikirize WA, Ekwaru JP, Mohammed K, Ogwal-Okeng JW and Aupont O (2004) Proceeding of the International Conference on Improving Use of Medicines. 2nd International Conference on improving Use of Medicines, Chiang Mia, Thailand.

16. Dimitrov MD and Rumrill PD (2003) Pretest-posttest designs and measurement of change. WORK: A Journal of Prevention, Assessment, & Rehabilitation 20: 159-165.

17. Abiola OO (2007) Procedures in Educational Research: Hanijam Publications Kaduna, Nigeria.

18. Cohen J (1998) Statistical power analysis for the behavioral sciences. (2ndedn), Hillsdale, NJ, United States.

19. Guyon AB, Barman A, Ahmed JU, Ahmed AU and Alam MS (1994) A baseline survey on use of drugs at the primary health care level in Bangladesh. Bull World Health 72: 265-271.

20. Krause G, Borchert M, Benzler J, Heinmuller R, Kaba I, et al. (1999) Rationality of drug prescriptions in rural health centers in Burkina Faso. Health Policy Plan, 14: 291-298.

21. Chareonkul C, Khun VL and Boonshuyar C (2002) Rational drug use in Cambodia: study of three pilot health centers in Kampong Thom Province. Southeast Asian J Trop Med Public Health 33: 418-424.

22. Rishi RK, Sangeeta S, Surendra K and Tailang M (2003) Prescription audit: experience in Garhwal (Uttaranchal), India. Tropical Doctor, 33: 76-79.

23. McMahon SR, Rimsza ME and Bay RC (1997) Parents can dose liquid medications accurately. Pediatrics 100:330-333.

8

Hypoglycemia and Hyperglycemia in Hospitalized Patients Receiving Insulin

Leblond J[1]*, Beauchesne MF[1-4], Bernier F[3,5,6], Lanthier L[5,6], Garant MP[3], Blais L[2,4], Frédéric Grondin RN[7] and B Cossette B[1,6]

[1]Department of Pharmacy, Centre hospitalier universitaire de Sherbrooke, Sherbrooke, Canada

[2]Faculty of Pharmacy, Université de Montréal, Montréal, Canada

[3]CR-CHUS, Centre hospitalier universitaire de Sherbrooke, Sherbrooke, Canada

[4]Research Center, Hôpital du Sacré-Coeur de Montréal, Montréal, Canada

[5]Department of Medicine, Centre hospitalier universitaire de Sherbrooke, Sherbrooke, Canada

[6]Faculty of Medicine and Health Sciences, Université de Sherbrooke, Sherbrooke, Canada

[7]Department of Nursing, Centre hospitalier universitaire de Sherbrooke, Sherbrooke, Canada

Abstract

Background: Insulin is commonly prescribed to treat hyperglycemia in the hospital setting, but is associated with a risk of hypoglycemia. The objective of this study was to determine the incidence rate and risk factors for hypoglycemia and hyperglycemia in hospitalized patients receiving insulin.

Method: Retrospective cohort study analysing 58,496 patient-days of insulin exposure from 7780 hospitalizations of 5537 adult subjects at a teaching hospital between July 2009 and June 2011. The incidence rate of hypoglycemia (glycemia ≤ 3.9 mmol/L) and hyperglycemia (glycemia >16.7 mmol/L) were evaluated. Glycemia was measured by point-of-care blood-glucose. The association between risk factors and hypoglycemia/hyperglycemia events was determined using a Cox model.

Results: The incidence rates for days with hypoglycemia were 11.1 per 100 patient-days for subcutaneous (s.c.) insulin and 10.4 per 100 patient-days for continuous intravenous insulin (CII). The incidence rates for days with hyperglycemia were 10.2 and 4.6 per 100 patient-days for s.c. insulin and CII, respectively. Clinically relevant risk factors associated with hypoglycemia for subjects on s.c. insulin were: creatinine clearance ≤ 60 mL/min: adjusted hazard ratio (HR) 1.14 [95% CI: 1.03-1.27]; surgery: HR 1.23 [95% CI: 1.04-1.46]; and diabetes: HR 1.79 [95% CI: 1.44-2.23]. For hyperglycemia, the risk factors were diabetes: HR 5.10 [95% CI: 3.65-7.12]; use of systemic corticosteroids: HR 2.13 [95% CI: 1.90-2.38]; and prescription of scheduled with sliding scale insulin: HR 1.89 [95% CI: 1.62-2.21].

Conclusion: The identified risk factors indicate areas for targeted improvement initiatives for glycemic control and should help reduce the rate of hyperglycemic and hypoglycemic events, thereby decreasing the occurrence of adverse outcomes.

Keywords: Hospital; Insulin; Hypoglycemia; Hyperglycemia; Diabetes

Introduction

The worldwide prevalence of diabetes is predicted to rise from 371 million people in 2012 to 552 million by 2030 [1]. In 2011, the prevalence of diabetes among community-dwelling American adults was of 9%, and 30.8% of them were treated with insulin [2]. In a study at a teaching hospital in the United States, as many as 26% of the patients had a diagnosis of diabetes and 12% had undiagnosed diabetes or hyperglycemia [3]. Insulin is frequently used to treat hyperglycemia in the hospital setting because it controls rapidly changing glucose concentrations in patients with unstable clinical conditions (e.g., acute renal insufficiency) [4-6].

Poor glycemic control represents a major safety issue in hospitalized patients with diabetes [7-9]. Hyperglycemia is associated with increased mortality, a higher likelihood of complications (independent of illness severity), a greater risk of admission to an intensive care unit (ICU), and longer lengths of stay [3,6,10-15]. Severe hypoglycemia can lead to complications such as coma, paresis, convulsions, and encephalopathy [4]. Hypoglycemia is also associated with a higher risk of mortality and longer lengths of stay [6,16,17]. One study estimated the latter to 2.5 additional days for each day with hypoglycemia [6,16].

A study conducted across 575 hospitals in the United States with more than 49 million point-of-care (POC) blood-glucose measurements showed that 32% of the values were above 10 mmol/L in ICU and non-ICU patients combined [18]. Glycemic measurements were lower than 3.9 mmol/L for 6.3% of the values in ICU patients and 5.7% for non-ICU patients [18]. In a study of 1990 hospitalized non-ICU patients with diabetes receiving subcutaneous insulin, the following hypoglycemia risk factors were identified: insulin dosing (≥ 0.6 units/kg/day vs. 0.2 units/kg/day), prescription of sliding scale insulin (SSI), elevated serum creatinine, and a lower hematocrit level [19]. To the best of our knowledge, no study has evaluated risk factors for hyperglycemia among all hospitalized patients treated with insulin, whether they were diabetic or not.

*Corresponding author: Leblond J, Centre hospitalier universitaire de Sherbrooke, 3001, 12th Avenue North, Sherbrooke, Quebec, Canada
E-mail: jleblond.chus@ssss.gouv.qc.ca

Both the recent recommendations from the Endocrine Society [6] and from the American Society of Health-System Pharmacists expert panel [20] advocate for the monitoring of inpatient rates of hypoglycemia and hyperglycemia to improve glycemic control in the hospital setting. The purpose of this study was to estimate the incidence rates and determine the risk factors for hypoglycemic and hyperglycemic events in hospitalized patients prescribed insulin.

Method

Study design

A retrospective cohort study was conducted. It included all inpatients who received insulin between July 1, 2009 and June 30, 2011 at the Centre hospitalier universitaire de Sherbrooke, a teaching hospital in the province of Québec (Canada). Subjects had to meet the following inclusion criteria: (1) aged ≥ 18 years; (2) at least one day with an active insulin prescription (subcutaneous (s.c.) or continuous intravenous insulin (CII)), and measurement of at least one POC capillary glucose value. Patients hospitalized on psychiatric wards were excluded because they usually have longer lengths of stay and the purpose of this study was to evaluate glycemic control in the context of acute care.

Data sources

Variables of interest were extracted from a hospital database that includes information from (1) the hospital's electronic health record (EHR), containing information on demographic variables, medications, laboratory results, and surgical protocols; and (2) the Med-Echo database, comprising data on diagnosis related to the hospitalization (International Classification of Diseases-10 or ICD-10).

Measurement of blood glucose

POC capillary glucose values were measured using the Precision Xceed Pro glucometer (Abbott, Princetown, NJ, USA) with automatic transfer of the data to the hospital's EHR. Plasma glucose values (venous samples) were not included in the analysis since they are not as frequently monitored.

Hypoglycemia and hyperglycemia

The primary outcomes were the days with at least one hypoglycemic episode (i.e., glycemia ≤ 3.9 mmol/L) and the days with at least one hyperglycemic episode (i.e., glycemia>16.7 mmol/L) based on POC capillary glucose values only. These cut off values were chosen to allow comparison between our results and those previously published [21-23]. The number of episodes per 100 patient-days was determined.

Exposure to insulin

Exposure to insulin was categorized, per patient-day, according to all insulin regimens prescribed during that day: (1) scheduled s.c. insulin only; (2) SSI only; (3) scheduled s.c. insulin and SSI; and (4) CII with or without s.c. insulin (referred to as CII).

Risk factors for hypoglycemia and hyperglycemia

Secondary objectives include the assessment of potential risk factors for hypoglycemia and hyperglycemia grouped in four categories: demographic variables; concomitant medications; diagnoses; and medical specialty at discharge. A detailed description of the potential risk factors is provided in the online appendix.

Validation sub-study

A sub-study was conducted to assess agreement between the information on variables of interest in the hospital's database and the EHR (gold standard). A sample of 250 values was randomly selected for this validation process. Further details are provided in the online appendix.

Statistical analysis

Descriptive statistics were used to report the characteristics of patients and hospitalizations. The incidence rates of days with hypoglycemia (glycemia ≤ 3.9 mmol/L) and hyperglycemia (glycemia >16.7 mmol/L) were estimated. We also assessed the association between selected risk factors and these outcomes. Crude and adjusted HRs were estimated using the counting process model, an extended Cox model, that allows discontinuous time intervals between repeated outcomes, and a correlation structure at the hospitalization level [24]. Separate Cox models were used to examine time to hypoglycemia and hyperglycemia events in the s.c. insulin subgroup and the CII subgroup. We excluded days when POC capillary glucose values were less than 10 mmol/L and SSI was the only insulin prescribed, since patients were unlikely to receive insulin on those days. Statistical analyses were performed using SAS version 9.2 (SAS Institute Inc., Cary, NC, USA).

Ethics approval

This study was approved by the institution's Ethics Committee.

Results

The cohort was composed of 5,537 subjects who experienced a total of 7,899 hospitalizations. Overall, there were 58,496 patient-days during which insulin was prescribed and at least one POC capillary glucose measurement was available (Figure 1). Table 1 presents patient characteristics per hospitalization and patient-days. The mean age was 67.6 years (SD: 14.1 years), with men accounting for 58.9% of the hospitalizations. In 75.3% of the hospitalizations, subjects were considered to have diabetes, mostly based on a documented diagnosis of diabetes (71.8%). Regarding the type of insulin regimen prescribed, SSI was the most common, representing 32.7% of the patient-days. The overall incidence rates of days with hypoglycemia and hyperglycemia were 10.9 and 8.8 per 100 patient-days, respectively.

Exposure to s.c. insulin

There were 43,739 patient-days with exposure to s.c. insulin alone (without CII exposure). The crude incidence rates of days with hypoglycemia and hyperglycemia events were 11.1 and 10.2 events per 100 patient-days, respectively. Insulin was the only antihyperglycemic medication prescribed on 61.0% of the patient-days. Insulin was prescribed in combination with one, two, or more than two antihyperglycemic agents in 26.4%, 10.9% and 1.7% of the patient-days, respectively.

Exposure to one antihyperglycemic agent, in combination with insulin, was associated with a 24% increase in the risk of experiencing hypoglycemia (HR: 1.24; 95% CI: 1.11-1.38) compared to insulin alone. Exposure to insulin and two antihyperglycemic agents increased the risk by 92% (HR: 1.92; 95% CI: 1.67-2.21) compared to insulin alone. Finally, exposure to more than two antihyperglycemic agents in combination with insulin more than doubled the risk (HR: 2.12; 95% CI: 1.52-2.97) compared to insulin alone.

The mean number of POC capillary glucose measurements per

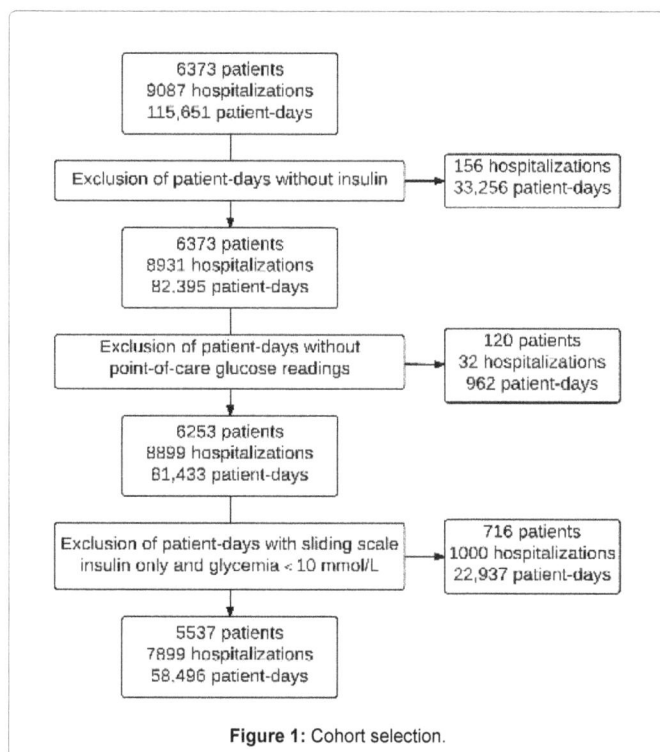

Figure 1: Cohort selection.

patient–day was 3.99 (SD: 1.0) for SSI only; 4.12 (SD: 1.6) for scheduled insulin only; and 4.39 (SD: 1.4) for scheduled insulin and SSI.

Table 2 provides the incidence rates as well as the crude and adjusted hazard ratios of days with hypoglycemia and hyperglycemia by risk factors. Subjects older than 45 years had lower risks of hypo- and hyperglycemia compared to 18-45 year-old. Having surgery increased the risk of hypoglycemia, while being in the ICU reduced this risk. Having diabetes significantly increased both the risks of hypo- and hyperglycemia. Lower renal function (eGFR ≤ 60 mL/min) increased the likelihood of hypoglycemia. Prescription of a SSI significantly reduced the risk of hypoglycemia, and was associated with a higher likelihood of hyperglycemia. Metformin was associated with a slightly higher risk of hypoglycemia and a lower risk of hyperglycemia. Use of insulin secretagogues (sulfonylurea or meglitinide) was associated with increased risks of hypo- and hyperglycemia. Finally, use of systemic corticosteroids significantly increased the risk of hyperglycemia.

Exposure to CII

There were 14,757 patient-days with exposure to CII insulin for which the crude incidence rates of days with hypoglycemia and hyperglycemia were 10.4 and 4.6 events per 100 patient-days, respectively.

Table 3 gives the incidence rates as well as the crude and adjusted hazard ratios of days with hypoglycemia and hyperglycemia by risk factor for the patients exposed to CII insulin. Older age was again associated with reduced risks of hypo- and hyperglycemia. Surgery reduced the risk of hypo- and hyperglycemia (while a greater risk of hypoglycemia was found for subjects on s.c. insulin). ICU stay reduced the risk of hyperglycemia (vs. a reduction in the risk of hypoglycemia with s.c. insulin). Diabetes and the use of corticosteroids were also associated with significantly higher risks of hyperglycemia. As seen with patients on s.c. insulin, lower renal function increased both risks of hypo- and hyperglycemia. Finally, parenteral nutrition was associated with hypoglycemia, which was not observed for patients on s.c. insulin.

Validation sub-study

Results from the validation substudy (Table A.1 of the online appendix) show an agreement ranging from 98.6% to 100% when

	Hospitalizations (n=7899)*	Patient–days (n=58,496)*
Age (years)		
18–44	535 (6.8)	-
45–54	710 (9.0)	-
55–64	1,720 (21.8)	-
65–74	2,437 (30.9)	-
≥75	2,497 (31.6)	-
Men	4,649 (58.9)	-
Weight, kg, Mean (SD)†	82.0 (21.9)	-
Hospitalization length (days)	9 (5–16)	-
Median (Q25–Q75)		
Patient–days with insulin and glycemia values	4 (2–9)	-
Median (Q25–Q75)		
Medical specialty at discharge		
Medical	3,680 (46.6)	-
Surgical	3,200 (40.5)	-
Family medicine	788 (10.0)	-
Other	231 (2.9)	-
Surgery	2,960 (37.5)	-
Intensive care unit	2,918‡ (36.9)	13 250 (22.7)
Diabetes	5,949 (75.3)	-
Treated infection	193 (2.4)	1378 (2.4)
Renal disorder		
<30 mL/min	848 (10.7)	9284 (15.9)
30-59 mL/min	1,868 (23.7)	16 561 (28.3)
≥60 mL/min	5,183 (65.6)	32 651 (55.8)
Hepatic disorder	245 (3.1)	-
Insulin regimens		
Scheduled s.c. only	-	8898 (15.2)
Sliding scale only§	-	19 133 (32.7)
Scheduled s.c. and sliding scale	-	15,708 (26.9)
Continuous intravenous insulin	-	14,757 (25.2)
Anti-hyperglycemic other than insulin		
Metformin	2,709 (34.3)	13,765 (23.5)
Sulfonylureas	1,437 (18.2)	7280 (12.5)
Meglitinides	500 (6.3)	3475 (5.9)
Thiazolidinediones	284 (3.6)	1303 (2.2)
Dipeptidyl peptidase-4 inhibitors	135 (1.7)	528 (0.9)
Alpha-glucosidase inhibitors	16 (0.2)	57 (0.1)
Parenteral nutrition	220 (2.8)	2800 (4.8)
Beta-blockers	3,843 (48.7)	27,541 (47.1)
Systemic corticostroids	2,083 (26.4)	14,695 (25.1)

Kg: Kilogram; Q25-Q75: Quartile 25% - Quartile 75%; s.c.: Sub-Cutaneous; SD: Standard Deviation.
*Figures are numbers (percentage) of hospitalizations or patient–days, unless stated otherwise.
†If no weight was available in the hospitalization, the most recent value observed during a hospitalization at our institution in the previous two years was assigned. No weight value was available during or in the two years prior to hospitalization for 442 hospitalizations.
‡Hospitalization
§Excludes days with sliding scale insulin only and POC capillary glucose values ≤ 10 mmol/L.

Table 1: Subjects' characteristics by hospitalization and patient-days.

Variables	Hypoglycemia (glycemia ≤ 3.9 mmol/L)			Hyperglycemia (glycemia >16.7 mmol/L)		
	IR[*]	Crude HR	Adjusted HR	IR[*]	Crude HR	Adjusted HR
Age in years ≥ 18–44	16.97	Reference	Reference	14.2	Reference	Reference
45–54	8.97	0.50 (0.38–0.65)	0.43 (0.33–0.54)	11.64	0.80 (0.55–1.15)	0.72 (0.53–0.98)
55–64	10.8	0.61 (0.49–0.76)	0.51 (0.43–0.62)	11.45	0.78 (0.55–1.11)	0.73 (0.54–1.00)
65–74	10.4	0.58 (0.48–0.71)	0.45 (0.38–0.53)	8.88	0.60 (0.43–0.85)	0.56 (0.41–0.75)
>75	11.53	0.64 (0.53–0.79)	0.53 (0.45–0.63)	9.93	0.67 (0.48–0.94)	0.61 (0.45–0.83)
Female vs. male	11.41	1.05 (0.95–1.15)	1.02 (0.93–1.11)	11.22	1.21 (1.07–1.36)	1.16 (1.03–1.30)
Surgery	11.6	1.03 (0.86–1.24)	1.23 (1.04–1.46)	9.37	0.83 (0.67–1.02)	0.97 (0.79–1.20)
Intensive care unit stay	4.32	0.35 (0.29–0.42)	0.54 (0.45–0.65)	9.12	0.85 (0.73–0.98)	1.02 (0.88–1.19)
Diabetes	11.83	2.87 (2.27–3.63)	1.79 (1.44–2.23)	10.96	3.94 (2.84–5.47)	5.10 (3.65–7.12)
Infection	7.02	0.62 (0.40–0.95)	0.74 (0.49–1.11)	9.98	0.98 (0.71–1.35)	0.95 (0.69–1.33)
eGFR, mL/min >60	9.42	Reference	Reference	9.33	Reference	Reference
30–60	12.68	1.36 (1.23–1.51)	1.14 (1.03–1.27)	11.34	1.23 (1.09–1.38)	1.15 (1.00–1.32)
<30	13.64	1.48 (1.32–1.67)	1.18 (1.04–1.34)	10.91	1.20 (1.02–1.40)	1.08 (0.91–1.28)
Hepatic disorder	9.65	0.86 (0.69–1.08)	0.76 (0.61–0.95)	13.57	1.43 (1.13–1.82)	1.25 (0.98–1.61)
Insulin regimen SSI only	5.06	0.28 (0.24–0.31)	0.27 (0.24–0.31)	9.32	1.42 (1.21–1.66)	1.24 (1.05–1.46)
Scheduled s.c. insulin only	16.49	Reference	Reference	6.52	Reference	Reference
Scheduled s.c. insulin and SSI	15.51	0.92 (0.84–1.02)	0.95 (0.87–1.05)	13.4	2.21 (1.88–2.60)	1.89 (1.62–2.21)
Metformin	11.61	1.05 (0.95–1.16)	1.17 (1.05–1.31)	8.78	0.78 (0.68–0.88)	0.67 (0.60–0.76)
Sulfonylurea	12.61	1.15 (1.02–1.30)	1.75 (1.55–1.98)	12.51	1.26 (1.10–1.44)	1.44 (1.26–1.63)
Meglitinides	13.61	1.25 (1.07–1.45)	1.56 (1.33–1.82)	13.28	1.37 (1.12–1.69)	1.37 (1.12–1.69)
Thiazolidinedione	11.61	1.03 (0.81–1.32)	1.00 (0.77–1.30)	13.63	1.34 (0.95–1.91)	1.30 (0.95–1.79)
DPP-4 inhibitor	6.52	0.56 (0.34–0.92)	0.55 (0.33–0.92)	11.09	1.05 (0.62–1.78)	1.01 (0.61–1.68)
Alpha glucosidase inhibitor	5.88	0.49 (0.13–1.80)	0.62 (0.16–2.38)	7.84	0.71 (0.25–1.97)	0.85 (0.34–2.11)
Parenteral nutrition	2.85	0.24 (0.10–0.59)	0.48 (0.21–1.09)	7.93	0.93 (0.57–1.50)	1.39 (0.86–2.26)
Beta-Blockers	12.52	1.31 (1.19–1.44)	1.14 (1.04–1.26)	9.83	0.93 (0.82–1.04)	0.93 (0.83–1.05)
Systemic corticosteroids	8.53	0.69 (0.61–0.78)	0.85 (0.76–0.95)	15.52	1.95 (1.73–2.20)	2.13 (1.90–2.38)

DPP4 inhibitor: Dipeptidyl Peptidase-4 Inhibitor; Egfr: Estimated Glomerular Filtration Rate; HR: Hazard Ratio; IR: Incidence Rate; s.c.: Sub-Cutaneous; SSI: Sliding Scale Insulin
[*]IR per 100 patients-days

Table 2: Incidence rate and hazard ratios of days with hypoglycemia (glycemia ≤ 3.9 mmol/L) and hyperglycemia (glycemia >16.7 mmol/L) by potential risk factors for subcutaneous insulin use.

Variables	Hypoglycemia (glycemia ≤ 3.9 mmol/L)			Hyperglycemia (glycemia >16.7 mmol/L)		
	IR[a]	Crude HR	Adjusted HR	IR[a]	Crude HR	Adjusted HR
Age in years ≥ 18–44	11.42	Reference	Reference	5.63	Reference	Reference
45–54	9.54	0.82 (0.59–1.15)	0.74 (0.55–1.00)	3.96	0.71 (0.43–1.17)	0.55 (0.36–0.84)
55–64	9.85	0.85 (0.63–1.13)	0.75 (0.57–0.99)	4.65	0.86 (0.55–1.35)	0.60 (0.42–0.86)
65–74	9.73	0.83 (0.62–1.10)	0.70 (0.53–0.92)	4.28	0.78 (0.51–1.21)	0.43 (0.30–0.62)
>75	11.90	1.05 (0.79–1.41)	0.90 (0.68–1.18)	5.14	0.94 (0.61–1.45)	0.49 (0.34–0.70)
Female vs. male	11.31	1.19 (1.04–1.37)	1.19 (1.05–1.36)	5.10	1.15 (0.94–1.41)	1.09 (0.90–1.33)
Surgery	9.33	0.83 (0.73–0.94)	0.86 (0.75–0.97)	3.34	0.45 (0.37–0.56)	0.54 (0.44–0.66)
Intensive care unit stay	10.14	0.90 (0.79–1.03)	0.91 (0.79–1.05)	3.22	0.47 (0.38–0.58)	0.57 (0.46–0.69)
Diabetes	11.10	1.21 (1.06–1.38)	1.11 (0.96–1.29)	7.13	5.01 (3.77–6.64)	3.98 (2.92–5.42)
Infection	13.11	1.25 (0.89–1.75)	1.27 (0.88–1.83)	1.91	0.46 (0.19–1.07)	0.46 (0.18–1.14)
eGFR, mL/min >60	9.30	Reference	Reference	3.13	Reference	Reference
30–60	11.66	1.25 (1.09–1.44)	1.20 (1.04–1.38)	6.94	2.43 (1.98–2.99)	2.31 (1.90–2.80)
<30	13.89	1.48 (1.23–1.77)	1.43 (1.18–1.73)	8.85	3.03 (2.37–3.88)	2.68 (2.11–3.41)
Hepatic disorder	13.61	1.32 (0.95–1.83)	1.33 (0.95–1.87)	7.56	1.67 (1.01–2.78)	1.53 (1.00–2.35)
Parenteral feeding	7.05	0.50 (0.37–0.67)	0.48 (0.36–0.65)	2.53	0.68 (0.40–1.16)	0.83 (0.51–1.35)
Beta-Blockers	10.87	1.08 (0.96–1.23)	1.03 (0.90–1.17)	5.48	1.43 (1.17–1.77)	1.25 (1.03–1.53)
Systemic corticosteroids	10.60	1.00 (0.86–1.17)	0.96 (0.82–1.12)	5.92	1.69 (1.34–2.14)	1.84 (1.47–2.29)

eGFR: Estimated Glomerular Filtration Rate; HR: Hazard Ratio; IR: Incidence Rate
[*]IR per 100 patients-days.

Table 3: Incidence rate and hazard ratios of days with hypoglycemia (glycemia ≤ 3.9 mmol/L) and hyperglycemia (glycemia >16.7 mmol/L) by potential risk factors for intravenous insulin use.

comparing values from the database to those recorded in the EHR. Of the excluded patient-days with glycemia <10 mmol/L and SSI as the only prescribed insulin, 35.6% of patients were exposed to insulin. Agreement values obtained from the EHR compared to nursing administration sheets ranged from 95.6% to 98.0% for the insulin categories. The agreement was 89.0% for concomitant medications.

Discussion

In our study on hospitalized subjects receiving s.c. insulin, the incidence rate of days with hypoglycemia (11.1 events per 100 patient-days) was in the range previously reported (5.9 to 17.6 events per 100 patient-days), but the incidence rate of days with hyperglycemia (10.2 events per 100 patient-days) was lower than previously reported (14.8 to 22.8 events per 100 patient-days for hyperglycemia) [21-23]. This could be explained by the fact that subjects with hyperglycemia but without a known diagnosis of diabetes at admission were included. SSI only was the insulin regimen most frequently used (32.7% of patient-days). For many physicians, SSI is simpler to prescribe than scheduled s.c. insulin dosage, but recent guidelines on hospital management of hyperglycemia advocate the use of scheduled s.c. insulin over prolonged SSI use, since the latter is associated with worst glycemic control [6].

The assessment of risk factors shows that patients older than 45 years were at lower risk of hypo- and hyperglycemia. This could be explained by the fact that 18-45 year-old were receiving scheduled s.c. insulin (with and without SSI) more frequently than older patients (data not shown). Another explanation might be that younger patients are more likely to have a previous diagnosis of diabetes. Patients with diabetes were at higher risk of hypoglycemia, an association previously documented [25,26]. Surgery was associated with a higher likelihood of hypoglycemia in subjects on s.c. insulin, which could be explained by the lower intake of food and vomiting in the perioperative period. Surgery was, however, associated with lower risks of hypo- and hyperglycemia in subjects on CII. This could be explained by the fact that these subjects were on an insulin protocol for CII and therefore monitored more closely.

An ICU stay was associated with a lower risk of hypoglycemia while on s.c. insulin and a lower risk of hyperglycemia while on CII. This is probably related to the heightened monitoring of patients in the ICU and common use of a standardized CII protocol. Insulin protocols with demonstrated safety and efficacy may result in lower rates of hypoglycemia in critically ill patients [27].

Lower renal function was associated with higher risks of hypoglycemia and hyperglycemia for s.c. insulin and CII. This finding is consistent with other studies in which higher creatinine levels were independently associated with hypoglycemia [19,28,29]. The higher risk of hyperglycemia could be explained by the fact that it is harder to reach glycemic control is these patients, since they experience hypoglycemia more frequently. Moreover, many antihyperglycemic drugs are contraindicated with chronic kidney disease. Change in kidney function might result in accumulation of the drugs leading to hypoglycemia. Change in medication to avoid these issues might result in temporary hyperglycemia.

Patients on SSI had a lower risk of hypoglycemia and a higher risk of hyperglycemia, which is expected since SSI is less effective than scheduled s.c. insulin to control glycemia, while decreasing the risk of hypoglycemia [6]. The association of insulin with metformin increased the risk of hypoglycemia and decreased the risk of hyperglycemia, which may be explained by improvement in insulin sensitivity. The use of secretagogues increased the risk of hypoglycemia in subjects on s.c. insulin, which was expected since these drugs promote the release of insulin. The higher risk of hyperglycemia observed in these patients could be explained by the fact that uncontrolled subjects were more likely prescribed an oral agent in addition to insulin. Patients on corticosteroids were at a higher risk of hyperglycemia (for both CII and s.c. insulin), which is consistent with this treatment's adverse effects. Parenteral nutrition was associated with a lower risk of hypoglycemia in patients on CII possibly due to the constant supply of calories (e.g., dextrose).

Our study has some limitations that should be considered when interpreting the results. We did not take into account the doses of insulin or the doses of other prescribed antihyperglycemic medications. When the subjects were prescribed CII, we could not differentiate between the patient-days with exposure to CII only and the "transition days" during which the subjects were exposed to CII and s.c. insulin. Therefore, the CII days were grouped as exposure to CII with and without s.c. insulin. Data on eGFR was collected during hospitalization, which may be inaccurate in patients with severe illnesses. Glucagon-like peptide-1 medications were not on the hospital formulary at the time of the study and thus, not readily retrievable from the EHR. The validation process indicated that subjects were exposed to insulin in 35.6% of the excluded patient-days with glycemia <10 mmol/L and prescriptions of SSI only. However, the daily amount of insulin given was minimal with an average of 3.9 units and a standard deviation of 2.4 units. This cutoff was based on a review of the SSI prescriptions. The inclusion of a single academic center limits the generalizability of our results, although this academic center consists of two sites with different patient populations and many different specialties prescribing and managing patients with hyperglycemia.

Despite these limitations, this cohort study included a large number of hospitalized (intensive care and other units) patients with and without diabetes receiving insulin (s.c. or CII) and an important number of variables to identify risk factors for hypoglycemia and hyperglycemia. The Cox model takes into account the correlation between the patient-days of a hospitalization and a patient's possible multiple hospitalizations. This study also highlights significant risk factors related to hypoglycemic and hyperglycemic events, which could lead to poorer outcomes. To the best of our knowledge, this is the first study looking at risk factors for hyperglycemia in hospitalized patients receiving insulin. Finally, the analysis structure (data extraction from the hospital's database and analysis with SAS software) put in place for this study can easily be replicated for different time periods, allowing our institution to assess the impact of new measures implemented to improve glycemic control such as a new standard order set for insulin or new directives for nursing on the timing of measurement of POC capillary glucose in relation to meal time.

In conclusion, clinicians should be aware of the risk factors associated with hypoglycemia and hyperglycemia in hospitalized subjects prescribed insulin. The risk factors identified target areas for improvement initiatives in order to reduce the rate of hyperglycemic and hypoglycemic events. The analysis structure put in place in this study will allow our institution to monitor glycemic control on a regular basis.

Acknowledgment

We thank Amélie Jourdain and Jean-Michel Gagnon for assistance with the data extraction and Tania Fayad for assistance with manuscript revision.

References

1. www.idf.org/diabetesatlas.

2. http://www.cdc.gov/diabetes/data/

3. Umpierrez GE, Isaacs SD, Bazargan N, You X, Thaler LM, et al. (2002) Hyperglycemia: an independent marker of in-hospital mortality in patients with undiagnosed diabetes. J Clin Endocrinol Metab 87:978-982.

4. Canadian Diabetes Association Clinical Practice Guidelines Expert Committee (2013) Canadian Diabetes Association 2013 Clinical Practice Guidelines for the Prevention and Management of Diabetes in Canada. Can J Diabetes 37:S1-S212.

5. Clement S, Braithwaite SS, Magee MF, Ahmann A, Smith EP, et al. (2004) Management of diabetes and hyperglycemia in hospitals. Diabetes care 27:553-591.

6. Umpierrez GE, Hellman R, Korytkowski MT, Kosiborod M, Maynard GA, et al. (2012) Management of hyperglycemia in hospitalized patients in non-critical care setting: an endocrine society clinical practice guideline. J Clin Endocrinol Metab 97:16-38.

7. Hellman R (2004) A systems approach to reducing errors in insulin therapy in the inpatient setting. Endocr Pract.10:100-108.

8. Hellman R (2006) Patient safety and inpatient glycemic control: translating concepts into action. Endocr Pract12:49-55.

9. Korytkowski M, Dinardo M, Donihi AC, Bigi L, Devita M (2006) Evolution of a diabetes inpatient safety committee. Endocr Pract 12:91-99.

10. Capes SE, Hunt D, Malmberg K, Gerstein HC (2000) Stress hyperglycaemia and increased risk of death after myocardial infarction in patients with and without diabetes: a systematic overview. Lancet.355:773-778.

11. Moghissi ES (2010) Reexamining the evidence for inpatient glucose control: new recommendations for glycemic targets. Am J Health Syst Pharm.67:S3-S8.

12. Capes SE, Hunt D, Malmberg K, Pathak P, Gerstein HC (2001) Stress hyperglycemia and prognosis of stroke in nondiabetic and diabetic patients: a systematic overview. Stroke 32:2426-2432.

13. Falciglia M, Freyberg RW, Almenoff PL, D'Alessio DA, Render ML (2009) Hyperglycemia-related mortality in critically ill patients varies with admission diagnosis. Crit Care Med 37:3001-3009.

14. Kosiborod M, Inzucchi SE, Spertus JA, Wang Y, Masoudi FA, et al. (2009) Elevated admission glucose and mortality in elderly patients hospitalized with heart failure. Circulation119:1899-907.

15. Kosiborod M, Rathore SS, Inzucchi SE, Masoudi FA, Wang Y, et al. (2005) Admission glucose and mortality in elderly patients hospitalized with acute myocardial infarction: implications for patients with and without recognized diabetes. Circulation111:3078-3086.

16. Turchin A, Matheny ME, Shubina M, Scanlon JV, Greenwood B, et al. (2009) Hypoglycemia and clinical outcomes in patients with diabetes hospitalized in the general ward. Diabetes care.32:1153-1157.

17. American Diabetes Association (2015) Glycemic Targets. Diabetes care 38:S33-S40.

18. Swanson CM, Potter DJ, Kongable GL, Cook CB (2011) Update on inpatient glycemic control in hospitals in the United States. Endocr Pract 17:853-861.

19. Rubin DJ, Rybin D, Doros G, McDonnell ME (2011) Weight-based, insulin dose-related hypoglycemia in hospitalized patients with diabetes. Diabetes Care 34:1723-1728.

20. Cobaugh DJ, Maynard G, Cooper L, Kienle PC, Vigersky R, et al. (2013) Enhancing insulin-use safety in hospitals: Practical recommendations from an ASHP Foundation expert consensus panel. Am J Health Syst Pharm 70:1404-1413.

21. Cheung NW, Cinnadaio N, O'Neill A, Koller L, Pratt HL, et al. (2011) Implementation of a dedicated hospital subcutaneous insulin prescription chart: effect on glycaemic control. Diabetes Res Clin Pract 92:337-341.

22. Juneja R, Golas AA, Carroll J, Nelson D, Abad VJ, et al. (2008) Safety and effectiveness of a computerized subcutaneous insulin program to treat inpatient hyperglycemia. J Diabetes Sci Technol 2:384-391.

23. Schnipper JL, Liang CL, Ndumele CD, Pendergrass ML(2010) Effects of a computerized order set on the inpatient management of hyperglycemia: a cluster-randomized controlled trial. Endocr Pract 16:209-218.

24. Guo Y, Bowman FD (2008) Modeling dose-dependent neural processing responses using mixed effects spline models: with application to a PET study of ethanol. Neuroimage.40:698-711.

25. Waeschle RM, Brauer A, Hilgers R, Herrmann P, Neumann P, et al. (2014) Hypoglycaemia and predisposing factors among clinical subgroups treated with intensive insulin therapy. Acta Anaesthesiol Scand 58:223-234.

26. Arabi YM, Tamim HM, Rishu AH (2009) Hypoglycemia with intensive insulin therapy in critically ill patients: predisposing factors and association with mortality. Crit Care Med.37:2536-2544.

27. Moghissi ES, Korytkowski MT, DiNardo M, Einhorn D, Hellman R, et al. (2009) American Association of Clinical Endocrinologists and American Diabetes Association consensus statement on inpatient glycemic control. Diabetes Care.32:1119-1131.

28. Kosiborod M, Inzucchi SE, Goyal A, Krumholz HM, Masoudi FA, et al. (2009) Relationship between spontaneous and iatrogenic hypoglycemia and mortality in patients hospitalized with acute myocardial infarction. JAMA 30:1556-1564.

29. Kagansky N, Levy S, Rimon E, Cojocaru L, Fridman A, et al. (2003) Hypoglycemia as a predictor of mortality in hospitalized elderly patients. Arch Intern Med163:1825-1829.

9

Intake of the First-Generation Anti-Histamines in Early Childhood may have an Adverse Effect on Cognitive Function. Population based Pharmacoepidemiologic Study in Non-Asthamtic Children

Wieslaw A Jedrychowski[1]*, Elżbieta Flak[1], Elzbieta Mroz[1], Maria Butscher[2] and Agata Sowa[1]

[1]Chair of Epidemiology and Preventive Medicine, Jagiellonian University Medical College in Krakow, Poland
[2]Polish-American Institute of Pediatrics, Jagiellonian University Medical College in Krakow, Poland

Abstract

As the allergic diseases increase steadily worldwide, the main goal of the study was to assess the association between the early intake of the first-generation sedative antihistamines in young non-asthmatic children and their cognitive function at the age of 7. The size of the exposure effect was measured by the Wechsler intelligence Scale for Children (WISC-R) and adjusted in multivariable models for major confounders known to be important for children cognitive development. The study included 212 children who were non-asthmatic and completed the monitoring of antihistamines intake over 3 years preceding the WISC-R intelligence testing.

While the first-generation drugs were used by 36.7% children and the newer generation by 39.6%, both categories of drugs were taken by 17.8% children. The analysis showed the deficit of 12 points on the verbal WISC-R IQ scale only in children who used the first- generation antihistamines for a longer time (beta coeff.=-11.7, 95% CI: -19.6, -3.7) compared to non-users. Out of the covariates included in the multivariable regression models, maternal education (beta coeff.=0.92, 95% CI: 0.37, 1.46) and breastfeeding at least for 6 months (beta coeff.=3.29; 95% CI: 0.34, 6.23) showed a significant positive impact on the verbal IQ. Intake of the newer generation antihistamines were associated neither with verbal nor performance IQ scores.

Concluding, the results suggest that the "sedative antihistamines" have a negative impact on the verbal but not performance IQs of young children if drugs were used over a longer period. The weaker verbal communication ability of young children may hinder the cognitive development of children and be associated with relatively poor school academic achievements.

Keywords: Epidemiologic study; Children; Antihistamines; Cognitive function

Introduction

Drugs with antihistamine action are among the commonly prescribed medicines in pediatrics for the symptomatic treatment of various allergic disorders such as, seasonal and perennial allergic rhinitis, conjunctivitis, atopic dermatitis or chronic urticaria. Antihistamines presently available on the market have been classified as first, second or third generation drugs and they differ in the chemical structures, pharmacodynamics, pharmacokinetics and adverse health events [1-5]. First-generation antihistamines used traditionally (diphenhydramine, chlorpheniiramine, clemastine, hydroxyzine, triprolidine and promethazine) are highly lipid soluble, have a low molecular weight and a high affinity for cerebral H1 receptors. They easily cross the blood brain barrier and show highly sedating effect on central nervous system even at low therapeutic doses. Sedation reflects the impairment of cognitive functions such as attention, memory, language, coordination or psychomotor performance, which can hinder daily activities, where mental concentration and skill are required [6-11]. As children are more sensitive to the side-effects of drugs than adults, the side effects may have implications for their further long-term intellectual development.

The newer generation antihistamines (astemizole, terfenamide, loratanide, cetirizine, fexofenadine) known as "nonsedative antihistamines", like the first-generation antihistamines have a similar affinity for the H1 receptor. However, having greater molecular weight they do not easily cross the blood brain barrier and do not cause unwanted CNS side effects. Hence, most newer-generation antihistamines have a much more favourable therapeutic index [12-16].

Most of the studies to assess the sedative effect of the H1 antagonists were carried out in the groups of asthmatic children. Although asthma is not a disease that directly affects cognitive development, but the effect of the disease may delay a child's cognitive development since children in severe asthma attacks may not receive adequate care in an optimal way and experience anoxic episodes. Subsequently, a child experiencing many anoxic insults may suffer from a cognitive delay due to the insufficient supply of oxygen to the brain [17].

The main purpose of this prospective epidemiologic population based study was to establish whether an early use of the first-generation antihistamines by young non-asthmatic children could have affected their cognitive function measured at the age of 7. The size of the effect on the cognitive scores was measured by the Wechsler Intelligence Scale for Children (WISC-R) and adjusted for major confounders known to be important for children cognitive development such as, maternal

*Corresponding author: Wieslaw Jedrychowski, Department of Epidemiology and Preventive Medicine, Jagiellonian University Medical College, 7, Kopernika Street, Krakow, Poland, E-mail: myjdryc@cyf.krakow.pl

education, the child's gender, breastfeeding practice, the presence of older siblings, and environmental tobacco smoke (ETS).

Material and Methods

This is part of an ongoing comparative longitudinal investigation on the health impact of prenatal exposure to outdoor/indoor air pollution in infants and children being conducted in Krakow, Poland. As described previously [18], between January 2001 and February 2004, we recruited a total of 484 womens between 8 and 13 weeks pregnant, who had born term babies (>36 weeks of gestation) and were registered at prenatal healthcare clinics in the central area of Krakow, where they had also lived for at least a year before screening. Pregnant women visiting the prenatal clinic received a letter of introduction and answered a short screening questionnaire to determine whether they met the eligibility criteria-age ≥ 18 years, non-smoking, singleton pregnancy, no current occupational exposure to known developmental toxicants and no history of illicit drug use, pregnancy-related diabetes, or hypertension. All participants received verbal and written information about the study. Ethical permission for the study was granted by the Bio-ethical Committee of Jagiellonian University Medical College.

The present study included 212 term babies who were non-asthmatic and completed the monitoring of intake of antihistamine drugs over 3 years preceding the WISC-R intelligence testing at the age 7. Estimated daily intake of oral antihistamines by children over the 3-years period preceding WISC-R testing were based on regular face-to-face interviews performed every 6 months by the trained field workers with mothers. Name(s) of the drug(s) reported by mothers had to be supported by showing the interviewer original packagings or containers of the drug(s) used. Detailed data on maternal education was used as a proxy for social class, intellectual ability and quality of parenting. Mothers were also asked whether the infant had ever been breastfed, and, if so, the age of the baby (in months) when exclusive breastfeeding was stopped. Exclusive breastfeeding was assumed if the child received only breast milk, and no other liquids or solids with the exception of medicine, or mineral supplements. Mixed feeding was assumed when the child received both breast milk and formula or only formula since birth. As maternal intelligence is a known correlate of child cognitive development, we administered the Test of Nonverbal Intelligence (TONI-3) to the mothers at the 4th year of follow-up. Data on the presence of tobacco smoking household members was used to define environmental tobacco smoke (ETS) at home.

Mental development testing of children

At age 7, the WISC-R was used, which is the most widely used intelligence and neuropsychological assessment and is considered to be a valid and reliable measure of general intelligence in children [19,20]. It has also been found to be a good measure of both inductive and deductive reasoning but it also measures knowledge and skills primarily influenced by biological and socio-cultural factors. The WISC-R includes questions of general knowledge, traditional arithmetic problems, vocabulary, completion of mazes, and arrangements of blocks and pictures and yields three IQ (intelligence quotient) scores, based on an average of 100, as well as subtests and index scores. WISC-R subtests measure specific verbal and performance abilities. The child's verbal IQ score (VIQ) is derived from scores on six of the subtests: information, digit span, vocabulary, arithmetic, comprehension, and similarities. The information subtest is a test of general knowledge, including questions about geography and literature. The digit span subtest requires the child to repeat strings of digits recited by the examiner. The vocabulary and arithmetic subtests are general measures

of the child's vocabulary and arithmetic skills. The comprehension subtest asks the child to solve practical problems and explain the meaning of simple proverbs. The similarities subtest asks the child to describe the similarities between pairs of items, for example that apples and oranges are both fruits. The child's performance IQ score (PIQ), which is a measure of non-verbal intellectual abilities is derived from scores on the seven subtests: picture completion, picture arrangement, block design, object assembly, coding, mazes, and symbol search. In the picture completion subtest, the child is asked to complete pictures with missing elements. The picture arrangement subtest entails arranging pictures in order to tell a story. The block design subtest requires the child to use blocks to make specific designs. The object assembly subtest asks the child to put together pieces in such a way as to construct an entire object. In the coding subtest, the child makes pairs from a series of shapes or numbers. The mazes subtest asks the child to solve maze puzzles of increasing difficulty. The symbol search subtest requires the child to match symbols that appear in different groups. Scores on the performance subtests are based on both the speed of response and the number of correct answers. The Wechsler scales were standardized for Polish children and are meant to be representative of the Polish population. The practical standardization of these tests was done during team practice sessions with Ms. Maria Butscher, a psychologist from the Jagiellonian University Medical College, who subsequently evaluated the IQ scoring.

Statistical data analysis

In the descriptive analysis, the distribution of various parameters related to the women and newborns under study were presented. Chi-square statistics (nominal variables) and analysis of variance (numerical variables) tested differences between subgroups included in the study and that who did not fully participate in the monitoring of the drug intake. The relationship between IQ scores of children and the exposure to antihistamines was evaluated by linear multivariable regression models. The models computed regression coefficients of the dependent variable (intelligence IQ scores) on the main predictor variable (antihistamines) accounting for potential confounders or modifiers (gender of child, maternal education, parity, breastfeeding practice and ETS). As the correlation coefficients between cognitive scores achieved by children and maternal education (number of schooling years) and maternal IQ assessed by TONI test did not differ, we have chosen to consider only maternal education as a proxy for maternal intellectual ability and quality of parental care. All statistical analyses were performed with STATA 12.1 version software for Windows.

Results

General characteristics of the study were presented in Table 1. As the characteristics of the subjects included in the analysis did not reveal significant differences compared with the group of children who dropped out of the study, except for the children's gender, we may assume that the material included in the analysis was representative of the population sample recruited initially (Table 2).

Overall mean VIQ scores in the study population was a little lower (mean=119.8; 95% CI: 118.4-121.3) than that for PIQ scores (mean=124.6; 95% CI: 122.9-126.3), but the difference was statistically insignificant. Out of the whole study sample, 56% children took antihistamines of various generations over shorter or longer period. The first-generation drugs were used by 36.7% children and the newer generation drugs by 39.6% children; both categories of drugs were taken by 17.8% children. The average use of the first generation drugs

Variables		Total N=225	Use of antihistamine drugs		P for difference
			(-) N=147	(+) N=78	
Maternal age:	mean	27.83	28.24	27.06	0.0157
	SD	3.481	3.415	3.495	
Maternal education: (years of schooling)	mean	15.80	15.90	15.62	0.4580
	SD	2.711	2.754	2.635	
Parity: 1	n (%)	146 (64.9)	91 (61.9)	55 (70.5)	0.2540
≥ 2	n (%)	79 (35.1)	56 (38.1)	23 (29.5)	
Gender: Boys	n (%)	104 (46.2)	64 (43.5)	40 (51.3)	0.3328
Girls	n (%)	121 (53.8)	83 (56.5)	38 (48.7)	
Gestational age: (weeks) >36	mean	39.44	39.49	39.36	0.3975
	SD	1.101	1.043	1.206	
Birth weight (g):	mean	3424.7	3438.8	3398.1	0.5033
	SD	432.89	438.67	423.29	
Length at birth (cm):	mean	54.82	54.93	54.60	0.3690
	SD	2.611	2.691	2.457	
Head circumference (cm):	mean	33.90	33.94	33.83	0.5972
	SD	1.420	1.406	1.454	
Breastfeeding exclusive >6 months	n (%)	62 (27.6)	45 (30.6)	17 (21.8)	0.2106
Postnatal ETS (1-7 age)	n (%)	32 (14.4)	22 (15.2)	10 (13.0)	0.8099
	Missing date	3	2	1	

Table 1: Characteristics of the study sample and the intake of the first-generation antihistamines by non asthmatic children.

Variables		Total N= 484	Monitoring N=225	Monitoring was not completed N=259	P for difference
Maternal age:	mean	27.55	27.83	27.31	0.1069
	SD	3.580	3.481	3.653	
Maternal education: (years of schooling)	mean	15.56	15.80	15.36	0.0795
	SD	2.759	2.711	2.790	
Parity: 1	n (%)	307 (63.4)	146 (64.9)	161 (62.2)	0.5985
≥ 2	n (%)	177 (36.6)	79 (35.1)	98 (37.8)	
Gender: Boys	n (%)	248 (51.2)	104 (46.2)	144 (55.6)	0.0492
Girls	n (%)	236 (48.8)	121 (53.8)	115 (44.4)	
Gestational age: (weeks)>36	mean	39.54	39.44	39.62	0.0955
	SD	1.141	1.101	1.170	
Birth weight (g):	mean	3443.0	3424.7	3459.0	0.3880
	SD	435.90	432.89	438.71	
Length at birth (cm):	mean	54.75	54.82	54.69	0.5956
	SD	2.615	2.611	2.622	
Head circumference (cm):	mean	33.91	33.90	33.91	0.9437
	SD	1.391	1.420	1.368	
Breastfeeding exclusive >6 months	n (%)	133 (27.5)	62 (27.6)	71 (27.4)	1.0000

Table 2: Characteristics of the children who completed the drug monitoring and those who failed to complete it.

was 9 days (95% CI: 8.9-9.7 days), and the newer generation drugs were used much longer i.e., 48 or more days (95% CI: 46.8-48.6).

While there was a significant negative trend of the verbal IQ scores with the use of the first-generation antihistamines, no such pattern was noticed in children who used the second or third generation drugs (Table 3). The distribution of verbal IQ scores was markedly shifted to lower values in the group of children who were longer exposed to antihistamines of the first- generation (Figure 1).

In order to assess the adjusted impact of the first-generation antihistamines on IQ WISC-R scales, multivariable linear regression

models were used, where a set of potential confounding variables (maternal education, gender of child, parity, breastfeeding practice, ETS, and co-exposure to the newer generation drugs) were included (Tables 4-6). The significant deficit of 12 points on the verbal IQ scale attributable to the first- generation antihistamines was noticed if used longer (beta coeff.=-11.7, 95% CI: -19.6, -3.7) (Table 4). Out of the confounders inserted in the regression models, maternal education (beta coeff.=0.92, 95% CI: 0.37, 1.46) and breastfeeding for 6 months or longer (beta coeff.=3.29; 95% CI: 0.34, 6.23) showed a significant positive impact on cognitive function.

Table 5 and 6 show that the negative effects of the first-generation antihistamines on the performance and full Wechsler IQ scales were insignificant and the beneficial impact of education and breastfeeding

IQ scores	Intake of the first generation drugs*				Nonparametric test for trend
	No-users exposure N=173	Short intake N=35	Moderate intake N=9	Long intake N=7	
IQ verbal scale	120.6 119.0-122.1	120.9 116.8-124.9	118.1 111.2-125.0	110.9 104.2-117.5	Z=-2.21 P=0.027
IQ non-verbal scale	124.2 122.3-126.2	125.7 121.4-130.0	124.8 114.4-135.1	125.9 110.7-140.9	Z=0.62 0.538
IQ full scale	124.7 123.1-126.4	125.7 121.8-129.6	123.4 114.7-132.2	122.6 113.3-131.9	Z=-0.85 P=0.393
IQ scores	**Intake of the second and/or third generation drugs****				**Nonparametric test for trend**
	No-users exposure N=136	Short intake N=44	Moderate intake N=32	Long intake N=13	
IQ verbal scale	120.7 118.9-122.5	118.1 114.2-122.0	119.7 118.1-123,3	116.2 105.6-126.8	Z=-0.51 P=0.611
IQ non-verbal scale	124.5 122.4-126.6	124.2 120.0-128.3	125.6 121.1-130.1	126.0 116.0-136.0	Z=0.23 P=0.818
IQ full scale	124.9 123.1-126.6	123.2 119.3-127.0	125.0 121.9-128.1	125.4 117.4-133.3	Z=0.21 P=0.832

Intake of the first generation drugs*
Short-term intake: 8-28 days (mean 15 days)
Moderate-term intake: 28-42 days (mean 35 days)
Long-term intake: 43-140 days (mean 74 days)

Intake of the second and/or third generation drugs**
Short-term intake: <189 days (mean 53 days)
Moderate-term intake: 190-364 days (mean 285 days)
Long-term intake: >364 days (mean 728 days)

Table 3: Trends for cognitive function of children at age 7 and the intake of the antihistamine drugs over three years preceding IQ testing.

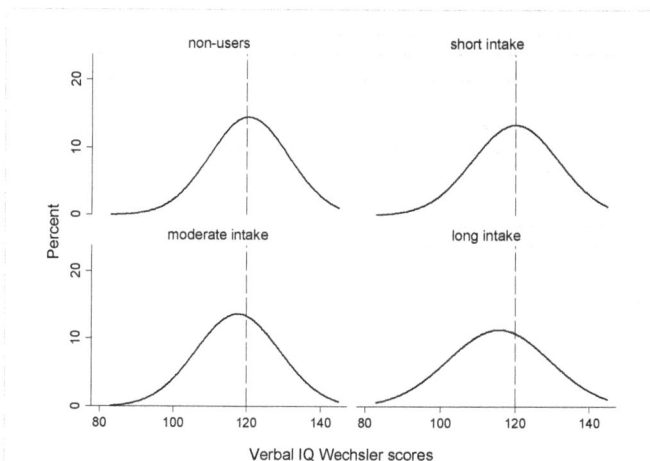

Figure 1: Distribution patterns of WISC-R scores and the intake of the first generation antihistamines (dash line: mean score in non-users).

Predictors	Coef.	T	P>t	[95% Conf.	Interval]
Gender of child (girls)	-1.73	-1.25	0.213	-4.48	1.06
Maternal education	0.92	3.34	0.001	.376	1.46
Parity (numer of older siblings)	-1.99	-1.78	0.077	-4.19	0.22
Exclusive breastfeeding	3.29	2.20	0.029	0.34	6.23
Postnatal exposure to ETS	-2.39	-1.09	0.277	-6.73	1.94
Intake of antihistamines (1st generation)					
1. Short intake	1.242	0.64	0.525	-2.60	5.08
2. Moderate intake	-4.25	-1.21	0.227	-11.16	2.67
3. Long intake	-11.65	-2.89	0.004	-19.60	-3.69
Intake of antihistamines (2nd or 3rd generation)					
1. Short intake	-0.65	-0.35	0.723	-4.27	2.97
2. Moderate intake	-0.73	-0.35	0.724	-4.78	3.33
3. Long intake	0.17	0.05	0.957	-5.97	6.30

Intake of the first generation drugs*
Short-term intake: 8-28 days (mean 15 days)
Moderate-term intake: 28-42 days (mean 35 days)
Long-term intake: 43-140 (mean 74 days)

Intake of the second and/or third generation drugs**
Short-term intake: <189 days (mean 53 days)
Moderate-term intake: 190-364 days (mean 285 days)
Long-term intake: >364 days (mean 728 days)

Table 4: Association between the verbal IQ scores and the intake of the first generation anti-histamines adjusted for potential confounders. Multivariable linear regression model.

Predictors	Coef.	T	P>t	[95% Conf.	Interval]
Gender of child (girls)	2.71	1.51	0.132	-0.83	6.24
Maternal education	0.31	0.88	0.381	-0.39	1.01
Parity (numer of older siblings)	1.97	1.37	0.173	-0.87	4.81
Exclusive breastfeeding	1.59	0.83	0.410	-2.21	5.39
Postnatal exposure to ETS	-2.87	-1.01	0.312	-8.46	2.72
Intake of antihistamines (1st generation)					
1. Short intake	2.20	0.88	0.382	-2.75	7.16
2. Moderate intake	-0.17	-0.04	0.970	-9.09	8.74
3. Long intake	1.63	0.31	0.755	-8.63	11.89
Intake of antihistamines (2nd or 3rd generation)					
1. Short intake	0.09	0.04	0.970	-4.57	4.75
2. Moderate intake	1.02	0.39	0.700	-4.20	6.25
3. Long intake	-1.48	-0.37	0.713	-9.39	6.43

Intake of the first generation drugs*
Short-term intake: 8-28 days (mean 15 days)
Moderate-term intake: 28-42 days (mean 35 days)
Long-term intake: 43-140 (mean 74 days)

Intake of the second and/or third generation drugs**
Short-term intake: <189 days (mean 53 days)
Moderate-term intake: 190-364 days (mean 285 days)
Long-term intake: >364 days (mean 728 days)

Table 5: Association between the performance IQ scores and the intake of the first generation anti-histamines adjusted for potential confounders. Multivariable linear regression model.

Figure 2 visualizes the patterns of relationship between the intake of the first and newer generation antihistamines and verbal IQ scores based on adjusted values estimated from multivariable regression models. While the exposure to the newer antihistamines did not affect verbal IQ scores, its level markedly decreased when the intake of the

first-generation drugs was reported over longer time (more than 60 days).

Discussion

Up to now the side-effects of the first-generation antihistamines on cognitive function of children have not been adequately studied. In contrast, the second-generation antihistamines have been subjected to many studies, which have provided a much better knowledge of their safety and optimal paediatric dosage in various allergic disorders. To our knowledge, this is the first pharmacoepidemiologic population based study performed in early childhood aimed at assessing the relationship between the intake of the first generation antihistamines and WISC-R test, which is the most widely used to measure intelligence of children and is considered to be a valid and reliable measure of general intelligence. The study revealed that the users of the first-generation

Predictors	Coef.	T	P>t	[95% Conf.	Interval]
Gender of child (girls)	0.43	0.30	0.767	-2.44	3.30
Maternal education	0.69	2.41	0.017	0.13	1.26
Parity (numer of older siblings)	-0.12	-0.10	0.921	-2.42	2.19
Exclusive breastfeeding	2.66	1.70	0.090	-.418	5.74
Postnatal exposure to ETS	-2.91	-1.26	0.207	-7.44	1.62
Intake of antihistamines (1st generation)					
1. Short intake	1.93	0.95	0.345	-2.09	5.95
2. Moderate intake	-2.59	-0.70	0.482	-9.82	4.65
3. Long intake	-5.98	-1.42	0.158	-14.30	2.34
Intake of antihistamines (2nd or 3rd generation)					
1. Short intake	-0.41	-0.21	0.832	-4.19	3.38
2. Moderate intake	0.26	0.12	0.903	-3.98	4.50
3. Long intake	-0.64	-0.20	0.844	-7.01	5.78

Intake of the first generation drugs*
Short-term intake: 8-8 days (mean 15 days)
Moderate-term intake: 28-42 days (mean 35 days)
Long-term intake: 43-140 (mean 74 days)

Intake of the second and/or third generation drugs**
Short-term intake: <189 days (mean 53 days)
Moderate-term intake: 190-364 days (mean 285 days)
Long-term intake: >364 days (mean 728 days)

Table 6: Association between the full IQ scores and the intake of the first generation anti-histamines adjusted for potential confounders. Multivariable linear regression model.

were not seen (Table 4). As for the full IQ scale (Table 6) the positive effect of maternal education remained significant (beta coeff. 0.69; 95% CI: 0.13, 1.26).

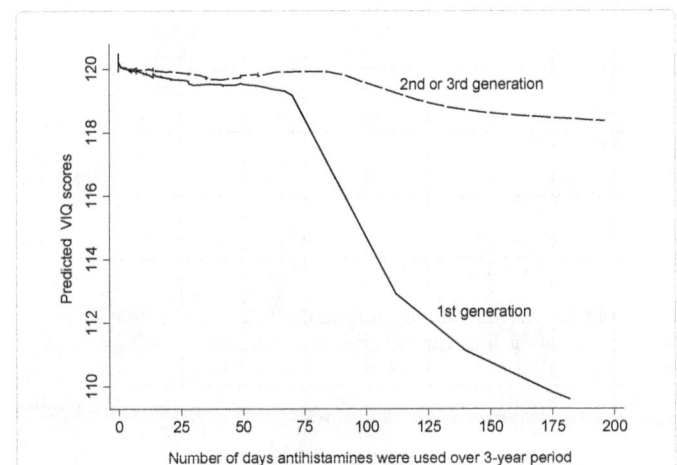

Figure 2: Predicted VIQ scores by the number of days the antihistamines were used over 3-years period.

antihistamines had achieved a significantly lower scoring on the verbal IQ scale (beta coeff.=-11.7, 95% CI: -19.6, -3.7) compared to non-users. All though the association between the first-generation antihistamines and the cognitive function of children was slightly attenuated in the multivariable regression model after accounting for major confounders, but the main effect remained stable and highly significant. Interestingly, the use of the first-generation drugs did not hinder the performance IQ scores.

The findings of the study are of interest as they may explain the communication problems of children and their worse potentials for academic achievements at school. Newer non-sedating second-generation H1-antihistamines appeared to be free from the unwanted side-effects and detrimental effects on mental functions. In this sense, our results strongly support earlier clinical observations suggesting an impairment of learning abilities of children under treatment of the first-generation antihistamine drug [6,7,9-12].

At present, there is no definitive and clear explanation for the positive association between maternal education and neurocognitive development of children, which has been shown in our study. Educational level of mothers is not only a good proxy for maternal cognitive capacity and socio-economic status of the family, but it may be an indicator of other relevant factors such as maternal behavior, life style, dietary habits before and during pregnancy, all of which are important for the study of children's health. With the exception of breastfeeding, none of the above-mentioned variables were considered in our analysis. Less educated mothers are possibly not as responsive to their infants' needs as better educated mothers or they may present some less favorable behavior during early childhood. Children living in a poor socio-economic environment are more likely to be exposed to environmental hazards and the adverse effects may be more pronounced in lower compared to higher socio-economic groups.

Moreover, studies carried out by Bellinger [21] suggest that social context also modifies the effects of chemical neurotoxins. For example, material hardship has been demonstrated to modify the neurotoxic effects of tobacco smoke in children in the study done by Rauh et al. [22]. The way in which maternal behavior may affect the development of children was discussed in a recently published paper by Surkan et al. [23].

Our study confirmed a positive effect of longer exclusive breastfeeding on the verbal IQ score, which by many authors is explained by the fact that breastfed and milk-formula-fed infants could have been influenced by omega-3 polyunsaturated fatty acids that are normally present in breast milk or other bioactive components essential for development [24,25]. However, there are other possible mechanisms that may explain the association between breastfeeding and child cognitive function since breastfeeding may be an indicator of a safe and sound maternal attachment status, which has been shown to have a positive influence on the child's psychological development into later age [26-29]. Breastfeeding may also be a marker of other unmeasured maternal characteristics such as maternal intelligence. In our analysis, we did not consider maternal intelligence as it was found that maternal education correlated significantly with maternal cognitive capacity.

Weakness of the study results from the small size of the study sample and the lack of precise information on pediatric antihistamines doses used in early childhood. Moreover, we could not perform verification of maternal reports with medical records. However, strength of our study is the prospective design, and assessment of individual intake of antihistamine drugs by interviews with mothers at regular 6-months

intervals preceding the health outcome measurement and controlling for several major confounding covariates. In addition, a set of relevant confounders of the relationship between the intake of drugs and cognitive development such as diagnosed asthma in children, chronic diseases of mothers or maternal active tobacco smoking, have been removed through entry criteria to the study. It is important to mention as well, that the assessment of the cognitive development of children was carried out by the trained staff using the Polish version of the Wechsler-R intelligence, adapted and standardized by the Polish Psychological Society.

Conclusions

The first-generation antihistamines negatively affect verbal but not performance IQs of young children when they are used over a relatively longer time. As language development is the part of the human communication system, the weaker verbal communication function may hinder the cognitive development of children and be associated with relatively poor school academic achievements.

Acknowledgements

This is part of an ongoing comparative longitudinal investigation on the health impact of prenatal exposure to outdoor/indoor air pollution in infants and children being conducted in New York City and Krakow. In part, the study received funding from an ROI grant entitled, "Vulnerability of the Fetus/Infant to PAH, PM2.5 and ETS" (5 ROI ES10165 NIEHS; 02/01/00-01/31/04) and from the NIEHS (ROI ES010165-0451) the Lundin Foundation and the Gladys T. and Roland Harriman Foundation. Principal investigator: Prof FP Perera; Co-investigator Prof WA Jedrychowski.

References

1. Simons FE, Fraser TG, Reggin JD, Roberts JR, Simons KJ (1996) Adverse central nervous system effects of older antihistamines in children. Pediatr Allergy Immunol 7: 22-27.

2. Emanuel MB (1999) Histamine and the antiallergic antihistamines: a history of their discoveries. Clin Exp Allergy 29 Suppl 3: 1-11.

3. Brown RE, Stevens DR, Haas HL (2001) The physiology of brain histamine. Prog Neurobiol 63: 637-672.

4. Simons FE (2002) H1-antihistamines in children. Clin Allergy Immunol 17: 437-464.

5. Del Cuvillo A, Sastre J, Montoro J, Jauregui I, Ferrer M, et al. (2007) Use of antihistamines in pediatrics. J Investig Allergol Clin Immunol 2: 28-40.

6. Gengo F, Gabos C, Miller JK (1989) The pharmacodynamics of diphenhydramine-induced drowsiness and changes in mental performance. Clin Pharmacol Ther 45: 15-21.

7. Meltzer EO (1990) Performance effects of antihistamines. J Allergy Clin Immunol 86: 613-619.

8. Vuurman EF, van Veggel LM, Uiterwijk MM, Leutner D, O'Hanlon JF (1993) Seasonal allergic rhinitis and antihistamine effects on children's learning. Ann Allergy 71: 121-126.

9. Kay GG, Berman B, Mockoviak SH, Morris CE, Reeves D, et al. (1997) Initial and steady-state effects of diphenhydramine and loratadine on sedation, cognition, mood, and psychomotor performance. Arch Intern Med 157: 2350-2356.

10. Kay GG (2000) The effects of antihistamines on cognition and performance. J Allergy Clin Immunol 105: S622-S627.

11. Church MK, Maurer M, Simons FE, Bindslev-Jensen C, van Cauwenberge P, et al. (2010) Risk of first-generation H(1)-antihistamines: a GA(2)LEN position paper. Allergy 65: 459-466.

12. Stevenson J, Cornah D, Evrard P, Vanderheyden V, Billard C, et al. (2002) Long-term evaluation of the impact of the h1-receptor antagonist cetirizine on the behavioral, cognitive, and psychomotor development of very young children with atopic dermatitis. Pediatr Res 52: 251-257.

13. Holgate ST, Canonica GW, Simons FE, Taglialatela M, Tharp M, et al. (2003)

Consensus Group on New-Generation Antihistamines (CONGA): present status and recommendations. Clin Exp Allergy 33: 1305-1324.

14. Simons FE (2004) Advances in H1-antihistamines. N Engl J Med 351: 2203-2217.

15. Tillement JP (2005) Pharmacologic profiles of the newer antihistamines. Clin Exp Allergy Rev 5: 7-11.

16. Banerji A, Long AA, Camargo CA Jr (2007) Diphenhydramine versus nonsedating antihistamines for acute allergic reactions: a literature review. Allergy Asthma Proc 28: 418-426.

17. Bass JL, Corwin M, Gozal D, Moore C, Nishida H, et al. (2004) The effect of chronic or intermittent hypoxia on cognition in childhood: a review of the evidence. Pediatrics 114: 805-816.

18. Jedrychowski W, Whyatt RM, Camann DE, Bawle UV, Peki K, et al. (2003) Effect of prenatal PAH exposure on birth outcomes and neurocognitive development in a cohort of newborns in Poland. Study design and preliminary ambient data. Int J Occup Med Environ Health 16: 21-29.

19. Wechsler D (1974) Manual of the Wechsler Intelligence Scale for Children-Revised. New York: Psychological Corporation.

20. Wechsler D (2004) Wechsler Intelligence Scale for Children-fourth edition. London, Pearson Assessment, Manual of the Wechsler Intelligence Scale for Children-Revised. New York: Psychological Corporation.

21. Bellinger DC (2008) Lead neurotoxicity and socioeconomic status: conceptual and analytical issues. Neurotoxicology 29: 828-832.

22. Rauh VA, Whyatt RM, Garfinkel R, Andrews H, Hoepner L, et al. (2004) Developmental effects of exposure to environmental tobacco smoke and maternal hardship among inner city children. Neurotoxicol Teratol 26: 373-385.

23. Surkan PJ, Schnaas L, Wright RJ, Téllez-Rojo MM, Lamadrid-Figueroa H, et al. (2008) Maternal self-esteem, exposure to lead, and child neurodevelopment. Neurotoxicology 29: 278-285.

24. Neuringer M, Connor WE (1986) n-3 fatty acids in the brain and retina: evidence for their essentiality. Nutr Rev 44: 285-294.

25. Lundqvist-Persson C, Lau G, Nordin P, Strandvik B, Sabel KG (2010) Early behaviour and development in breast-fed premature infants are influenced by omega-6 and omega-3 fatty acid status. Early Hum Dev 86: 407-412.

26. Morley R, Cole TJ, Powell R, Lucas A (1988) Mother's choice to provide breast milk and developmental outcome. Arch Dis Child 63: 1382-1385.

27. Jansen J, deWeerth C, Riksen-Walraven M (2008) Breastfeeding and the mother infant relationship: a review. Dev Rev 28: 503-521.

28. Meedya S, Fahy K, Kable A (2010) Factors that positively influence breastfeeding duration to 6 months: a literature review. Women Birth 23: 135-145.

29. Whitehouse AJ, Robinson M, Li J, Oddy WH (2011) Duration of breast feeding and language ability in middle childhood. Paediatr Perinat Epidemiol 25: 44-52.

10

Evaluation of Antibiotic Use in Medical Ward of Fitche District Hospital, North Showa Zone, Oromia Region, Ethiopia

Addisu Alemayehu Gube[1]*, Rufael Gonfa[2] and Tarekegn Tadesse[2]

[1]Department of Nursing, College of Medicine and Health Sciences, Arbaminch University, Arbaminch, Ethiopia
[2]Department of Pharmacy, College of Medicine and Health Sciences, Ambo University, Ambo, Ethiopia

Abstract

Background: Antibiotic are among the most prescribed drug in medical ward. Because of the rise in health care cost lack of uniformity in drug prescribing and the emergency of antibiotic resistance monitoring and control of antibiotic use are growing concern and strict antibiotic policies should be warranted. Inappropriate use of antibiotic can increase morbidity, mortality, patient cost and bacterial antibiotic resistance.

Objective: To evaluate antibiotic use practice in medical ward of Fitche hospital, North Showa Zone, Oromia region, Ethiopia.

Methodology: Institution based cross sectional study was conducted by collecting data retrospectively from 200 patient cards drawn by Simple random sampling using balloting from Medical ward of Fitche hospital from March 10-May 30, 2016. After checking for completeness and consistency, data was entered in SPSS (IBM 20) and descriptive statistics was carried.

Result: Out of the total 200 patient cards, 110 (55%) were of male and 90 (45%) were of female. Most antibiotics were prescribed for empirical treatment 163 (81.5%) and least for prophylactic treatment 5 (2.5%). In this study, of the total 340 drugs prescribed in Medical ward, the prevalence of antibiotics use was 220 (64.7%). In this study, 65% received more than one antibiotic. And the most commonly prescribed groups of antibiotic were Cephalosporin 32.5% and the most commonly prescribed antibiotic was ceftriaxone 27.5%.

Conclusion: This study revealed that of the total of 340 drugs prescribed for 200 patients in Medical Ward of Fitche District Hospital, 64.7% were antibiotics and the most commonly prescribed groups of antibiotic were Cephalosporin and the most commonly prescribed antibiotic was ceftriaxone. And majority of patients in Medical ward 65% received more than one antibiotic.

Keywords: Drug; Medical ward; Fitche hospital; Antibiotics

Introduction

Antibiotics are powerful medicines that fight bacterial infections. Used properly, antibiotics can save lives. They either kill bacteria or keep them from reproducing. Your body's natural defences can usually take it from there [1]. They are one of the pillars of modern medical care and play major role in prophylaxis and treatment of infectious disease. The issue of their availability, selection and proper use are of critical importance to the community antibiotic miser use: however, worldwide with the extent of the problem being greater in the developing countries, through their purchase in local pharmacies and drug stores and through inappropriate prescribing habit and an overzealous desire to treat every infection [2]. They are one of the most common drugs prescribed in hospital today. It has been estimated that up to third of all patients receive at least one antibiotic during hospitalization. The cost involved is there for correspondingly high and up to 40% of a hospital's drug expenditure may be devoted to the purchase of antibiotics [3,4]. Antimicrobial therapy is administered to 25% to 40% of hospital inpatient, and, in 50% of cases, is inadequate in terms of dosage, rout of administration, or indication Realties such as this strengthen the notion that rational and therefore adequate use of antimicrobial agents plays an essential role in insuring patient safety, particularly in the intensive care setting above all because antibiotic misuse fosters bacterial resistance and increasing the cost of health system [5-7].

In the past decade, there has been an alarming trend towards increase in antimicrobial resistance; there are different factors for the development of antimicrobial resistance: among these; human pathogens, the overuse and inappropriate prescribing of broad spectrum antibiotics has been implicated [8-10]. In the hospital, use of antibiotic drug has been major concern in the last few decades for several reasons for the purchasers of health care service and administration. Antibiotics drugs account for a major proportions of the escalating drug budget. To a greater extent particularly in hospital, the overuse and misuse of antibiotic drug considered to be one of the reasons for increasing resistance among various photogenes: these worries have led to the implementation of strict antibiotic policies in hospital in many countries with different strategies and different outcomes.

Monitoring of drug use is essential in order to follow the effect and adherence to the hospital's antibiotic policies: patient medical record may be reviewed for this purpose. But this method can be quite exhaustive [10]. Excessive and inappropriate use of antibiotic is highly associated with the emergence of antibiotic resistance which presents major threat to global public health. Antibiotic resistance reduce the

*Corresponding author: Addisu Alemayehu Gube, Department of Nursing, College of Medicine and Health Sciences, Arbaminch University, Ethiopia, E-mail: addis166@gmail.com

effectiveness of and number of option for antibiotic treatment, leading to increased morbidity, mortality, and health care expenditure [11,12]. Growing misuse of antibiotics has been reported in hospitals, causing toxic effects and various infections due to resistant microorganisms that increase the cost and duration of hospitalization. Increased cost of health care will definitely jeopardizes the capacity of the poor population to seek the modern health care. There is a pressing need to develop appropriate measures to curtail misuse of drugs in general and antibiotics in particular. Besides; a drug use in hospitals has a considerable influence on further drug use outside the hospitals [13].

Several strategies for controlling antibiotic usage have been proposed. Such as formulary replacement or restriction, introduction order form, health care provider education, feedback activates, and approval requirement from infectious disease specialist for drug prescription [14,15]. Drug Use Evaluation (DUE) is an ongoing systematic process designed to maintain the appropriate and effective use of drug. It incorporates qualitative measure and emphasizes outcome. Including pharmacoeconomics assessment. DUE can identify problem in drug use, reduce adverse drug reaction, optimize drug therapy and minimize drug related expense it often include intervention to ensure appropriate drug use [16]. Drug use evaluation focuses on the area that show greater potential for improvements. It involve on compressive review of patient prescription and medication data, during and after dispensing in order to ensure appropriate therapeutic decision making and promote positive outcome [17].

In Ethiopia, particularly in Fitche, there are no sound studies conducted about the evaluation of antibiotics use in hospital wards. Therefore, this study was designed to evaluate use of antibiotics in medical ward of Fitche hospital, North Showa Zone, Oromia region, Ethiopia.

Methods and Materials

Study are and period

The study was conducted in Fitche hospital North Showa Zone, Oromia region, which is found 115 km from Addis Ababa. Its total population is 27,493 in numbers of which 12, 933 are males and 14,560 are females. The town has many governmental and privet organization such as Government hospital and health center. Fitche hospital has different departments and wards like OPD, medical, gynecology, pediatrics, and surgical ward. And the study focused in Medical ward of the hospital. The study was conducted from March 10 to May 30, 2016.

Study design

Institution based cross sectional study was conducted by collecting data retrospectively from patient card in Medical ward of Fitche hospital.

Source population

All patients who are admitted/referred/discharged/died in Medical Ward of Fitche hospital.

Study population

All patients who are admitted in medical ward and who have taken at least one antibiotic with or without concurrent medication and admitted, referred, discharged, or died in the study period.

Sampling size and sampling technique

The sample size for this study was calculated using single population proportion formula based on the following Assumptions: p=50%, with 95% confidence level and 5% level of precision. So, total of 384 was calculated and since, the number of population was less than 10,000, the correction formula was used and the sample size became: 200 patient cards.

From the total cards of patients who admitted to a medical ward from September 10, 2015 to May 10, 2016 and fulfill the inclusion criteria, 200 patient cards were selected by Simple random sampling using balloting.

Data processing and analysis

After checking for completeness and consistency, data was entered in SPSS (IBM 20) and descriptive statistics was carried. And data were presented using narratives, tables and figure.

Ethical consideration

A formal letter was written from Ambo University, College of Medicine and Health Sciences, department of Pharmacy to Fiche Hospital in order to get permission to conduct the study. And Fitch Hospital Administrators were notified about the objective of the study and the confidentiality of patient cards.

Results

Socio demographic characteristics

The most age group treated by antibiotics were 15-25 year of age which accounts 61 (30.5%). While the least age group treated by antibiotics were those of greater than 70 year of age. Of the patients, 110 (55%) were males and 90 (45%) were females (Table 1).

Patterns of antibiotic prescribing

In this study, the total of 340 drugs including antibiotics were prescribed to the total of 200 patients; out of which 220 (64.7%) were antibiotics. From the total of antibiotics, Ceftriaxone 55 (27.5%) was the most frequently prescribed antibiotics followed by doxycycline 40 (20%); Ciprofloxacin 23 (11.5%) and Cephalexin was prescribed for only 2 (1%) patient (Tables 2 and 3).

In this study, from the total of 200 patients, many of the patients are treated by two antibiotics: 84(42%), 70(35%) receive one antibiotics and the rest 46(23%) receive three antibiotics (Figure 1).

With regard to purpose of antibiotic prescribing, this study revealed that majority of antibiotics were prescribed for empirical treatment 163 (81.5%), followed by kinetic treatment 32 (16%) and prophylactic use accounted the least 5(2.5%) (Figure 2).

Variables	Frequency	Percentage
Sex		
Male	110	55%
Female	90	45%
Age		
15-25	61	30.5%
26-36	43	21.5%
37-47	35	17.5%
48-58	25	12.5%
59-69	21	10.5%
70-80	15	7.5%

Table 1: Socio demographic characteristics of patients in Medical ward of Fiche District Hospital.

Antibiotics Groups	Frequency	Percentage (%)
Cephalosporin	65	32.5%
TTC	40	20%
Flour quinolone	37	18.5%
Metronidazole	21	10.5%
CAF	17	8.5%
Cotrimoxazole	6	3%
Aminoglycoside	7	3.5%
Penicillin	4	2%
Augmentin	3	1.5%
Total	200	100%

Table 2: Most commonly prescribed group of antibiotics in medical ward of Fitche District Hospital.

Antibiotics	Frequency	Percentage (%)
Ceftriaxone	55	27.5%
Doxycycline	40	20%
Ciprofloxacin	23	11.5%
Metronidazole	21	10.5%
Chloramphenicol	17	8.5%
Norfloxacine	14	7%
Cloxacillin	8	4%
Cotrimoxazole	6	3%
Gentamycin	4	2%
Ampicillin	4	2%
Clarithromycin	3	1.5%
Augmentin	3	1.5%
Cephalexin	2	1%
Total	200	100%

Table 3: Most commonly prescribed antibiotics in medical ward of Fitche District Hospital.

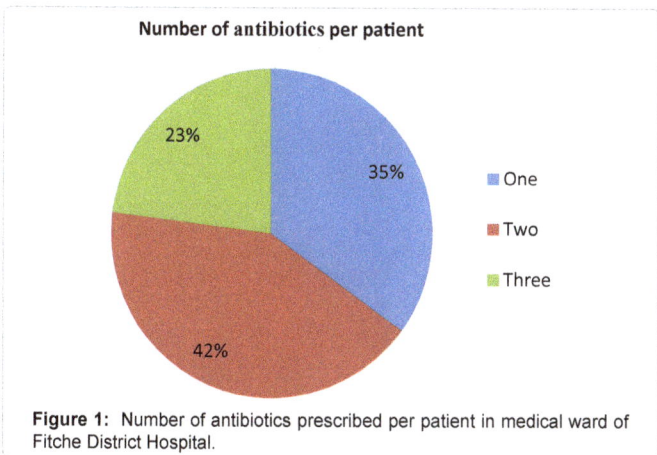

Figure 1: Number of antibiotics prescribed per patient in medical ward of Fitche District Hospital.

According to this study Community Acquired Pneumonia (CAP) was the most commonly distributed disease which account 61 (30%) followed by meningitis 38 (19%) and Acute Gastroenteritis (AGE) 25(12%) (Table 4).

In this study, when we see the duration of hospitalization for 200 patients, 80 (40%) stay for 1-4 days, 65 (32.5%) for 5-9 days, 30 (15%) for 10-14 days, 20 (10%) stay for 15-19 days and 5 (2.5%) stay for greater than 20 days in hospital.

Route of administration and potential drug-drug interaction

In this study out of 220 prescribed antibiotics for 200 patients, most of them prescribed in IV route which account 76(38.2%), followed by PO 68(34.1%) and IM 16 (6.3%) (Table 5).

Appropriateness of antibiotic use

When we see the appropriateness of the antibiotic use with respect to dose, frequency and duration, the study revealed that 181 (90.5%), 194(97%) and 186(93%) were corresponds to appropriate dose, frequency and duration respectively and 14(7%), 5(1.5%) and 10(5%) were inappropriate dose, frequency and duration respectively.

Discussion

This institution based cross sectional study has investigated antibiotic use in Medical ward of Fitche District Hospital, North Showa Zone, Oromia Region, Ethiopia.

The use of antibiotics in medical ward is justifiable practice even though it requires a regular review of the chosen regimen to maximize the benefit of the patient. In this study, of the total 340 drugs prescribed in Medical ward, the prevalence of antibiotics use was 220 (64.7%). This finding is lower than the finding of the study conducted

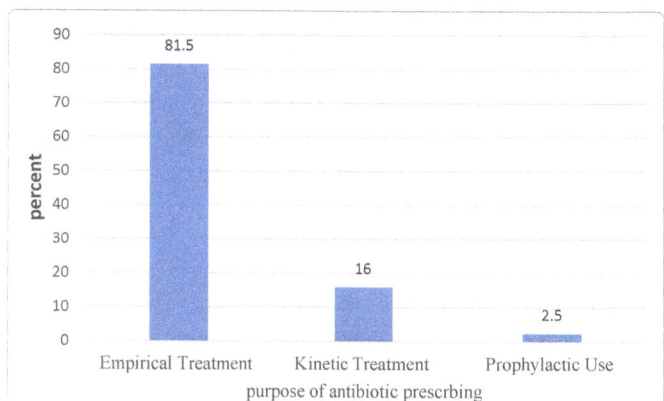

Figure 2: Antibiotic treatment types in medical ward of Fiche District Hospital.

S. No.	Disease	Frequency	Percentage
1	CAP	61	30%
2	Meningitis	38	19%
3	AGE	25	12%
4	UTI	23	11.5%
5	AFI	13	6.5%
6	Typhoid	9	4.5%
7	Septic arthritis	8	4%
8	Cellulitis	7	3.5%
9	PUD	6	3%
10	Rheumatic arthritis	6	6%
11	Other	4	2%
	Total	200	100%

Table 4: Distribution of common disease for which antibiotics were prescribed in medical ward of Fitche District Hospital.

Route	Frequency	Percentage
IV	84	38.2%
IV+PO	31	14.1%
PO	75	34.1%
IM	16	7.3%
IM+PO	14	6.3%

Table 5: Route of administration of antibiotics in medical ward of Fitche Hospital.

in Debremarkos Referral Hospital, Northwest Ethiopia where the prevalence of antibiotics use was 71.36% [18]. This might be because the study carried out in Debremarkos was carried in the whole Referral hospital and shows the findings from all departments where as our study only focused in medical ward of Fitche district hospital.

The finding of this study is higher than the finding of the study conducted in Dessie Referral hospital, Northeast Ethiopia, where the prevalence of antibiotics use was 24.37% [19]. This might be because this study is carried out in outpatient pharmacies and the time gap between the two studies. In this study, of the total 200 patients treated at Medical ward of Fitche district hospital, majority of them 65% received more than one antibiotic. This finding is almost comparable with the finding of the study conducted in Ayder Referral hospital, Mekelle Ethiopia, where majority of patients 58.8% in the hospital received more than one antibiotic. Although the simultaneous use of two or more antibiotics has a certain rational, indiscriminate or routine use of antibiotic combination may have several negative consequences: primarily, the patient Risk of toxicity from two or more antibiotics, increased cost and the emergence of drug resistance.

In this study, the most commonly prescribed groups of antibiotic were Cephalosporin 32.5% and the most commonly prescribed antibiotic was ceftriaxone 27.5%. This findings is almost similar with the finding of the study conducted in Ayder Referral hospital, Mekelle Ethiopia, where the most commonly prescribed groups of antibiotics and the most commonly prescribed antibiotic were Cephalosporin 32.7% and ceftriaxone 28.7% respectively.

Conclusion and Recommendations

Conclusion

This study revealed that of the total of 340 drugs prescribed for 200 patients in Medical Ward of Fitche District Hospital, 64.7% were antibiotics and the most commonly prescribed groups of antibiotic were Cephalosporin and the most commonly prescribed antibiotic was ceftriaxone. And majority of patients in Medical ward 65% received more than one antibiotic.

Recommendations

District health office and Fitche Hospital should work together in order to oversee and control antibiotics use in the hospital, Medical ward in particular. They have to make sure whether standard and national guidelines are being followed during using antibiotics in the hospital.

Acknowledgement

The authors' sincere thanks go to Ambo University for provision of the opportunity to conduct the research. They also like to give their deepest gratitude for Fitche District hospital staffs for their cooperation in providing basic information. Lastly their thanks go to Medical Record Room workers and all research participants who took part in the study.

References

1. Antibiotics (2016) U.S. National Library of Medicine.

2. Ibewuchi R, Mbata T (2002) Rational and irrational use of antibiotics. Africa Health 24: 16-18.

3. Lim VK, Cheong YM, Suleiman AB (1993) Pattern of antibiotic usage in hospitals in Malaysia. Singapore Med J 34: 525-528.

4. http://apps.who.int/medicinedocs/en/d/Js2289e/

5. Correa L (2007) Restriction to the use of antimicrobials in the hospital environment. Einstein: Continuing Education in Health 5: 48-52.

6. Eickhoff T (1992) Antibiotics and nosocomial infections. In: Bennet J, Brachman P (eds.) Hospital Infections (3rd edn.). Brown and Company, Boston pp: 245-264.

7. Neu H (1993) Antimicrobialagent: role in prevention and control nosocomial infections. In: Wenzel R (ed.) Prevention and Control of Nosocomial Infection (2nd edn.). Williams and Wilkins, Baltimore pp: 406-441.

8. Dranitstaris G, Brook's J, McGeer A, landry L, Loeb M (1998) Assessment in health care Meeting. InSocTechnol.

9. http://www.who.int/drugresistance/infosharing/AMR_WS_WERNIGERODE_ REPORT_EURO.pdf

10. Kivert R, Dahl M, Llerena A, Maimets M, Wettermark B et al. (1998) Antibiotic use in 3 European University Hospital. Scand J infects Dis 30: 277-280.

11. Fishman N (2006) Antimicrobial stewardship. Am J Med 119: S62-S70.

12. Smith RD, Coast J (2002) Antimicrobial resistance: A global response. Bull World Health Org 80: 126-133.

13. Gyssen IC, Blok W, vanden Broek PJ, HeksterYA, vander Meer JW (1997) Implementation of an educational program and an antibiotic order form to optimize quality of antimicrobial drug use In a department Internal medicine. Eur J Clin Microbiol Infect Dis 16: 904-912.

14. Guglielemo BJ (1995) Practical strategies for the appropriate use of antimicrobial. Pharm World Sci 17: 96-102.

15. Phillips MS, Gayman JE, Todd MW (1996) ASHP guidelines on medication-use evaluation. American Society of Health-system Pharmacists. Am J Health Syst Pharm 53: 1953-1955.

16. Robert J, Pean Y, Varon E, Bru JP, Bedos JP, et al. (2012) Point prevalence survey of antibiotic use in French hospitals in 2009. J Antimicrob Chemother 67: 1020-1026.

17. Tigestu AD, Tesfahun CE (2014) Assessment of drug use pattern using World Health Organization core drug use indicators at Debremarkos Referral Hospital, Northwest Ethiopia. Int J Innovat Pharmaceut Sci Res 2: 2347-2154.

18. Endale G, Solomon A, Wuletaw A, Asrat A (2013) Antibiotic prescribing pattern in a referral hospital in Ethiopia. Afr J Pharm Pharmacol 7: 2657-2661.

19. Solomon A, Rahel A, Fantahun M, Melkam W, Assen A, et al. (2015) Antibiotics utilization and their cost in Ayder Referral Hospital, Mekelle, Ethiopia. Glob J Med Res 15.

11

Myrica rubra Fruit Drink Sub-Chronic Toxicity and Hepatoprotective Effect in Rats

Badraddin Mohammed Al-Hadiya[1], Mohamed Fahad AlAjmi[2]* and Kamal Eldin Hussein El Tahir[3]

[1]Departments of Pharmaceutical Chemistry, College of Pharmacy, King Saud University, Riyadh, Saudi Arabia
[2]Departments of Pharmacognosy, College of Pharmacy, King Saud University, Riyadh, Saudi Arabia
[3]Departments of Pharmacology, College of Pharmacy, King Saud University, Riyadh, Saudi Arabia

Abstract

Background: This study dealt with the effect of the subchronic toxicity of *Myrica rubra* fruit beverage drink (MRD) in rats and its hepatoprotective effect against carbon tetrachloride (CCl_4)-induced hepatotoxicity.

Methodology: Different groups of normal male and female Wistar rats were treated with 50% MRD as drinking vehicle (13 weeks), as substitution of the normal drinking water. Coulter Counter was used for red blood corpuscles (RBCs) and white blood corpuscles (WBCs) count. The Reflotron instrument and Reflotron haemoglobin kit used for determination of haemoglobin content, while the Reflotron strips for determination of blood glucose, total triglycerides and cholesterol contents, blood enzymatic levels, and bilirubin. Atomic absorption spectroscopy was used for determination of blood Na^+, Mg^{++} and Ca^{++} concentrations.

Principal findings: Treatment induced significant increases in the red blood corpuscles (RBCs) count, haematocrit and haemoglobin content. It also significantly decreased plasma levels of total cholesterol and the low-density lipoproteins (LDL) without affecting the levels of high-density lipoproteins (HDL), glucose, triglycerides and bilirubin, together with the significant decrease in hepatic malonaldehyde production. The treatment resulted in significant reductions in the enzymes alanine transiminase (ALT), aspartate aminotransferase (AST) and Alkaline phosphatase (ALP) and a significant diuretic effect.

Conclusion: The results of the study point to the potential of *Myrica rubra* fruit drink to act as a new functional food.

Keywords: *Myrica rubra* drink; Hepatoprotection; Hepatotoxicity; Hepatic enzymes

Introduction

Myrica rubra or Bayberry, Yumberry, Waxberry or Chinese strawberry tree is usually cited as *Myrica rubra* by Siebold and Zuccarini (1846).

Myrica rubra sieb et zucc. fruits, family Myricaceae, are stony red fruits with berry-like edible portions. The fruit is grown in China, India, Japan and some other south eastern Asian countries such as, Vietnam, Burma and Thailand. It is known by various other names such as Yangmei, Bayberry and Chinese arbutus. It is also known as Waxmytle and Yamamoto in Japan.

Phytochemical investigations of the fruit juice revealed the presence of high concentrations of polyphenols and proanthocyanidins [1]. The latter are condensed tannins (polymers) composed of various flavan-3-ol or catechin units. The most available are the reddish procyanidins [2]. In addition to the fruits both of the leaves and the bark of the tree constituents were analyzed [3-5].

The proanthocyanidins were reported to possess various actions that included antioxidant [6,7], anti-viral [7,8], hypolipidemic [9], anti-cancer [10], and anti-inflammatory actions [11].

Myrica rubra juice is now widely distributed world-wise as a 50% refreshing drink and also as a carbonated beverage - under the trade name Yumberry. Thus, it was thought of interest to investigate the outcomes of the sub-chronic toxicity (treatment for 13 weeks) of this refreshing drink. When it was observed that it decreases some hepatic enzymes, it was thought to investigate the effect of short term treatment of rats (4 weeks) with the drink as a sole source of drinking vehicle.

Materials and Methods

Yumberry juice drink

Yumberry juice bottled drink was purchased from the local market in Riyadh city, Kingdom of Saudi Arabia. The bottled drink is a product of China (Zhejiang Yumberry Juice Co.).

Animals

In this study male Wistar rats (body weight 250 ± 10 g) and females (220 ± 8 g) were used. The animals were provided with standard chow diet, supplied by Silo and Flour Mills Organization, Feed Mill, Riyadh, Saudi Arabia. All animals were housed at a temperature of 22° ± 1°C and relative humidity of 50 ± 5%. The light: dark cycle was 12 hours each. The animals' treatment was conducted in accordance with the Guide for the Care and Use of Laboratory Animals. The protocol of the current study was approved by the ethics Committee of the College of Pharmacy, King Saud University, Riyadh, KSA.

*Corresponding author: Mohamed Fahad AlAjmi, Departments of Pharmacognosy, College of Pharmacy, King Saud University, Riyadh, Riyadh 11451, P.O. Box 2457, Saudi Arabia, E-mail: malajmii@ksu.edu.sa

Treatment of the animals

The control group was allowed tap water ad lib. The treatment group was administered *Myrica rubra* juice refreshing drink (50% Yumberry drink) as the sole source of drinking vehicle for 13 weeks in case of the sub-chronic toxicity and for 4 weeks in the case of the Hepatoprotective activity.

To investigate the hepatoprotective effects, carbon tetrachloride CCl_4 was used as an inducer of hepatotoxicity. For this purpose, it was administered as a mixture of CCl_4: paraffin oil in the ratio of 1:1 at a dose of 1 ml/kg intraperitoneally (i.p). Male Wistar rats were divided into 3 groups (N=8 animals per group). Group No. 1 was injected with paraffin oil only (1 ml/kg intraperitoneally) as a single dose. Group 2 was injected with the mixture of CCl_4 and paraffin oil. Group 3-the one given Yumberry drink for 4 weeks-was administered the mixture of CCl_4 and paraffin oil as a single dose (1 ml/kg i.p.) in the morning following the 4-week-treatment period. Blood was collected on the third day.

Collection of blood from the sub-chronically-treated and control animals

On days 90 and 91 following the start of the treatment, the animals were anaesthetized with diethyl ether and blood (7 ml) was collected from each control and treated animal using cardiac puncture employing a 23-gange needle fitted to a 10-ml plastic syringe. 1 ml from each animal was used for determination of the various blood cell counts, the hemoglobin content and the clotting times. The remaining blood (6 ml each) was mixed with 3.6 (w/v) aqueous trisodium citrate solution in the ratio of 1:9 (citrate:blood) to prevent blood clotting. The blood was then centrifuged at 3000 rpm (EMS Centrifuge) for 20 minutes to obtain platelets and blood cells-free plasma and to calculate the haematocrit value for each animal. The latter were corrected for the added trisodium citrate. The plasma was then stored at -20°C until used within the next few days for the determination of the various parameters indicated below.

Determination of blood cell counts

The numbers of RBCs and WBCs per µl whole blood obtained from each control or treated rat was determined using Coulter Counter, Model S8 90 (Coulter Electronics, Lubon beds, U.K.). The volume of blood used was 125 µl/test.

Determination of haemoglobin content

The haemoglobin content was determined using the Reflotron Instrument and Reflotron haemoglobin kit (Roche Diagnostic GmbH, D-68298, Mannheim, Germany). The test depends upon conversion of haemoglobin to methaemoglobin in presence of potassium ferricyanide as outlined by Van Assendelft [12].

Determination of the haematocrit value

The haematocrit value of each blood sample was calculated following the centrifugation of the collected blood in graduated centrifuge tubes at 3000 rpm (EMS Centrifuge) for 20 minutes.

Determination of blood glucose level

The concentration of glucose was determined in each cell-free plasma using the Reflotron Instrument and the Reflotron Glucose strip (Roche Diagnostics). It depends upon the principle of conversion of glucose in the sample in presence of molecular oxygen and the enzyme GOD (Glucose Oxidase Dehydrogenase to S-D-gluconolactone and H_2O_2. The latter in presence of the indicator 3,3,5,5-tetramethyl benzidine and the enzyme POD (peroxidase 'horseradish') gives a color which was measured as outlined by Trasch [13].

Determination of blood total cholesterol

The cholesterol contents in the different plasmas were determined using the Reflotron instrument and the Reflotron strips (Roche Diagnostics) depending upon the principle of conversion of the blood cholesterol esters to cholesterol in presence of the enzyme cholesterol esterase. The produced cholesterol is then converted in presence of molecular oxygen and cholesterol Oxidase to cholestenone and H_2O_2. The latter in presence of the indicator 3,3,5,5-tetramethyl benzidine and the enzyme POD (peroxidase 'horseradish') gives a color which was measured as outlined by Braun [14].

Determination of blood total triglycerides

The triglycerides contents of the different plasmas were determined using the Reflotron Instrument and the provided strips (Roche Diagnostics). The method depends upon the principle of conversion of the blood triglycerides in presence of the enzyme esterase to glycerin and fatty acids. The produced glycerin in presence of ATP and the enzyme glycerin kinase I is then converted to glycerin-3-phosphate and ADP. The glycerin-3-phosphate is then acted on by the enzyme glycerin phosphate Oxidase and molecular oxygen to produce dihydroxyacetone phosphate and H_2O_2. The latter in presence of the indicator 4-(4-dimethylaminophenyl) 5-methyl-2-(3,5-dimethoxy-4-hydroxyphenyl) imidazole dihydrochloride and the enzyme POD (Peroxide 'horse radish') produces a color which can be measured as outlined by Carstensen et al. [15].

Determination of blood GOT (AST) (Glutamic oxaloacetic acid transiminase or Aspartate aminotransferase)

The levels of AST in the different plasmas were determined using Reflotron Instrument and the provided strips (Roche Diagnostics, Germany). The principle depends upon the ability of the enzyme GOT to act on ketoglutarate and alanine sulfinate to produce glutamate and pyruvate. The latter in presence of molecular O_2, phosphate ions and water is acted on by the enzyme pyruvate Oxidase to CO_2, acetyl phosphate and H_2O_2. The latter in presence of the peroxidase enzyme and the indicator 4-(4-dimethyl aminophenyl) 5-methyl-2-(3, 5-di-t-butyl-4-hydroxyphenyl) imidazole dihydrochloride gives a blue color which intensity can be measured as outlined by Denake [16].

Determination of blood ALT (Alanine Transiminase) or GPT (Glutamate- Pyruvate Transiminase)

The concentrations of the ALT in the different plasmas were determined using the Reflotron Instrument and the provided strips (Roche Diagnostics, Germany). The principle depends upon the ability of ALT to convert ketoglutarate and alanine to glutamate and pyruvate. The latter in presence of PO_4^{2-}, water and molecular oxygen is then converted by the enzyme pyruvate Oxidase to acetyl phosphate, CO_2 and H_2O_2. The latter in presence of the enzyme peroxidase and the indicator 4-(4-dimethyl aminophenyl) 5-methyl-2-(3, 5-di-t-butyl-4-hydroxyphenyl) imidazole dihydrochloride produces a blue color, which color intensity, can be measured as outlined by Denake and Rittersdorf [17].

Determination of blood alkaline phosphatase

The contents of alkaline Phosphatase in the different plasmas were determined using Reflotron Instrument and the provided strips (Roche Diagnostics). The principle depends upon the ability of the enzyme alkaline Phosphatase to convert o-cresophthalein phosphate and methylglucamine to methylglucamine phosphate and the colored compound o-cresophthalein that can be measured at 567 nm as outlined by Rosalki and Heins [18,19].

Determination of blood K⁺

The concentrations of K^+ in the different plasmas were determined using Reflotron Instrument and the provided strips (Roche Diagnostics). The principle depends upon the interaction and complexation of K^+ in the plasmas with valinomycin and the indicators 4-[(2,6-dibromo-4-nitrophenyl) azo]-2-naphthol to give a colored complex that can be measured as outlined by Lum and Cambizzino [20].

Determination of blood bilirubin

The concentrations of bilirubin in the different plasmas were determined using the Reflotron Instrument and provided strips (Roche Diagnostics). The principle depends upon the interaction of blood bilirubin with the indicator 2-methoxy-4-nitrophenyl diazonium tetrafluroborate to produce the colored product azobilirubin as outlined by Freitag [21].

Determination of blood Na⁺, Mg⁺⁺ and Ca⁺⁺

The concentrations of Na^+, Mg^{++} and Ca^{++} in the different plasmas were determined using atomic absorption spectroscopy using Varian AA775, atomic absorption spectrophotometer. For the determination of Na^+ the fixed working conditions were: Lamp current 5 mA, fuel: acetylene support air and flame stoichiometry: oxidizing. In the flame emission the wavelength used was 589.0 nm, the spectral band pass was 0.1 nm, the fuel: acetylene and the support: air.

For the determination of magnesium (Mg^{++}) the fixed working conditions were: lamp current 3.5 mA, fuel: acetylene, support: air and flame stoichiometry: oxidizing. The working flame emission conditions were: wavelength 285.2 nm, spectral band pass 0.1 nm, fuel: acetylene and support: nitrous oxide.

For the determination of Ca^{++}, the fixed working conditions were: lamp current 3.5 mA, fuel: acetylene, support: nitrous oxide and flame stoichiometry: reducing: red cone 1-1.5 cm high. The flame emission conditions were: wavelength 422.7 nm, spectral band pass 0.1 nm, fuel: acetylene and support: nitrous oxide [22,23].

Determination of urinary Na⁺, K⁺ and Ca⁺⁺ contents

The concentrations of Na^+ and Ca^{++} in urine were determined using atomic absorption spectrophotometry as described above. The concentrations of K^+ were determined using Reflotron Instrument and specific strips as described above. It should be noted that following collection of urines, they were acidified immediately after collection by the addition of concentrated HCl (1 ml acid+3 ml urine) to prevent the precipitation of calcium oxalate and phosphate [24].

Statistical analysis

All values reported were the mean ± standard error (s.e.) of mean. Statistical differences were examined using ANOVA techniques using the least significant difference criterion or the 't' test as appropriate.

Results

General observations during the sub-chronic study regarding the general health of the animals

All animals treated with Myrica rubra drink (MRD) as the sole drinking vehicle for the whole 13 weeks were healthy. There were no any toxicological signs in the respiratory, cardiovascular, central and autonomic nervous system. There were no changes in the eyes.

Water and food consumption

Table 1 depicts the mean ± s.e. mean drinking vehicles and food/kg/week in the control and treated groups (males and females). The food and MRD consumed by the treated animals (both male and female rats) were significantly greater than that consumed by the corresponding control animals (P<0.05, N=8).

Effect on blood cells, haematocrit and haemoglobin

Table 2 depicts the effects of MRD treatment on total erythrocytes, leukocytes, platelets, haematocrit and haemoglobin content.

Effect on blood glucose, blood lipids and bilirubin

Treatment of both sexes of rats with MRD induced significant decreases in both total cholesterol and LDL (P<0.01, N=8) without any effect on glucose, HDL, triglycerides and bilirubin. Table 3 shows the cumulative results.

Effect on liver enzymes

Treatment of rats (both sexes) with MRD as the sole drinking

Animal group (Sex)	Mean Consumption/kg/week	
	Drinking Vehicle (ml)	Food (g)
Control (Male)	708 ± 17.3	541.3 ± 12.6
Control (Female)	661 ± 13.9	480 ± 16.3
MRD (Male)	879.9 ± 15.1*	639.5 ± 9.7*
MRD (Female)	830 ± 11.9*	576 ± 9.3*

*P<0.05, N=8, compared with the corresponding control.

Table 1: Water and Food Consumption by Rats during Treatment with MRD.

Treatment (sex)	No. of Cells/µl Blood			Haematocrit	Haemoglobin g %
	RBC×10⁶	WBC×10³	Platelets×10³		
Control (male)	9.1 ± 0.07	13.6 ± 0.1	301 ± 0.2	43.5 ± 0.6	14.1 ± 0.1
Control (female)	7.8 ± 0.03	11.6 ± 0.08	285 ± 0.1	39.6 ± 0.2	13.5 ± 0.08
MRD (male)	10.08 ± 0.1*	13.9 ± 0.2	310 ± 0.3	48.3 ± 1*	15.7 ± 0.04*
MRD (female)	8.75 ± 0.07*	11.4 ± 0.1	291 ± 0.2	44.9 ± 0.7*	14.8 ± 0.05*

*P<0.01, N=8, compared with the corresponding control.

Table 2: The effects of MRD treatment on total erythrocytes, leukocytes, platelets, haematocrit and haemoglobin content.

Parameter	mg %					
Treatment (sex)	Glucose	Total Cholesterol	LDL	HDL	Triglyceride	Bilirubin
Control (Male)	109 ± 6.7	99 ± 5.3	31.3 ± 1.7	49.6 ± 2.3	88.7 ± 3.9	0.3 ± 0.01
Control (Female)	102 ± 4.9	86 ± 3.9	33.1 ± 3.1	41 ± 3.5	78 ± 1.7	0.25 ± 0.02
MRD (Male)	116 ± 9.1	87.9 ± 3.4*	25.9 ± 2.1*	48.9 ± 1.9	85.1 ± 2.3	0.29 ± 0.02
MRD (Female)	108 ± 7.3	75.1 ± 4.2*	28 ± 1.3*	43 ± 1.7	80 ± 2.5	0.23 ± 0.01

*P<0.01, N=8, compared with the corresponding control.

Table 3: Effect of MRD on Blood Lipids, Glucose, Triglycerides and Bilirubin.

Parameter	U/litre Plasma		
Treatment (sex)	ALT	AST	Alkaline Phosphatase
Control (Male)	27.4 ± 1.3	65.0 ± 3.9	95.0 ± 1.6
Control (Female)	24.9 ± 0.9	55.0 ± 4.1	83.0 ± 0.9
MRD (Male)	21.1 ± 0.7*	51.5 ± 3.2*	79.8 ± 4.2*
MRD (Female)	21.5 ± 1.1*	44.5 ± 1.7*	68.9 ± 2.9*

P<0.05, N=8 compared with its respective control

Table 4: Effect of MRD on hepatic enzymes in rats.

Parameter	U/Litre (Plasma)			mg % (Plasma)	µmole/g liver tissue
Treatment	ALT	AST	Alkaline Phosphatase	Bilirubin	Malon-aldehyde
Control (paraffin oil)	29.3 ± 0.9	70.0 ± 3.8	90.0 ± 6.1	0.3 ± 0.1	1.1 ± 0.09
CCl_4	91.7 ± 3.1	190.0 ± 6.9	261.0 ± 7.3	0.8 ± 0.2	3.7 ± 0.2
MRD	52.1 ± 2.9*	133.2 ± 11.3*	188.0 ± 4.9*	0.58 ± 0.1*	1.6 ± 0.15*

*P<0.01, N=8 compared with CCl_4-treated animals.

Table 5: Effect of MRD on carbon tetrachloride-induced hepatotoxicity in male rats.

vehicle for 13 weeks induced significant decreases in ALT, AST and alkaline phosphatase enzymes (P<0.05, N=8). Table 4 depicts the cumulative results.

Effect on blood ions

The blood levels of Na^+, K^+, Ca^{++} and Mg^{++} in the control male rats were 142 ± 0.9, 4.8 ± 0.03, 2.45 ± 0.03 and 0.9 ± 0.1 mmole/litre, respectively. The corresponding values in female rats were 133 ± 1.9, 4.6 ± 0.1, 2.3 ± 0.1 and 0.8 ± 0.07 mmole/litre. Treatment with MRD did not induce any significant changes in these levels.

Effect on urine production and the urinary concentrations of Na^+, K^+ and Ca^{++} ions

Treatment of both sexes of rats with MRD significantly increased the volume of urine voided from 3.95 ± 0.07 ml (male control) to 5.1 ± 0.1 ml and from 3.36 ± 0.04 ml (female control) to 4.51 ± 0.08 ml (P<0.05, N=8). The treatment increased the excretion of Na^+ from 0.128 ± 0.01 (control male) to 0.139 ± 0.02 mmole/litre and from 0.114 ± 0.03 (control female) to 0.123 ± 0.04 mmole/litre. These were insignificant increases (P>0.05, N=8). There were no significant changes in both K^+ and Ca^{++} excreted in urine. The treatment also decreased the urinary pH from 8.0 ± 0.3 (control male) and 8.1 ± 0.4 (control female) to 7.0 ± 0.5 and 6.9 ± 0.3, respectively. These changes were not significant (P>0.05, N=8).

Effect on carbon tetrachloride-induced hepatic damage in male rats

Treatment of male Wistar rats with a mixture of CCl_4 and paraffin (50:50) in a dose of 1 ml/kg (i.p.) induced severe damage to the liver on the third day following treatment of the animals (Table 5) as revealed by the significant increases in the hepatic enzymes ALT, AST, alkaline Phosphatase and in the hepatic level of malonaldehyde and the plasma level of bilirubin (P<0.01, N=8). MRD treatment significantly protected the animals against these increases (P<0.01, N=8).

Discussion

The results of this study clearly demonstrated the functional activity of *Myrica rubra* fruit juice that is formulated in form of a beverage drink. One of the first observed effects is its stimulant effect on the RBCs and their content of haemoglobin. Such actions were not followed in detail

in this study. They may be due to stimulation of erythropoietin. The second observed clear effect is the ability of the drink to decrease both of the total cholesterol and the LDL. The metabolism of these lipids is generally regulated by a family of membrane-bound transcription factors called sterol regulatory element binding proteins, e.g., SREBP-1 [25] and SREBP-2 is reported to regulate the genes involved in cholesterol synthesis [26]. Furthermore, peroxisome prolifertor activated receptors, e.g., PPAR-alpha are involved in the lipids metabolism [27].

MRD is known to contain high concentration of proanthocyanidins [1]. These are condensed tannin polymers composed of various flavan-3-ol catechin units. The most available are the reddish procyanidins [2]. MRD constituents may act to suppress lipid metabolism regulatory proteins. Indeed, in a recent study, [7] revealed the ability of oligomeric proanthocyanidins to suppress SPEBP-2 [7] and to increase PPAR-α expression. Another possibility is that the proanthocyanidins and the various poly phenols present in MRD [1,2] may act to suppress fat absorption in the intestine. Previous studies revealed the inherent ability of proanthocyanidins to decrease hyperlipidemia in mouse model type 2 diabetes [9] and in streptozotocin-induced type 1 diabetes in rats [7]. The observed ability of MRD to decrease the levels of the hepatic enzymes during the subchronic treatment may be related to the ability of its proanthocyanidins to elevate the level of the Hepatoprotective glutathione. Indeed, these substances have been shown to elevate the level of glutathione in diabetic rats and mice.

Part of this study revealed the potential of MRD to act as a hepatoprotective against CCl_4-induced elevations in the plasma levels of ALT, AST, alkaline Phosphatase, bilirubin and malonaldehyde. The hepatotoxicity of CCl_4 is very well studied and is believed to occur as a result of generation of free radicals within the liver [28]. The initial step in this hepatotoxicity is the production of the trichloromethyl radical (-•CCl_3) via the enzyme cytochrome P450 subtypes (2E1, 2B1, 2B2 and 3A) [29,30]. The latter radical then interacts with molecular oxygen resulting in the production of the trichloromethyl peroxyl radical (-•O-O-CCl_3) [30]. This radical then initiates the peroxidation of the membrane phospholipids and the unsaturated fatty acids. All these peroxides act to damage the cellular components (e.g. mitochondria, endoplasmic reticulum and plasma membranes) with the resultant hepatotoxicity [28,30,31]. In addition, CCl_4 is reported to release various destructive cytokines such as TNFα [32]. Thus, the observed hepatoprotective effect of MRD may be highly related to the ability of some of its constituents to act as free radical scavengers. Indeed such antioxidant action has been observed for its constituents polyphenols, flavonoids and proanthocyanidins [6,7,33,34].

On a broad basis, the results of this study point clearly to the property of *Myrica rubra* fruit drink as an anti-anemic, a hypocholesterolemic and a hepatoprotective pointing to its potential as a new functional food.

Acknowledgement

This project was funded by a grant from Deanship of Research under the number RGP-VPP- 50. This funding is highly appreciated.

References

1. Fang Z, Zhang M, Tao G, Sun Y, Sun J (2006) Chemical composition of clarified bayberry (Myrica rubra Sieb. et Zucc.) juice sediment. J Agric Food Chem 54: 7710-7716.

2. Saito M, Hoshiyama H, Ariga T, Kataoka S, Yamaji N (1998) Antiulcer activity of grape seed extract and procyanidins. J Agric Food Chem 46: 1460-1464.

3. Tao J, Morikawa T, Toguchida I, Ando S, Matsuda H, et al. (2002) Inhibitors of nitric oxide production from the bark of Myrica rubra: structures of new biphenyl

type diarylheptanoid glycosides and taraxerane type triterpene. Bioorg Med Chem 10: 4005-4012.

4. Tong Y, Zhou XM, Wang SJ, Yang Y, Cao YL (2009) Analgesic activity of myricetin isolated from Myrica rubra Sieb. et Zucc. leaves. Arch Pharm Res 32: 527-533.

5. Wang SJ, Tong Y, Lu S, Yang R, Liao X, et al. (2010) Anti-inflammatory activity of myricetin isolated from Myrica rubra Sieb. et Zucc. leaves. Planta Med 76: 1492-1496.

6. Dixon RA, Xie DY, Sharma SB (2005) Proanthocyanidins--a final frontier in flavonoid research? New Phytol 165: 9-28.

7. Yokozawa T, Cho EJ, Park CH, Kim JH (2012) Protective Effect of Proanthocyanidin against Diabetic Oxidative Stress. Evid Based Complement Alternat Med 2012: 623879.

8. Cheng HY, Lin TC, Ishimaru K, Yang CM, Wang KC, et al. (2003) In vitro antiviral activity of prodelphinidin B-2 3,3'-di-O-gallate from Myrica rubra. Planta Med 69: 953-956.

9. Lee YA, Cho EJ, Yokozawa T (2008) Effects of proanthocyanidin preparations on hyperlipidemia and other biomarkers in mouse model of type 2 diabetes. J Agric Food Chem 56: 7781-7789.

10. Kuo PL, Hsu YL, Lin TC, Lin LT, Lin CC (2004) Induction of apoptosis in human breast adenocarcinoma MCF-7 cells by prodelphinidin B-2 3,3'-di-O-gallate from Myrica rubra via Fas-mediated pathway. J Pharm Pharmacol 56: 1399-1406.

11. Lee YA, Kim YJ, Cho EJ, Yokozawa T (2007) Ameliorative effects of proanthocyanidin on oxidative stress and inflammation in streptozotocin-induced diabetic rats. J Agric Food Chem 55: 9395-9400.

12. Van Assendelft OW (1970) Spectrophotometry of haemoglobin derivatives. Ed. Royal Van Gorem Ltd., Assen. The Netherlands.

13. Trasch H (1984) Quantification of glucose in plasma. Clin Chem 30: 969-972.

14. Bruan HP (1984) Quantitation of total cholesterol in serum and plasma. Clin Chem 30: 991-996.

15. Cartensen CA, Murawaki R, Koller PU (1985) Determination of triglycerides in plasma. J Clin Chem Clin BioChem 30: 608-612.

16. Deneke U (1985) Quantification of G.O.T. (Glutamate oxalo transaminase) in blood and plasma. Clin Chem 31: 921-929.

17. Deneke U, Ritterdorf W (1984) Quantitative determination of ALT (Alanine Transaminase). Clin Chem 30: 1009-1014.

18. Rosalki SB (1993) Multicenter Evaluation of Iso-ALP Test Kit for Measurement of Bone Alkaline Phosphatase Activity in Serum and Plasma. Clin Chem 39: 648-652.

19. Heins M, Heil W, Withold W (1995) Storage of serum or whole blood samples? Effects of time and temperature on 22 serum analytes. Eur J Clin Chem Clin Biochem 33: 231-238.

20. Lum G, Cambizzino R (1974) Determination of total bilirubin. Clin Pathol 61: 108-112.

21. Freitag H (1987) Determination of bilirubin in plasma. Clin Chem 33: 1011-1017.

22. Hwang JY, Sandonato L (1969) Determination of calcium using atomic absorption. Anal Chem Acta 48: 183-196.

23. Adams PB, Passmore WO (1966) Quantitation of calcium and Na+ by atomic absorption spectrophotometry. Anal Chem 38: 630-639.

24. Pybus J (1969) Determination of calcium and magnesium in serum and urine by atomic absorption spectrophotometry. Clin Chim Acta 23: 309-317.

25. Yahagi N, Shimano H, Hasty AH, Matsuzaka T, Ide T, et al. (2002) Absence of sterol regulatory element-binding protein-1 (SREBP-1) ameliorates fatty livers but not obesity or insulin resistance in Lep(ob)/Lep(ob) mice. J Biol Chem 277: 19353-19357.

26. Shimano H, Yahagi N, Amemiya-Kudo M, Hasty AH, Osuga J, et al. (1999) Sterol regulatory element-binding protein-1 as a key transcription factor for nutritional induction of lipogenic enzyme genes. J Biol Chem 274: 35832-35839.

27. Ferré P (2004) The biology of peroxisome proliferator-activated receptors: relationship with lipid metabolism and insulin sensitivity. Diabetes 53 S43-S50.

28. Ruch RJ, Klaunig JE, Schultz NE, Askari AB, Lacher DA, et al. (1986) Mechanisms of chloroform and carbon tetrachloride toxicity in primary cultured mouse hepatocytes. Environ Health Perspect 69: 301-305.

29. Slater TF (1981) Free radicals as reactive intermediates in tissue injury. Adv Exp Med Biol 136: 575-589.

30. Brattin WJ, Glende EA Jr, Recknagel RO (1985) Pathological mechanisms in carbon tetrachloride hepatotoxicity. J Free Radic Biol Med 1: 27-38.

31. Younes M, Siegers CP (1984) Interrelation between lipid peroxidation and other hepatotoxic events. Biochem Pharmacol 33: 2001-2003.

32. Weber LW, Boll M, Stampfl A (2003) Hepatotoxicity and mechanism of action of haloalkanes: carbon tetrachloride as a toxicological model. Crit Rev Toxicol 33: 105-136.

33. Xie DY, Dixon RA (2005) Proanthocyanidin biosynthesis--still more questions than answers? Phytochemistry 66: 2127-2144.

34. Yang Z, Zheng Y (2009) Effect of high oxygen storage on quality, enzymes and DPPH-RADI activity of Chinese bay. J Agr Food Chem.

12

National Drug Information Center Services through Ministry of Health Hotline Calling Center (937) in Saudi Arabia

Alomi YA[1]*, AL- Mudaiheem H[2], Alsharfa A[3], Albassri H[4], Alonizi K[5], Alothaian M[6], Alreshidi M[7] and Alzahrani T[8]

[1]National Clinical Pharmacy and Pharmacy Practice Programs, Pharmacy R&D Administration, Riyadh, Saudi Arabia
[2]National Drug Information Center, General Administration of Pharmaceutical Care Department, Ministry of Health, Saudi Arabia
[3]Drug Information Center, Pharmaceutical Care Department, Ras Tanoura Hospital, East Province, Ministry of Health, Saudi Arabia
[4]Drug Information Center, Pharmaceutical Care Department, Saud Bin Jalawi Hospital, Alahasa, Ministry of Health, Saudi Arabia
[5]Regional Drug Information Center, Pharmaceutical Care Administration, Tabouk, Ministry of Health, Saudi Arabia
[6]Drug Information Center, Pharmaceutical Care Department, King Fahad Hospital, Alahasa, Ministry of Health Saudi Arabia
[7]Pharmaceutical Care Administration, Hail, Ministry of Health, Saudi Arabia
[8]Training and Education Administration, Almadina Amonaoura, Ministry of Health, Saudi Arabia

Abstract

Objective: National drug information center (NDIC) has started providing services since January 2013, and answering public and professional inquiries through MOH-Hotline Calling Services (937) since December 2013. The objective of this study to explore the analysis of national drug information inquiries by the hotline services in Saudi Arabia.

Method: Simulation including all 12-month 2014 of receiving adults and pediatrics drug information inquiries; through MOH-hotline calling services (937). Ten on-call clinical pharmacists and expert trained pharmacists were receiving calls from public and professional asking about drug information, through manual documentation system of drug information inquiries by drug information data collecting form.

Results: The total number answered calls were 976 calls through the entire study period. Of them, 264 (27%) calls were documented. The question most asked was on dose standardization (27%) followed by drug Administration (15.3%). Medications were the most asked about (83.3%). Antibacterial was the most frequent question (19.80%) followed by Vitamins and supplements (11.68%) then antidiabetic by (4.87%).

Conclusion: National drug information center was providing new first-time hotline services by answering drug information inquiries from professional and public. Targeting to educate professional and public about drug therapy of common diseases will decrease drug related problems. Expanding drug information hotline services with electronic documentation, expansion of clinical pharmacist with advanced training will improve patient outcomes and avoid the unnecessary cost.

Keywords: National drug information; Hotline; Clinical pharmacist; Pharmacist; Saudi Arabia

Introduction

The first drug information center was founded in the world and located in United Sate of America (USA) at begging of the 1960s, and in the United Kingdom in 1977 [1,2], the services expanded over years in the USA and other countries [3-13]. In Saudi Arabia, the first drug information center was established at King Saud University college of pharmacy in early 1978 [14], then in late 1980s King Khalid University Hospital (KKUH) and King Faisal Specialist Hospital and Research Center (KFSHRC) had established drug information and poisoning information center [15,16].The first drug and poisoning information center at MOH was founded in 1989 at very public 500 beds-hospital King Saud Medical City previously known as " Riyadh Central Hospital". It was operated by a pharmacist, and supervised by a clinical pharmacist who had a master degree in clinical pharmacy from the University of Pacific from United Sate of America. The center had started with a limited scope service of answering drug information inquiries, with available of an old version of references British National Formulary, and Micromedex Drugdex in Microfiche version, and provided eight hour's morning duty. In 1994, the number of pharmacists increased and expanded the scope of services by participating in the Pharmacy and Therapeutic committee and sharing in 4th Edition of MOH Drug Formulary. In 2008, the local drug and poisoning information center converted to be regional coverage and expanded the scope of services in Riyadh area, and headed by the

critical care clinical pharmacist certified board of pharmacotherapy. The number staff increased to 10 clinical pharmacists and new services had been started as clinical pharmacy programs including medication safety program, anticoagulation program, pain management program, and drug utilization evaluation program. An electronic documentation and workload analysis system had been started to measure pharmacist impact on patient outcome and cost avoidance. In 2013 the regional center converted to national drug information center (NDIC) at General Administration of Pharmaceutical Care at Ministry of Health (GAPC-MOH) to cover all 21 regions in the kingdom of Saudi Arabia with expanded scope of services based on American Society Health-Syst Pharmacist (ASHP) updating guidelines and recommendations, and International Pharmaceutical Federation (FIP) [17,18]. It was

*Corresponding author: Alomi YA, Former General Manager of General Administration of Pharmaceutical Care Head, National Clinical pharmacy and Pharmacy Practice Programs Head, Pharmacy R&D Administration, Riyadh, Saudi Arabia, E-mail: yalomi@gmail.com

running with a network of more than ten drug information centers at MOH hospitals with hotline calling services started in late of 2013; and then expanded services to all more than 250 hospitals and 2500 primary care centers, with five years strategic plan of services [19].

Method

Ministry of Health started providing 937 hotline services in January 2013 through the general administration of emergency. These services were answering the call by a physician or may be the calls were transferred according to specialty (e.g. number of collaborative departments; Corona, Poisoning, Drug Information and Neonate and Pediatrics…etc.), the center can receive several calls at same time, it capable to get up to 20 calls at the same time. The call center is receiving 500 calls monthly. NDIC had started providing hotline services with collaboration with the general administration of emergency in December 2013. It's a 24/7 active service throughout the year covering holidays as well, receiving calls from the public and professional health care providers from all around the Kingdom. This service was operated with an eleven Clinical Pharmacist and trained Pharmacist who provided Drug Information to professional and public. All pharmacists either holding Pharm D degree or Master in clinical pharmacy or pharmacist trained in a short course in basic drug information and 5 weeks practical training at accredited drug information center and accredited by general administration of pharmaceutical care. We provided all pharmacists with a collection of online references as showed in Table 1. All pharmacists provided over all 21 regions at Saudi Arabia. All clinical pharmacists and trained pharmacists who work as a drug information pharmacist in the site were scheduled to cover calls from 937 at any time transferred to their phones. Schedules were divided into five shifts covers 24 hrs/day in each shift covered by a clinical Pharmacist as a supervisor, the updating monthly schedule sent to all participants and a follow-up report was sent daily to evaluate the process. The study period was from December 2013–November 2014, excluding all Poisoning calls and any calls, were not documented was also excluded in this study.

A drug information request form was used in a manual documentation consistent of four parts; fist part: questioner data (name, ID#, nationality, gender, profession, qualification, contacts information). Second part: patient data (name, ID#, nationality, gender, weight, height, diagnosis). Third part: question documentation (the type of question, the question, and its answer, reference of the answer). Fourth part: drug information inquiries cost avoidance based on American model [20]. By the end of the study, the authors found very poor documentation in the references section. To overcome this problem the authors present again as in Table 1, and asked the pharmacist arrange the references from 1 to 20 numbers based more frequent to least one, the pharmacists filled the table separately and return it back to the authors. Then references were rearranged based on their answers with average member. All the medications were asked it will be categorized grouping based on British National Formulary 64th edition. All data were later entered and analyzed by using excel sheet (Microsoft Office 2007).

Results

A total of 1479 calls were received during the period of 12 months. A number of drug information calls had been answered 976 (67.13%), poisoning calls had been answered 17 (1%), missed calls 421 (28.46%), and the number of calls was closed 65 (4.49%). Of answered calls only 264 (27%) calls were documented and including a total of 300 inquiries (each call contains more than one inquiry). Most inquiries were from by public 180 (60%) and 120 (40%) were from by professionals. Of professional sector; the most inquiry was pharmacists 48 (48%), then 45 (37.5%) from by physicians, 7 (5.8%) made by Nurses, and 20 (16.6%) not specified. The most frequent inquiry was asked about dose standardization by (27), followed by drug administration (15.3%) and adverse drug reaction (11.66%) and the center helped in detecting 75 cases of ADRs throughout this period as showed in Table 2. Comparison between professional and public as a type of inquiries showed Table 3. The most inquiries were about drugs (81 -83.8%) and food supplement (13.3-11.1%) from both professional and publics respectively. The medications most frequent was asked about Antibacterial by (19.80%) followed by vitamins (11.68%), anti-diabetic (4.87) antihypertensive with (4.54%), Analgesia and anticonvulsant both were (4.22%), rheumatic disease and gout and antihistamine both were asked by (3.89%), followed by contraceptives (3.57%), Antidepressant, immunosuppressant agent, and corticosteroid were least frequent by (2.92%). Comparison between professional and public as most medications were asked showed Table 4. The most frequent reference used was Lexi-comp, Up-to-date, and Micromedex to answer all type of inquiries both professional and public as showed in Table 5. The average costs avoidance per call was (415.78 USD), and total cost avoidance was (109,768 USD) with partial documentation, the estimated total cost with complete documentation was (405,801 USD) per year, cost avoidance of answering public inquiries were (80,806.5 USD) and Professional inquires were (28,961.5 USD) for more detail the reader can refer to published reference [21].

Discussion

GAPC-MOH started drug information centers program based on strategic planning of pharmaceutical care as part of national pharmacy practice program [22]. The program had started since December 2013 and coordinated by national drug information center located at MOH. The program should cover more 250 hospital and 2500 primary care centers over all Kingdom of Saudi Arabia. The program headed by 1st author Alomi YA as expert critical care clinical pharmacist with two boards; Board Certified of Pharmacotherapy Specialist (BCPS) and Board Certified of Nutrition Support Pharmacy (BCNSP). He had more 15 years experiences in clinical pharmacy and pharmacy practice. The program coordinated by 2nd author AL- Mudaiheem H with Pharm/MSc. Clin Pharm degree and more than 5 years' experience in pharmacy practice. The national drug information center established the scope of services based on ASHP and FIP recommendations. By the end of the 1st year of starting services, the center expanded their services and participated in MOH 937 call center.

National drug information center in Saudi Arabia resembled what had been done to USA, UK, and recently Germany as worldwide [1,2]. The center also resembles two countries in the Middle East including Iran and Palestine as providing services national wide to the entire public country [12-24]. However, our national drug information center more specialized on drug information with excluding poisoning information. In 2013 MOH established new general administration by the name of General Administration of Poison Control center and forensic chemical which specialized in all poisonous related issues. This reason made us exclude all poison questions from our analysis, this is not our scope of services but the pharmacist should answer the question if he received as part of ethical pharmacy practice.

In the study, the number missed call was high due to sometimes technical reason. Call center used equipment received several call at a time, sometimes the pharmacist during answering the inquiry another call was transferred to the same pharmacist. The computer

Resources	Resources
Tertiary Resources	
Medicine Complete	Lexi-Comp
Access Medicine	Up-to-date
Access Pharmacy	Pharmacy Online Library
Sanford Guide to Antimicrobial Therapy	Natural Medicine Comprehensive Database
Compounding Today	
Secondary Resources	
Micromedex	IDIS
AIDS Journals	
Primary Resources	
The Medical letter	Hospital pharmacy Journal
Annals of Pharmacotherapy	Pharmacist Letter
American Journal of Hospital System Pharmacist	Value in Health
Clinical Toxicology	Medical Teacher

Table 1: Collection of pharmacists.

Inquiry classification	%
Dose standardization	27
Drug Administration	15.33
ADR	11.66
Drug Identification	10.33
Drug availability/ formulary	9.66
Drug-drug interaction	7.66
Drug in pregnancy	7
Others	6
Drugs in breast feeding	2
Compounding	1.33
Compatibility	1
Drug- Nutrition interaction	0.66
pharmacokinetic	0.33
Total	100

Table 2: Percentage of inquiry classification.

Inquiry classification	Both	Public %	Professional %
Dose standardization	27	27.77	25.83
Drug Administration	15.33	16.11	14.16
Drug in pregnancy	7.66	12.7	8.33
ADR	11.66	9.47	15
Drug availability/ formulary	9.66	9.4	5
Drug Identification	10	7.22	9.16
Drug-drug interaction	7.33	6.66	10.83
Others	6	5	5
Compatibility	1	1.66	1.66
Drugs in breast feeding	2	1.11	2.5
Compounding	1.33	0.55	2.5
Drug- Nutrition interaction	0.66	0.55	0
Pharmacokinetic	0.33	0.55	0
Total	100	100	100

Table 3: Percentage of inquiry classification public and professional.

will consider it as missed call. In addition, on-call pharmacist busy with his work during morning hours or the phone is silent or closed. All technical related issued will be corrected by general call center. National drug information during the period of study was using manual documentation system, this procedure is very bothersome and boring issue to all pharmacists, and it is not strange to find a very low percentage of drug information inquiries documentation. General Drawbacks of our services was the manual documentation system which has been overcome in our current phase II, all documentation process was converted into an online system. Today's we are using an electronic documentation system through monkey survey subscription on MOH website. The new system will help the pharmacist for quick documentation and make as a dashboard for any time of data analysis [23].

In similar data which involved receiving inquiries from public and professionals as explored in Table 6, looking into each class of question inquiry and compare it with our current study on dose standardization in arrange of (14-34%) with a similarity results of Entezari-Maleki T et al., Rosenberg JM et al., Pohjanoksa-Mäntylä, Schwarz UI et al., and Assiri YA et al. studies [1,6,11,13,14]. In drug Administration inquiries having a range of (7.5-16.11%) resemble results with Entezari-Maleki T et al., Schwarz UI et al., and Assiri YA et al. studies [1,13,14]. Moving to Adverse drug reaction ranges from (9.47-28%) also within range of previous studies Entezari-Maleki T et al, Rosenberg JM et al., Pohjanoksa-Mäntylä, Schwarz UI et al., and Assiri YA et al. studies [1,6,11,13,14]. The range of Drug Identification from previous studies (7.22-20.4%) our data fit with this range [1,13,14]. The drug availability/ formulary inquiries type similar with previous studies (4.2-26%) as in Pohjanoksa-Mäntylä, Schwarz UI et al., and Assiri YA et al. studies [11,13,14]. Drug in pregnancy with a range of (3.3-16%) also within range of previous data as showed in Rosenberg JM et al. and Assiri YA et al. studies [6,14].

Here, we discussed professional related type of questioner; only one study found a very old date by Leach FN in the United Kingdom [3]. Our study was the only updated one that's discussed this professional type. It is normal to find a lot of differences between our study and the old one. For instant; the authors found dose standardization the highest type of inquiries while adverse drug reaction was the highest type of inquiries. Previously most of the physician focused on drug-related problems while nowadays with a huge number of medications all health care professional cannot memorize all the doses and any pharmacokinetics related calculation, it is normal for find this results in our study due to this reason. The second in the list of professional related type was adverse drug reaction, drug administration, and drug-drug interaction while in the previous study was drug identification, drug in pregnancies, drug compounding the reason behind that the number of references were not existing in old age while today we a lot of references discussed and answer this type of inquiries like Micromedex and Lexi-comp, etc., in addition the internet resources was not available, and most of the drug available readymade and rarely needed for compounding, therefore, it is normal to find those results.

The public related type of questioner; it is only one study discussed this issue by Maywald U et al. [9] in Germany and another studies the majorities of questioners were public type Shadnia Sh et al. in Iran [12]. There are several differences in type of inquiries in our study the top in the list were dose standardization, and drug administration while in Germany and Iran study was adverse drug reaction this can be found due to our population had poor knowledge background of medication and patient education program did not exist in most of the hospitals,

Drug categories	Total Number of inquiries from Public and Professional	Number of inquiries from Public	Percentage of inquiries from Public	Number of inquiries from Professional	Percentage of inquiries from Professional
Antibacterial	61(19.8)	42	23.2	19	14.84
Antifungal	4 (1.29)	2	1.1	2	1.56
Antiviral	1 (0.32)	1	0.55	0	0
Anthelmintics	2 (0.64)	2	1,1	0	0
Antihypertensive	14 (4.54)	10	5.52	4	3.13
Antidiabetic	15 (4.87)	10	5.52	5	3.91
Immunosuppressant Agent and Corticosteroid	9 (2.92)	0	0	9	7.03
Anticonvulsants	13 (4.22)	5	2,76	8	6.25
Antipsychotics	3 (0.97)	0	0	3	2.34
Antidepressant	9 (2.92)	6	3.31	3	2.34
Anticoagulants	13 (4.22)	12	6.63	1	0.78
Antiplateletes	2 (0.64)	1	0.55	1	0.78
Antilipemic	3 (0.97)	1	0.55	2	1.56
Antihistamine	12 (3.89)	9	4.97	3	2.34
Anesthesia	3 (0.97)	0	0	3	2.34
Analgesia	13 (4.22)	5	2.76	8	6.25
Bronchodilators	5 (1.62)	1	0.55	4	3.13
Thyroid products	1 (0.32)	0	0	1	0.78
Rheumatic disease and gout	12 (3.89)	8	4.42	4	3.13
Parkinsonism and related disorder	2 (0.64)	2	1,1	0	0
Antisecretory drugs and mucosal protectant	8 (2.59)	7	3.87	1	0.78
Blood disorder	2 (0.64)	1	0.55	1	0.78
Genito-urinary disorder	1 (0.32)	0	0	1	0.78
Antifoaming agent	1 (0.32)	0	0	1	0.78
Neuromuscular disorder	1 (0.32)	1	0.55	0	0
Laxative	1 (0.32)	0	0	1	0.78
Dermatology	6 (1.94)	5	2.76	1	0.78
Contraceptives	11 (3.57)	2	1,1	9	7.03
Antiflatulents	1 (0.32)	0	0	1	0.78
fluids and electrolytes	6 (1.94)	5	2.76	1	0.78
Bone metabolism	3 (0.97)	2	1,1	1	0.78
drugs used in substance dependence	2 (0.64)	0	0	2	1.56
Baby formula	3 (0.97)	1	0.55	2	1.56
Diuretics	2 (0.64)	1	0.55	1	0.78
Treatment of obesity	4 (1.29)	3	1.66	1	0.78
CNS stimulants	1 (0.32)	1	0.55	0	0
Sex hormones	2 (0.64)	2	1,1	0	0
Cough preparation	6 (1.94)	3	1.66	3	2.34
Vitamins	36 (11.68)	20	11.05	16	12.5
Vaccines	3 (0.97)	2	1,1	1	0.78
Antispasmodics	9 (2.92)	6	3.31	3	2.34
Intestinal secretion	3 (0.97)	2	1,1	1	0.78
Total	309 (100%)	181	100%	128	100%

Table 4: Comparison between professional and public.

and this reflects the system in the country of obtaining medications without prescription from private pharmacies adding to this no patient counseling program active throughout the kingdom and finally, there are no label standards applied into MOH hospitals and PHC yet. Also; we can't negligent the fact of internal resources available to everyone that may send a wrong or biased information which leads to confusion by most of the callers. In addition the awareness by Saudi Food and Drug Authority of adverse drug reaction reporting system did not exist,

while in Germany and Iran the second one was drug-drug interaction and drug identification respectively, it could be the good background of medication in Germany and the dilution of professional involved Iran study. In our study the third type of inquiries from our public was drug in pregnancy, this reflects patient perception on his health care and drug related problem. This perception encourages the entire pharmacist to start patient medication education program as soon as possible overall health care institution in Saudi Arabia

Resources	Arrangement	Resources	Arrangement
Tertiary Resources			
Lexi-Comp	1.57	Natural Medicine Comprehensive Database	9.43
Up-to-date	2.71	Access Pharmacy	9.85
Medicine Complete	7	Access Medicine	10.85
Sanford Guide to Antimicrobial Therapy	7.43	Compounding Today	12.43
Pharmacy Online Library	8.71		
Secondary Resources			
Micromedex	2.29	AIDS Journals	15.86
IDIS	14.43		
Primary Resources			
The Medical letter	10.14	American Journal of Hospital System Pharmacist	13.29
Annals of Pharmacotherapy	11.43	Hospital pharmacy Journal	14.43
Clinical Toxicology	11.57	Value in Health	16.857
Pharmacist Letter	12.43	Medical Teacher	17.29

Table 5: Frequent reference used was Lexi-comp, Up-to-date, and Micromedex.

Inquiry classification	Present study. Rosenberg JM, et.al. 2015 Saudi Arabia			Shadnia Sh et al. Assiri YA, et.al. 2011 Iran [12]		Entezari-Maleki T et al. Pohjanoksa-Mäntylä MK, 2014 Iran [13]		Leach FN Schwarz Ul et.al. 1978 UK [3]		Maywald U et al. 2004 Germany [9]	Rosenberg JM, et.al. 2004 USA [1]		Assiri YA, et.al. 2007 Saudi Arabia [15]		Pohjanoksa-Mäntylä MK, 2008 Finland. [11]	Schwarz Ul et.al. 1999 Germany [6]	
	Drug Information Center			**Drug and Poisoning Information Center**		**Drug and Poisoning Information Center**		**Regional Drug information**		**Public Health Saxony in Germany**	**Most of DIC in the US**		**University DIC**		**Helsinki University DIC**	**DI Regional center in Germany**	
	60% Public	40% Professional	total	97.14% Public	2.86% Professional	57.63% Public	42.37% Professional	3.62% Public	96.37% Professional	100% Public	15% Public	85% Professional	% 17.50% Public	82.50% Professional	Not Written	Others 33%	Professional 67%
Dose standardization	27.77	25.83	27	6.06		19.32				5	17 10.1		21.7		14	34	
Drug Administration	16.11	14.16	15.33	13.21		7.58		8.4					7.5				
Drug in pregnancy	12.7	8.33	7.66	4.44				11.2					3.3			16	
ADR	9.47	15	11.66	20.14		15.05		19.3		23.9	16.2		13.3		11	28	
Drug availability/ formulary	9.4	5	9.66	0		15.87							4.2		26		
Drug Identification	7.22	9.16	10	17.64		18.74		17.4			14.3		20.4				
Drug-drug interaction	6.66	10.83	7.33	5.23				6		7.1	9.1		7.3				
Drug-Nutrition interaction	0.55	0	0.66	0													
Compatibility	1.66	1.66	1	0.68				7.9			4.2		1.8				
Drugs in breast feeding	1.11	2.5	2	2.31													
Compounding	0.55	2.5	1.33	0				8.6									
Pharmacokinetic	0.55	0	0.33	0				5.7			4					15	
Others	5	5	6														
Total	100	100	100														

Table 6: Percentage of Inquiry Classification public and professional.

This is the first study found discussed the national drug information center at MOH in Saudi Arabia, this is piloting epidemiologic prospective analysis of drug information inquiries. Although of poor documentation from pharmacist answered the inquiries especially the references used, lack of skills of answering drug information inquiries, and time lack of answering the question the pharmacists are not full-time staff, in addition to the technical system of 937.

Currently, we changed drug information documentation from manual to online through our website at MOH portal, all technical related issued well be corrected by 937 general administration. We are planning to increase drug information education courses to all pharmacist, and increase the number of pharmacists who answering the questions, and repeat the study again on a yearly basis.

In similar data which involved receiving inquiries from public and professionals together, looking into drug category and compare it with our current study with the consideration that's our classification based on BNF database, more detail and specific information which was found in any previous studies. The 1st class of inquiries was about antibacterial. It is was out of range results for Entezari-Maleki T et al., Pohjanoksa-Mäntylä and Schwarz UI et al., studies [6,11,13] in the range of (7.58-19%), most of our community pharmacies break pharmacy law by dispensing antibiotics without prescriptions. CNS medications fit within results in a range of (15-20%) by Schwarz UI et.al and Pohjanoksa-Mantyla studies [6,13]. Coming to the cardiovascular medications also it was out of range of previous studies ranges (8-20%) by Schwarz UI et al., Pohjanoksa-Mäntylä et al., and Entezari-Maleki T et al. studies [6,11,13]. The 2nd public disease in Saudi Arabia is cardiovascular diseases, it is normal to find it as more percentages of inquiries than previous studies. In analgesia which was the fourth class of inquiries was almost the same as only one study by Shadnia Sh et al. [12] and had no comparative data found in any of others studies. The results of Antidiabetic was within the range of previous studies (1.73-18.74%) by Shadnia Sh et al. [12] and Entezari-Maleki T et al. [13].

The public inquiries related to drug category; the 1st class of inquiries was Antibacterial compared in just only one study Maywald U et al. [9], our result was lower reasoning that to poor documentation of drug information inquiries, in Gastrointestinal drugs a mostly resemble while in Cardiovascular range our result lower than Maywald U et al. study [9] due to poor drug information inquiries documentation. The CNS medications related inquiries was lower that Maywald U et al. [9], because very restricted law, policy and procedures for narcotics and controlled medications, in addition to our traditional behavior of rejection CNS diseases from the public.In regards to references of answering of drug information inquiries, there were four studies [1,12,13,14] had a documentation of drug information inquiry documentation process ending with the reference in answering each question. All those studies discussed inquiries from both professional and public, and no existing studies discussed either professional or nor public even our study. Our center used frequently Lexi-Comp as it was with Shadnia Sh et al. [12]. The reason of that's being inquiries were higher in public asking about dose standardization, drug administration in our study, and adverse drug reaction Shadnia Sh study; so the search supposed to be direct, with no details. In addition, Lexi-Comp came as an application makes it more convenient to use even without internet connection. The 2nd resource used Up-to-date, this normal to find that being understanding the question were derived from professionals and more than 40% of total inquiries asking about dose standardization. Moreover, the new version of Up-to-date has an application which is friendlier in use; this resembles what found in Entezari-Maleki T et al. [13]. The 3rd reference was in our study the Micromedex, while the

previous studies by Rosenberg JM, et.al. [1], Assiri YA et al. [14] And Entezari-Maleki T et al. [13] were being 1st and 2nd common reference respectively. More than 80% of inquiries derived from professionals Rosenberg JM et al. [1], Assiri YA et al. [14] And more than 40% of inquiries in regards to dose standardization and more in depth detail of information. Our study been 3rd reference due to most of our consumers were public with different demands. Meanwhile, in general, all five data shows that the most frequent resource been used are Lexi-Comp, Micromedex and up-to-date.

Limitations

Although this is the first study founded about national drug information center at MOH in Saudi Arabia, with more detail comparisons of professional and public inquiries, there are some limitations in the study including poor documentation of drug information inquiries, using manual documentation, and founding of new services at MOH with little experiences toward public answering inquiries.

Conclusion

Despite that the national drug information center provided 1st new services to the huge population of professional and public. The study should be repeated gain with an electronic documentation system in order to get all data clearly, using hand application of entering data, expansion of clinical pharmacist answering inquiries with comprehensive advanced training in drug information skills. Moreover, get international accreditation of the center and services, make this service as part of accreditation for local drug information center at MOH, involve Pharm D student and residents at their clinical rotation, and an incentive payment to all participants to encourage our staff for excellent performances.

References

1. Rosenberg JM, Koumis T, Nathan JP, Cicero LA, McGuire H (2004) Current status of pharmacist-operated drug information centers in the United States. Am J Health-Syst Pharm 61:2023-2032.

2. Davies DM, Ashton CH, Rao JG, Rawlins MD, Routledge PA, et al. (1977) Comprehensive clinical drug information service: first year's experience. Br Med J 1: 89-90.

3. Leach FN (1978) The regional drug information service: a factor in health care? Br Med J 1: 766-768.

4. Calder G, Davies JS, McNulty H, Smith JC (1981) Drug information network in the United Kingdom National Health Service. Am J Hosp Pharm 38: 663-666.

5. Markind JE, Stachnik JM (1996) European drug information centers. J Hum Lact 12: 239-242.

6. Schwarz UI, Stoelben S, Ebert U, Siepmann M, Krappweis J, et al. (1999) Regional drug information service. Int J Clin Pharmacol Ther 37: 263-268.

7. Joshi MP (1997) University hospital-based drug information service in a developing country. Eur J Clin Pharmacol 53: 89-94.

8. Lassanova M, Tisonova J, Bozekova L, Kriska M (2001) Drug information center. Bratisl Lek Listy 102: 305-306.

9. Maywald U, Schindler C, Krappweis J, Kirch W (2004) First patient-centered drug information service in Germany--a descriptive study. Ann Pharmacother 38: 2154-2159.

10. Hall V, Gomez C, Fernandez-Llimos F (2006) Situation of Drug Information Centers and Services in Costa Rica. Pharm Pract 4: 1-7.

11. Pohjanoksa-Mäntylä MK, Antila J, Eerikäinen S, Enäkoski M, Hannuksela O, et al. (2008) Utilization of a community pharmacy-operated national drug information call center in Finland. Res Social Adm Pharm. 4: 144-152.

12. Shadnia Sh, Soltaninejad K, Sohrabi F, Rezvani M, Barari B, et al. (2011) The Performance of Loghman-Hakim Drug and Poison Information Center from 2006 to 2008. Iran J Pharm Res 10: 647-652.

13. Entezari-Maleki TE, Taraz M, Javadi MR, Hajimiri MH, Eslami K, et al. (2014) A two year utilization of the pharmacist operated drug information center in Iran. J Res Pharm Pract 3: 117-122.

14. Asiri YA, AlArifi MN, Alsultan MS, Gubara OA (2007) Evaluation of drug and poison information center in Saudi Arabia during the period 2000-2002. Saudi Med J 28:617-719.

15. Timm DM, Swartz KM, Amoh KN (1991) King Khalid University Hospital Drug and Poison Information Service. A descriptive report and comparison with the University of Minnesota Drug Information Center. J Pharm Technol 7:179-183.

16. Al-Jedai A (2011) International Pharmacy Residency Accreditation: The Saudi Experience. ACCP International Clinical Pharmacist 1: 1-2.

17. Ghaibi S, Ipema H, Gabay M (2015) ASHP Guidelines on the Pharmacist's Role in Providing Drug Information. Am J Health-Syst Pharm 72:573-577

18. FIP Pharmacy Information Section, Requirements for Drug Information Centres (2005) International Pharmaceutical Federation.

19. http://www.moh.gov.sa/endepts/Pharmacy/Affiliated-Departments/Pages/NDPICD.aspx

20. Kinky DE, Erush SC, Laskin MS, Gibson GA (1999) Economic Impact of a Drug Information Service. Ann Pharmacother 33:11-16.

21. Alomi YA, AL-Mudaiheem H, Alreshidi M, Alarnous T, Alsharafa A, et al. (2015) Cost-Efficiency of National drug information center through Ministry of Health hotline calling services (937) in Saudi Arabia application of American model. Value in Health 18: A735.

22. Alomi YA (2015) National Pharmacy Practice Programs at Ministry of Health in Saudi Arabia. J Pharm Pharm Scien 1: 17-18.

23. http://www.moh.gov.sa/endepts/Pharmacy/Pages/eFormes.aspx

24. Sawalha AF (2008) Poison Control and the Drug Information Center: The Palestinian Experience. Isr Med Assoc J 10: 757-760.

13

Non Adherence and Contributing Factors among Ambulatory Patients with Anti Diabetic Medications in Adama Referral Hospital

Gelaw BK*, Mohammed A, Tegegne GT, Defersha AD, Fromsa M , Tadesse E, Thrumurgan G and Ahmed M

Department of Pharmacy, College of Medicine and Health Science, Ambo University, Oromia, Ethiopia

Abstract

Background: The term diabetes mellitus describes metabolic disorders of multiple etiologies characterized by hyperglycemia with disturbances of carbohydrates, fat and protein metabolism resulting from defects in insulin secretion, insulin action or both. Anti-diabetic medications are integral for glycemic control in diabetes. Non adherence to drugs can alter blood glucose levels, resulting in complications. The objective of this study was to determine the magnitude of non-adherence and its contributing factors among diabetic patients attending the diabetic clinic in Adama hospital.

Methods: This descriptive cross-sectional study was carried out among patients with diabetes mellitus attending the diabetes mellitus clinic of Adama referral hospital. Every other patient was selected and data regarding their medication adherence was collected using a structured interview. Data analysis was carried out using SPSS-16.

Result: The response rate from this study was 98.3%. A total of 270 patients were interviewed; 51.5% were males. A total of 68.1% of the patients included in the study were married. 14% were younger than 40 years of age, 50% were between 40 and 60 years of age. 21.8% of the participants ascribed their non-adherence to forgetting to take their medications. Patients with duration of diabetes ≤ 5 years (82.07%) were more compliant to their medication than those with >5 years 60.8%, which was found to be statistically significant (P=0.003). Insulin 47% and glibenclamide plus metformine 43.7% were the most commonly prescribed mono and combination therapies respectively. Common co morbid conditions include, Hypertension 148(54.82%), Visual impairment 89(32.96%). The proportion of male patients adherent to their anti-diabetic medications was found to be lower 69.78% compared to the female patients (74.81%), but the difference was not statistically significant (p>0.05).

Conclusion: Most diabetic patients are currently being managed with the most effective available drugs. However as the result from this study indicates the desired blood sugar level could not be controlled and maintained adequately. This was because of poor adherence with the prescribed drug regimen and poor knowledge and practice of successful self management.

Keywords: Diabetes mellitus; Non adherence; Anti diabetic medications; Diabetic patients

Acronyms and Abbreviations: DM: Diabetes Mellitus; OHA: Oral Hypoglycemic Agents; T2D: Type 2 Diabetes; SPSS: Statistical Package for Social Science; CSA: Central Statistics Agency; UAE: United Arab Emirates; ARH: Adama Referral Hospital; FPG: Fasting Plasma Glucose; HbA1C: Glycated Hemoglobin; ADA: American Diabetic Association; SD: Standard Deviation; SNNP: Southern Nations Nationalities and Peoples Region; WHO: World Health Organization; JUSH: Jimma University Specialized Hospital; GP: General Practitioner

Introduction

Background

Diabetes mellitus refers to a group of common metabolic disorders that share the phenotype of hyperglycemia. The prevalence of diabetes mellitus is growing rapidly worldwide and is reaching epidemic proportions. It is estimated that there are currently 285 million people with diabetes worldwide and this number is set to increase to 438 million by the year 2030 [1]. Epidemiological data indicate that all nations, rich and poor, are suffering the impact of the diabetes epidemic. The impact is worse in those countries that are socially and economically disadvantaged. In Africans 80% of diabetes patients are undiagnosed. Most of them may be asymptomatic or have mild symptoms which they ignore or attribute to other myths. Some may not present in hospital out of poverty even when symptomatic [2].

Information on chronic complications of diabetes in sub-Saharan Africa is scarce; however, its incidence has gone hand in hand with the growing disease prevalence, demonstrating the importance of assessing complications [3].

Factors contributing to optimum disease management included age, complexity of treatment, duration of disease, and psychosocial issues [4].

Ethiopia is the second most populous country in Sub- Saharan Africa where more than 80% of the population lives in the country side. In Ethiopia, national data on prevalence and incidence of diabetes are lacking. However, patient attendance rates and medical admissions in major hospitals are rising. The estimated prevalence of Diabetes Mellitus (DM) in adult population of Ethiopia is 1.9% [5].

---

*Corresponding author: Gelaw BK, Department of Pharmacy, College of Medicine and Health Science, Ambo University, Oromia, Ethiopia, E-mail: belayneh.kefale@yahoo.com

Management of diabetes mellitus involves both pharmacological and non pharmacological approaches. Non pharmacological approaches include life style modification, dietary modification and physical exercise. The pharmacological approach is used when the non pharmacological approach fails to achieve the desired outcome. Pharmacotherapy for type 2 DM has changed dramatically in the last few years with the addition of several new drug classes and recommendations to achieve more stringent glycemic control. Recently initiation of metformine in all patients with T2D at diagnosis along with appropriate life style modification has been introduced where there is no contraindication. In addition to metformine, OHA, injectable insulin, amylin analogs and inhaled insulin are other options for treatment of T2D [6]. The choice of therapy for type 1 DM is simple: All patients need insulin. However, how that insulin is delivered to the patient is a matter of considerable practice difference among patients and clinicians [7].

Non-adherence rates are relatively high across disease states, treatment regimens, and age groups. The drop in adherence is noted to be most dramatic after the first six months of therapy among patients with chronic conditions such as diabetes mellitus. A systematic review of studies on adherence to medication among diabetes patients showed that average adherence to oral anti diabetes medications ranges from 36% to 93%, while adherence to other treatment recommendations especially dietary adherence among these patients remains poor. Medication may contribute to non-adherence secondary to its side effects and cost, while poor patient-healthcare provider relationships may also be a major determinant of non-adherence [8].

Poor adherence to medication regimens is common, contributing to substantial worsening of disease, death and increased health-care costs. Hence, practitioners should always look for poor adherence and can enhance adherence by emphasizing the value of a patient's regimen, making the regimen simple and customizing the regimen to the patient's lifestyle.

Statement of the problem

The prevalence of diabetes mellitus is growing rapidly worldwide and is reaching epidemic proportions. Non-adherence, poverty, lack of knowledge and poor follow ups are the main factors observed in poor glycemic control. Non adherence to prescribed medication schedule has been and continuous to be a major problem in the world. In chronic disease, it has been described as taking less than 80% of the prescribed treatment. Previous studies have found adherence to diabetes treatment generally to be sub optimal ranging (23%-77%) [9].

In Ethiopia, national data on prevalence and incidence of diabetes are lacking. However, patient attendance rates and medical admissions in major hospitals are rising. The World Health Organization (WHO) estimated the number of diabetic cases in Ethiopia to be 800,000 by the year 2000, and the number is expected to increase to 1.8 million by 2030 [10].

There is a continuing need to routinely assess the likely reasons for non adherence among patients with diabetes in clinical practice. This is especially important in developing countries such as Ethiopia where economic instability and inadequate access to health care facilities might have led to the increased incidence of medication non adherence. In resource-limited countries like Ethiopia, the preponderance of economic instability, low literacy level, and restricted access to health care facilities might have led to the increase incidence of medication non-adherence. To the best of our knowledge, evidence-based research that evaluate medication adherence among patients with diabetes in Ethiopia is scanty.

In addition to this;

1. Most of previous studies were done in developed countries, leaving the gaps in knowledge about the prevalence and factors that may be associated with adherence to diabetic patient in Ethiopia.

2. Few studies on anti-diabetic medication adherence have been reported from Ethiopia.

3. The sample size used in some of the studies is very small and the method of selection of participants in some cases has lead to highly selective samples that are not representatives of the population from which they are picked.

Therefore the purpose of this study is to fill the gap in knowledge of the adherence and contributing factors and the association between them in diabetic patients in Adama hospital.

Structural frame work

The structural frame work is shown in Figure 1.

Significance of the study

Determining the significance of non adherence and identification of the factors leading to non adherence to a prescribed treatment through a continued research can assist in planning interventions to overcome the barriers. Hence, this study will be carried out to;

1. Give information on patient non-adherence and related factors that may help for the health care system to whom it concerns.

2. Give information based on the respondent's responses on different aspect of the disease that may help for further study of policy makers and some concerned governmental bodies.

3. Design an interventional method that can solve problems related to non adherence.

4. Give recommendations on how to manage problems associated with non adherence in diabetic patients.

5. It can help as a base line for further study on patient's adherence and to determine various adherence and non-adherence issues.

Objective

General objective: The aim of this study was to determine the magnitude of non-adherence and its contributing factors among diabetic patients attending DM clinic in Adama referral hospital.

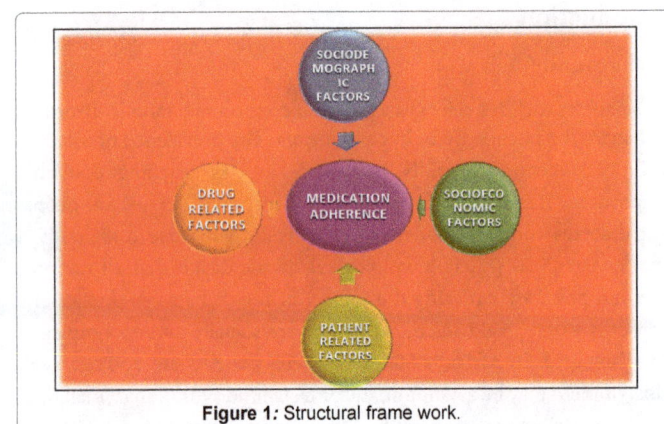

Figure 1: Structural frame work.

Specific objectives:

1. To assess adherence to medication among ambulatory patients with diabetes,

2. To identify the probable reasons for non adherence with a view to develop intervention to improve adherence.

3. To determine the relationship between non-adherence and various socio demographic and other drug and patient related factors.

4. To describe the prevalence of different perceived problems of respondents with disease or the medication and on the health care system,

5. To provide the base line data for future study.

Study Method

Study area and period

The study setting was Adama referral hospital, East Showa, Oromia National Regional State, Ethiopia. Adama is located 99 km south east of Addis Ababa, (the capital city of Ethiopia). It was established in 1946 by Italian Missionaries and formerly called "Haile Mariam Mammo memorial hospital". It is a medical college and teaches Accelerated Medicine, Emergency Surgery and Anesthesia Nurses. The hospital gives services for about 5 million people East and Southern parts of Oromia, Afar, Somali and Southern Nation Nationalities and People (SNNP). Now the hospital has 465 different workers to who different services, of which 194 are administration workers. The other 271 workers are health professionals. There are specialist in different field (23), Practitioners (GP) 36, Nurses (116), Laboratory Workers (20), X-Ray (5), Physiotherapy (2), Sanitarians (2), Biomedical (1), Midwifery (16), Anesthesia (9), Health Officers (9), Psychiatry Nurses (3) And Masters in different fields(14).

The data obtained from the hospital shows that averages of 723 ambulatory diabetes patients attend the clinic for follow up. There are two formal diabetes clinic days per week "Wednesday and Thursday ". This study was done for a period of one month from 15th April to 15th May 2014.

Study design

A prospective cross-sectional study was conducted at the ambulatory diabetic clinic of Adama Referral Hospital (ARH).

Inclusion criteria:

1. Ambulatory patients who are

1.1 On anti-diabetic medications for greater than six months.

1.2 Consented to participate in the study.

1.3 Will attend the diabetic clinic during the study period

Exclusion criteria:

1. Unconscious patients

2. Patient age less than 18 years and

3. Very ill patients were excluded

Population:

1. Source population

Diabetic patients being treated at adama referral hospital.

2. Study population

All diabetic patients receiving anti diabetic medication in the ambulatory diabetic clinic during the study period.

Sample size determination: The sample size was calculated using single population proportion formula as follows

$$n = \frac{Z^2 P(1-P)}{W^2}$$

where,

n=desired sample size for population>10,000

Z=standard normal duration usually set as 1.96 (which corresponds to 95% confidence level)

P=we use positive prevalence estimated. To maximize sample size.

Negative prevalence =1-0.5=0.5

W=degree of accuracy desired (marginal error is 0.05 then the sample size is

$$n = \frac{(1.96)^2\, 0.5(1-0.5)}{(0.05)^2} = 384.16 = \sim384$$ - Since the total population is

<10,000 that is 723; we use the Correction formula to determine final sample size.

$$nf = \frac{n}{1+\frac{n}{N}} \quad = \quad nf = \frac{384}{1+\frac{384}{723}} \quad nf = 250$$

N=final sample size when a population is <10,000

n=initial sample size when the population is >10,000

nf=estimated study population

Then 10% contingency was added on 250

250×10%=25

$$nf + contingency = 275$$

Sampling technique

A systematic random sampling technique was used.

Data collection procedure: The study involves cross-sectional interview of consecutive diabetic patients who visit the DM clinic during the study period. The interview was conducted with pre-tested adherence tool. Patients included in the pretest were subsequently excluded from the study. After the pilot testing, some question-items in the questionnaire were modified and reframed to ensure validity of the instrument.

Instruments: The questionnaire, which was the instrument of the study, was pre tested on diabetes patients.

This tool consists of information about the socio demographic characteristics of the respondents, the pattern of drug adherence and factors contributing to non-adherence. It also consists of information related to drugs prescribed, dose, frequency and Patients' mean fasting plasma glucose reading at the last clinic visit. Each questionnaire containing 25 questions that took an average of 5 to 10 minutes to fill was used in the interview. It was designed to have two sections; the first section elucidate the socio-demographic characteristics of diabetic patients while the second section contained questions that assess the adherence patterns and the likely reasons for patients' non adherence to prescribed medications.

Study variables

Independent variables:

1. Age

2. Religion

3. Educational level (class year)

4. Marital status

5. Income

6. Residence

Dependent variables:

1. Knowledge about the medications

2. Knowledge about the disease

3. Outcomes of treatment with anti-diabetic drugs.

Data analysis

Data quality assurance and interpretation: Data were sorted, coded and entered into Predictive Analytics Software (PASW) (formerly SPSS) window version 16 for management and analysis. Descriptive statistics including frequency, mean, range, and standard deviation were used to summarize patients' baseline socio-demographic data and evaluate distribution of responses. Correlation and logistic analysis was employed.

Ethical considerations: Before data collection to conduct this study ethical approval was obtained from Ambo University College of medicine and health science research team leader and the letter was submitted to Adama referral hospital medical director office prior to the beginning of undertaking the study in the area. All the study participants were informed about the purpose of the study; their right to refuse was maintained. Ethical conduct was maintained during data collection and throughout the research process. Verbal consent was obtained from each patient before the interview. Patients were assured of their anonymity. The confidentiality of the data obtained was assured and the name and address of the patient was omitted from the questioner.

Result

The response rate from this study was 98.3%. A total of 270 patients were interviewed; One hundred thirty one (48.5%) were females. The mean age for the studied population was 55.11 (SD=14.24) years (range 19 to 85 years). The education profile of these patients revealed that 74 (27.4) had no formal or informal education while 99 (36.7%) have secondary or post secondary education. Sixty six (24.4%) were retirees from private and public establishments and 33 (12.2%) were government employees. A total of 184 (68.1%) of the patients included in the study were married. Thirty eight (14%) of the patients were younger than 40 years of age, one hundred and thirty five (50%) were between 40 and 60 years of age and 97 (35.9%) were older than 60 years of age. This and other socio demographic characteristics are given in Table 1.

Approximately 195 (72.2%) of patients self-reported adherence to their anti diabetic drug regimens. In the pattern of drug use, 170 (62.96%) of patients have excellent adherence, 25 (9.26%) have good and 75(27.8%) have poor adherence (Figure 2).

A total of 59 (21.8%) of the participants ascribed their non-

Variable	Frequency	percentage	Variable	Frequency	Percentage
Age (years)			**Occupation**		
18-30	22	8.1	Government employee	33	12.2
31-40	16	5.9	NGO employee	20	7.4
41-50	50	18.5	Self-employee	75	27.8
51-60	85	31.5	Student	54	20
>60	97	35.9	House wife	6	2.2
			Retired	66	24.4
			Dependent	16	5.9
Sex			**Monthly in come**		
Female	131	48.5	<500	94	34.8
Male	139	51.5	501-1000	75	27.8
			1001-2000	49	18.1
			>2000	37	13.7
			No income	15	5.6
Marital status			**Place of residence**		
Married	18	6.7	Rural	51	18.9
Divorced	184	68.1	Urban	219	81.1
Separate	33	12.2			
Widowed/er	3	1.1			
	32	11.9			
Educational level			**Religion**		
Never went	74	27.4	Orthodox	149	55.2
Primary school	97	35.9	Muslim	63	23.3
Secondary school	50	18.5	Protestant	43	15.9
Post-secondary	49	18.1	Waqefeta	9	3.3
			Others	6	2.2

Table 1: Socio-demographic characteristics of patients, Adama Ethiopia, 2014.

Non Adherence and Contributing Factors among Ambulatory Patients with Anti Diabetic Medications...

67

FREQUENCY

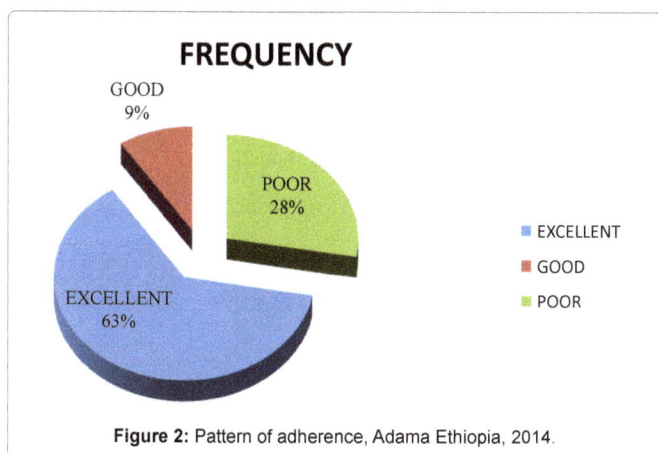

Figure 2: Pattern of adherence, Adama Ethiopia, 2014.

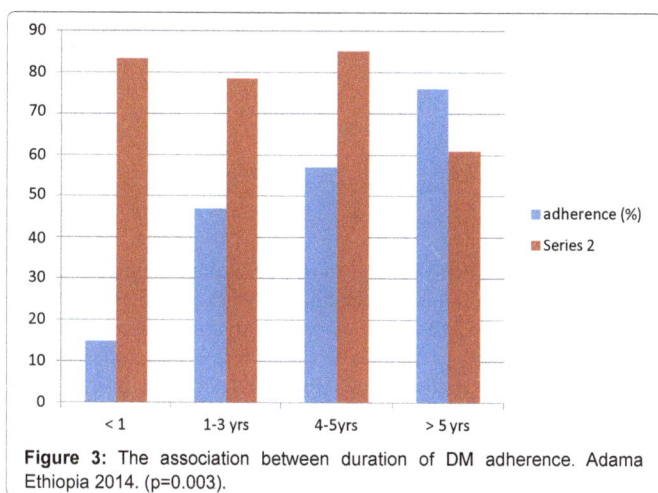

Figure 3: The association between duration of DM adherence. Adama Ethiopia 2014. (p=0.003).

p value

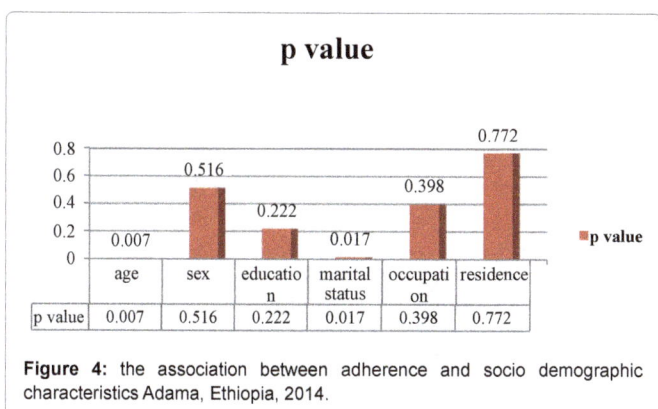

	age	sex	education	marital status	occupation	residence
p value	0.007	0.516	0.222	0.017	0.398	0.772

Figure 4: the association between adherence and socio demographic characteristics Adama, Ethiopia, 2014.

adherence to forgetting to take their medications. Other factors include use of traditional and/or religious medicines 48 (17.8%), lack of finances 39 (14.4%). Of the total population, 248 (91.85%) of the patients reported that they monitored their blood glucose levels monthly at the DM clinic of the Hospital on a regular basis. The proportion of male patients adherent to their anti-diabetic medications was found to be lower 97 (69.78%) compared to the female patients (74.81%), but the difference was not statistically significant (p>0.05). Adherence to anti-diabetic drugs was found to be higher among graduates (post secondary e.g. college (80.77%) and university (73.91%)) compared to those with illiterate and up to secondary school (71.04%), but this finding was not statistically significant (p>0.05). It was also noted that patients with a

duration of diabetes ≤ 5 years (82.07%) were more compliant to their medication than those with diabetes >5 years (60.8%), which was found to be statistically significant (P=0.003) (Figure 3).

Investigation of association between respondents' socio-demographic characteristics and estimates of non adherence, such as and forgetfulness of medication doses, showed that age and marital status seemed to have statistically significant influence (p<0.05) on respondents' tendencies to have good adherence (Figure 4).

The duration of diabetes from first diagnosis indicates that eighteen (6.7%) had been diagnosed for less than one year, 60 (22.2%) diagnosed 1 to 3 years, 67 (22.2%) for 4 to 5 years and 125 (46.3%) patients diagnosed before five years. Co morbid conditions include, Hypertension 148 (54.82%), Visual impairment 89 (32.96%), Nephropathy 37 (13.71%), Limb paralysis 30 (11.1%) and 44 (16.3%) have no co morbidity. The profile of prescribed anti diabetic medications among the patients indicated that a combination of sulfonylurea mostly glibenclamide, and metformine as co-administered products 118 (43.7%) was the most commonly prescribed combination therapy. Insulin alone, 127 (47%); glibenclamide alone was used by 19 (7%); and metformine alone, 1 (0.4%). Combination of glibenclamide and insulin were used by 4 (1.5%). Only 12 (4.4%) monitor their blood glucose level on regular basis using their glucose measuring device at home. All the respondents, 270 (100%) agree that they needed to continue taking their hypoglycemic medications throughout their lifetime and inappropriate use of medications will lead to development of more problems. Fifty nine (21.8%) forget to take the prescribed medication(s). Some of the approaches reported to be adopted, once they remembered included; taking the required dose of medication as soon as remembered or skip it if it is close to the next dose 66 (24.4%), doubling the next dose to make up for the forgotten dose 16 (5.9%), and 17 (6.3) forget it completely (Tables 2-4).

Discussion

The management of diabetes mellitus involves both pharmacologic and non pharmacologic approaches. For the patient both approaches need a strict compliance to the agreements reached with the physician in order to achieve the desired goals of treatment. Despite this fact most patients were found to be non adherent to their recommended treatments and this is caused by several factors. As a result assessment adherence of patients to their respective treatments through continued researches is crucial.

This is a research done on patients with diabetes to evaluate the patients' self-reported adherence to their anti-diabetic drug therapy. The prevalence of adherence to anti-diabetic medications in this study was 72.2%. In comparison to this finding, two studies conducted in India showed that the patients' self-reported adherence rate to anti-diabetic medications was 66.9% and 57.5% [11-16]. In this regard most

Factors	Frequency	Percentage (%)
Forgetfulness	59	21.8
High cost of the drug	39	14.4
Lack of trust in the efficacy of the drug	9	3.3
Nature or schedule of my work	9	3.3
Traditional and/or religious belief	48	17.8
Side effect of the drug	14	5.2
Feeling better	23	8.5
Feeling worse	9	3.3

Table 2: Patients' opinions on factors that prevent optimal medication adherence Adama Ethiopia 2014.

QUESTIONS	Adherence score (frequency [%])				Mean score
	1	2	3	4	
1. How often do you forget to take your medicine?	0	6 (2.2%)	53 (19.6%)	211 (78.1%)	3.76
2. How often do you stop taking your medicine because you feel better?	0	1 (0.4%)	22 (8.1%)	247 (91.5%)	3.91
3. How often do you stop taking your medicine because you feel worse?	0	0	9 (3.3%)	261 (96.7)	3.97
4. How often do you stop taking your medicine because you feel they are ineffective?	0	1 (0.4%)	8 (3%)	261 (97.7%)	3.96
5. How often do you stop taking your medicine because you fear side effects or have caused side effects?	0	0	14 (5.2%)	256 (94.8%)	3.95
6. How often do you stop taking your medicine because you are using traditional medicine or religious belief?	0	5 (1.9%)	43 (15.9%)	222 (82.2%)	3.77

Note: Adherence Scores Scales: 4, Never; 3, Rarely; 2, Frequently; 1, Daily.

Table 3: Adherence scores, Adama Ethiopia, 2014.

Adherence Score	Adherence Status	Frequency	Percentage (%)
24 (Full Score)	Adherent	170	62.96
23 (One Point Missed From Question 1)	Adherent	25	9.26
23 (One Point Missed From Other Question)	Non Adherent	27	10
20-22	Non Adherent	45	16.67
<20	Nonadherent	3	1.11
Total		270	100

Note: Adherers were those that scored a full score of 24 or score of.

Table 4: Frequency distribution of adherers and no adherers, Adama Ethiopia, 2014.

patients in the present study are resides in a big city and benefit from the widely disseminated information concerning their disease and directly from their physician.

A systematic review on the compliance to medication among diabetic patients, showed that the average compliance to the oral hypoglycemic agents ranged from 36%-93% [17].

Study from UAE reported a relatively higher over all adherences of 84% [12].

The adherence rates differed across gender and females were more compliant 74.81% than males 69.79% in the present study. This was in contrast to the result of study from India and and UAE [11,12]. Women spent most of their time at home and they might benefit from this to taking their medications as prescribed.

With regard to the educational level, higher adherence rates were noted among graduated patients (diploma) 80.77% and secondary school 80% were found to be the most compliant to the prescribed treatment in this study. This was supported by previous researches done in Saudi Arabia and UAE [12,15]. And it is consistent with the assumption that as the complexity of the diabetes drug therapy increases, patients are required to understand the prescribed drug therapy to adhere to treatment; hence it would be better understood by those with higher educational profiles. The duration of diabetes plays an important role in management of diabetes. This study showed that most of the patients (53.7 %) had a diabetic history of 1-5 years and the longer the duration of diabetes, the lower the rate of adherence (82.07% vs. 60.8%) in duration ≤ 5 years and >6 years respectively. This finding was consistent with the study from UAE and India indicating a negative relationship between the duration of diabetes and patient adherence to drug therapy [11,12]. During the early stage of the disease patients tend to be more committed to their disease, but their commitment do not lasts long since they adapt the burden and deterioration continues.

The most common reasons for non adherence to medications were modifiable factors that could be overcome by adopting suitable measures. Forgetfulness was the most commonly mentioned reason for non-compliance, similar to the findings from of studies from UAE, Nigeria, and India [12,13,17]. In contrast, a study from India reported self decision 35.08% as the main causal factor for non-adherence to anti-diabetic medications [16]. This barrier can be overcome by assisting patients in organizing their medications with pillboxes and dosing alarms and family members can assist in medication adherence in the elderly and in those taking multiple medications.

The high cost of medication agreed by majority of the patients as the most important reason preventing optimal adherence.

In this study, the main external challenge of adherence is financial problem (61.90%) This is in agreement with study done in Nigeria in which around 2/3, 37.1% in Ethiopia where the non-adherence is due to financial difficulty [8,14]. Ethiopia is a developing country in which most of the population has a lower income and this is one factor that contribute the limited health service in general and DM management in particular. The identified causes of non-adherence to taking anti-diabetic medications as prescribed were nature of work /busy schedule of work, patient dissatisfaction, cost of drug and forgetfulness were found to be 13.85%, 10.77%, 21.54% and 53.85% , respectively in this study. Similarly, non-adherence to appointment keeping was caused by forgetfulness 9.53%, nature of work and busy schedules 42.86%, travelling away from home 42.86%, intentional 4.76%. Patients who come from rural areas and those elderly patients who don't have care giver have difficulty of keeping clinic appointments. Similar study identified busy work schedules especially for patients in the working population as one of the reasons why some patients do not take their anti-diabetic medications 16.19% [14].

The majority of the patients were on mono therapy the same result as with study from Ethiopia [14]. But the mono therapy mostly prescribed in this case was Insulin (47%) unlike the above study in which glibenclamide (74.3%) was used. The present study includes both type one and type two diabetes patients and it is not surprising that insulin is used in most patients that it is used in both type I and II (when necessary) and also the prevalence of the types of DM should be considered in this two areas. The most commonly used combination therapy was Glibenclamide and metformine (43.7%). This is in agreement with the Study in Nigeria that showed the same combination therapy in 36.8% of patients.

The practice of self-monitoring of blood glucose levels by patients is indicative of their commitment to diabetes management. The study showed that 41.1%. Of the patients had adequate glycemic control and it is consistent with other study who reported adequate glycemic control in 41.8% of type-2 diabetic patients. Although, HbA1c is the established gold standard, FPG level is being used to assess and monitor glycemic control in this hospital. The glycosilated hemoglobin (HbA1c) test was not routinely recommended for patients probably on account of the high cost of the test in the hospital or because it may not be part of the established guideline within the hospital.

Conclusion and Recommendation

Conclusion

This study was able to show the main factors that can undermine the desired outcomes of diabetes pharmacotherapy in diabetic patients by decreasing adherence to their medications. This factors can be patient related such as (forgetfulness, intentional omission of dose) and drug related (cost, side effects and multiple drug therapy especially in those with co morbidity), all of which are modifiable factors. Most diabetic patients are currently being managed with the most effective available drugs. However as the result from this study indicates the desired blood sugar level could not be controlled and maintained adequately. This was because of poor adherence with the prescribed drug regimen and poor knowledge and practice of successful self management.

Recommendation

1. Adequate, clear and quality information regarding diabetes and anti diabetic medications should be provided to all diabetic patients in order to make the patient aware of future complications of the disease and the benefits of drug therapy as the factors related to non adherence in this area are modifiable and associated with low knowledge about the disease and treatment.

2. The practice of cost free medication service to the patients that cannot afford to buy in this hospital is appreciable as cost of drug is among the factors hindering adherence but the inclusion of other needy patients should be considered since there are still large number of poor patients who are losing hope of their future.

3. The role of health professionals at this point should be considerable in providing a cost effective, safest and the most effective available medication.

4. Patients should be encouraged to appropriately use anti diabetic drugs and a regular awareness should be created regarding the benefits of using them there by preventing the intentional non adherences.

5. The medication adherence rate in this study was 72.2%. Although the exact estimate of adherence may not be accurately depicted, as this is a small cross-sectional study; future large-scale studies are needed for further understanding of the problem and development of more effective interventions

Acknowledgement

We are very grateful to our college staff members for unreserved guidance and constructive suggestions and comments from the stage of proposal development to this end. We would like to thank Ambo University for supporting the budget which required for this research. Finally our deepest gratitude goes to Adama referral hospital staff workers who helped and allowed us in collecting and gathering data from the hospital.

References

1. Anjana RM, Ali MK, Pradeepa R, Deepa M, Datta M, et al. (2011) The Need for Obtaining Accurate Nationwide Estimates of Diabetes Prevalence in India-Rationale for a National Study on Diabetes. Indian J Med Res April 133: 369-380.

2. Oputa RN, Chinenye S (2012) Diabetes Mellitus: A Global Epidemic with Potential Solutions Afr J Diabetes Medicine.

3. Majaliwa ES, Elusiyan BE, Adesiyun OO, Laigong P, Adeniran AK, et al. (2008) Type 1 diabetes mellitus in the African population: epidemiology and management challenges. Acta biomed 79: 255-259.

4. Cramer JA (2004) A systematic review of adherence with medications for diabetes. Diabetes Care 27: 1218-1224.

5. Solomon AF, Chalachew MA, Hawult TA (2013) Assessment of the Level and Associated Factors with Knowledge And Practice Of Diabetes Mellitus Among Diabetic Patients Attending At Felegehiwot Hospital, Northwest Ethiopia. Clinical Medicine Research 2: 110-120.

6. Rwegerera GM (2014) Adherence to anti-diabetic drugs among patients with Type 2 diabetes mellitus at Muhimbili National Hospital, Dar es Salaam, Tanzania- A cross-sectional study. Pan Afr Med J 17: 252.

7. JT Dipiro, RL Talbert, GC Yee (1229) Pharmacotherapy: A Pathophysiologic Approach; Seventh Edition; Section 8.

8. Adisa R, Fakeye T, Fasanmade A (2011) Medication Adherence among Ambulatory Patients with Type 2 Diabetes in a Tertiary Healthcare Setting In Southwestern Nigeria. Pharmacy Practice 9:72-81.

9. Kalyango JN, Owino E, Nambuya AP (2008) Non-adherence to diabetes treatment at Mulago Hospital in Uganda: prevalence and associated factors. Afr Health Sci 8: 67-73.

10. Tamiru S, Alemseged F (2010) Risk Factors for Cardiovascular Diseases among Diabetic Patients In Southwest Ethiopia. Ethiop J Health Sci 20: 121-128.

11. Manjusha S, Madhu P, Atmatam P, Modi A, Sumariya R (2014) Medication Adherence to Antidiabetic Therapy in Patients with Type 2 Diabetes Mellitus. Int J Pharm Pharm Sci 6:564-570.

12. Arifulla M, John LJ, Sreedharan J, Muttappallymyalil J, Basha SA (2014) Patients' Adherence to Anti-Diabetic Medications in a Hospital at Ajman, UAE. Malays J Med Sci 21: 44-49.

13. Adisa R, Alutundu M, Fakeye TO (2009) Factors Contributing to Nonadherence to Oral Hypoglycemic Medications among Ambulatory Type 2 Diabetes Patients in Southwestern Nigeria. Pharmacy Practice 7:163-169.

14. Wabe NT, Angamo MT, Hussein S (2011) Medication adherence in diabetes mellitus and self management practices among type-2 diabetics in Ethiopia. N Am J Med Sci 3: 418-423.

15. Khan AR, Al-Abdul Lateef ZN, Al Aithan MA, Bu-Khamseen MA, Al Ibrahim I, et al. (2012) Factors Contributing to Non Compliance among Diabetics Attending Primary Health Center at Al Hasa District of Saudi Arabia. J Family and Community Med 19:26-32.

16. Kumar P A Study on Medication Non-Adherence in Ambulatory Diabetic Patients and Need for Pharmacist Intervention for Improving Patient Adherence. Indian Journal of Research in Pharmacy and Biotechnology 1: 446.

17. Mukherjee S, Sharmasarkar B, Das KK, Bhattacharyya A, Deb A (2013) Compliance to anti-diabetic drugs: observations from the diabetic clinic of a medical college in kolkata, India. J Clin Diagn Res 7: 661-665.

14

Perceptions of Doctors and Pharmacists towards Medication Error Reporting and Prevention in Kedah, Malaysia: A Rasch Model Analysis

Teoh BC[1], Alrasheedy AA[2]*, Hassali MA[3], Tew MM[1] and Samsudin MA[4]

[1]*Kuala Muda District Health Office, Kedah, Malaysia*
[2]*Pharmacy Practice Department, College of Pharmacy, Qassim University, Saudi Arabia*
[3]*School of Pharmaceutical Sciences, Universiti Sains Malaysia, Penang, Malaysia*
[4]*School of Educational Studies, Universitis Sains Malaysia, Penang, Malaysia*

Abstract

Objective: Reporting of medication errors in Malaysia is currently low. Consequently, the objective of the study is to explore the perceptions of doctors and pharmacists towards reporting of medication errors and to explore perceived factors that could cause or prevent medication errors.

Method: The study was a cross-sectional mail survey. All eight primary outpatient care clinics under Kuala Muda District Health Office, Kedah, Malaysia were included. The study targeted all doctors and pharmacists working in these clinics. The survey questionnaire consisted of two domains — perceptions of medication errors reporting and exploration of perceived preventive factors of medication errors. The Rasch model was used in data analysis.

Results: A total of sixty-seven questionnaires were received from the eight clinics, giving a response rate of 100%. Doctors believed that patients' knowledge about their medications and counselling by pharmacists are the most important preventing factors of medication errors. Pharmacists believed that compliance with the standard operating procedures, decreasing the heavy workload and patients' knowledge about their medications are the most important preventing factors. Regarding reporting of medication errors, both doctors and pharmacists had relatively the same perceptions. While they did not agree that their workload interferes with their ability to report medication errors, both pharmacists and doctors moderately agreed that individuals could be blamed when an error is reported in the department.

Conclusion: The study findings showed that the workload was not a barrier to medication error reporting. Moreover, both doctors and pharmacists stated that prevention of medication errors is a high priority in their work place. However, the fear of blame could prevent some doctors and pharmacists from reporting medication errors. Consequently, reporting medication errors needs be encouraged in the Malaysian primary care setting building on the current initiatives and activities in Malaysia. This could further promote the culture of medication safety and error reporting.

Keywords: Safety; Medication errors; Malaysia; Reporting

Introduction

Medication errors are not uncommon and can occur at any phase of the complex medication use process (prescription, transcription, dispensing and administration) [1-4]. In fact, medication errors can cause serious clinical consequences and represent a major concern for healthcare professionals and policy makers around the globe [2,4]. Moreover, medication errors can increase the healthcare cost and put a financial burden on the health system [5]. Therefore, one of the strategies to reduce medication errors is to encourage reporting of these errors so that suitable solutions can be made to prevent them from occurring. The analysis of reports and feedback can help to improve the medication safety and make changes at the level of the individual practitioner or the team, at the level of the institution/employer and at the national level [5].

In Malaysia, Ministry of Health — as the health policy maker — has started initiatives and programs to further promote the medication safety. Now, medication error reporting system is in place and health care professionals can report online via the national medication error reporting system (MERS) [6]. Also, medication errors can be reported using the medication error report form and sent via the mail to the National Medication Safety Center (MedSC) [7]. In fact, medication safety is promoted as "Medication safety is Everyone's Responsibility" [7]. Furthermore, a guideline on medication error reporting was published by Ministry of Health in 2009 to facilitate the reporting process and provide detailed information regarding medication errors, scope of error reporting, procedures of reporting, types of medication errors, classification of the medication error severity [8].

A medication error is defined by the National Coordination Council for Medication Error Reporting and Prevention (NCCMERP) as "A medication error is any preventable event that may cause or lead to inappropriate medication use or patient harm while the medication is in the control of the health care professional, patient, or consumer. Such events may be related to professional practice, health care products, procedures, and systems, including prescribing, order communication, product labelling, packaging, and nomenclature, compounding, dispensing, distribution, administration, education, monitoring, and use" [9]. Most medication errors involve dose error,

*Corresponding author: Alrasheedy AA, PhD, BCPS Pharmacy Practice Department, College of Pharmacy, Qassim University, Saudi Arabia, E-mail: alian-a@hotmail.com

frequency error, unavailable drug, unavoidable delay, administration error, drug-drug interaction and drug-allergy interaction [10,11].

Healthcare providers particularly physicians and pharmacists are the key players in safe use of medications in primary outpatient care [12,13]. However, medication errors still occur and often go undetected [8]. In Malaysia, medication error reporting is currently on a voluntary basis [8]. With voluntary reporting systems, fears of recrimination or heavy workloads might prevent the reporting of medication errors [11]. Moreover, one study which included 12 Ministry of Health (MOH) primacy care clinics from four states in Malaysia showed that medication errors were the most common clinical management errors (41.3% of all management errors) [14]. Another Malaysian study from outpatient pharmacy department in Kelantan state showed that the prevalence of medication errors in prescriptions for geriatric patients was 25.17% [15]. Therefore, exploring pharmacists' and physicians' perceptions is an important step towards developing an effective medication error reporting system as medication errors reporting is dependent on healthcare providers in most cases [16]. Also, it is vital to investigate the preventing factors and the medication safety culture via assessment of prescribers' perceptions to ease the development of a mechanism that could be integrated with the current health system.

To date, healthcare organizations had implemented various programs to improve medication error reporting system. World Health Organization (WHO) stated that patient safety in primary care is an important topic and should be addressed in all countries. Moreover, medication safety incidents are prevalent in primary care setting [17]. Since some medication errors may cause morbidity and mortality, it is needed to further strengthen the current healthcare system with an effective mechanism for monitoring and reporting of errors [8]. As there is paucity of data in this field in Malaysia, therefore, the objective of the study is to explore the perceptions of doctors and pharmacists practising in primary clinics regarding reporting of medication errors and to explore perceived preventing factors of these errors.

Methods

Study design

This is a cross-sectional questionnaire-based mail survey.

Questionnaires development

The survey instrument was developed from the literature relevant to medication safety [12,16,18]. Modifications were done to make it suitable to the local setting. The survey instrument consisted of 2 domains which included respondents' perceptions on preventive factors of medication errors and respondents' perceptions on culture of medication errors reporting. The questionnaire was prepared in English language. The scale used in this study was a five point Likert type rating (1 - Strongly Disagree, 2 - Disagree, 3 - Neither agree nor disagree, 4 - Agree and 5- Strongly Agree). The survey instructions stated that there are no correct or incorrect responses and instructed participants to rate the response that best reflects their perceptions. The survey instrument was reviewed for its validity by a group of experts in the field of medication safety. Moreover, a pilot study was conducted with15 pharmacists and 15 doctors from outpatient care clinics, Federal Provincial Health Department Kuala Lumpur. Some minor revisions were made based on the comments during the pilot study.

Study setting, population and sampling

All 8 primary outpatient care clinics under Kuala Muda District Health Office, Kedah, Malaysia were included. The targeted population was all pharmacists and doctors working under primary outpatient care of Kuala Muda District Health Office. This is a census study as data is gathered on every member of the population (52 doctors and 15 pharmacists). Inclusion criteria were all registered pharmacists and doctors working in primary outpatient care clinics in Kuala Muda District Health Office. The exclusion criteria were provisional registered pharmacists (PRP), pharmacy students attached to the relevant health facilities, doctors under housemanship and doctors or pharmacists on long leave/sick leave.

Survey administration

A mail survey was sent in November 2013 to all the participants. The survey instrument was accompanied by an addressed envelope (for returning the completed questionnaire) and a cover letter explaining the aim of the study, definition of medication error and confidentiality of all responses from participants. The participants were asked to complete the questionnaires and return them in two weeks time. The first reminder was sent to each pharmacist and doctor approximately after first week. The second reminder was sent after one week of the first reminder.

Data analysis

All the data received from this survey were entered in the SPSS version 18. Appropriate descriptive statistics were used for data analysis. The Rasch model was used to examine pharmacists and doctors' perception toward preventive factors of medication errors and culture of medication errors reporting.

Rasch model analysis

Rasch measurement, a form of item response theory, was selected as the primary method of data analysis because it provides advantage over traditional statistical approaches. According to Royal (2010), page 23, Rasch models are "are logistic, latent trait models of probability for monotonically increasing functions. Unlike statistical models that are developed based on data, Rasch measurement models are static models that are imposed upon data. Rasch models assume the probability of a respondent agreeing with a particular item is a logistic function of the relative distance between the person and item location on a linear continuum" [19]. Winsteps measurement software was used to perform the Rasch analysis.

According to Zain et al (2010), "the Rasch model transforms raw item difficulties and raw person scores to equal interval measures of logits on a line in a "meter stick". The idea of a line helps us to determine item positions by considering each item relative to the items already positioned on the line" [20]. Hence, placing logits scale on a meter stick provides equal and standard interval data [20]. Thus, in Rasch model, raw scores are converted into standardized units which are then aligned on a ruler that measures each component of the model [21]. In principle, according to Hardigan and Carvajal (2007), Likert scale data can be used as a basis for obtaining interval level estimates on a continuum by applying the Rasch Model [21]. Results of Rasch models are linear, independent and objective. Hence, inferences can be drawn from them [22].

The equal interval measures transformed by Rasch Model are used to map persons and items onto a linear (interval) scale. Item maps are useful for identifying meaningful constructs, as the graphical illustrations visually display any potential relationships among item responses. The maps showed person distributions on the left and item distributions on the right, along a hierarchy on a common scale. The numbers along the left column indicate logits, which are the interval level measures produced from ordinal level raw scores when data were computed via Rasch model. The measures essentially serve as a ruler with truly equidistant values. Placing both persons and items on the same scale allows for easy and meaningful interpretation of the results. Such mapping (called person-item maps) produce useful tools for evaluating perceptions towards medication errors and culture of medication errors reporting. The person-item maps provided ways for evaluating and interpreting the data. Items order in the maps illustrates the level of item difficulties. This means that items which more difficult to agree with or items which easier to agree with can be identified.

Markers denoted on the map showed important statistics such as mean (M), one standard deviation (SD) and two standard deviations (T), for both persons and items. Prior to analysing the data, overall collected data were diagnosed in order to provide a precise and productive measurement, same like process of calibrating an instrument [20]. The responses of the 67 doctors and pharmacists were analysed using Ministeps 3.81.0 (Rasch-model computer program). In order the items can be used in the Rasch model, the item infit mean square and outfit mean square should be distributed between 0.7 and 1.4 [23]. These indicators provide evidence of unidimensionality in the data and present evidence of strong content validity [19]. After diagnosing data, the raw data were transformed using Rasch analysis to order pharmacists and doctors along the continuum of the measure of perceptions towards medication errors and culture of reporting.

Results

Demographic characteristics of the respondents

A total of 67 questionnaires were received from the clinics under Kuala Muda District Health Office (PKDKM), with a response rate of 100%. The majority of the respondents were female (82.1%) with an average age of 31.8 ± 5.70 years and working experience of 5.2 ± 4.36 years. Of the respondents, 52 were doctors (three of them were family medicine specialists and the rest were general practitioners) while 15 respondents were pharmacists. The total prescriptions per month ranged from 850 to 15,000 prescriptions for all the 8 clinics under PKDKM. Table 1 showed the characteristics of the respondents in details (Table 1).

Findings

Table 2 and 3 showed the items statistics for perception of preventive factors of medication errors and culture of medication error reporting respectively. For Table 2, the difficulty of items is distributed from -1.64 Logits to 1.76 Logits. The infit mean squares of the items are between 0.65 and 1.40 while the outfit mean squares are between 0.67 and 1.46. For Table 3, the difficulty of items distributed from -1.93 Logits to 2.18. The infit mean squares of the items are between 0.65 and 1.22 while the outfit mean squares are between 0.67 and 1.19. Thus, this data exhibited good fit and supported the uni-dimensionality requirement of the model. The Cronbach alpha coefficients are above 0.7 indicating the questionnaire is reliable.

Respondents' perceptions of preventive factors of medication errors

The distribution of doctors according to their perception of preventing factors of medication errors and the distribution of items according to difficulty are shown in Figure 1. On the left side, the distribution of doctors was represented. Items located below the participants are the items that doctors were more likely to agree with.

Variable	n (%)
Profession	
Doctors	52 (77.6)
Pharmacists	15 (22.4)
Total	67 (100)
Working experience in current position (years)	
0-4	40 (59.7)
5-9	15 (22.4)
10-14	9 (13.4)
15-19	2 (3)
≥ 20	1 (1.5)
Total	67 (100)
Age (years)	
<30	37 (55.2)
30-39	22 (32.8)
40-49	7 (10.4)
≥ 50	1 (1.5)
Total	67 (100)
Average number of prescriptions per month in respective settings	
850	3 (4.5)
1800	4 (6)
2400	8 (11.9)
2600	2 (3)
2800	4 (6)
3200	3 (4.5)
7300	13 (19.4)
15000	30 (44.8)
Total	67 (100)

Table 1: Characteristics of the respondents (n=67).

The items located above the participants are the items that the doctors were unlikely to agree with. The items distribution on the map has valuable information on doctors' current perception. Figure 1 shows an item-person map in which doctors are placed relative to the hierarchy of items. On the right side, items are listed in order of difficulty, with the hardest to agree with at the top and the easiest item to agree with at the bottom. The same scenario happened to pharmacists as shown in Figure 2.

Regarding doctors' perception, from the item person map in Figure 1, the statement "patients' knowledge about their own medications helps to reduce medication errors" has the lowest difficulty as it was located at the bottom of the scale (-1.82 Logits). In other words, this statement was the most easily agreed on or highly perceived by doctors. The second most easily agreed preventive factor was patient counselling by pharmacists help to decrease the number of medication errors (-1.60 Logits). These two statements were followed by others statements as shown in Figure 1. Statement of "generic substitution has no influence on medication errors" has the highest level of difficulty (1.71 Logits) (located at the top of the scale). In doctors' perception, this statement was the hardest to be agreed on.

Regarding pharmacists' perceptions of preventive factors of medication errors, from the item person map in Figure 2, there were three statements where pharmacists most easily to agree with (-1.32 Logits). These included "It is important to comply with the standard operating procedures to decrease the number of medications errors", "A heavy workload will increase the number of medication errors" and "Patients' knowledge about their own medications helps to reduce medication errors". Pharmacists had the same perception of doctors towards the statement "generic substitution has no influence on medication errors" as it was the hardest to be agreed on (2.06 Logits).

Perception towards preventive factors of Medication Errors	Measure	Infit mean square	Outfit mean square
Generic substitution has no influence on medication errors	1.76	1.35	1.40
Medication error is a result of an error made by an individual professional	1.53	1.11	1.23
Medication error is a result of insufficient standard operating procedures	0.85	0.81	0.83
Prescription with generic name of drugs help to reduce medication errors	0.62	1.41	1.44
It is not necessary to report to superior if a medication error occurs but it does not harm the patient	0.62	1.12	1.26
It is embarrassing to discuss medication errors with colleagues	0.54	1.13	1.24
There is need to change working routines based on the errors that have been observed to decrease the number of medication errors	0.48	0.89	0.95
Seamless information flow between health care units decreases the number of medication errors	0.33	0.67	0.74
Internal reporting of the medication errors prevents the same medication errors to reoccur	-0.34	0.70	0.73
Collaboration between different health care providers and settings helps to decrease medication errors	-0.6	0.82	0.83
It is important to comply with the standard operating procedures to decrease the number of medications errors	-0.74	0.65	0.67
A heavy workload will increase the number of medication errors	-0.92	1.40	1.46
Long working hours (more than 8 hours a day) increase risk of medication errors	-1.12	1.26	1.25
Patient counselling by pharmacists help to decrease the number of medication errors	-1.37	0.73	0.75
Patients' knowledge about their own medications helps to reduce medication errors	-1.64	0.85	0.85

Table 2: Measures and Validity Indices for perception towards preventive factors of medication errors

Perceptions towards culture of medication errors reporting	Measure	Infit mean square	Outfit mean square
My workload interferes with my ability to report medication errors	2.18	1.22	1.19
I afraid of negative consequences associated with medical errors reporting	1.22	1.13	1.12
Individuals will be blamed when an error is reported in my department	0.59	0.55	0.57
Staffs are supported for reporting medication errors	-0.86	0.96	1.02
My department takes an action on reported medication errors (near miss/ incident) to improve medication safety	-1.19	1.17	1.11
Senior officers/managers at my workplace stated that patient safety/prevention of medication error is a high priority	-1.93	0.76	0.75

Table 3: Item statistic for perception towards culture of medication errors reporting.

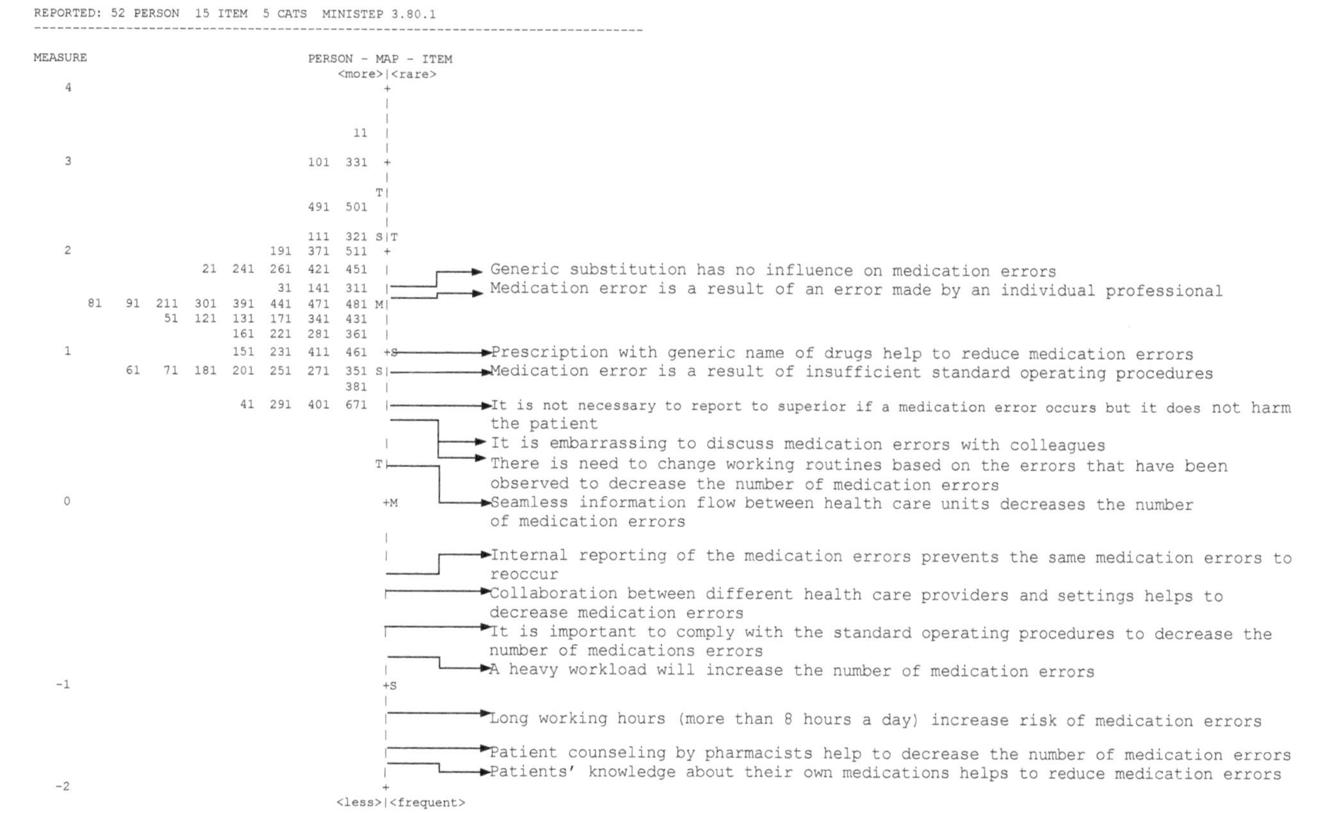

Figure 1: Person-item map for doctors' perception towards preventive factors of medication errors.

```
REPORTED: 15 PERSON  15 ITEM  5 CATS  MINISTEP 3.80.1
--------------------------------------------------------------------------------

MEASURE         PERSON - MAP - ITEM
                    <more>|<rare>
    3        522   622 T+
                       |
                       |
                       |
                     S |
                 602  |T
    2            662   +        ┌──► Generic substitution has no influence on medication errors
       532  562  582  592 M|
                 572  612   |
                 642  652   |    ┌──► Medication error is a result of an error made by an individual professional
                       |
                     S |
    1        552  632  +S   ┌──►It is not necessary to report to superior if a medication error occurs but it does not harm the
                       |       patient
                       |    ┌──►It is embarrassing to discuss medication errors with colleagues
                       |    ►Seamless information flow between health care units decreases the number of medication errors
                 542 T|──────►Medication error is a result of insufficient standard operating procedures
                       |    ►There is need to change working routines based on the errors that have been observed to decrease
                       |       the number of medication errors
                       |
    0                 +M──────►Internal reporting of the medication errors prevents the same medication errors to reoccur
                       |    ► Prescription with generic name of drugs help to reduce medication errors
                       |    ►Patient counseling by pharmacists help to decrease the number of medication errors
                       |    ►Collaboration between different health care providers and settings helps to decrease medication
                       |       errors
                       |    ►Long working hours (more than 8 hours a day) increase risk of medication errors
                       |
   -1                 +S
                       |
                       |    ┌──► A heavy workload will increase the number of medication errors
                       |    ┌──► Patients' knowledge about their own medications helps to reduce medication errors
                       |    └──► It is important to comply with the standard operating procedures to decrease the number of
                       |       medications errors
                       |
   -2                 +
                   <less>|<frequent>
```

Figure 2: Person-item map for pharmacists' perception towards preventive factors of medication errors.

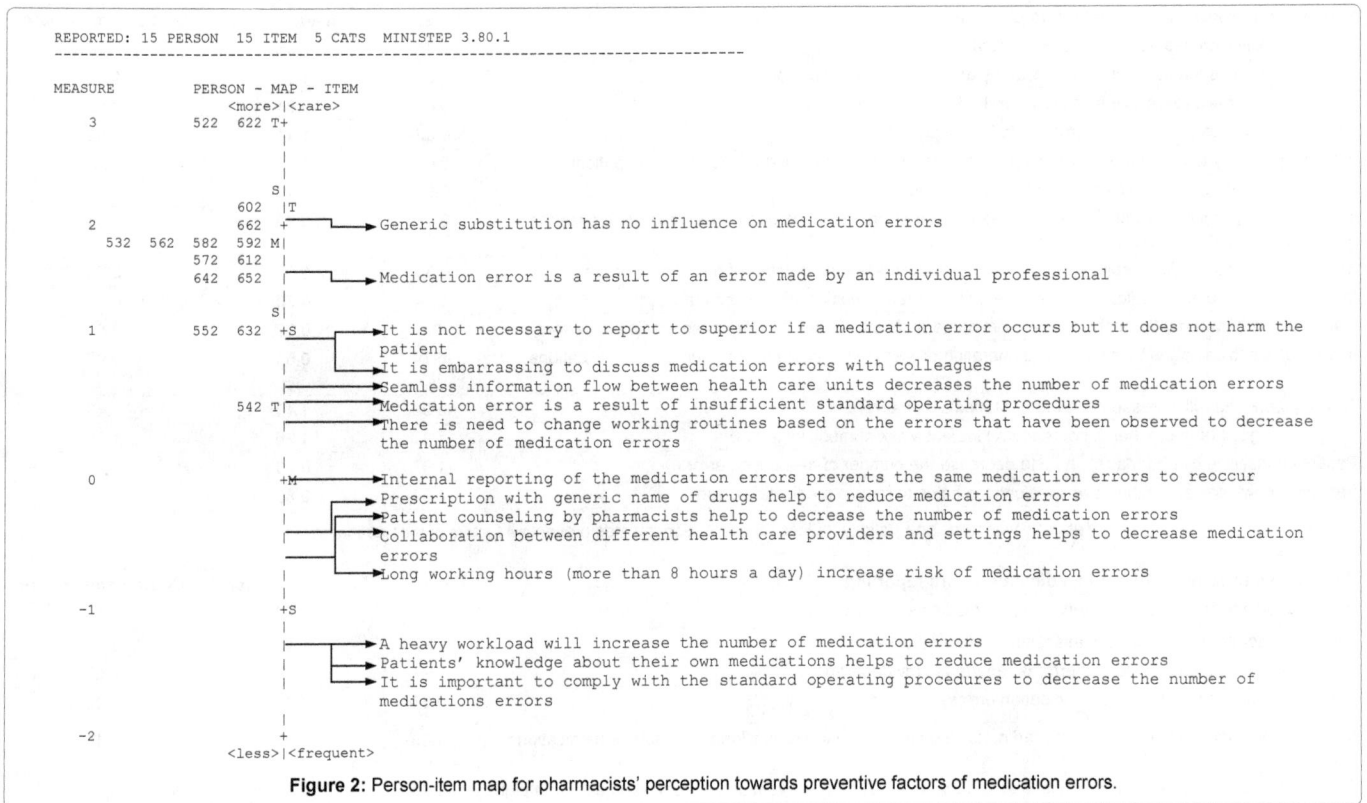

Both pharmacists and doctors most easily agreed that patients' knowledge about their medications helps to reduce medication errors (-1.32 Logits and -1.82 Logits, respectively). Meanwhile, pharmacists easily agreed that prescriptions with generic names help to reduce medication errors but this was hardly agreed with by doctors (-0.61 Logits and 0.94 Logits respectively).

Table 4 summarizes the comparison of perceptions towards preventive factors of medication errors between pharmacists and doctors from the hardest to agree with (at the top) to the most easily to agree with (at the bottom).

Perceptions of medication error reporting

For reporting of medication errors, both pharmacists and doctors had the same perceptions. From Figure 3 and 4, item person map showed that they most easily agreed that senior officers/managers at their workplace stated prevention of medication error is a high priority (-1.89 Logits and -2.04 Logits respectively) while it was most difficult to agree that their workload interferes with their ability to report medication errors (2.24 Logits and 2.21 Logits respectively)

Table 5 summarizes the comparison of perceptions towards medication errors reporting between doctors and pharmacists.

Discussion

Perceptions of preventive factors of medication errors

Both pharmacists and doctors in PKDKM most easily agreed that patients' knowledge about their own medications helps to reduce medication errors. This was contradicting with some studies in literature in which they reported that the most highly perceived factor for medication errors was heavy workload [16,24,25]. In our study, heavy workload was the third and fourth factor to be easily agreed on by pharmacists and doctors, respectively. Thus, it was not the most highly perceived factor for medication errors.

In fact, human factors can limit the healthcare safety and contribute to medication errors. These factors include inattention, memory lapse, lack of knowledge and interruptions and other several personal and environmental factors [26]. Moreover, poor communication between patients and health care professionals is a major contributing factor to medication errors and adverse drug events [27]. Communication issues include both written and verbal issues. Written communication issues include for example wrong doses and wrong medicines. Verbal communication issues include miscommunication between patients and pharmacists [27].

Generally, if patients are more knowledgeable, errors in treatment may be prevented. This is because anxiety about the uncertainty of treatment can be reduced or alleviated by adequate knowledge [28]. Therefore, patients should learn the name of the medicines that are prescribed to them, as well as dosage, strength and frequency in order to avoid medication errors [29].

For both pharmacists and doctors, the most difficult statement to agree with was that generic substitution has no influence on medication errors. According to Hakonsen et al. (2010) study that was conducted in a large Norwegian hospital to explore the nurses experiences with generic substitution, the nurses in the wards felt insecure about the generic substitution. They also indicated that the large number of generic medications and frequent generic substitutions can lead to medication errors. Moreover, 42% reported that they have experienced errors due to generic substitution primarily because of five reasons that included difficult medicine names, frequent changes in the drug inventory, and the large number of generic medicines, heavy workload and inadequate training [30]. Our study showed that perceptions of doctors and pharmacists were similar to that of nurses on the effect of generic substitution on medication safety.

Perceptions of Doctors and Pharmacists towards Medication Error Reporting and Prevention...

75

```
REPORTED: 52 PERSON  10 ITEM  5 CATS  MINISTEP 3.80.1
-----------------------------------------------------------------------

MEASURE                                    PERSON - MAP - ITEM
                                             <more>|<rare>
    4                                            +
                                                 |
                                                 |
                                                 |
    3                                    11      +
                                                 |
                                                 |
                                                 |
    2                                   111   |T +
                                     151  331    +
                                               T|
                                                 |
                                        21       |
    1                          91     181   S|
                    61   71   81   251   281  +S
                       241  431  451  461    |
    31   41  171  191  321  351  391  411  421  441  491 M|
        51  161  201  221  231  271  371  501    |
        101  341  361  381  471  481  671      |
    0       121  131  211  291  301  311  401  +M
                    141  261  511  S|
   -1                               +S
                                     |
                                   T
                                     |
                                     |
   -2                                +
                                   <less>|<frequent>
```

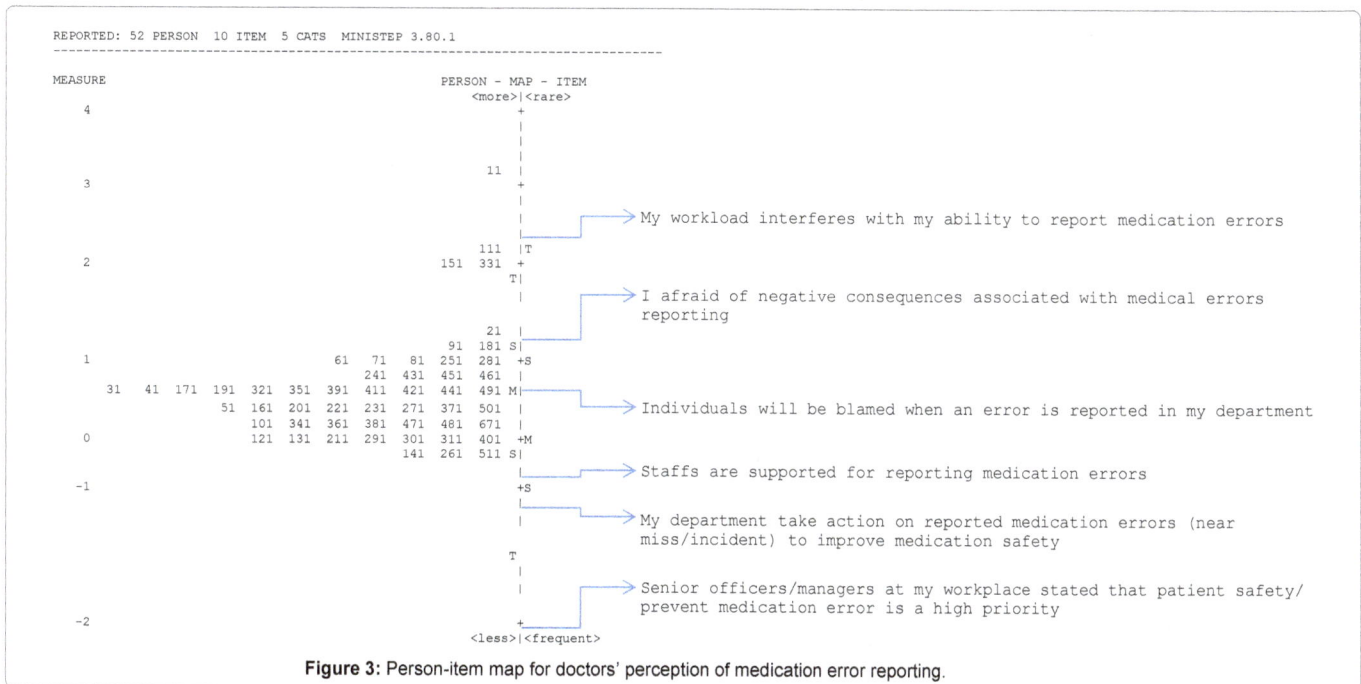

Figure 3: Person-item map for doctors' perception of medication error reporting.

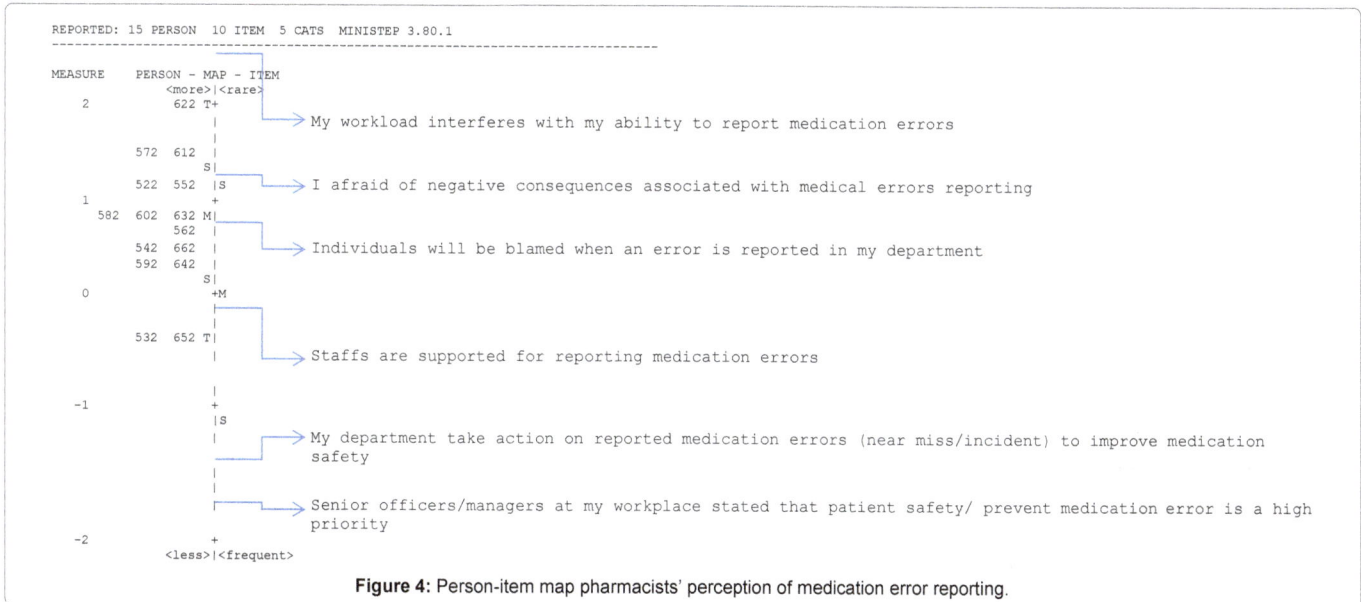

- My workload interferes with my ability to report medication errors
- I afraid of negative consequences associated with medical errors reporting
- Individuals will be blamed when an error is reported in my department
- Staffs are supported for reporting medication errors
- My department take action on reported medication errors (near miss/incident) to improve medication safety
- Senior officers/managers at my workplace stated that patient safety/ prevent medication error is a high priority

```
REPORTED: 15 PERSON  10 ITEM  5 CATS  MINISTEP 3.80.1
-----------------------------------------------------------------------

MEASURE     PERSON - MAP - ITEM
              <more>|<rare>
    2          622 T+
                     |
             572  612 |
                   S|
             522  552 |S
    1                 +
        582  602  632 M|
             562      |
             542  662 |
             592  642 |
                   S|
    0              +M
                     |
             532  652 T|
                     |
                     |
   -1              +
                   |S
                     |
                     |
                     |
   -2          +
         <less>|<frequent>
```

Figure 4: Person-item map pharmacists' perception of medication error reporting.

- My workload interferes with my ability to report medication errors
- I afraid of negative consequences associated with medical errors reporting
- Individuals will be blamed when an error is reported in my department
- Staffs are supported for reporting medication errors
- My department take action on reported medication errors (near miss/incident) to improve medication safety
- Senior officers/managers at my workplace stated that patient safety/ prevent medication error is a high priority

Pharmacists easily agreed that prescription with generic name help to reduce medication errors but this was hardly agreed on by doctors. Ashcroft et al. suggested that misreading of prescription—a main factor of medication errors is mainly experienced by the pharmacist who received the prescription form the doctor. It might involve the similarity in drugs names [24]. According to American Society of Health-System Pharmacists (ASHP) guidelines on preventing medication errors, prescribers should use generic names of medications in prescriptions to avoid misreading of prescriptions [28]. Thus, writing in generic name could reduce the medication errors from the pharmacists' side.

Perceptions of medication error reporting

Both pharmacists and doctors in PKDKM had almost the same perceptions towards reporting medication errors. They most easily agreed that senior officers/managers at workplace stated that patient safety or prevention of medication errors is a high priority. This was followed by statement 'my department take action on reported medication errors to improve medication safety and staff are supported for reporting medication errors. These findings were consistent with the fact that patient safety is seen as high priority by governments throughout the world [31]. To date, the main approaches that have been examined for improving patient safety in primary care that had been done included campaign and education, incident reporting, audit and safety culture surveys [32]. Although there is no consensus about the best ways to improve patient safety in primary care, it is considered an important issue that needs to be addressed and investigated [32]. Reporting of medication errors set up a process so that errors can be communicated to key stakeholders. Once data are collected and

Doctors (n=52)	Pharmacists (n=15)
• Generic substitution has no influence on medication errors	• Generic substitution has no influence on medication errors
• Medication error is a result of an error made by an individual professional	• Medication error is a result of an error made by an individual professional
• Prescription with generic name of drugs help to reduce medication error	• It is not necessary to report to superior if a medication error occurs but it does not harm the patient
• Medication error is a result of insufficient standard operating procedures	• It is embarrassing to discuss medication errors with colleagues
• It is not necessary to report to superior if a medication error occurs but it does not harm the patient	• Seamless information flow between health care units decreases the number of medication errors
• It is embarrassing to discuss medication errors with colleagues	• Medication error is a result of insufficient standard operating procedures
• There is need to change working routines based on the errors that have been observed to decrease the number of medication errors	• There is need to change working routines based on the errors that have been observed to decrease the number of medication errors
• Seamless information flow between health care units decreases the number of medication errors	• Internal reporting of the medication errors prevents the same medication errors to reoccur
• Internal reporting of the medication errors prevents the same medication errors to reoccur	• Prescription with generic name of drugs help to reduce medication errors
• Collaboration between different health care providers and settings helps to decrease medication errors	• Collaboration between different health care providers and settings helps to decrease medication errors
• It is important to comply with the standard operating procedures to decrease the number of medications errors	• Long working hours (more than 8 hours a day) increase risk of medication errors
• A heavy workload will increase the number of medication errors	• Patient counselling by pharmacists help to decrease the number of medication errors
• Long working hours (more than 8 hours a day) increase risk of medication errors	• A heavy workload will increase the number of medication errors
• Patient counseling by pharmacists help to decrease the number of medication errors	• Patients' knowledge about their own medications helps to reduce medication errors
• Patients' knowledge about their own medications helps to reduce medication errors	• It is important to comply with the standard operating procedures to decrease the number of medications errors

Table 4: Comparison between Doctors' and Pharmacists' Perceptions towards the Preventive Factors of Medication Errors (from the hardest to agree with on top to the most easily to agree with at the bottom).

Doctors (n=52)	Pharmacists (n=15)
• My workload interferes with my ability to report medication errors	• My workload interferes with my ability to report medication errors
• I afraid of negative consequences associated with medical errors reporting	• I afraid of negative consequences associated with medical errors reporting
• Individuals will be blamed when an error is reported in my department	• Individuals will be blamed when an error is reported in my department
• Staffs are supported for reporting medication errors	• Staffs are supported for reporting medication errors
• My department take action on reported medication errors (near miss/incident) to improve medication safety	• My department take action on reported medication errors (near miss/incident) to improve medication safety
• Senior officers/managers at my workplace stated that patient safety/prevent medication error is a high priority	• Senior officers/managers at my workplace stated that patient safety/prevent medication error is a high priority

Table 5: Comparison between Doctors' and Pharmacists' Perceptions of reporting of Medication Errors (from the hardest to agree with on top to the most easily to agree with at the bottom).

analysed, relevant authorities/agencies can evaluate causes and revise or create processes to reduce the risk of errors [33]. Therefore, staffs should be encouraged to report medication errors. This is because underreporting prevents efforts to avoid future errors. Hence, no changes or improvement in medication safety without efficient reporting of errors.

Both pharmacists and doctors moderately agreed that individuals could be blamed when an error reported in the department. This might be a barrier to error reporting as healthcare professionals reported feeling worried as well as fearful of being blamed or disciplinary actions following an error would be taken against them [34,35]. Fear of these negative consequences can lead to reporting of errors only when the error could no longer be hidden [36]. Fears of punishment have led to a norm of silence, where silence kills. To eliminate this barrier, individuals and organizations must be able to move from individual blame toward a culture of safety, where the blame of errors is eliminated and reporting is rewarded in order to increase reporting of all types of errors [33].

Both pharmacists and doctors most difficult to agree that workload interferes with their ability to report medication errors. This is different from the findings of previous studies where the barriers to error reporting were due to being busy, extra work needed to do report and incident reports take time to complete [35,37,38]. The difference could be explained that work load might be less in the primary clinics in our study compared to the other studies. In some clinics, the total patients and prescriptions per day was less than 200 and thus it might be not too many for them to deal with. Alternatively, it could be explained that pharmacists and doctors are willing to report errors regardless of the workload. In the year of 2013, only two medication error reports were submitted from pharmacists, with a total prescription of four hundred thirty thousand for that year. Studies on medication errors in Malaysia appeared to be very few in literature. One study which included 12 MOH primacy care clinics from four states in Malaysia showed that that medication errors were the most common clinical management errors (41.3% of all management errors) [14]. Another study from outpatient pharmacy department in Kelantan showed that the prevalence of medication errors in prescriptions for geriatric patients was 25.17% [15]. Since workload was not a barrier for error reporting in PKDKM, the low medication error reporting rate might due the fear of blame or disciplinary action when an error is reported. To avert underreporting and to effectively learn from errors, there is a need for the health policy makers to develop policies that support routine reporting of errors, so that increased numbers of reports of actual and near misses errors are rewarded. By easing the transition of an institution to a culture of safety and eliminating the potential blame, error reporting will most likely increase [13]. Finally, the current culture in safety is that it is neither wholly punitive nor wholly blame-free when errors happen [39]. In fact, it is necessary to create a reporting environment in which reporting errors are rewarded and valued. At the same time, a well-established system of accountability should be in place to confront those individuals who wilfully and repeatedly make unsafe practices or knowingly disregard a risk that would most likely cause a bad outcome to the patient [40].

Limitations

The study was conducted in one Malaysian state (i.e., Kedah). Therefore, its findings cannot be generalized to the whole country. However, given the paucity of data regarding medication error reporting in Malaysia, we believe these preliminary findings are useful for future guidance for health authorities. Moreover, the current findings warrant a large scale study to further study this medication errors reporting practices.

Conclusion

Both doctors and pharmacists highly perceived patients' knowledge about their medications help to reduce medication errors and that generic substitution will have influence on medication errors. Pharmacists believed that prescriptions with generic name help to reduce medication errors while doctors did not have this perception. Both doctors and pharmacists indicated that senior officers/managers at work place stated that prevention of medication errors is a high priority. They did not consider workload as barrier to their ability to report medication errors. However, the fear of blame could prevent some doctors and pharmacists from reporting medication errors. Consequently, reporting medication errors should be encouraged in the primary care setting building on the current initiatives and activities in Malaysia to further promote the culture of medication safety.

Acknowledgement

The authors would like to acknowledge the Director General of Health Malaysia for the permission to publish this study.

References

1. Belén Jiménez Muñoz A, Muiño Miguez A, Paz Rodriguez Pérez M, Dolores Vigil Escribano M, Esther Durán Garcia M, et al. (2010) Medication error prevalence. Int J Health Care Qual Assur 23: 328-338.

2. Alsulami Z, Conroy S, Choonara I (2013) Medication errors in the Middle East countries: A systematic review of the literature. Eur J Clin Pharmacol 69: 995-1008.

3. Salmasi S, Khan TM, Hong YH, Ming LC, Wong TW (2015) Medication Errors in the Southeast Asian Countries: A Systematic Review. PLoS ONE 10: e0136545.

4. Saghafi F, Zargarzadeh AH (2014) Medication error detection in two major teaching hospitals: What are the types of errors? J Res Med Sci 19: 617-623.

5. Glavin RJ (2010) Drug errors: Consequences, mechanisms, and avoidance. Br J Anaesth 105: 76-82.

6. http://mers.moh.gov.my/MERS/

7. http://www.pharmacy.gov.my/v2/sites/default/files/document-upload/medication-error-reporting-form-final.pdf

8. Ministry Of Health Malaysia (2009) Guideline on medication error reporting.

9. National Coordinating Council for Medication Error Reporting and Prevention (2015) What is a medication error.

10. O'Shea E (1999) Factors contributing to medication errors: AA literature review. J Clin Nurs 8:496-504.

11. Seeley CE, Nicewander D, Page R, Dysert PA 2nd (2004) A baseline study of medication error rates at Baylor University Medical Center in preparation for implementation of a computerized physician order entry system. Proc Bayl Univ Med Cent 17:357-361

12. Teinila T, Kaunisvesi K, Airaksinen M (2011) Primary care physicians' perceptions of medication errors and error prevention in cooperation with community pharmacists. Res Social Adm Pharm 7:162-179.

13. Aljadhey H, Mahmoud MA, Hassali MA, Alrasheedy A, Alahmad A, et al. (2014) Challenges to and the future of medication safety in Saudi Arabia: A qualitative study. Saudi Pharm J 22: 326-332.

14. Khoo EM, Lee WK, Sararaks S, Samad AA, Liew SM, et al. (2012) Medical errors in primary care clinics--a cross sectional study. BMC Fam Pract 13:127.

15. Abdullah DC, Ibrahim NS, Ibrahim MI (2004) Medication errors among geriatrics at the outpatient pharmacy in a teaching hospital in Kelantan. Malays J Med Sci 11:52-58.

16. Teinila T, Gronroos V, Airaksinen M (2008) A system approach to dispensing errors: A national study on perceptions of the Finnish community pharmacists. Pharm World Sci 30:823-833.

17. World Health Organization (2012) Safer Primary Care: A Global Challenge.

18. Institute for Safe Medication Practices (2002) Pathways for medication safety.

19. Royal K (2010) Evaluating faculty perceptions of student learning outcomes: A rasch measurement analysis. J Multidiscip Eval 6:18-31.

20. Zain A, Samsudin MA, Rohandi, Jusoh A (2010) Using Rasch Model to measure students' attitudes toward science in low performing secondary schools in Malaysia. Int Educ Stud 3:56-63.

21. Hardigan P, Carvajal M (2007) Job satisfaction among practicing pharmacists: A Rasch Analysis. The Internet J Allied Health Sci Pract 5:1-9.

22. Wright B, Stone M (1979) Best Test Design.

23. Bond T, Fox C (2001) Applying the Rasch model: Fundamental measurement in the human Sciences.

24. Ashcrof D, Quinlan P, Blenkinsopp A (2005) Prospective study of the incidence, nature and causes of dispnesing errors in community pharmacies. Pharmacoepidemiol Drug Saf. 14: 327-332.

25. Dean B, Schachter M, Vincent C, Barber N (2002) Causes of prescribing errors in hospital inpatients: A prospective study. Lancet 359:1373-1378.

26. Improving medication safety (2012) Committee opinion No. 531.American College of Obstetricians and Gynecologists. Obstet Gynecol 120: 406-410.

27. Hickner J, Zafar A, Kuo GM (2010) Field test results of a new ambulatory care Medication Error and Adverse Drug Event Reporting System--MEADERS. Ann Fam Med 8: 517-525.

28. (1993) ASHP guidelines on preventing medication errors in hospitals. Am J Hosp Pharm. 50: 305-314.

29. Davis N, Cohen JM (1981) Medication errors: Causes and Prevention.

30. Hakonsen H, Hopen HS, Abelsen L, Ek B, Toverud EL (2010) Generic substitution: A potential risk factor for medication errors in hospitals. Adv Ther 27: 118-126.

31. Scott I (2010) What are the most effective strategies for improving quality and safety of healthcare? Intern Med J 39: 389- 400.

32. The Health Foundation (2011) Research scan: Improving safety in primary care.

33. Wolf Z, Hughes R (2008) Error reporting and disclosure. Rockville: Agency for Healthcare Research and Quality, US.

34. Wolf ZR, Serembus JF, Smetzer J, Cohen H, Cohen M (2000) Responses and concerns of healthcare providers to medication errors. Clin Nurse Spec 14: 278-287

35. Wakefield DS, Wakefield BJ, Uden-Holman T, Blegen MA (1996) Perceived barriers in reporting medication administration errors. Best Pract Benchmarking Healthc 1: 191-197.

36. Cook AF, Hoas H, Guttmannova K, Joyner JC (2004) An error by any other name. Am J Nurs Jun 104: 32-43.

37. Elder NC, Graham D, Brandt E, Hickner J (2007) Barriers and motivators for making error reports from family medicine offices: A report from the American Academy of Family Physicians National Research Network (AAFP NRN). J Am Board Fam Med 20: 115-123.

38. Uribe CL, Schweikhart SB, Pathak DS, Dow M, Marsh GB (2002) Perceived barriers to medical-error reporting: An exploratory investigation. J Healthc Manag 47: 263-279.

39. Institute for Safe Medication Practices (2006) Our long journey towards a safety-minded Just Culture Part II: Where we're going.

40. Institute for Safe Medication Practices (2006) Our long journey towards a safety-minded Just Culture Part I: Where we've been.

15

Prevalence and Pattern of Potential Drug-Drug Interactions in the Critical Care Units of a Tertiary Hospital in Alexandria, Egypt

Sarah Mahmoud Abd El Samia Mohamed[1], Zahira Metwaly Gad[2], Nessrin Ahmed El-Nimr[3]* and Ahmed Abdel Hady Abdel Razek[4]

[1]*Pharmacist, Alexandria Main University Hospital, Egypt*
[2]*Professor of Epidemiology, Epidemiology Department, High Institute of Public Health, Alexandria University, Egypt*
[3]*Lecturer of Epidemiology, Epidemiology Department, High Institute of Public Health, Alexandria University, Egypt*
[4]*Lecturer of Critical Medicine, Faculty of Medicine, Alexandria University, Egypt*

Abstract

Background: The complexity of the pharmacotherapy involved in the simultaneous use of several drugs and various therapeutic classes makes critically ill patients at an increased risk for potential DDIs. The objectives were to estimate the prevalence of potential DDIs in the critical care units (CCUs) at a main trtiary hospital, to analyze their clinical significance, onset, documentation and severity and to identify their possible determinants.

Materials and methods: Using a cross sectional design, 750 patients, admitted to the CCUs, whose medical prescriptions contain 4 or more drugs were included. A pre-designed structured questionnaire and a record review sheet were used to collect the following data: sociodemographic, smoking habits, medical history, long term used medications, the presence of hospital aquired infections, APAHE II score, length of stay, organ impairment, number of drugs per prescription and the number of prescribing physicians. Calculating the number of interactions for each patient was performed. The list of prescribed drugs for patient was analyzed using different software.

Results: The prevalence of potential DDIs among patients admitted to CCUs was 53.07%. The mean number of interactions occurred per patient was 2.98 ± 1.91. The highest proportion of interactions had a significance number 1.0, possible and suspected documentation, delayed onset and moderate severity. Age of the patient and the number of prescribed drugs were the two independent factors found to be significantly affecting the prevalence of potential DDIs.

Conclusion: Critically ill patients are at risk of DDIs and the patients' age and the number of drugs prescribed increases this possibility.

Keywords: Critical care; Drug-drug interaction

Introduction

A drug-drug interaction (DDI) may be defined as the pharmacologic or clinical response to the administration of a drug combination different from that anticipated from the known effects of the two agents when given alone [1]. Stockley's drug interaction definition declares that an interaction is said to occur when the effects of one drug are changed by the presence of another drug, food, drink or by some environmental or chemical agent [2,3]. The clinical result of a DDI may manifest as antagonism, synergism or idiosyncratic. According to Drug Interaction Facts, each drug interaction pair has a monograph that includes the following sections: significance, type, mechanism, effect, management and monitoring of each DDI [3].

Drug-drug interactions are a preventable cause of morbidity and mortality [4,5]. Previous studies showed that DDIs significantly increased risk of hospitalization, significantly prolonged length of hospital stay, cost of treatment and elevated the risk of death [6-8]. The incidence and degree of severity of an interaction depend on both patient-related factors and information about the effects of the interaction. Patient-related factors include age, genetics, disease process, impairment of organ function, diet, alcohol consumption and smoking [1,9,10]. One of the risk factors for the occurrence of DDIs is the number of prescribed drugs. A positive correlation between polypharmacy and DDIs have been demonstrated in several studies [9,10]. The risk of DDIs can increase from approximately 6% in patients taking only two medications to 50% in those taking five medications and 100% in those taking ten medications [11]. Other determinants for the occurrence of a DDI include the pharmacokinetic profile and the pharmacological characteristics of the medications [4].

Critical care medicine is a multidisciplinary subspecialty that has realized remarkable growth over the last 40 to 50 years, paralleling advances in life support technologies [12]. Common features among the majority of critically ill patients are their acuity, complex pathophysiologic states and the use of a large number of pharmacologic agents in their management. On average, these patients have six to nine drugs prescribed per day while being cared for in the critical care unit (CCU) [12,13]. Due to the complexity of the pharmacotherapy involved in the simultaneous use of several drugs and various therapeutic classes, critically ill patients are at an increased risk for DDIs [4].

Recognition of the drug therapy selection, dosing and monitoring demands within the CCU by pioneering clinical pharmacists caused the development of critical care as a specialty within the pharmacy profession [12,13]. The number of adverse drug events and the subsequent cost of these events can be reduced by pharmacist intervention. Monitoring for adverse drug reactions was an importance

*Corresponding author: Nessrin Ahmed El-Nimr, Lecturer of Epidemiology, Epidemiology Department, High Institute of Public Health, Alexandria University, Egypt, E-mail: dr.elnimr@gmail.com

responsibility of the pharmacist. Many medications taken by CCU patients have significant adverse effect profiles and multiple known drug drug interactions [13].

The prevalence of potential DDIs among critically ill patients was studied by many authors in different countries [4,5,14-17]. In a study conducted to assess the role of pharmacist in identification of medication related problems in the ICU of a teaching hospital in Egypt, potential DDIs were detected among 8.4% of patients [18]. To our knowledge, no studies have been conducted in this field in our city. The objectives of the present study were to estimate the prevalence of potential DDIs in the CCUs at a main trtiary hospital in Alexandria, Egypt, to analyze their clinical significance, onset, documentation and severity and finally to identify their possible determinants.

Materials and Methods

A cross-sectional study was conducted throughout the second half of 2011 in the 1st and 3rd Critical Care Units (CCUs) at a main tertiary hospital in Alexandria, Egypt. The study was approved by the ethics committee at the High Institute of Public Health, Alexandria University. In addition, an approval to conduct the study was obtained from the hospital director and the head of the critical care department.

The inclusion criteria included patients (all ages and both sexes) admitted to the CCUs whose medical prescriptions contain 4 or more drugs. Patients using topical drugs (ointments, creams, ear drops or eye drops) were not included. The sample size was calculated using Epi info 6 program. Based on a prevalence of potential DDI of 8.4%, [19] level of significance 95% and level of precision 2%, the minimum required sample size was 750 patients. Patients were consecutively included in the study from both units till the completion of the sample size.

The required data were collected by interviewing patients (if conscious) or one of their relatives (during the official times for the visit) using a pre-designed structured questionnaire. The collected data included socio-demographic characteristics as age, sex, marital status, education and occupation as well as the social habitual risk factors as smoking cigarettes and shisha (local waterpipe).

A record review sheet was prepared to collect data about the presence of co-morbidities, the long-term used medications, the presence of hospital acquired infections, Acute Physiology and Chronic Health Evaluation II score (APACHE II score), length of stay in the CCUs, renal and hepatic impairments. In addition, a 24 hours prescription was reviewed for each patient [15,16]. Information regarding the number of drugs per prescription and the number of prescribing physicians during the patient's stay at the CCUs were also obtained.

Calculating the number of interactions between the prescribed drugs for each patient was performed. A to Z Drug Facts was used for classification of drug groups [20]. The list of drugs for each prescription was analyzed using each of the following: Drug interaction checker software "Drug Interaction Facts" (iFacts-AZ) Version: 13.5.0/2010.5.28, [21]. Stockley's Drug Interactions [2] and the British National Formulary [22]. Free online drug interaction checker programs were also used to identify the clinical value (level of significance), documentation (level of evidence or records), onset of effect (rapid or delayed) and the severity of the interaction (minor, moderate or major) [23-26].

Data management

The collected data were coded, entered and cleaned using SPSS

for Windows version 16.0 (SPSS Inc., Chicago, IL, USA). Descriptive statistics using frequency distribution tables and graphs was carried out. For quantitative variables, mean and standard deviation were calculated, while percent was used to describe categorical data. Pearson's chi square was used for analysis of categorical data. Multiple logistic regression analysis was used to estimate the strength of association between the exposure and a binary outcome. All statistical analyses were done using two tailed tests and a p value <0.05 was considered to be statistically significant.

Results

From a total of 750 patients studied, with the mean age of 44.46 ± 21.29 years, 54.8% were males, 69.62% were married and 34.17% were illiterate. The mean length of stay was 9.02 ± 12.70 days, the mean number of prescribed drugs per patient was 7 ± 2 and the mean number of prescribing physicians was 3 ± 2 for each patient. The principle conditions for admission of patients to the CCUs included cardiovascular diseases (44.53%), respiratory diseases (19.6%), external causes for morbidity and mortality such as: road traffic accidents, near drowning, gun shooting and explosion injury (14.13%) and injuries and poisoning (12.13%). About 62% of patients had co-morbid conditions including cardiovascular diseases (46.46%), endocrinal and metabolic diseases (26.25%), respiratory and genitourinary diseases (6.97% and 6.16% respectively).

The prevalence of potential DDIs among patients admitted to CCUs was 53.07%, figure 1. The majority of patients (67.34%) had 1-3 interactions among their medications, while 28.39% had 4-6 interactions. Only 4.27% of patients had 7 or more l potential DDIs among their prescribed medications. The mean number of interactions occurred per patient was 2.98 ± 1.91 interactions (range, 1-12 interactions). There were 89 different potential DDI pairs. The total number of potential DDIs was 1183 interactions.

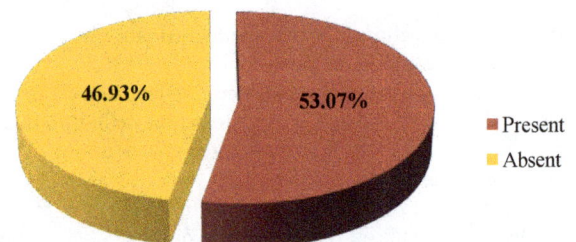

Figure 1: Prevalence of potential DDIs among patients admitted to CCUs (Alexandria, 2011).

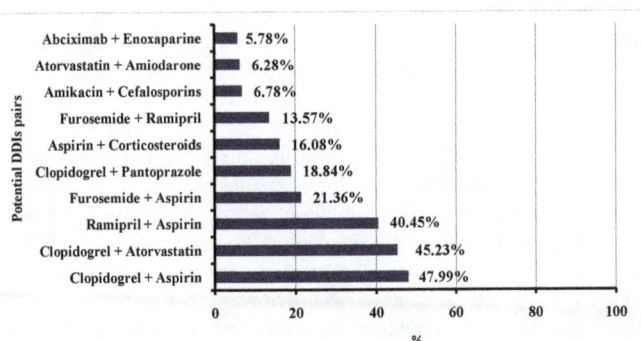

Figure 2: Top 10 potential DDIs among patients admitted to the CCUs (Alexandria, 2011).

Figure 2 illustrates the top ten potential DDIs that occurred among patients admitted to the CCUs. Interactions from the co-administration of Clopidogrel with Aspirin ranked first (47.99%), followed by the co-administration of Clopidogrel with Atorvastatin (45.23%) and the co-administration of Ramipril with Aspirin (40.45%). The proportion of interactions that resulted from the co-administration of Furosemide with Aspirin, Clopidogrel with Pantoprazole, Aspirin with Corticosteroids and Furosemide with Ramipril ranged from 13.57% to 21.36%, while 5.78% to 6.78% of patients had interactions that resulted from the co-administration of Amikacin with Cephalosporins, Atorvastatin with Amiodarone, and the co-administration of Abciximab with Enoxaparine.

Figure 3 shows the distribution of the detected 1183 potential DDIs according to their clinical value, documentation, onset and severity. As regards the clinical value (Figure 3a), the highest proportion of interactions (30.52%) had a significance number 1.0, followed by significant numbers 4.0 and 2.0 (27.13% and 25.71%, respectively). The highest proportion of interactions had possible and suspected documentation, followed by probable documentation (35.76%, 31.87% and 26.63%, respectively). Interactions with unlikely documentations were the least common (1.52%), as shown in figure 3b. Regarding onset of effect (Figure 3c), 77.09% of the potential DDIs detected had a delayed onset (after 24 hours) and 18.85% had a rapid onset (within the 24 hours). Considering severity, nearly half of the interactions (52.83%) had moderate effects (worsening of the clinical condition) and 32.21% had major effects (potential risk of life or irreversible damage). Only 14.96% had minor effects (imperceptible or light), figure 3d.

Table 1 shows that of the age of patients admitted to the CCUs ranged between 9 months to 99 years. It is obvious from the table that as the age of patients increased, the prevalence of potential DDIs increased. This association was statistically significant (X^2=100.1, p=0.000). Males had a slightly higher prevalence of potential DDIs than females. However, this difference was not statistically significant. Married and widowed patients had higher rates of potential DDIs, while single patients had the least rate of potential DDIs. This association was statistically significant (X^2=52.6, p=0.000). It is clear from the table that the higher the level of education, the lower the proportion of potential DDIs. This association was statistically significant (X^2=35.9, p=0.000). Patients who were retired, housewives or non skilled workers had higher rates of potential DDIs, followed by skilled workers. Students had the least proportion of potential DDIs. This association was statistically significant (X^2=41.9, p=0.000). As regards smoking habits, higher rates of potential DDIs were found among patients who smoked cigarettes and shisha, compared to those who did not smoke. The association between smoking and the presence of potential DDIs was statistically significant (X^2=11.1, p=0.000 and X^2=28.3, p=0.001, respectively).

Table 2 shows that the mean length of stay of patients at the CCUs was 9.02 ± 12.7 days (range, 1-125 days). Patients who stayed in the CCUs between 25 to <30 days had the highest prevalence of potential DDIs, followed by those who stayed from 5 to <10 days, while those who stayed for 30 days or more had the lowest proportion of potential DDIs, with a statistically insignificant difference. Patients who had renal or hepatic impairments had a higher prevalence of potential DDIs. This association was statistically significant (X^2=5.1, p=0.024). The table also shows that the mean APACHE II score of patients admitted to CCUs was 18 ± 10 (range, 2-45). The highest prevalence of potential DDIs was found among patients who had an APACHE II score that ranged from 31 to <41, followed by those who had a score that ranged from 11 to <21. The least prevalence was found among patients with a score range of 41 to 51. This association was statistically significant (X^2= 13.4, p=0.010).

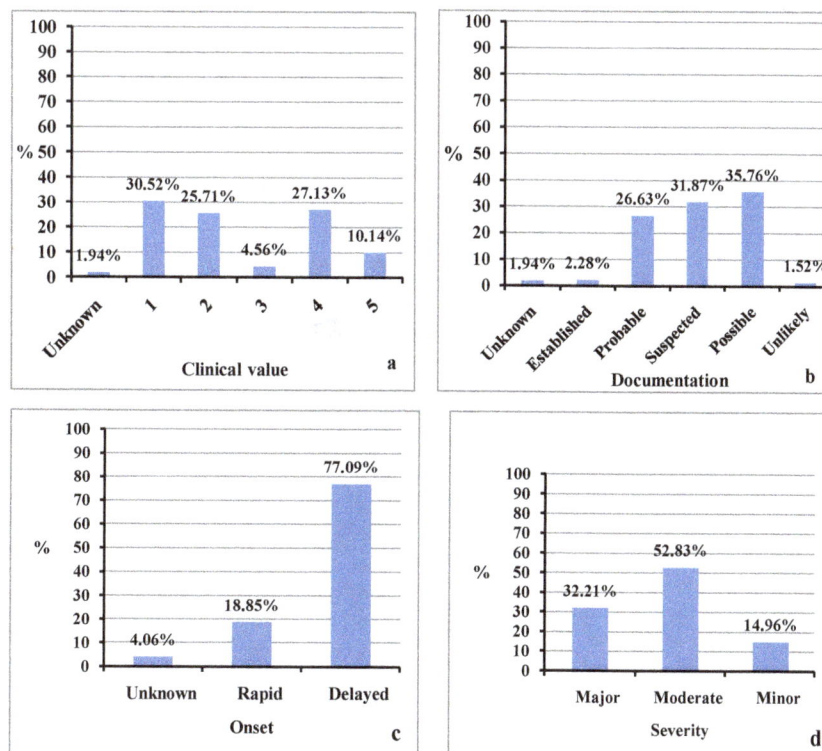

Figure 3: Distribution of potential DDIs among medications prescribed to patients admitted to CCUs according to the a) clinical value, b) documentation, c) onset and d) severity of the interactions (Alexandria, 2011).

Personal characteristics and smoking habits	Potential DDIs		X^2
	Present (n=398) No. (%)	Absent (n=352) No. (%)	
1- Personal characteristics:			
Age in years:			
<20	32 (24.6)	98 (75.4)	
20-	49 (33.8)	96 (66.2)	
40-	166 (64.6)	91 (35.4)	100.1* p=0.000
60-	133 (68.6)	61 (31.4)	
80+	18 (75.0)	6 (25.0)	
Mean ± SD (range)	44.46 ± 21.29 (9 months-99 years)		
Sex:			
Male	226 (55.0)	185 (45.0)	1.3
Female	172 (50.7)	167 (49.3)	p=0.246
Marital status:			
Single	34 (27.2)	91 (72.8)	
Married	298 (62.2)	181 (37.8)	52.6*
Widowed	39 (66.1)	20 (33.9)	p=0.000
Divorced	12 (48.0)	13 (52.0)	
Education:			
Illiterate	158 (64.8)	86 (35.2)	
Read and write	92 (62.2)	56 (37.8)	
Primary or preparatory	45 (55.6)	36 (44.4)	35.9*
Secondary	51 (42.1)	70 (57.9)	p=0.000
University	45 (37.8)	74 (62.2)	
Post graduate	0 (0.0)	1 (100.0)	
Occupation:			
Don't work	26 (45.6)	31(54.4)	
Housewife	146 (62.1)	89 (37.9)	
Retired	55 (67.9)	26 (32.1)	41.9*
Student	21 (26.3)	59 (73.8)	p=0.000
Skilled worker	39 (58.2)	28 (41.8)	
Non skilled worker	60 (60.0)	40 (40.0)	
2- Smoking habits:			
Smoking cigarettes			
Yes	179 (63.0)	105 (37.0)	11.1*
No	205 (50.2)	203 (49.8)	p=0.001
Smoking shisha			
Yes	124 (63.6)	71 (36.4)	28.3*
No	260 (52.3)	237 (47.7)	p=0.000

*Significant (p<0.05)

Table 1: Distribution of potential DDIs among patients admitted to CCUs according to their personal characteristics and smoking habits (Alexandria, 2011).

The mean number of prescribed medications per prescription was 7 ± 2 medications (range, 4-15 medications). It is clear from table 2 that as the number of medications prescribed increased, the prevalence of potential DDIs also increased. This association was statistically significant (X^2= 101.2, p=0.000). The number of prescribing physicians per patient ranged from 1-14 physicians (mean=3 ± 2 physicians). Unexpectedly, the prevalence of potential DDIs decreased as the number of prescribing physicians increased, except for patients who had 13 to 15 physicians, where all of them had potential DDIs. No statistically significant association was found. An almost equal prevalence of potential DDIs was found among both patients with and without hospital acquired infections, with a statistically insignificant difference. The proportion of potential DDIs was higher among patients who had co-morbid conditions, with a statistically significant difference (X^2=25.9, p=0.000). Finally, table 2 shows that patients with long term use of medications had a higher proportion of potential

DDIs. This association was statistically significant (X^2=19.6, p=0.000).

Table 3 shows the logistic regression analysis of the factors affecting the prevalence of potential DDIs among patients admitted to the CCUs as the dependent variable. Only two independent factors were found to be significantly affecting the prevalence of potential DDIs. The first factor was the patient's age (OR=1.023, 95% CI=1.012-1.034). The second was the number of prescribed drugs (OR=1.762, 95% CI=1.584-1.960). The model correctly classified 74.9% of cases.

Parameter	Potential DDIs		X^2
	Present (n=398) No. (%)	Absent (n=352) No. (%)	
Length of stay in days:			
Age in years:			
<5	196 (53.6)	170 (46.4)	
5-	102 (58.0)	74 (42.0)	
10-	46 (52.9)	41 (47.1)	
15-	15 (37.5)	25 (62.5)	9.7
20-	10 (35.7)	18 (64.3)	p=0.139
25-	6 (66.7)	3 (33.3)	
30+	23 (52.3)	21 (47.7)	
Mean ± SD (range)	9.0 2 ± 12.7 (1-125)		
Renal or hepatic impairment:			
Yes	285 (55.9)	225 (44.1)	5.1*
No	172 (50.7)	167 (49.3)	p=0.024
APACHE II score:			
≤10	109 (47.2)	122 (52.8)	
11-	192 (57.5)	142 (42.5)	
21-	56 (48.3)	60 (51.7)	13.4*
31-	34 (68.0)	16 (32.0)	p=0.010
41-45	7 (36.8)	12 (63.2)	
Mean ± SD (range)	18 ± 10 (2-45)		
Number of prescribed medications/prescription:			
4-6	101 (28.0)	260 (72.0)	
7-9	209 (72.8)	78 (27.2)	101.2*
10-12	79 (84.9)	14 (15.1)	p=0.000
13-15	9 (100.0)	0 (0.0)	
Mean ± SD (range)	7 ± 2 (4-15)	74 (62.2)	
Number of prescribing physicians/patient:			
4-6	78 (52.3)	71 (47.7)	
7-9	18 (46.2)	21(53.8)	3.9
10-12	3 (37.5)	5 (62.5)	p=0.268
13-15	3 (100.0)	0 (0.0)	
Mean ± SD (range)	3 ± 2 (1-14)		
Presence of hospital acquired infection:			
Yes	131 (51.6)	123 (48.4)	0.34
No	267 (53.8)	229 (46.2)	p=0.558
Presence of co-morbidities:			
Yes	281 (60.3)	185 (39.7)	25.9*
No	117 (41.2)	167 (58.8)	p=0.000
Long term use of medications:			
Yes	243 (60.6)	158 (39.4)	19.6*
No	155 (44.4)	194 (55.6)	p=0.000

*Significant (p<0.05)
APACHE, Acute Physiology and Chronic Health Evaluation

Table 2: Distribution of potential DDIs among patients admitted to CCUs according to certain parameters (Alexandria, 2011).

Independent variables	Coefficient B	p. value	Odds ratio	95% Confidence Interval
Age	.022	0.000	1.023	1.012-1.034
Number of prescribed drugs	.567	0.000	1.762	1.584-1.960
Constant	-4.567			

Sensitivity of the model was 74.9%

Table 3: Logistic regression analysis of the factors affecting the prevalence of potential DDIs among patients admitted to CCUs (Alexandria, 2011).

Discussion

Drug interaction is a very important issue in drug therapy, especially in pediatric and geriatric patients. Patients admitted at the CCU are at higher risk for the development of DDIs. Patients in the CCU often are aged and have physiological alteration, summing up to unfavorable clinical conditions for drug metabolism such as shock, renal failure and hepatic disease [14]. The study highlighted a 53.07% prevalence of potential DDIs that would have resulted from the combinations of the prescribed drugs. This finding was comparable with those reported in other studies [5,27]. Higher rates were reported from Brazil in 2008 [14] and 2011 [4] and from Switzerland in 2010 [28], while lower rates were reported from Canada in 2007 [29] and Egypt in 2009 [18]. One important reason for discrepancies among studies is different classification and inclusion/exclusion of potential DDIs. Others reasons may include the decisions used to provide drug therapy, hospital pharmacists' work and the availability of electronic drug information system in the hospital.

The present study showed that interactions with significant levels 1.0 and 2.0 were among the most prevalent types, accounting for more than half of the potential DDIs observed. This means that in most cases the patient's life could be at risk and in such cases the physician and nursing staff should keep the patient under close observation. On the other hand, type 4.0 accounted for about one quarter of all potential DDIs, meaning that the drugs prescribed for patients will not cause any serious or fatal interactions [1]. Similar results were reported in other studies [15,29]. In contrast, other studies declared that the most prevalent type of interactions observed were types 4.0 and 5.0 [14,30].

Most of the potential DDIs observed in the current study were of the delayed type, which could take up to several days or weeks to occur, needing no immediate concern or medical intervention [1]. Lower percentages of delayed onset potential DDIs, ranging from 48.7% to 61%, were reported by many other studies [5,14,15,27,30]. On the other hand, higher percentages of delayed onset potential DDIs were reported by Iranmanesh et al., in 2012 (89.2%) [31].

Considering the severity of interactions, the current study found that about one third of the potential DDIs observed were major interactions, and in such cases the patient's life could be threatened and immediate medical intervention is required [1]. Much lower rate was reported by Bertolia et al. (2010) [28]. About half of the potential DDIs in the present work had a moderate severity of action. In such case, patients should be kept under close observation to prevent any complications [1]. Other studies reported that nearly half of the interactions of moderate severity [14,30]. Higher percentages were found in several studies [5,15,27,29,31].

Several studies reported that the most prevalent interactions were of possible and probable documentation, [5,14,15,29-31] which was in accordance with the current results. It should be noted that proper monitoring of patients, a reduction in the dosage regimen and increasing the dosing intervals could help to reduce risks of severe drug interactions which are well documented. Most of the observed potential DDIs counted for probable, suspected and possible documentation.

Regarding the top ten potential DDIs, interactions of oral anticoagulants (clopidorel) and low dose aspirin/statins/proton pump inhibitors (pantoprazole) ranked 1st, 2nd and 5th, respectively. This finding was comparable with that reported by Bertolia et al. (2010) [28]. Interactions of low dose aspirin and ACE inhibitors and the interaction of aspirin and corticosteroids ranked 3rd and 6th interactions, respectively. Similar findings were reported by Riechelmann et al. (2007) [29] and Hammes et al., (2009) [14]. The 7th potential DDI resulted from the co-administration of furosemide with ramipril. Other studies reported comparable findings [4,15]. The 8th potential interaction resulted from the concurrent use of aminoglycoside antibiotics as amikacin with cephalosporin antibiotics as cefoperazone. This finding was similar to that reported in another study [4].

The factors that had a significant association with the occurrence of DDIs in the present work included the patient's age, marital state, level of education, occupation, smoking cigarettes, smoking shisha, presence of renal or hepatic impairment, APACHE II score, number of prescribed medications per prescription, number of prescribing physicians per patient, presence of comorbidities and the long term use of medications. These findings were comparable with those reportd in several studies [4-6,13,14,28,31].

Logistic regression analysis for the possible risk factors of DDIs among patients admitted to the CCUs in the present work showed that the age of patient and the number of prescribed drugs were the only significant factors. These findings were in accordance with other studies which showed that both variables were indeed two of the major, if not the most important, risk factors for DDIs [6,14,27-29]. Other risk factors for the occurrence of DDIs identified by other studies included sex [27] and length of hospital stay [4,6]. Although the current findings showed that DDIs were not preventable, awareness of the medical team on the prevalence, risk factors and mechanisms involved in the occurrence of potential DDIs can help in the reduction of the real occurrence of potential DDIs among hospitalized patients in general and the critically ill patients in specific.

In conclusion, critically ill patients are at risk of DDIs (53.07%). Potential DDIs with a clinical value 1, possible documentation, delayed onset or moderate severity were the most frequently identified. Patients' age and the number of drugs prescribed were the independent risk factor for increase of this possibility. So, to avoid DDIs and improve the treatment of patients in the CCUs, continued education, computer system for prescriptions, pharmacotherapy monitoring of patients and the pharmacist participation in the multidisciplinary team are essential.

References

1. Tatro DS (2009) Drug interaction facts. St. Louis, MO: Wolters Kluwer Health, Inc.

2. Stockley IH (2005) editor. Stockley's Drug Interactions. 9th ed. London: Pharmaceutical Press.

3. Bista D, Palaian S, Shankar PR, Prabhu MM, Paudel R, et al. (2007) Understanding the essentials of drug interactions: a potential need for safe and effective use of drugs. Kathmandu Univ Med J (KUMJ) 5: 421-430.

4. Reis AM, Cassiani SH (2011) Prevalence of potential drug interactions in patients in an intensive care unit of a university hospital in Brazil. Clinics (Sao Paulo) 66: 9-15.

5. Bista D, Saha A, Mishra P, Palaian S, Shankar PR (2009) Pattern of potential drug-drug interactions in the intensive care unit of a teaching hospital in Nepal: a pilot study. JCDR 3: 1713.

6. Moura CS, Acurcio FA, Belo NO (2009) Drug-drug interactions associated with length of stay and cost of hospitalization. J Pharm Pharm Sci 12: 266-272.

7. Vonbach P (2009) Drug-drug interactions in the hospital. Basel: Südwestdeutscher Verlag Für Hochschulschriften AG.

8. Ernst FR, Grizzle AJ (2001) Drug-related morbidity and mortality: updating the cost-of-illness model. J Am Pharm Assoc (Wash) 41: 192-199.

9. Gennaro AR (2000) Remington: The science and practice of pharmacy. 20th ed. Philadelphia: Lippincott Williams & Wilkins.

10. World Health Organization (2008) WHO Model Formulary. Geneva: WHO Press 634.

11. Lin P (2003) Drug interactions and polypharmacy in the elderly. The Canadian Alzheimer disease review 10-4.

12. Helms RA (2006) Textbook of therapeutics: Drug and disease management. 6th ed. Philadelphia, Pa: Lippincott Williams & Wilkins.

13. Saokaew S, Maphanta S, Thangsomboon P (2009) Impact of pharmacist's interventions on cost of drug therapy in intensive care unit. Pharmacy Practice 7: 81-87.

14. Hammes JA, Pfuetzenreiter F, Silveira F, Koenig A, Westphal GA (2008) Potential drug interactions prevalence in intensive care units. Rev Bras TerIntensiva 20: 349-354.

15. Nazari MA, Moqhadam NK (2006) Evaluation of pharmacokinetic drug interactions in prescriptions of intensive care unit in a teaching hospital. Iran J Pharm Res 3: 215-218.

16. Rafiei H, Arab M, Ranjbar H, Sepehri GR, Arab N, et al. (2012) The prevalence of potential drug interactions in Intensive Care Units. J Crit Care 4: 191-196.

17. Lima RE, De Bortoli Cassiani SH (2009) Potential drug interactions in intensive care patients at a teaching hospital. Rev Lat Am Enfermagem 17: 222-227.

18. Sabry NA, Farid SF, Abdel Aziz EO (2009) Role of the pharmacist in identification of medication related problems in the ICU: A preliminary screening study in an Egyptian teaching hospital. Aust J Basic appl sci 3: 995-1003.

19. World Health Organization (2006) WHO Model Formulary. London: Royal Pharmaceutical Society of Great Britain 501.

20. Tatro DS (2007) A to Z drug facts. 8th ed. Lippincott Williams & Wilkins, Facts & Comparisons.

21. Skyscape.com [Internet]. Boston: Facts and comparisons; ©2010 [cited Jul 2011]. Skyscape.com, Inc.

22. Joint Formulary Committee. (2009) British national formulary. London: British Medical Association and Royal Pharmaceutical Society of Great Britain 978.

23. MIMS [Internet]. USA: Drug interaction checker; ©2013 [cited 2013 Jan 9].

24. Drugs.com [Internet]. New Zealand: Drug interactions checker. Wolters Kluwer Health, Physicians' Desk Reference, Cerner Multum and Thomson Micromedex; ©2000-2010 [updated 2010 May 1; cited 2013 Jan 4].

25. Healthline [Internet]. Drug interaction checker. New York; ©2005 – 2010 [updated 2010 May 1; cited 2012 Dec 12].

26. Medscape drug interaction checker [Internet]. New York: The American Society of Health-System Pharmacists; ©1994-2010 [updated 2010 May 1; cited 2012 Nov 21].

27. Cruciol-Souza JM, Thomson JC (2006) A pharmacoepidemiologic study of drug interactions in a Brazilian teaching hospital. Clinics (Sao Paulo) 61: 515-520.

28. Bertoli R, Bissig M, Caronzolo D, Odorico M, Pons M, et al. (2010) Assessment of potential drug-drug interactions at hospital discharge. Swiss Med Wkly 140: w13043.

29. Riechelmann RP, Tannock IF, Wang L, Saad ED, Taback NA, et al. (2007) Potential drug interactions and duplicate prescriptions among cancer patients. J Natl Cancer Inst 99: 592-600.

30. Hajebi G, Mortazavi SA (2002) An investigation of drug interactions in hospital pharmacy prescriptions. Iran J Pharm Res 1: 15-19.

31. Iranmanesh S, Rafiei H, Aein F (2011) The study of potential drug-drug interactions among older patients admitted to the intensive care unit in Kerman, Iran. Middle East J Age Ageing 7: 37-41.

16

Prevalence, Determinants, and Reasons for the Non-Reporting of Adverse Drug Reactions by Pharmacists in the Miyagi and Hokkaido Regions of Japan

Obara T[1,2]*, Yamaguchi H[1], Satoh M[1], Iida Y[1], Sakai T[3], Aoki Y[4], Murai Y[1,5], Matsuura M[1], Sato M[1], Ohkubo T[6], Iseki K[7] and Mano N[1]

[1]Department of Pharmaceutical Sciences, Tohoku University Hospital, Sendai, Japan
[2]Department of Preventive Medicine and Epidemiology, Tohoku Medical Megabank Organization, Tohoku University, Sendai, Japan
[3]Pharmaceutical Information Center, Faculty of Pharmacy, Meijo University, Nagoya, Japan
[4]National Institute of Health Sciences, Tokyo, Japan
[5]Pharmacy Education and Research Center, Tohoku University Graduate School of Pharmaceutical Sciences, Sendai, Japan
[6]Department of Hygiene and Public Health, Teikyo University School of Medicine, Tokyo, Japan
[7]Department of Pharmacy, Hokkaido University Hospital, Sapporo, Japan

Abstract

Little is known about the potential of adverse drug reaction (ADR) non-reporting by Japanese pharmacists. The aim of the present study was to clarify the prevalence, determinants, and reasons for ADR non-reporting by pharmacists in the Miyagi and Hokkaido regions of Japan. In this cross-sectional, self-administered questionnaire-based study, we contacted 3,164 pharmacists who belonged to the Miyagi Prefecture Hospital Pharmacists Association or the Hokkaido Society of Hospital Pharmacists during the 3-month period between January to March 2013. Of the 1,795 respondents 22.4% were <30 years of age, 25.6% were ≥ 50 years of age, and 42.1% were female. A total of 77.6% of the respondents did not have a personal history of ADR reporting. The multivariate logistic regression analysis showed that female sex (odds ratio, 1.52; 95% confidence interval, 1.17-1.97), having <10 years of practical experience (2.59, 1.39-4.82 for 5-9 years; 7.03, 2.94-16.83 for <5 years), working at a community pharmacy or drugstore (1.90, 1.16-3.12), having <5 pharmacists in the workplace (2.01, 1.48-2.75), and not understanding the ADR reporting system (5.93, 4.23-8.33) were significantly and independently associated with not having a personal history of ADR reporting. The most common reason for ADR non-reporting was "It was a well-known adverse drug reaction" (43.0%) followed by "Association between the drug and adverse reaction was not clear" (38.0%), "It was a minor adverse drug reaction" (29.0%), "Did not know how to make a report" (17.4%), and "Never been consulted about ADRs" (17.2%). As an understanding the ADR reporting system was strongly associated with ADR reporting, a more aggressive promotion of the ADR reporting system among pharmacists is warranted.

Keywords: Adverse drug reaction; Pharmacist; Questionnaire

Abbreviations

ADR: Adverse Drug Reaction; JADER: The Japanese Adverse Drug Event Report Database; PMDA: The Pharmaceutical and Medical Devices Agency

Introduction

A spontaneous adverse drug reaction (ADR) reporting system is traditionally used for postmarketing drug safety surveillance in many countries. There are several reports from various countries that have demonstrated both knowledge and attitudes of health professionals are associated with spontaneous ADR reporting [1,2]. However, ADR reporting systems can differ depending upon the particular region, with the guidelines for determining relevant cases and reporting methods found to vary from country to country. Japan first began collecting information on adverse reactions to drugs after the enactment of a law in 1961. Since then, there has been an accumulation of information on serious adverse events from individual case and study reports from industries, direct voluntary reports from medical institutions, and study results from treatment outcome studies (all-case surveillance), as well as postmarketing clinical trials.

As a result, information from approximately 350,000 adverse event cases has been reported. Events that occurred after 2004 have been compiled in the Japanese Adverse Drug Event Report database (JADER), with this information becoming available for download through the Pharmaceutical and Medical Devices Agency (PMDA) website starting in 2012 (http://www.pmda.go.jp/safety/reports/hcp/0001.html). Within the clinical setting, pharmacists have the professional responsibility for pharmacovigilance. However, little is known regarding the potential non-reporting of ADRs by Japanese pharmacists. Therefore, the aim of the present study was to clarify the prevalence, determinants, and reasons for ADR non-reporting by pharmacists in the Miyagi and Hokkaido regions of Japan.

Methods

This study was a cross-sectional, self-administered questionnaire-based study involving pharmacists who belonged to the Miyagi Prefecture Hospital Pharmacists Association or the Hokkaido Society of Hospital Pharmacists. The questionnaire was developed based on previous studies [1,3,4] and was pre-tested on a sample group that consisted of ten pharmacists and five pharmacovigilance professionals to whom the purpose of the study was explained. Based on the comments received during the pilot testing, slight modifications to the wording of the questionnaire were made prior to its use in this study. Data from the pilot study were not included in the final analysis.

*Corresponding author: Obara T, Department of Pharmaceutical Sciences, Tohoku University Hospital, 2-1 Seiryou-cho, Aoba-ku, Sendai 980-8574, Japan, E-mail: obara-t@hosp.tohoku.ac.jp

The final questionnaire consisted of five sections: (a) Characteristics of the pharmacists (age, sex, workplace, experience as a pharmacist, postgraduate degree, and the number of pharmacists in the workplace); (b) Knowledge of the ADR reporting system; (c) Personal history of ADR reporting; (d) Reasons for not having reported an ADR; (e) Personal opinion on pharmacovigilance (preference for receiving information on pharmacovigilance, and who was responsible for pharmacovigilance within the clinical practice); and (f) Knowledge of recent developments in pharmacovigilance in Japan and terminology related to pharmacovigilance (payment system for medical services, database for pharmacovigilance, 'pharmacovigilance per se', and 'regulatory science'). The questionnaire was distributed and collected by mail, with the study conducted over the 3-month period between January to March 2013. Parts of the responses to the questionnaire were used for this paper.

Pharmacists who did not know about the ADR reporting system or who knew about it but did not understand how the ADR reporting system worked were defined as the 'not understanding the ADR reporting system' group. After classifying the participants, a chi-square test was used to compare the prevalence of pharmacists who did not understand the ADR reporting system and who did not have a personal history of ADR reporting (ADR non-reporting) in each category (age, sex, level of education, years of practical experience, workplace, number of pharmacists within the workplace, and region).

Determinants of 'not understanding the ADR reporting system' and 'ADR non-reporting' were identified through the use of multilevel and multivariate logistic regression analyses to estimate odds ratios (ORs) with 95% confidence intervals (CIs) for not understanding the ADR reporting system and ADR non-reporting. Multivariate logistic regression analysis was adjusted for variables that were significantly related to not understanding the ADR reporting system and ADR non-reporting on univariate analyses. Data are shown as means ± standard deviation (SD). A p-value less than 0.05 were defined as significant. All statistical analyses were conducted with SAS version 9.4 (SAS Institute Inc., Cary, NC, USA).

Results

Of the 3,164 pharmacists who were sent questionnaires, 1,877 (59.3%) responded. The analysis excluded those pharmacists who did not completely answer the questions about age, sex, knowledge of the ADR reporting system, and personal history of ADR reporting. Characteristics of the 1,795 pharmacists who were eligible for the analysis was shown in Table 1. 22.4% were <30 years of age, 25.6% were ≥ 50 years of age, and 42.1% were women. The analysis showed that 3.0% of the pharmacists had a doctorate, 35.2% had ≥ 20 years of experience as a pharmacist, ≥88.1% worked in a hospital, and 43.3% worked at a place where there were ≥ 10 pharmacists. The prevalence of pharmacists who did not understand the ADR reporting system and who did not have a personal history of ADR reporting was shown in Figure 1. The percentages of pharmacists who did not understand the ADR reporting system and who did not have a personal history of ADR reporting were 38.7% and 77.6%, respectively. The analysis revealed that not understanding the ADR reporting system and ADR non-reporting were significantly associated with being female, younger, not having a postdoctoral degree, having a shorter period of experience, working in a community pharmacy, and having fewer pharmacists in their workplace.

Results of the multivariate logistic regression analyses for not understanding the ADR reporting system and not having a personal

history of ADR reporting were shown in Table 2. The multivariate logistic regression analysis showed that having a master's degree (OR, 2.80; 95% CI, 1.19-6.63), bachelor's degree (3.02, 1.30-7.01), <20 years of practical experience (1.63, 1.12-2.35 for 10-19 years; 3.13, 1.96-4.97 for 5-9 years; 2.60, 1.50-4.48 for <5 years), and having 5-9 other pharmacists in the workplace (1.41, 1.10-1.81) were significantly associated with not understanding the ADR reporting system. The multivariate logistic regression analysis also showed that the female sex (1.52, 1.17-1.97), having <10 years of practical experience (2.59, 1.39-4.82 for 5-9 years; 7.03, 2.94-16.83 for <5 years), working at a community pharmacy or drugstore (1.90, 1.16-3.12), having <5 pharmacists in the workplace (2.01, 1.48-2.75), and not understanding the ADR reporting system (5.93, 4.23-8.33) were significantly and independently associated with not having a personal history of ADR reporting.

Reasons for ADR non-reporting among pharmacists who did not have a personal history of ADR reporting are shown in Table 3. Overall, the most common reason for ADR non-reporting was "It was a well-known ADR" (43.0%) followed by "Association between the drug and adverse reaction was not clear" (38.0%), "It was an insignificant ADR" (29.0%), "Did not know how to make a report" (17.4%), and "Never been consulted about ADRs" (17.2%). Among pharmacists who selected 'Other' as the reason for ADR non-reporting, the most common response was "Report was sent to the pharmaceutical company". A significantly greater proportion of pharmacists who did not understand the ADR reporting system selected "Did not know how to make a report," "Did not have time to make a report," "Believe reporting is the responsibility of the physician," and "Did not understand the significance of reporting" as the reasons for ADR non-reporting compared to the pharmacists who did understand the ADR reporting system.

Discussion

The present study found that 1) 77.6% of pharmacists did not have a personal history of ADR reporting; 2) the determinants of ADR non-reporting included being female, having <10 years of practical experience, working at a community pharmacy or drugstore, and having <5 pharmacists in the workplace; and 3) the most common reason for ADR non-reporting was "It was a well-known ADR."

This is the first report to examine the awareness and practice of Japanese pharmacists with respect to the ADR reporting system. The voluntary ADR reporting system is a method of collecting information on adverse events that has already been implemented in many countries globally. In order to obtain information on adverse events and achieve proper usage of pharmaceutical products, it is essential to assess the awareness of the ADR reporting system among healthcare providers including pharmacists.

Prevalence

Although there were some variations with regard to the age, sex, level of education, years of practical experience, workplace, and number of pharmacists in the workplace, the present study demonstrated that 38.7% of the pharmacists did not understand the ADR reporting system and that 77.6% did not have a personal history of ADR reporting. In particular, the percentage of pharmacists who did not understand the ADR reporting system or did not have experience with reporting was highest among pharmacists who were women, were younger, did not have a doctorate degree, had less experience as a pharmacist, worked at

Sex	
Female, %	42.1
Male, %	57.9
Age	
<30 years, %	22.4
30-39 years, %	30.4
40-49 years, %	21.6
≥ 50 years, %	25.6
Highest level of education	
Bachelors, %	65.4
Masters, %	17.0
Doctorate, %	3.0
No answer, %	14.6
Years of practical experience as a pharmacist	
<5 years, %	16.0
5-9 years, %	22.0
10-19 years, %	25.0
≥ 20 years, %	35.2
No answer, %	1.8
Workplace	
Hospital, doctor's office, or clinic, %	88.1
Community pharmacy or drugstore, %	9.8
Other, %	2.0
No answer, %	0.2
Number of pharmacists in the work place	
<5, %	31.8
5-9, %	24.7
≥ 10, %	43.3
No answer, %	0.1
Region	
Miyagi, %	25.4
Hokkaido, %	74.7
Understanding the ADR reporting system	
I understand what it is, %	61.3
I have heard of it, but do not understand what it is, %	35.2
I do not know what it is, %	3.5
Personal history of ADR reporting	
No, %	77.6
Yes, %	22.4
Understanding the ADR reporting system for patients and their family	
I understand what it is, %	34.5
I have heard of it, but do not understand what it is, %	28.4
I do not know what it is, %	36.8
No answer, %	0.2

ADR: Adverse Drug Reaction

Table 1: Characteristics of participants (n=1,795).

a community pharmacy, and had fewer pharmacists in their workplace. Previously published studies have shown that the percentage of pharmacists without experience in making reports ranged between 75.0% and 85.4% [1,3-5], which indicates that the understanding and the specific measures pursued with regard to ADR reporting among pharmacists may be similar between Japan and other countries. Since the role of pharmacists and the ADR reporting systems is known to differ slightly between countries, it may not be appropriate to directly compare the present results with the findings from these previous studies. However, at a fundamental level, the role of pharmacists in drug safety evaluations is most likely quite similar countries of the developed world.

Factors related to not understanding the reporting system and non-reporting

The present study found that the determinants of not understanding the reporting system were: having a master's or bachelor's degree as the highest level of education (vs. doctorate degree), <20 years of practical experience, and 5-9 pharmacists in the workplace. Furthermore, the determinants for the non-reporting included: female sex, <10 years of practical experience, working at a community pharmacy or drugstore, and <5 pharmacists in the workplace. Factors that reflected an inadequate education or information presentation were extracted as the determinants for not understanding the system. It has been previously reported that enrichment of the pharmacy education and a continuing

a. Percentage of pharmacists who did not understand the ADR reporting system.

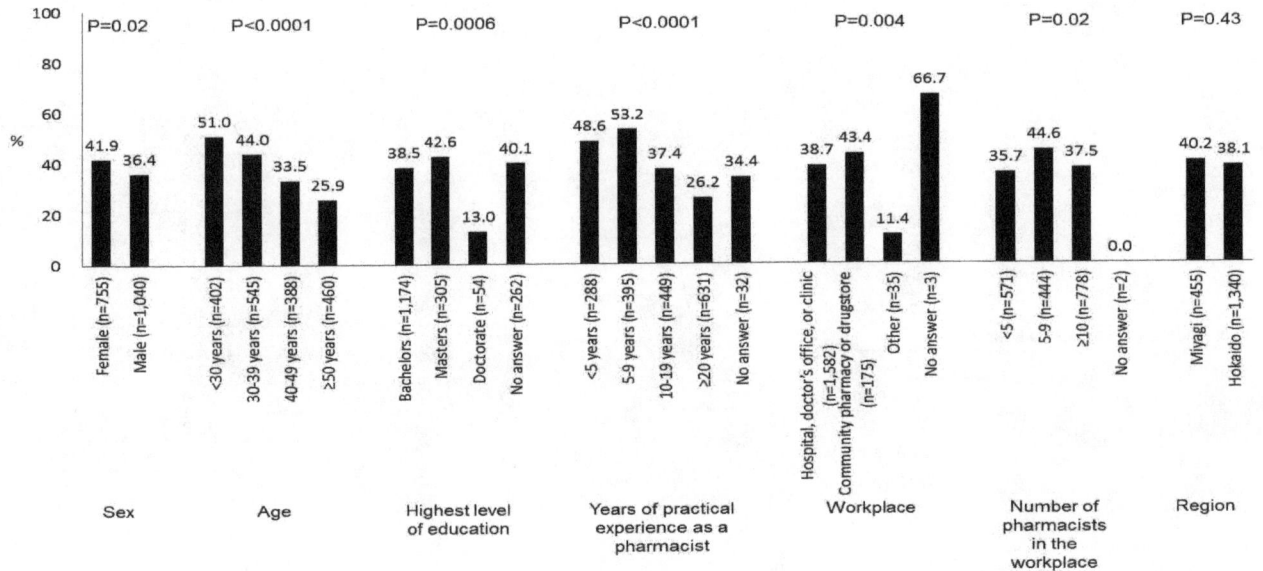

b. Percentage of pharmacists who did not have a personal history of ADR reporting.

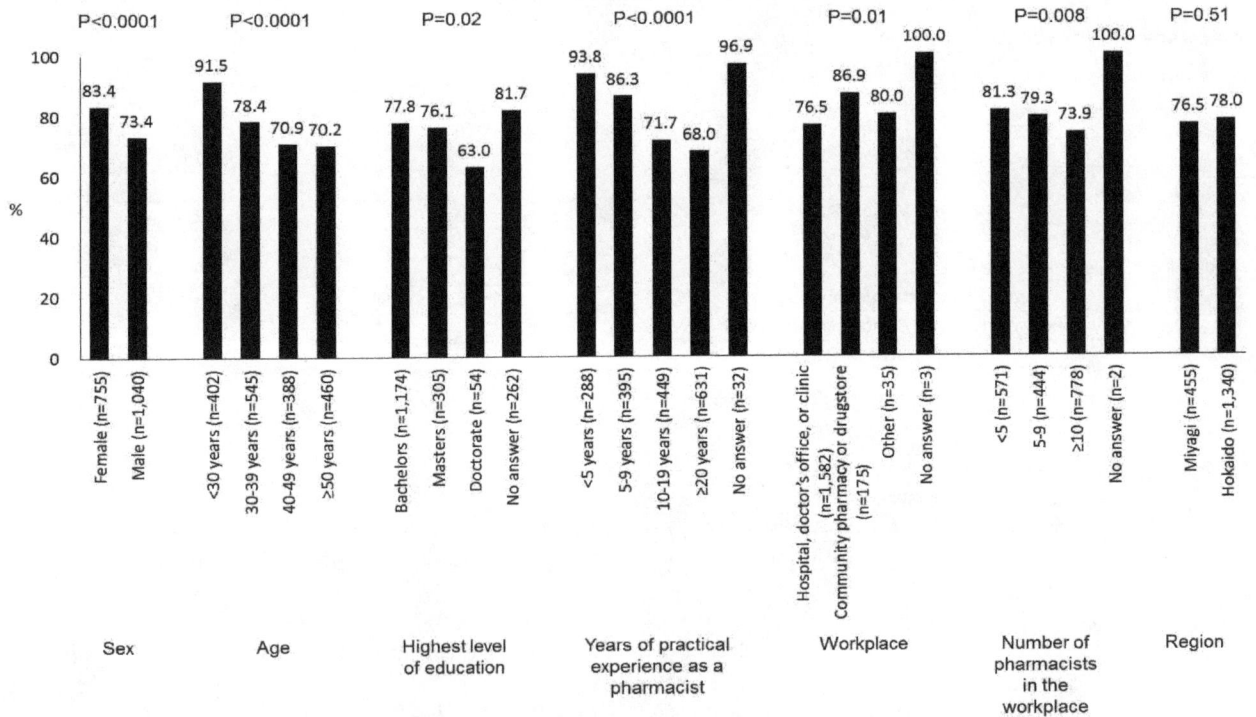

Figure 1: The prevalence of pharmacists who did not understand the ADR reporting system and who did not have a personal history of ADR reporting.

	Not understanding the ADR reporting system				Not having a personal history of ADR reporting			
Variables	OR	95%CI			OR	95%CI		
Sex								
Female	1.12	0.92	-	1.38	1.52	1.17	-	1.97
Male	1				1			
Age								
<30 years	1.25	0.73	-	2.14	12.0	0.55	-	2.62

30-39 years	1.18	0.76	-	1.83	1.09	0.64	-	1.86
40-49 years	1.27	0.92	-	1.75	1.05	0.74	-	1.49
≥ 50 years	1				1			
Highest level of education								
Bachelors	3.02	1.30	-	7.01	1.42	0.73	-	2.80
Masters	2.80	1.19	-	6.63	0.96	0.47	-	1.95
Doctorate	1				1			
Years of practical experience as a pharmacist								
<5 years	2.60	1.50	-	4.48	7.03	2.94	-	16.83
5-9 years	3.13	1.96	-	4.97	2.59	1.39	-	4.82
10-19 years	1.63	1.12	-	2.35	1.16	0.75	-	1.80
≥ 20 years	1				1			
Workplace								
Hospital, doctor's office, or clinic	1				1			
Community pharmacy or drugstore	1.37	0.98	-	1.93	1.90	1.16	-	3.12
Other	0.36	0.12	-	1.06	2.10	0.84	-	5.23
Number of pharmacists in the workplace								
<5	1.19	0.92	-	1.54	2.01	1.48	-	2.75
9-May	1.41	1.10	-	1.81	1.36	0.99	-	1.87
≥ 10	1				1			
Understanding the ADR reporting system								
Not understanding	-	-	-	-	5.93	4.23	-	8.33
Understanding	-	-	-	-	1		-	

ORs for 'no answer' to each question are not shown. ADR: Adverse Drug Reaction; OR: Odds Ratio; CI: Confidence Interval

Table 2: The multivariate logistic regression analyses for not understanding the ADR reporting system and not having a personal history of ADR reporting.

	Total	Understanding the ADR reporting system		
		No	Yes	
	n=1,393	n=649	n=744	P
It was a well-known ADR	43.0	41.6	44.2	0.32
Association between the drug and adverse reaction was not clear	38.0	36.2	39.5	0.2
It was an insignificant ADR	29.0	25.6	32.0	0.009
Did not know how to make a report	17.4	29.6	6.9	<.0001
Never been consulted about ADRs	17.2	15.1	19.0	0.06
Sufficient information could not be obtained from patients	8.3	8.6	8.1	0.7
ADR reporting system is very complicated	6.8	6.8	6.9	0.96
Did not have time to make a report	6.3	7.9	4.8	0.02
Believe reporting is the responsibility of the physician	4.2	5.4	3.2	0.045
Did not understand the significance of reporting	0.7	1.4	0.1	0.008
There was a concern of possibly being legally responsible	0.1	0	0.3	0.5
Other	8.1	5.7	10.2	0.002

ADR: Adverse Drug Reaction

Table 3: Reasons for ADR non-reporting among the 1,392 pharmacists who did not have a personal history of ADR reporting.

postgraduate education dealing with general adverse event reporting enhanced the understanding the ADR reporting system [5-9]. Although pharmacists have the legal and social responsibilities in ADR reporting, the opportunity of systematic learning ADR reporting system has been limited only at the pharmacy school curriculum in Japan. Therefore, we ought to provide for Japanese pharmacists the opportunity to receive education and hands on training in ADR reporting. Factors that reflect less experience and were extracted as determinants of non-reporting included, medical work environments with difficulties in obtaining detailed patient information, fewer opportunities to see patients with serious illnesses, or fewer patients likely to have ADRs. This study showed that being a pharmacist with both <10 years of practical experience and having contact with <10 pharmacists in the workplace were common factors for not understanding and for non-reporting the ADR. Thus, in the future it will be necessary to proactively provide information regarding the ADR reporting system to these individuals who have had less experience and limited access to other pharmacists. Female sex was one of the determinants for the ADR non-reporting. Sex difference might reflect the difference of factors that we could not evaluate in this study such as employment status.

Reasons for ADR non-reporting

Pharmacists who understand the ADR reporting system but have had no experience in ADR reporting responded that the reasons for ADR non-reporting were "It was a well-known ADR" (43%), "Association between the drug and adverse reaction was not clear" (38%), and "It was an insignificant ADR" (29%). These responses were similar to those reported in other previous studies [4,6,7,10,11]. In Japan, the information (or cases) that the government views as being appropriate to report includes "the onset of adverse reaction, infection, or malfunction through the usage of pharmaceutical products, medical devices, or regenerative medicine products, that is determined to require a report from the perspective of preventing the onset or spreading of health and hygiene hazards." However, since the definition of what the government requires is somewhat complicated and open to different interpretations, the results from our current study may more closely reflect the actual situation, with the decision on whether or not to report ADR information made at the discretion of the healthcare worker. By clarifying the definition of what cases are appropriate for reporting, it is anticipated that this should lead to a further accumulation of adverse event information, as well as improvements in the usability of this database system in the future.

Limitations

Limitations of current study may include making generalizations from the present study results that are based on information from pharmacists from only two regions of forty-seven prefectures in Japan. We need to examine whether or not there are big differences in the pharmacovigilance among different states of Japan. In addition, pharmacists who have an interest in this study subject have been the ones who are proactively providing responses. Thus, the proportion of pharmacists who understand the ADR reporting system or have experience in ADR reporting may be even lower in the actual overall pharmacist population. Nonetheless, since the response rate of this study survey was approximately 60%, this presumably indicates that these results do largely reflect the pharmacists' viewpoint within the overall study region.

Perspectives

In 2012, the ADR database containing the reports collected since 2004 became available on the PMDA website. This has helped facilitate the effective usage of the adverse event information collected by pharmacists in clinical settings. With continued education and training, in the future, both researchers and pharmacists working in a clinical setting will be able to compile and analyze the information contained in this database. Furthermore, over time it is also anticipated that pharmacists will be able to better contribute to the appropriate usage of pharmaceutical products in Japan.

Conclusion

This study examined the prevalence of pharmacists who had a personal history of ADR reporting and clarified the determinants and reasons for ADR non-reporting. As a better understanding the ADR reporting system was strongly associated with the ADR reporting, this indicates that a more aggressive promotion of understanding the ADR reporting system among pharmacists is warranted.

Acknowledgement

The authors would like to thank the Miyagi Prefecture Hospital Pharmacists Association and the Hokkaido Society of Hospital Pharmacists and pharmacists and pharmacovigilance professionals who helped to develop the questionnaire. This research was partially supported by the Research on Regulatory Harmonization and Evaluation of Pharmaceuticals, Medical Devices, Regenerative and Cellular Therapy Products, Gene Therapy Products, and Cosmetics from Japan Agency for Medical Research and Development, AMED.

References

1. Toklu HZ, Uysal MK (2008) The knowledge and attitude of the Turkish community pharmacists toward pharmacovigilance in the Kadikoy district of Istanbul. Pharm World Sci 30: 556-562.

2. Bäckström M, Mjörndal T, Dahlqvist R, Nordkvist-Olsson T (2000) Attitudes to reporting adverse drug reactions in northern Sweden. Eur J Clin Pharmacol 56: 729-732.

3. Aziz Z, Siang TC, Badarudin NS (2007) Reporting of adverse drug reactions: Predictors of under-reporting in Malaysia. Pharmacoepidemiol Drug Saf 16: 223-228.

4. Vessal G, Mardani Z, Mollai M (2009) Knowledge, attitudes, and perceptions of pharmacists to adverse drug reaction reporting in Iran. Pharm World Sci 31: 183-187.

5. Su C, Ji H, Su Y (2010) Hospital pharmacists' knowledge and opinions regarding adverse drug reaction reporting in Northern China. Pharmacoepidemiol Drug Saf 19: 217-222.

6. Irujo M, Beitia G, Bes-Rastrollo M, Figueiras A, Hernández-Díaz S, et al (2007) Factors that influence under-reporting of suspected adverse drug reactions among community pharmacists in a Spanish region. Drug Saf 30: 1073-1082.

7. Granas AG, Buajordet M, Stenberg-Nilsen H, Harg P, Horn AM (2007) Pharmacists' attitudes towards the reporting of suspected adverse drug reactions in Norway. Pharmacoepidemiol Drug Saf 16: 429-434.

8. Green CF, Mottram DR, Rowe PH, Pirmohamed M (2001) Attitudes and knowledge of hospital pharmacists to adverse drug reaction reporting. Br J Clin Pharmacol 51: 81-86.

9. Sweis D, Wong IC (2000) A survey on factors that could affect adverse drug reaction reporting according to hospital pharmacists in Great Britain. Drug Saf 23: 165-172.

10. Eland IA, Belton KJ, van Grootheest AC, Meiners AP, Rawlins MD, et al (1999) Attitudinal survey of voluntary reporting of adverse drug reactions. Br J Clin Pharmacol 48: 623-627.

11. Hasford J, Goettler M, Munter KH, Müller-Oerlinghausen B (2002) Physician's knowledge and attitudes regarding the spontaneous reporting system for adverse drug reactions. J Clin Epidemiol 55: 945-950.

17

Preventive Prescribing of Laxatives for Opioid-induced Constipation Using Electronic Clinical Rule Implementation by Cinical Pharmacists

Anne-Marie J W Scheepers-Hoeks[1]*, Rene J E Grouls[1], Cees Neef[2], Anne-Marie J Doppen[3] and Erik H M Korsten[4,5]

[1]Department of Clinical Pharmacy, Catharina Hospital, Eindhoven, The Netherlands
[2]Department of Clinical Pharmacy and Toxicology, Maastricht University Medical Centre, CAPHRI, Maastricht, The Netherlands
[3]Department of Pharmacy, Rivas Zorggroep, Gorinchem, The Netherlands
[4]Department of Signal Processing Systems, Faculty of Electronic Engineering, Eindhoven University of Technology, Eindhoven, The Netherlands
[5]Department of Anaesthesiology, Catharina Hospital, Eindhoven, The Netherlands

Abstract

Objective: The objective of this study was: (1) to develop and validate an electronic clinical rule for 'Opioid-Laxative Use' and to implement this rule in clinical pharmacy practice; (2) to improve guideline compliance by using this refined clinical rule; and (3) to investigate if opioid-induced constipation (OIC) can be reduced in hospitalised patients by the application of this clinical rule.

Methods: Interventions using clinical rule alerts were performed between June and September 2009. We compared guideline compliance before and after the intervention to determine the difference. Interventions consisted of telephone consultations by a clinical pharmacist advising physicians to add a laxative to opioid therapy. Patient files were matched to a historical control group using an opioid without a laxative to examine the difference between intervention- and control patients in the presence of OIC.

Results: Prospective validation of the rule resulted in several refinements. In the intervention period, 140 alerts were generated, 60 of which (43%) led to co-prescription of a laxative. Therefore, guideline compliance increased from 70% to 83%. A significant difference in OIC was found between the intervention group (12%) and the control group (56%).

Conclusions: This study showed that pharmacy intervention based on an electronic clinical rule for 'Opioid-Laxative Use' led to more adequate co-prescription of opioids and laxatives. This led to a better compliance with the guideline as well as a better outcome, as measured by the significant decrease in the prevalence of OIC.

Keywords: Gastrointestinal tract; Computerised physician order entry; Opioid-induced constipation; Clinical decision support systems

Introduction

While opioids are the cornerstone of pain management for moderate to severe cancer pain and chronic non-cancer pain, the use of opioids is commonly associated with opioid-induced bowel dysfunction, which has a serious impact on patients' quality of life. The gastrointestinal (GI) tract is an important site of opioid-related adverse effects due to the presence of opioid receptors, whose activation by exogenous opioids disrupts GI motility and secretion, thereby inhibiting normal bowel function [1]. These adverse events include a range of different gastrointestinal symptoms, including straining, hard stools, incomplete evacuation, abdominal distension, bloating, increased gastroesophageal reflux and constipation [2].

Constipation is the most common and often most debilitating adverse event while using opioids, with a reported incidence of 41% in patients with chronic non-cancer pain treated with morphine [3]. Pappagallo found that 80% of patients receiving opioids required at least one treatment for constipation, while 58% needed two or more treatments [4]. In another study surveying 2,055 patients using opioids for non-cancer pain, 57% reported having constipation associated with opioid treatment [5]. Of these patients, 33% considered constipation to be the most bothersome adverse event associated with their opioid treatment.

Reducing or avoiding opioid-induced constipation (OIC) is an important objective for improving the management of patients with chronic pain. Opioid dose reduction or discontinuation of opioid therapy negatively affects pain management and severely impairs patients' quality of life [1]. Therefore, preventing the occurrence of OIC remains the best treatment. First, guidelines generally recommend non-pharmacological interventions, such as increasing dietary fibre and fluid intake and encouraging mobility. However, these interventions are usually insufficient to prevent or treat OIC, and most patients receiving long-term opioid therapy require pharmacological intervention. Several types of pharmacological agents are available for treating OIC, including stool softeners, bowel stimulants and bulk laxatives, which are all grouped as laxatives in this paper.

It is widely advised to start a laxative concurrently with opioids before OIC can occur. However, a study which assessed laxative prescription in patients receiving a strong opioid for the first time showed that only 37% of patients started taking laxatives within 5 days of starting opioid therapy [6-8]. In community practice in the Netherlands, a laxative is prescribed for only 15-50% of patients starting opioids [9].

*Corresponding author: Scheepers-Hoeks AMJW, Catharina Hospital Eindhoven, Post Box 1350, 5602 ZA Eindhoven, The Netherlands, E-mail: anne-marie.scheepers@catharinaziekenhuis.nl

Retrospective research in the Catharina Hospital in Eindhoven in 2008 showed that co-prescription of a laxative was omitted at the start of therapy in 67% of clinical patients receiving opioids [9,10]. A study by Bouvy et al. showed that pharmacy intervention can lead to better opioid and laxative combination therapy in the community setting [6].

To our knowledge, no research has been performed on pharmacy intervention to improve opioid and laxative combination therapy in a hospital setting, and the effects on clinical outcomes have not been studied. In clinical practice, problems like OIC may potentially be prevented with the help of electronic clinical decision support systems (CDSSs). These systems are computer-based information systems which integrate clinical information and patient information to support decision making in patient care [11]. For example, clinical information on drugs or laboratory values can be used to generate alerts when a patient is not treated according to the guidelines. This information from guidelines and protocols can be translated into clinical rules: decision support algorithms, which are integrated in the CDSS. In the Catharina Hospital, research on clinical rules started in 1998. Since then, many clinical rules have been developed and implemented in clinical practice: for example, the clinical rule 'NSAIDs and Prophylactic Gastro-Protection' or the clinical rule 'Renal Impairement' [10].

The objective of the present study consists of three parts:

- to develop and validate a clinical rule for 'Opioid-Laxative Use' and to implement this rule in clinical pharmacy practice;

- to improve guideline compliance by using this refined clinical rule;

- and to investigate if opioid-induced constipation can be reduced in hospitalised patients by the application of this clinical rule.

Methods

Study site

This study was conducted in the Catharina Hospital in Eindhoven, The Netherlands, which is a 600-bed university-affiliated hospital. The hospital uses an electronic health record (EHR) (CS-EZIS, Chipsoft BV, Amsterdam) with integrated computerised physician order entry (CPOE). In this system, most patient data (medication, laboratory data, therapy, microbiology, diagnosis, etc.) are recorded. The integrated CPOE includes basic drug-oriented decision support, such as drug-drug interactions and drug-dose checking, based on the nationally established electronic drug database (WinAp, G-standard, Den Haag, The Netherlands) [12]. Since 2004, the Department of Pharmacy at the Catharina Hospital has been involved in the development of a strategy for designing and validating clinical rules by means of an advanced clinical decision support system–the CDSS Gaston (Medecs BV, Eindhoven).

Decision support system

In this study, the CDSS Gaston was used. This system, which is commercially available worldwide, was developed in 1998 at the Technical University Eindhoven in collaboration with our hospital. Technical assistance during our research was supplied by Medecs BV. The CDSS Gaston is linked to our EHR, which allows the electronic data stored in the EHR to be used in clinical rules [13,14]. The CDSS consists of two modules: (1) a guideline editor for developing electronic guidelines and (2) a guideline execution engine. The editor is a user-friendly environment, in which clinical rules are built as flowcharts. The steps in the flowchart contain the selection definitions based on the

parameters that are available in the EHR. The engine is used for retro- and prospective database research and prospective alerting.

Clinical rule 'Opioid-Laxative Use'

In 2008, the clinical rule for 'Opioid-Laxative Use' was developed according to a strategy designed in our hospital. This strategy is based on the Plan-Do-Check-Act cycle and includes an expert team that optimises the quality and clinical relevance of clinical rules [10]. The 'Opioid-Laxative Use' rule was specifically selected for development based on a national study that identified high-risk patients with medication-related problems leading to hospital admission [15].

The first draft of the clinical rule was designed to generate an alert when a patient uses an opioid without a laxative. This clinical rule was designed and retrospectively validated in a previous study. Patients were included if a new prescription for a drug from the category 'opioid analgesics' had been made in the previous 24 hours. Piritramide and sufentanyl are mostly used for a short post-surgery period. Therefore, these drugs were only included in the rule if they were used for more than 72 hours. The clinical rule was prospectively validated according to the development strategy to fine-tune the clinical rule so that it leads only to relevant alerts [10]. The adaptations made to the clinical rule are shown in Figure 1 and described in the Results section.

Site setup and participants

The development of the clinical rule was carried out by the *research team,* consisting of a pharmacist who built the clinical rule, a hospital pharmacist/clinical pharmacologist and a research pharmacist experienced in decision support. Time investment for this rule was three months full time (spread over six months) for the pharmacist and one hour a week for six months for the other two members of the research team. Furthermore, the clinical relevance was monitored by an *expert team* that consisted of two specialised physicians (an anaesthesiologist and an oncologist) and an experienced hospital pharmacist, all of them experts on pain management.

From June until September 2009, the clinical rule 'Opioid-Laxative Use' was implemented in daily hospital practice (intervention phase). This clinical rule included all patients admitted to the hospital except for intensive care patients. If a patient met all criteria defined in the clinical rule, an alert was generated.

Once a day at noon, an (Excel) list of alerts was generated by the CDSS and placed on the electronic pharmacy desktop. The relevance of each alert was first evaluated by a hospital pharmacist, who then consulted the physician on duty by telephone to discuss the recommendation. Subsequently, the physician decided whether or not to follow the recommendation. In our hospital, we recommended that the physician start macrogol, as it was the laxative of first choice. Also, the physician was asked why a laxative had not been co-prescribed with the opioid initially.

Outcome values

The main outcome value in this study was the percentage of patients having OIC. During the intervention phase from June 2009 until September 2009, the first 50 consecutive patients with a successful intervention were collected. A successful intervention was defined as the start of a prescription for a laxative within 24 hours after the hospital pharmacist consulted the physician. These 50 patients were matched to 50 controls collected in the period January 2009 until June 2009 (control phase), in which the clinical rule had not been used. These control patients were selected for using an opioid without a

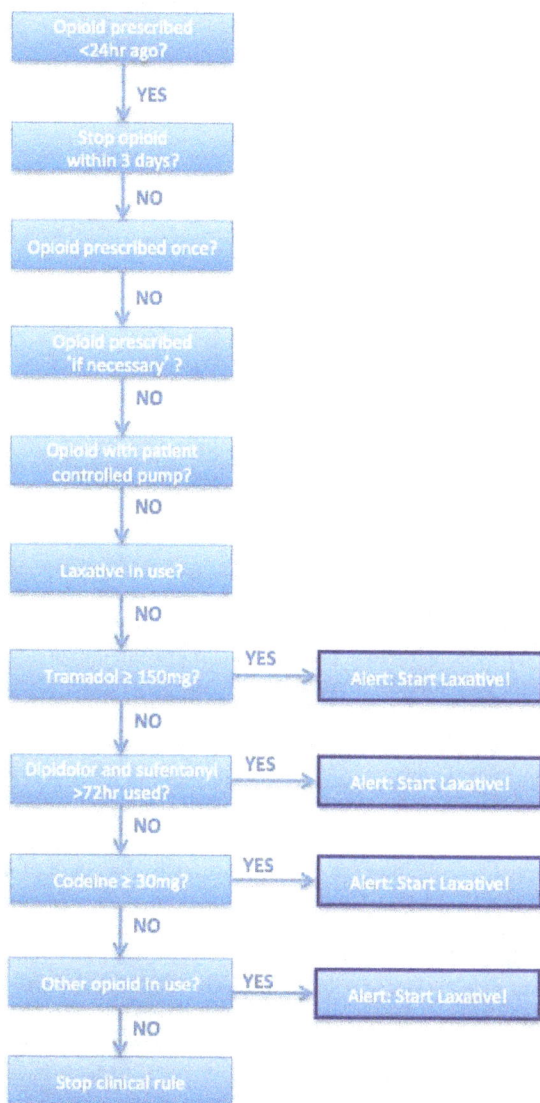

Figure 1: Schematic flowchart of the clinical rule for 'Opioid-Laxative Use'.

prescription for a laxative. Patients were matched for sex, age (± 10 years), opioid and department (surgery vs. non-surgery). To assess the presence of OIC, all patient files were investigated by three independent researchers. In case of uncertainty, the patient file was evaluated by all three researchers. OIC was scored binomially as a combined outcome parameter: no defecation for 3 or more days and/or a notification of constipation in the patient file and/or the start of a laxative during treatment with opioids. We also evaluated the combined use of an opioid and laxative at the moment of discharge from the hospital.

Secondly, the percentage of guideline compliance was measured before and after the intervention phase and the results were compared to determine the difference. According to the guideline, every patient using an opioid needs a co-prescription of a laxative. The percentage of patients using opioids and a co-prescription of a laxative was measured in the control phase as well as in the intervention phase.

This study was approved by the independent Medical Research Ethics Committee of the Catharina Hospital, indicating that the

Medical Research Involving Human Subjects Act does not apply for this study.

PSS (Version 19) was used to analyse the results using an ANOVA test for continuous variables and a two-sided chi-square test for categorical variables at a significance level of $\alpha=0.05$ and $1-\beta=0.80$.

Results

Refinement of the clinical rule 'Opioid-Laxative Use'

Prospective validation of the clinical rule using the validation strategy with the expert team led to the following refinements:

• Patients using opioids as a component of self-manufactured products of our hospital pharmacy were included.

• Patients using stool hardeners (e.g loperamide) were excluded.

• Patients using an opioid planned to stop within 3 days were excluded.

• Patients using opioids in a patient-controlled analgesia pump who used an opioid only once or only when necessary were excluded.

• Patients using the weak opioids tramadol or codeine in a dosage equal to or below 150 mg a day or 30 mg a day respectively were excluded. This choice was based on the registered doses for pain management.

Figure 1 shows the final schematic flowchart of the clinical rule. The expert team found that all alerts generated by the CDSS during prospective validation were clinically relevant, expressed as a positive predictive value of 100% [10].

Guideline compliance

The first draft of the clinical rule for 'Opioid-Laxative Use' showed that 67% of the patients using opioids had no co-prescription of a laxative [10]. Refinement through the validation strategy (Plan-Do-Check-Act) showed that the clinical rule could be adjusted to select only patients who actually need intervention according to the expert team. The refined rule was tested retrospectively on 50 patients from the control group and this showed that for 30% of the patients using opioids, a laxative was omitted. This percentage of non-compliance with the rule could be further reduced to 17% by pharmacy intervention using the alerts generated by the CDSS.

Intervention study

During 100 days of intervention, 140 alerts were generated by the CDSS. First the physicians were asked why a laxative had not yet been prescribed; in most cases the laxative had been forgotten (Figure 2a). Secondly, the advice to start a laxative was given, which in 43% of the cases (60/140) led to a successful intervention (Figure 2b). For 57% of patients, consultation did not lead to an intervention. Fourteen patients (10%) had already been discharged at the time of intervention. For 44 patients, the physician made the deliberate choice not to prescribe a laxative, and for 22 patients, the physician forgot the prescription after consultation by telephone (Figure 2). Reasons for deliberately not starting a laxative were that patients were receiving terminal care with opioids (28 times), patients had diarrhoea (eight times), patients had already used the opioid without a laxative and without OIC before admission (five times), and the physician was not persuaded to start a laxative before OIC occurred (three times).

Of the 60 patients with a successful intervention, 10 were excluded

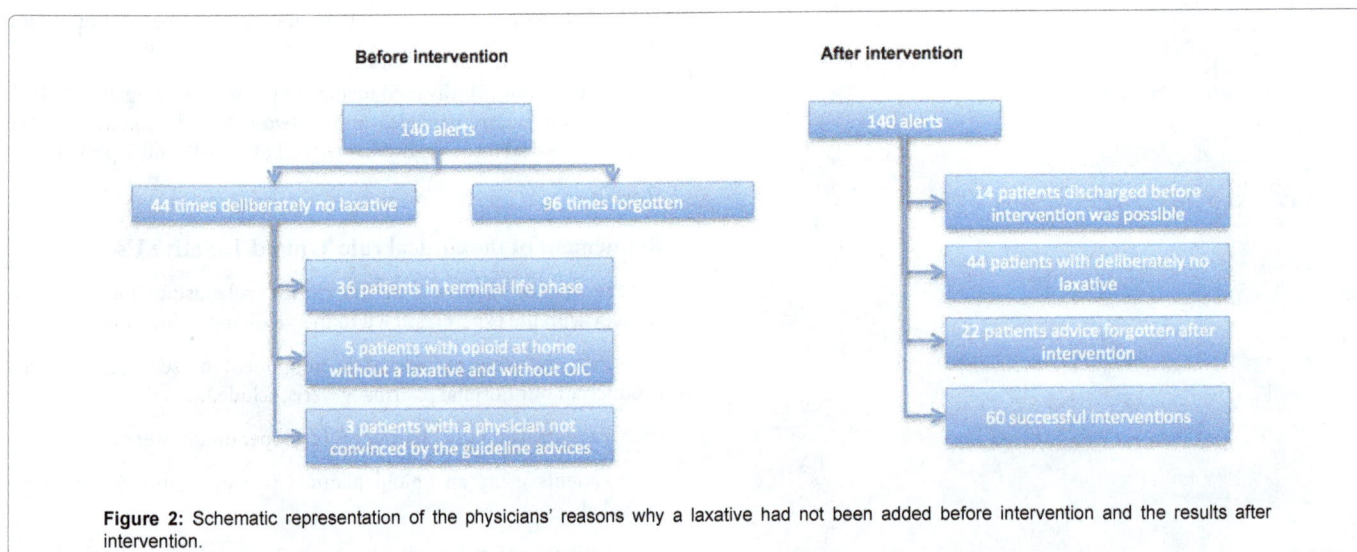

Figure 2: Schematic representation of the physicians' reasons why a laxative had not been added before intervention and the results after intervention.

	Interventions (n=50)	Controls (n=50)	P-value
Average age (yr ± SD)	65.7 (±2.0)	65.6 (±11.2)	n.s.
Gender male/female	26/24	26/24	n.s.
Non-surgery vs. surgery department	32 vs.18	33 vs.17	n.s.
Constipation developed during stay	6	28	<0.001
Opioid use <5 days	15	12	n.s.
Laxative prescribed within 5 days	50	16	<0.001
Discharged with opioid, with laxative	27	13	0.04
Discharged with opioid, without laxative	5	22	<0.001
Discharged without opioid, with laxative	4	2	n.s.
Discharged without opioid, without laxative	14	15	n.s.

n.s.=not significant

Table 1: General study characteristics and results of the intervention study.

for having an incomplete patient record. Therefore, 50 patients with a successful intervention and a complete dossier were matched to 50 controls with a complete dossier showing the defecation status during admission.

In the matched control group without intervention, 28 patients (56%) developed OIC compared to six patients (12%) in the intervention group (Table 1). This result is statistically significant (p<0.001). Also, the two groups showed a significant difference in the number of patients discharged with an active opioid prescription.

Discussion

This study validated and refined the clinical rule for 'Opioid-Laxative Use' and investigated the effect of the refined rule on guideline compliance after implementation in daily hospital practice. It demonstrated that this clinical rule can be optimised to select only those patients who need a laxative prescription in combination with their opioid therapy. Also, it showed that implementation of this rule led to a significant decrease in the prevalence of opioid-induced constipation. A key strength of this study was that, to our knowledge, it was the first to investigate clinical outcomes of adding a laxative to opioid therapy. Despite the fact that this advice is widely given in current guidelines and is mandatory according to Dutch Health Authority, we did not find other studies reporting on a reduction of OIC after increasing guideline compliance.

Before implementation of the clinical rule, 30% of the patients using opioids had no co-prescription of a laxative. By applying the clinical rule to our admitted patients, guideline non-compliance was reduced to 17%. Although this was an improvement in guideline compliance, we found that the follow-up of the interventions remained low (43%). However, in many cases the physician had a valid reason for not prescribing a laxative: for example, for patients with diarrhoea or in a terminal phase of life. For 22 patients the intervention was forgotten, so there is still room for improvement. Further research is needed to find a solution for increasing guideline and alert compliance.

Prospective validation is an important step in the development of a clinical rule [10,16,17]. Despite the consultation of an expert team in the earlier phases of validation, many changes were still required to optimise the clinical rule during prospective validation. This confirms that structured development and validation of clinical rules are crucial before widespread implementation in clinical practice [10,16,17]. In the near future, the rule will be further optimised: for instance, when data on the bowel elimination (e.g., diarrhoea) of patients have been added to the EHR.

The importance of adding a laxative to opioid therapy is evident. Constipation occurred even in the intervention group, which reinforces the recommendation to add a laxative in opioid therapy. However, little is known about which opioid leads to OIC most often and whether or not this is a dosage-related side effect. For this reason, the content of the rule is partly based on expert opinion rather than on evidence from literature. Further literature research might clarify this issue [18].

Several types of pharmacologic agents are used to treat opioid-induced constipation, including osmotic or lubricant laxatives, stimulant laxatives and prokinetics. Newer studies in this area suggest that the effects of these 'older' therapies are non-specific and generally unpredictable, often generating diarrhoea or cramps. In our study, these newer therapies were not included, as they were not available in our hospital during the study period.

This study showed a significant effect on OIC in a relatively small group of patients. A larger number of patients is needed to address the difference in effect in relation to different opioids, sex or age differences or differences between hospital departments.

This study showed that pharmacy intervention is a suitable method for implementing a clinical rule in daily practice. However, this method was not compared with other possible alerting methods. Currently, we are investigating the options to make the co-prescription of the laxative more transparent. We found that it was not always clear to the physicians that the laxative was started only for prevention of OIC. For example, this study showed that three patients in the intervention group were discharged with a prescription for a laxative but not for an opioid. A solution could be the development of pre-defined combination prescriptions that are easy for a physician to prescribe. An important subject for further investigation will be how to integrate these new and promising systems into clinical workflow.

Conclusion

This study showed that pharmacy intervention based on an electronic clinical rule for 'Opioid-Laxative Use' led to better co-prescription of opioids and laxatives. This led to a better compliance with the guideline as well as a better outcome, as measured by the significant decrease in the prevalence of OIC. Therefore, we conclude that the use of this electronic rule increases medication safety. As a co-prescription is not always indicated, the addition of a laxative to opioid therapy should always be prescribed in consultation with the physician.

Acknowledgements

We thank Medecs BV, Eindhoven, The Netherlands for their technical support during the study. We thank the physicians of the expert team for their collaboration in the development of the clinical rule. We thank the research students of the Department of Pharmacy of the University of Utrecht for their help in the development of the clinical rule.

References

1. Reimer K, Hopp M, Zenz M, Maier C, Holzer P et al. (2009) Meeting the challenges of opioid-induced constipation in chronic pain management–a novel approach. Pharmacology 83:10-17.

2. Panchal SJ, Muller-Schwefe P, Wurzelmann JI (2007) Opioid-induced bowel dysfunction: prevalence, pathophysiology and burden. Int J Clin Pract 61:1181-1187.

3. Moulin DE, Iezzi A, Amireh R, Sharpe WK, Boyd D (1996) Randomised trial of oral morphine for chronic non-cancer pain. Lancet 347:143-147.

4. Pappagallo M (2001) Incidence, prevalence, and management of opioid bowel dysfunction. The American Journal of Surgery 182:11S-18S.

5. Cook SF, Lanza L, Zhou X, Sweeney CT, Goss D et al. (2008) Gastrointestinal side effects in chronic opioid users: results from a population-based survey. Aliment Pharmacol & Ther 27:1224-1232.

6. Bouvy ML, Buurma H, Egberts TCG (2002) Laxative prescribing in relation to opioid use and the influence of pharmacy-based intervention. Journal of Clinical Pharmacy and Therapeutics 27 107-110.

7. Dutch Oncology Centre (2009) (Integraal Kankercentrum Nederland). National guideline constipation (Dutch) version 2.0 [Internet; cited 2010 Jun 16] 2009 Sep 28.

8. Verduijn MMFH (2010) Pharmacotherapeutic guideline painmanagement (Dutch). Utrecht, The Dutch College of General Practitioners (Nederlands Huisartsen Genootschap).

9. Dik EDB (1999) Laxatives during morfineclass drugs. Suggestions for therapy improvement (Dutch). Pharmaceutisch Weekblad 134: 1348-1352.

10. Scheepers-Hoeks AMJW, Grouls RJE, Neef C, Ackerman EW, Korsten HHM (2013) Strategy for development and pre-implementation validation of effective clinical decision support. Eur J of Hosp Pharm 20: 155-160.

11. Medical Subject Headings (MeSH) (2010) US National Library of Medicine.

12. Dutch drug database G-standard. (2008) Den Haag, The Netherlands.

13. De Clercq P, Hasman A (2004) Experiences with the development, implementation and evaluation of automated decision support systems. Stud Health Technol and Inform 107:1033-1037.

14. De Clercq PA, Hasman A, Blom JA, Korsten HHM (2001) Design and implementation of a framework to support the development of clinical guidelines. Int J Med Inform 64:285-318.

15. Leendertse AJ, Egberts ACG, Stoker LJ, van den Bemt PMLA, HARM Study Group (2008) Frequency of and risk factors for preventable medication-related hospital admissions in the Netherlands. Arch Intern Med 168:1890-1896.

16. Martins SB, Lai S, Tu S, Shankar R, Hastings SN et al. (2006) Offline testing of the ATHENA Hypertension decision support system knowledge base to improve the accuracy of recommendations. AMIA Annu Symp Proc 539-543.

17. McCoy AB, Waitman LR, Lewis JB, Wright JA, Choma DP et al. (2012) A framework for evaluating the appropriateness of clinical decision support alerts and responses. J Am Med Info Assoc 19:346-352.

18. Berde C, Nurko S (2008) Opioid side effects–mechanism-based therapy. New England Journal of Medicine 358:2400-2402.

Quercetin Curtails Obesity and Dyslipidemia, but Not Insulin Resistance in Long-Term Type 2 Diabetic Male Wistar Rats Fed the High-Fat, High-Sucrose Diet

Almass A Abuzaid[1], Mohamed A Osman[2]* and Abdalla O Elkhawad[3]

[1]Department of Public Health, University of Medical Sciences and Technology, Khartoum, Sudan
[2]Kirkwood Regional Center, University of Iowa, Coralville, IA, USA
[3]Department of Pharmacology, University of Medical Sciences and Technology, Khartoum, Sudan

Abstract

It is unclear whether the persistence of Type 2 Diabetes (T2D)-associated insulin resistance in Wistar rats is entirely dependent on obesity and dyslipidemia or other factors are involved. We wanted to reveal whether alleviation of obesity and dyslipidemia by quercetin would sufficiently cure the insulin resistance in diabetic Wistar rats. For this purpose, ninety, male Wistar rats were randomized into three experimental groups (n=30): Normal Control (NC) fed chow diet, Diabetic Control (DC) fed High-Fat, High-Sucrose Diet (HFHSD) and diabetic, Quercetin-Treated (QT) fed the HFHSD and gavaged with quercetin at 50 mg.kg^{-1} bw.day^{-1}. On Days 0, 60 and 120, Body Mass Index (BMI) and Abdominal Circumference:Thoracic Circumference (AC:TC) ratio were measured on ten rats from each group. Rats were then euthanized and fasting blood samples were withdrawn and used to quantify plasma glucose, Triacyclglycerols (TAG), LDL-cholesterol, total cholesterol, C-Reactive Protein (CRP) and insulin concentrations. Insulin resistance score, Relative Pancreatic Weight (RPW, %) and number of islet of Langerhans were also determined.

We show that quercetin normalized BMI, AC:TC ratio, RPW (%) and dyslipidemia, and enhanced the islets number of Langerhans in the QT rats on Day 120 relative to the NC rats. In the diabetic DC rats, AC:TC ratio correlated positively with hyperglycemia and negatively with RPW (%). Quercetin lowered, but failed to normalize hyperinsulinemia, insulin resistance score, hyperglycemia and CRP in the QT rats relative to the NC rats suggesting that other factors are involved in the insulin resistance pathogenesis in T2D Wistar rats. Our data also suggest that AC:TC ratio is a predictor of the obesity-induced T2D in Wistar rats.

Keywords: Type 2 Diabetes; Obesity; Dyslipidemia; Insulin resistance; Hyperglycemia; Quercetin

Introduction

Obesity is defined as an excess adipose tissue accompanying BMI ≥ 30 kg/m^2 and large waist circumference [1]. Obesity is caused by energy intake that exceeds energy expenditure leading to development of metabolic syndrome [2] wide-spread inflammation and chronic health disorders.

In obese individuals, proinflammatory molecules, such TNF-α, IL-1 and IL-6 are produced by the adipose tissue and thought to trigger β-cells injury and peripheral insulin resistance which culminate into Type 2 Diabetes (T2D) development [3]. Current interventions to lower obesity epidemic, such as consumption of nutrient-dense diet that provides less Calories, promotion of physical activity and use of anti-T2D medications and bariatric surgery have not been as efficient at down-regulating the upsurge of obesity [4]. Worldwide, more than 1 billion individuals are overweight, of whom 300 million are obese [1]. The huge number of afflicted individuals stimulated research that seeks an effective, safe dietary additive that cures the obesity-associated T2D and related chronic health disorders.

Quercetin is a phytochemical flavonoid that present in plants as hydrophilic glycosides. After hydrolysis of the glycosides, the average absorption of quercetin aglycone is estimated to be about 73% [5]. Several *in vivo* protective mechanisms limit the prooxidant and genotoxicant potential of quercetin. Oral administration of quercetin to rats [6] and to mice [7] at 30,300 or 3,000 mg.kg^{-1} bw.day^{-1} did not trigger mutagenic or genotoxic effects in somatic cells of treated rats and mice in comparison to untreated control. Quercetin mitigates hyperglycemia [8] and promotes energy expenditure via up-regulating PPAR-α gene expression [9]. Quercetin decreases visceral and liver fat in mice [10] and body weight in rats [11], dyslipidemia in mice [9] and rats [12] and oxidative stress metabolic disorders and risk factors of

T2D. In particular, obesity and dyslipidemia have been implicated with induction of insulin resistance. However, whether alleviation of T2D-associated obesity and dyslipidemia would entirely cure the insulin resistance is poorly understood and yet to be conclusively determined.

We hypothesized that long-term state of obesity and dyslipidemia although initially induce insulin resistance in T2D rats, but cure of obesity and dyslipidemia might not normalize the insulin resistance as other aberrant homeostatic alterations may have developed. Our objective was to elucidate whether cure of obesity and dyslipidemia by quercetin would lead to complete normalization of the insulin resistance in long-term T2D Wistar rats or other factors would block quercetin effect.

Materials and Methods

Kits and reagents

Quercetin was purchased from the Sigma Aldrich USA. Biochemical kits for lipids profiles were purchased from Biosystems S.A. Costa Brava 30, 08030 Barcelona, Spain. Insulin kits were purchased from BOSOH Company, Japan.

*Corresponding author: Mohamed A Osman, Academy of Sciences, Human Nutrition Section, Kirkwood Regional Center at the University of Iowa, Coralville, Iowa, USA, E-mail: mohamed.osman@kirkwood.edu

Animals

Healthy male Wistar rats (90 rats), six-week old, weighting 220-240 g, were used in the experiment. Each three rats were housed in a separate cage in the Restricted Animal Facility of the Faculty of Pharmacy, University of Khartoum. All rats were adapted for two weeks on stranded chow diet (Table 1) then randomized into three treatment groups (n=30): Normal Control (NC) fed the standard chow diet, Diabetic Control (DC) Fed High-Fat, High-Sucrose Diet (HFHSD; Table 2) and diabetic, Quercetin-Treated Group (QT) fed the HFHSD and gavaged with quercetin at 50 mg/kg bw^{-1}.day^{-1} until Day 120 of the study. All diets were fed *ad libitum* and rats were given free access to drinking water. The environment within the room was maintained to provide a temperature of 22-25°C, a relative humidity of 35-45%, and 12/12 h light/dark cycle.

Induction of obesity, type 2 diabetes and insulin resistance

To induce long-term obesity, T2D and insulin resistance, the rats in the DC and QT Groups were fed the HFHSD *ad libitum* for 12 months. By the end of the 12th month (Day 0), rats in the different groups were housed individually and the rats in the QT Group were gavaged quercetin at 50 mg.kg^{-1} bw.day^{-1} until the end of the study. The HFHSD constitutes 15% protein, 30% fat (20% of which was beef lard), 47% carbohydrates (35% of which was refined sugar), 5% fiber and 3% multivitamin multimineral complex (adopted from Srinivasan et al. [13] with modifications). The rats in the NC Group continued to consume the standard chow diet *ad libitum* until the end of the study.

Samples collection and analyses

Determination of the anthropometrical parameters: Following an overnight fast on Days 0, 60, and 120, the body weight was determined in grams, body length (from nose to anus) was measured in centimeters and BMI was calculated by dividing the body weight by squared body length. To determine the AC:TC ratio, AC was measured

	Weight %	Kcal %
Fat	11.4	13.103
Carbohydrates	51.4	59.877
Corns starch	28.6	-
Protein	23.2	27.020
Mineral-vitamin mix	10.1	-
Fiber	3.9	-
Total	100	100

Adopted from rat diet 5012 (LabDiet, St. Louis, MO)

Table 1: The macro- and micronutrients constituents and energy of the chow diet fed to the NC rats.

	Weight %	Kcal %
Fat	30	52.53
Carbohydrates	46	35.8
Sucrose	34%	-
Corn starch	13%	-
Protein	15	11.67
Mineral mix	3.0	-
Vitamin mix	1	-
Cellulose	5	-
Total	100	100

The fat constituent contained 20% beef lard. Values are calculated from ingredients mix

Table 2: The macro- and micronutrients constituents and energy (Calories) of the obesogenic, diabetogenic HFHSD fed to the DC and QT rats.

directly anterior to the forefeet in centimeters and TC was measured immediately behind the foreleg in centimeters [14].

Blood sample collection and dissection of pancreas: On days 0, 60 and 120 the rats were euthanized by decapitation under light halothane' anesthesia. Fasting blood samples were withdrawn by cardiac puncture and plasma was separated by centrifugation at 5,000 × g for 15 min in a refrigerating centrifuge and stored at -80°C until used for quantification of plasma glucose, triacyclglycerols (**TAG**), LDL-cholesterol, total cholesterol, CRP and insulin concentrations. The pancreas was dissected aseptically in a biosafety cabinet and processed for morphometric and histomorphometric analysis.

Determination of plasma metabolites, CRP and insulin

Plasma glucose concentration was determined by using the One Touch' Glucometer and confirmed spectrophotometrically. Plasma TAG, total cholesterol, LDL-cholesterol and CRP were determined spectrophotometrically by using commercial kits based on the manufacturers' instructions. Additionally, plasma insulin was analyzed by using immune-enzymatic assay TOSOH AIA-360 Chemistry Analyzer. Insulin resistance was calculated by using the homeostasis model assessment of insulin resistance (HOMA-IR=Insulin, μIU/mL × glucose, mg/dL)/405 as previously described [15].

Morphometric and histomorphometric analyses

The RPW (%) was determined after adipose tissue was precisely removed from the euthanized rats on Days 0, 60 and 120 using a sensitive digital scale. Pancreases tissues intended for histopathological works were rapidly fixed in 10% formalin in PBS, dehydrated in a graded ethanol series, cleared in xylene and embedded in paraffin wax. Pancreatic sections (5 μm thick) were stained with Hematoxylin and Eosin (H&E) and used for detection of islet of Langerhans [16]. Four sections were examined from each animal in the different experimental groups. The number of pancreatic islets of Langerhans per section was determined under 10 high power fields. The number of islets was assessed by counting all islets section of different non-overlapping fields for the same slide of each animal. The histopathological images were captured by using the SPOT idea™ CMOS|5.0 Mp digital camera mounted on Olympus CH20i (Olympus BX51) microscope equipped with grid and micrometer and hooked a SPOT idea™ CMOS software.

Statistical analysis

The data were analyzed by using the Two-way ANOVA procedure of the statistical software GraphPad Prism 5' (GraphPad Software Inc., La Jolla, CA, USA). Bonferroni test was used for the pairwise comparison of the means with significance set at α=0.05 and 95% confidence intervals. The Pearson Correlation Coefficient (r) was computed to determine the association between each two variables. Data were expressed as the means ± SEM. Statistical significance was declared when P<0.05. Means with superscript differ significantly at P<0.05.

Results

Anthropometrical analyses

Feeding the HFHSD to the DC and QT rats significantly (all P<0.001; Figur 1A) increased the BMI of the diabetic DC rats on Days 0, 60 and 120 and the QT rats on Day 0 only relative to the normal control NC rats. Interestingly, by Days 60 and 120, quercetin administration

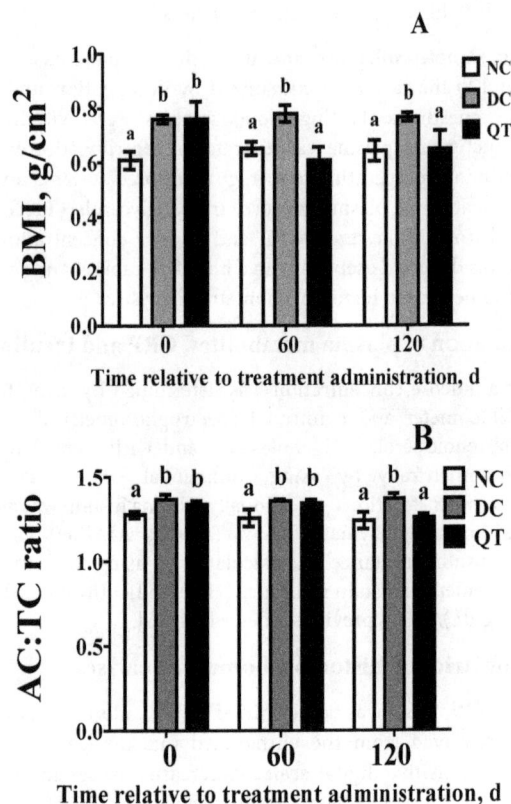

Figure 1: The BMI (g/cm²) and AC:TC ratio values on Days 0, 60 and 120 of male Wistar rats fed the standard chow diet (NC), fed the HFHSD (DC) or fed the HFHSD and gavaged with quercetin (QT) at 50 mg.kg⁻¹ bw.day⁻¹ until Day 120 of the study. Values are the means ± SEM. Means with different superscripts differ significantly. Statistical significance declared at $P \leq 0.05$. Panel A: The BMI (g/cm²) values. Feeding the HFHSD to the DC and QT rats significantly (all $P<0.001$; Figur 1A) increased the BMI of the diabetic DC rats on Days 0, 60 and 120 (0.7597 ± 0.02; 0.7795 ± 0.03; 0.7667 ± 0.02, respectively) and the QT rats on Day 0 only (0.7597 ± 0.02) relative to the normal control NC rats (0.6093 ± 0.01; 0.6511 ± 0.009; 0.6419 ± 0.01, respectively). On Days 60 and 120, quercetin administration normalized (both $P>0.05$) the BMI of the QT rats relative to the NC rats (0.6072 ± 0.01; 0.6472 ± 0.01 vs. 0.6511 ± 0.01; 0.6419 ± 0.02, respectively). Panel B: The AC:TC ratio of the DC rats became significantly greater ($P<0.0001$) on Days 0, 60 and 120 relative to NC rats (1.3683 ± 0.03; 1.3577 ± 0.01; 1.3708 ± 0.03 vs. 1.2774 ± 0.02; 1.2576 ± 0.05; 1.2418 ± 0.05 units, respectively). In contrast, the AC:TC ratio of the QT rats was greater ($P \leq$ 0.001) only on Days 0 and 60 (relative to the NC rats (1.3370 ± 0.02 and 1.3446 ± 0.02 vs. 1.2774 ± 0.02; 1.2576 ± 0.05 units, respectively). By Shown in Figure 1B, quercetin lowered ($P<0.0001$) AC:TC ratio of the QT rats compared with the DC rats and not different ($P>0.05$) relative to the NC rats (1.2599 ± 0.02 vs. 1.3708 ± 0.03 and 1.2418 ± 0.05 units, respectively) on Day 120.

normalized (both $P>0.05$) the BMI of the QT rats (Figure 1A).

The AC:TC ratio of the DC rats became significantly greater ($P<0.0001$) on Days 0, 60 and 120 relative to NC rats. In contrast, the AC:TC ratio of the QT rats was greater ($P \leq 0.001$) on Days 0 and 60. Quercetin, however, lowered ($P<0.0001$) AC:TC ratio of the QT rats compared with the DC rats, but not different ($P>0.05$) relative to the NC rats (Figure 1B). Illustrated in Table 3, BMI did not correlate with the AC:TC ratio in all the experimental rats.

Morphometric and histomorphometric analyses

The RPW (%) significantly (all $P<0.0001$) decreased in the DC rats on Days 0, 60 and 120 and in the QT rats on Day 0 compared to NC rats.

On Days 60 and 120, however, quercetin administration significantly (both $P<0.0001$) increased the RPW (%) in the QT rats to be greater compared with the DC rats, but not different ($P>0.05$) compared with the NC rats. Also, quercetin increased ($P<0.01$) the islets of Langerhans number in the QT rats relative to the DC rats, slightly ($P=0.08$; Table 4) compared with the NC rats on Day 120.

Correlation between the anthropometrical and morphometrical parameters

BMI did not correlate with AC:TC ratio (all $r \leq 0.2994$, $P>0.05$; Table 3), RPW (all $r \leq -0.4180$, $P>0.05$; Table 3) and hyperglycemia ($r \leq 0.3831$, $P>0.05$; Table 3), in all of our experimental groups (Table 3). We observed a strong inverse correlation between the AC:TC ratio and RPW in the QT and NC rats ($r=-0.7085$; $P \leq 0.05$ and $r=-0.8428$, $P \leq 0.01$, respectively). Also, plasma glucose significantly ($r \geq 0.665$; $P \leq 0.05$) correlated positively with AC:TC ratio in QT rats (Table 3).

Development of dyslipidemia

Under effect of the HFHSD, the dyslipidemia parameters plasma TAG, LDL-cholesterol and total cholesterol significantly (all $P<0.0001$) increased in the diabetic DC rats on Days 0, 60 and 120, and in the QT

Parameters	Statistics	Treatment groups		
		DC	QT	NC
BMI vs. AC:TC	r	0.1659	0.1400	0.2994
	P	0.6468	0.7187	0.4712
BMI vs. RPW	r	-0.4180	-0.3257	-0.4172
	P	0.1923	0.3312	0.2038
BMI vs. PG	r	0.2160	0.3831	0.3676
	P	0.5489	0.2745	0.3703
AC:TC vs. RPW	r	-0.4417	-0.7085	-0.8428
	P	0.0523	0.0049	0.0086
AC:TC vs. PG	r	0.7937	0.6650	0.5286
	P	0.0140	0.0361	0.0780

r=Pearson Correlation Coefficients (Prob>| r | under H0: Rho=0). BMI stands for body mass index, g/cm², AC:TC stands for abdominal circumference to thoracic circumference ratio, RPW stands for relative pancreatic weight and PG stands for plasma glucose concentration in mg/dL. DC stands for diabetic control group, QT for diabetic quercetin-treated group and NC for non-diabetic control group. Quercetin was gavaged at 50 mg.kg⁻¹ bw.day⁻¹ until Day 120 of the study. Values are the means ± SEM. Statistical significance declared at $P \leq 0.05$.

Table 3: The correlation among anthropometrical parameters, RPW, and plasma glucose concentration on Day 120 of male Wistar rats fed the standard chow diet (NC), fed the HFHSD (DC) or fed the HFHSD and gavaged with quercetin (QT).

Parameter	Statistics	Treatment groups		
		DC	QT	NC
PG vs. IRS	r	0.7000	0.8490	0.9473
	P	0.0500	0.007	0.0001
PG vs. IsL	r	- 0.5519	-0.5553	-0.6354
	P	0.0150	0.0790	0.0660
IRS vs. IsL	r	-0.6283	0.0129	0.0483
	P	0.0699	0.9738	0.6700

r=Pearson Correlation Coefficients (Prob>| r | under H0: Rho=0). DC stands for diabetic control group, QT stands for diabetic quercetin-treated group, NC stands for non-diabetic control group, PG stands for plasma glucose, IRS stands for insulin resistance score, and IsL stands for islets of Langerhans number. Quercetin was gavaged at 50 mg.kg⁻¹ bw.day⁻¹ until Day 120 of the study. Statistical significance was declared at $P \leq 0.05$.

Table 4: The correlation among plasma glucose concentration, insulin resistance score and the number of islets of Langerhans on Day 120 of male Wistar rats fed the standard chow diet (NC), fed the HFHSD (DC) or fed the HFHSD and gavaged with quercetin (QT).

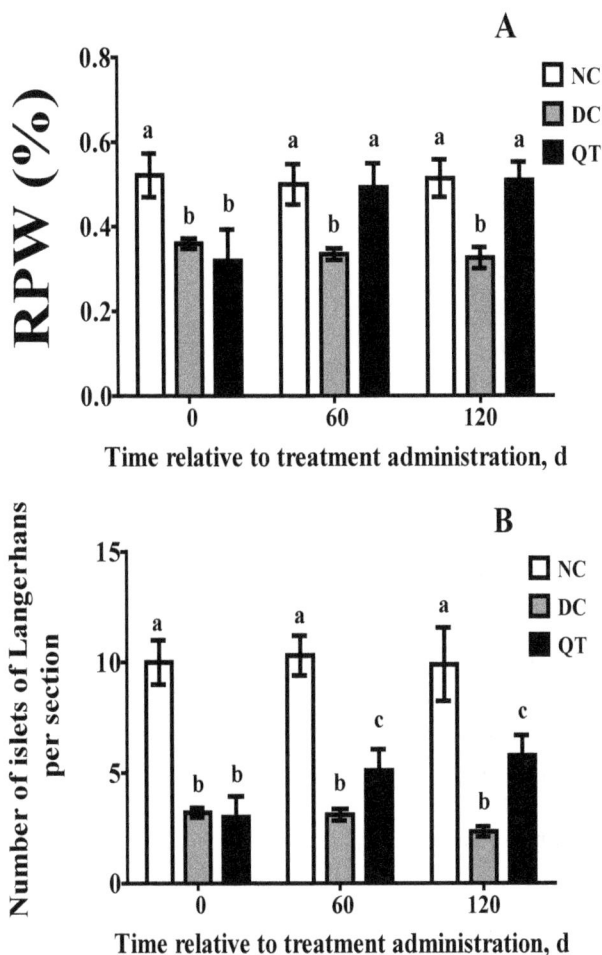

Figure 2: The RPW (%) and the number of islets of Langerhans per section Days 0, 60 and 120 of male Wistar rats fed the standard chow diet (NC), fed the HFHSD (DC) or fed the HFHSD and gavaged with quercetin (QT) at 50 mg.kg⁻¹ bw.day⁻¹ until day 120 of the study. Panel A: The RPW (%). Affected by HFHSD the RPW (%) of the DC significantly decreased ($P<0.0001$) relative to the NC control rats (0.3600 ± 0.01; 0.3350 ± 0.01; 0.3260 ± 0.03 vs. 0.5210 ± 0.02; 0.5000 ± 0.02; 0.5135 ± 0.01, respectively) on Days 0, 60 and 120. However, on Day 0, the QT rats demonstrated decreased ($P<0.0001$) RPW (%) relative to the NC rats (0.3190 ± 0.02 vs. 0.5210 ± 0.02, respectively). On Days 60 and 120, quercetin administration increased the RPW (%) in the QT rats to be greater ($P<0.0001$) compared with the diabetic DC rats (0.4920 ± 0.02; 0.5090 ± 0.02 vs. 0.3350 ± 0.01; 0.3260 ± 0.01, respectively), but not different in contrast with normal control NC rats (0.4920 ± 0.02; 0.5090 ± 0.01 vs. 0.5000 ± 0.02; 0.5135 ± 0.01, respectively). Panel B: The number of islets of Langerhans per section. Influenced by the HFHSD, the number of islets of Langerhans per section decreased significantly ($P \leq 0.0001$) in the DC and QT rats on Days 0 (3.2 ± 0.70 and 3.0 ± 0.94 vs. 10.0 ± 1.0), Day 60 (3.1 ± 0.81 and 5.10 ± 0.96 vs. 10.3 ± 0.90) and Day 120 (2.33 ± 0.75 and 5.76 ± 0.91 vs. 9.88 ± 1.66 islets, respectively). Under effect of quercetin, the QT rats demonstrated greater number of islets of Langerhans on Days 60 and 120 (5.10 ± 0.96 and 5.76 ± 0.91 vs. 3.1 ± 0.81 and 2.33 ± 0.75 islets, respectively). Values are means ± SEM. Means with different superscripts differ significantly. Statistical significance declared at $P \leq 0.05$.

Plasma glucose and insulin concentrations and the Insulin Resistance Score (IRS)

Influenced by the HFHSD plasma glucose concentration significantly ($P \leq 0.01$) increased in the DC and QT rats on Days 0, 60 and 120 to be greater relative to the NC rats (Figure 4A).

Feeding the HFHSD significantly ($P \leq 0.01$) increased plasma insulin concentrations in the DC and QT rats on Days 0, 60 and 120 relative to the control NC rats fed the chow diet (Figure 4B). By Days 60 and 120, however, administration of quercetin decreased ($P<0.01$) plasma insulin in the QT rats compared with the DC rats, yet higher ($P<0.01$) relative to the NC rats (Figure 4B).

Shown in Figure 4C, the DC and QT rats demonstrated significantly ($P \leq 0.001$) higher ISR relative to the NC rats on Days 0, 60 and 120. Administration of quercetin lowered ($P<0.0001$) the ISR of the QT rats relative to the diabetic control DC rats on Days 60 and 120 yet failed ($P<0.01$) to normalize it relative to the nondiabetic control NC rats (Figure 4C). As shown in Table 4, the hyperglycemia correlated positively ($r \geq 0.70$; $P \leq 0.05$) with IRS and negatively ($r=-0.5519$; $P \leq 0.02$) with the number of islets of Langerhans in the pancreas of the DC, QT and NC rats on Day120. But, the IRS correlated negatively with the number of islets of Langerhans in the DC rats only on Day 120 (Table 4).

The correlation between hyperglycemia and dyslipidemia

On Day 120, the hyperglycemia correlated significantly ($r \geq 0.7000$; $P<0.05$) positive with plasma TAG concentration in the DC and NC rats (Table 5). But, under the effect of quercetin, no correlation ($r=0.3014$; $P>0.05$) was detected between hyperglycemia and TAG concentrations in the QT rats (Table 5). In contrast, the hyperglycemia did not correlate ($r \leq 0.1411$; $P>0.05$) with the LDL-cholesterol and total cholesterol in the in all experimental rats (Table 5).

Development of inflammation

The inflammatory marker CRP elevated significantly ($P<0.001$) in the plasma of the diabetic DC and QT rats relative to the NC rats on Days 0, 60 and 120 (Figure 5). Affected by quercetin, the plasma CRP concentrations decreased ($P \leq 0.001$) in the QT rats on Days 60 and 120 relative to the DC rats. Despite this, quercetin failed ($P<0.0001$) to normalize plasma CRP in the QT rats compared to the control NC rats on Days 60 and 120 (Figure 5).

Parameters	Statistics	Treatment groups		
		DC	QT	NC
PG vs. TAG	r	0.7000	0.30141	0.7222
	P	0.0244	0.3974	0.0431
PG vs. T-ch	r	-0.0762	-0.0223	0.1411
	P	0.8343	0.9512	0.7388
PG vs. LDL-ch	r	-0.0849	-0.2714	-0.2455
	P	0.8156	0.4482	0.5579

r=Pearson Correlation Coefficients (Prob>| r| under H0: Rho=0). DC stands for diabetic control group, QT stands for diabetic quercetin-treated group, NC stands for non-diabetic control group, PG stands for plasma glucose, TAG stands for triacyclglycerols, T-ch stands for total cholesterol and LDL-ch stands for low-density lipoprotein cholesterol. Quercetin was gavaged at 50 mg.kg⁻¹ bw.day⁻¹ until Day 120 of the study. Statistical significance was declared at $P \leq 0.05$.

Table 5: The correlation among plasma glucose, TAG, total-cholesterol and LDL-cholesterol concentrations on Day 120 of male Wistar rats fed the standard chow diet (NC), fed the HFHSD (DC) or fed the HFHSD and gavaged with quercetin (QT).

rats on Day 0 compared with the normal control NC rats (Figures 2A-2C). Administration of quercetin significantly ($P<0.0001$) decreased TAG, LDL-cholesterol and total cholesterol in plasma of the QT rats on Days 60 and 120 relative to the diabetic DC rats and normalized ($P>0.05$) them relative to the NC rats (Figures 3A-3C).

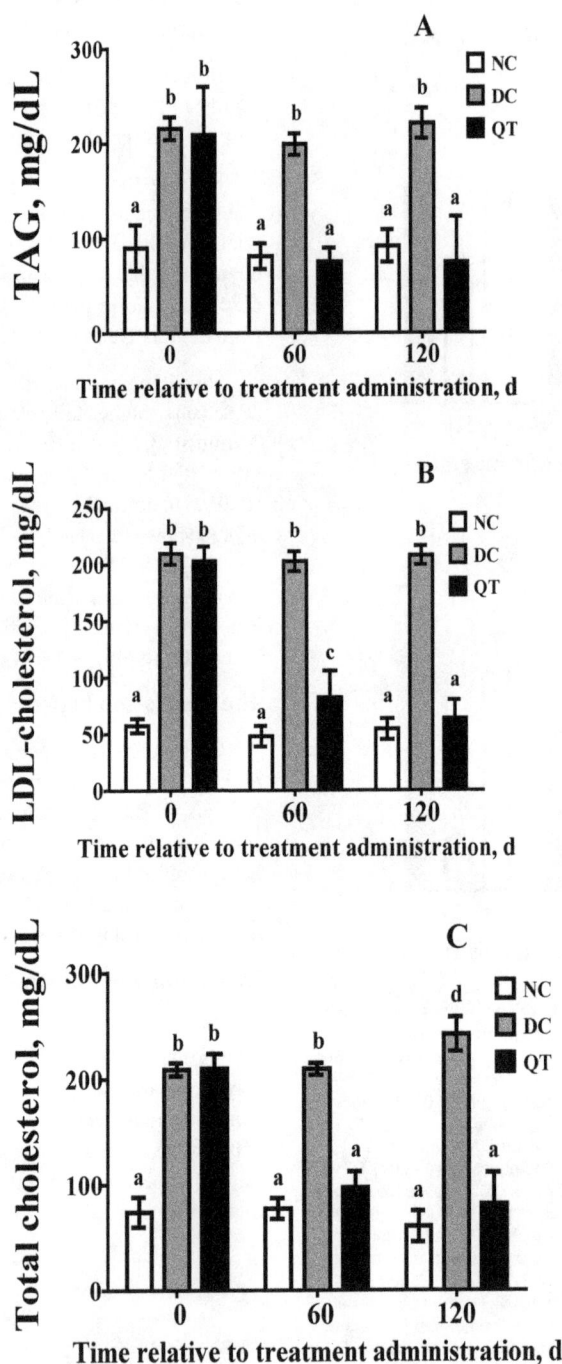

Figure 3: Plasma TAG, LDL-cholesterol and total cholesterol concentrations on Days 0, 60 and 120 of male Wistar rats fed the standard chow diet (NC), fed the HFHSD (DC) or fed the HFHSD and gavaged with quercetin (QT) at 50 mg.kg^{-1} bw.day^{-1} until day 120 of the study. Panel A: Plasma TAG concentrations, mg/dL. Plasma TAG concentrations significantly (all $P<0.0001$) increased in the diabetic DC rats on Days 0, 60 and 120 (216 ± 12.2; 199.2 ± 11.5; 221.1 ± 15.9) and in the QT rats on Day 0 (209.4 ± 16.0) compared with the normal control NC rats (90.3 ± 8.6; 81.2 ± 4.6; 91.9 ± 6.1 mg/dL, respectively). Administration of quercetin significantly ($P<0.0001$) decreased TAG in plasma of the QT rats on Days 60 and 120 relative to the diabetic DC rats (75.2 ± 4.6; 74.5 ± 15.2 vs. 216 ± 11.5; 199.2 ± 15.9 mg/dL) and normalized ($P>0.05$) it relative to the NC rats (75.2 ± 4.6; 74.5 ± 15.2 vs. 81.2 ± 4.8; 91.9 ± 6.1 mg/dL, respectively). Panel B: Plasma LDL-cholesterol, mg/dL. Plasma LDL-cholesterol concentrations significantly (all $P<0.0001$) increased in the diabetic DC rats on Days 0, 60 and 120 (239.6 ± 12.8; 202.6 ± 9.0; 207.8 ± 11.7) and in the QT rats on Day 0 (232.7 ± 23.5) compared with the normal control NC rats (57.3 ± 6.2; 48.0 ± 3.7; 54.1 ± 9.2 mg/dL, respectively). Quercetin significantly ($P<0.0001$) decreased LDL-cholesterol in the QT rats on Days 60 and 120 relative to the diabetic DC rats (82.7 ± 4.6; 63.1 ± 16.8 vs. 202.6 ± 9.0; 207.8 ± 11.7 mg/dL) and normalized ($P>0.05$) it relative to the NC rats (82.7 ± 4.6; 63.1 ± 16.8 vs. 202.6 ± 9.0; 207.8 ± 11.7 mg/dL, respectively). Panel C: Plasma total-cholesterol, mg/dL. Plasma total cholesterol, mg/dL. Influenced by HFHSD, plasma total cholesterol concentrations significantly (all $P<0.0001$) increased in the diabetic DC rats on Days 0, 60 and 120 (208.9 ± 6.2; 209.4 ± 5.5; 241.9 ± 6.2) and in the QT rats on Day 0 (209.7 ± 4.5) compared with the normal control NC rats (74.3 ± 4.9; 77.6 ± 3.5; 60.8 ± 5.2 mg/dL, respectively). On Days 60 and 120, quercetin significantly ($P<0.0001$) decreased total cholesterol in the QT rats on compared with the diabetic DC rats (97.0 ± 4.9; 81.6 ± 9.5 vs. 209.4 ± 5.5; 241.9 ± 16.3 mg/dL) and normalized ($P>0.05$) it relative to the NC rats (97.0 ± 4.9; 81.6 ± 9.5 vs. 77.6 ± 3.5; 60.8 ± 5.2 mg/dL, respectively). Values are the means $\pm$ SEM. Means with different superscripts differ significantly. Statistical significance declared at $P \leq 0.05$.

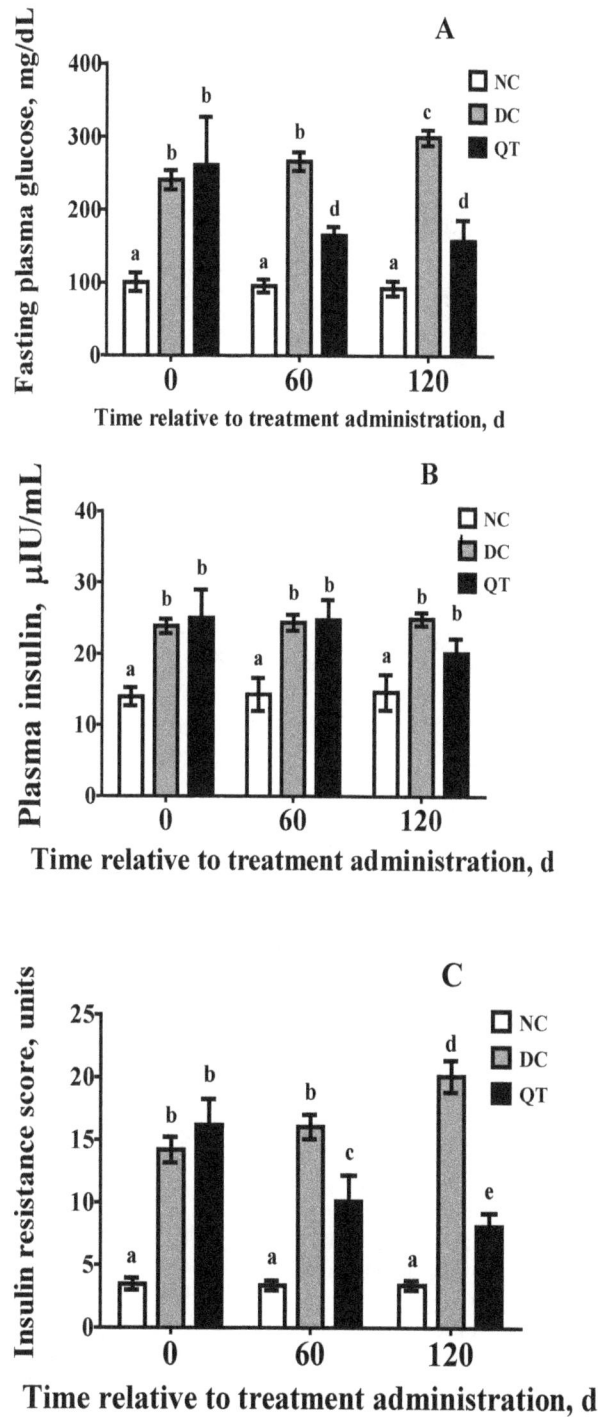

Figure 4: Plasma glucose, plasma insulin and the insulin resistance score values on Days 0, 60 and 120 of male Wistar rats fed the standard chow diet (NC), fed the HFHSD (DC) or fed the HFHSD and gavaged with quercetin (QT) at 50 mg.kg^{-1} bw.day^{-1} until day 120 of the study. Panel A: Plasma glucose concentrations, mg/dL. Feeding the HFHSD significantly ($P \le 0.01$) increased plasma glucose concentration in the DC and QT rats on Days 0, 60 and 120 to be greater relative to the NC rats (240. 7 ± 13.1 and 260.7 ± 21.0 vs. 100.5 ± 4.6) on Day 0, (266.2 ± 12.7 and 165.2 ± 3.7 vs. 95.3 ± 3.2) on Day 60 and (299.3 ± 10.7 and 157.6 ± 9.0 vs. 92.0 ± 3.2 mg/dL, respectively) on Day 120. Panel B: Plasma insulin concentrations, µIU/mL. Influenced by the HFHSD plasma insulin concentrations significantly ($P \le 0.01$) increased in the DC and QT rats on Day 0 (23.9 ± 3.20 and 25.0 ± 4.0 vs. 14.0 ±1.31), Day 60 (24.4 ± 3.60 and 24.7 ± 2.84 vs. 14.3 ± 2.35) and Day 120 (24.6 ± 0.71 and 20.1 ± 0.47 vs. 14.6 ± 0.41 µIU/mL, respectively) relative to the control NC rats fed the chow diet. By Day 120, however, administration of quercetin decreased ($P<0.01$) plasma insulin in the QT rats compared with the DC rats, yet higher ($P<0.01$) relative to the NC rats (20.1 ± 2.07 vs. 24.9 ± 2.96 and 14.6 ± 2.51 µIU/mL, respectively). Panel C: Insulin resistance score (ISR), units. The DC and QT rats demonstrated significantly ($P \le 0.001$) higher ISR relative to the NC rats on Day 0 (14.2 ± 3.22 and 16.1 ± 3.1 vs. 3.47 ± 0.46), Day 60 (16.0 ± 2.01 and 10.1 ± 1.08 vs. 3.36 ± 0.30) and Day 120 (20.1 ± 1.10 and 8.14 ± 1.65 vs. 3.38 ± 0.05 units, respectively). Administration of quercetin lowered ($P<0.0001$) the ISR of the QT rats relative to the diabetic control DC rats on Days 60 and 120 yet failed to normalize it relative to the nondiabetic control NC rats (10.1 ± 2.08; 8.14 ± 1.02 vs. 16.0 ± 3.10; 20.1 ± 4.0 and 3.36 ± 0.39; 3.38 ± 0.39 units, respectively).

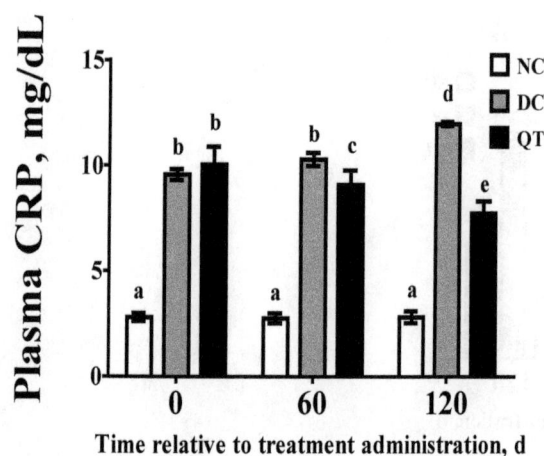

Figure 5: CRP elevated significantly (*P*<0.001) in the plasma of the diabetic DC and QT rats relative to the NC rats on Days 0 (9.58 ± 0.81 and 10.04 ± 0.86 vs. 2.81 ± 0.19), Day 60 (10.30 ± 0.97 and 9.10 ± 0.68 vs. 2.76 ± 0.23) and Day 120 (12.0 ± 0.30 and 7.75 ± 0.57 vs. 2.82 mg/dL, respectively). But, quercetin administration lowered (*P* ≤ 0.001) in the QT rats on Days 60 and 120 relative to the DC rats (9.10 ± 0.68 and 7.75 ± 0.57 vs. 10.30 ± 0.97 and 12.0 ± 0.30 mg/dL, respectively). Despite this, quercetin failed (*P*<0.0001) to normalize plasma CRP in the QT rats compared to the control NC rats on Days 60 and 120 (.10 ± 0.68 and 7.75 ± 0.57 vs. 2.76 ± 0.23 and 2.82 mg/dL, respectively).

Discussion

This study describes the ability of quercetin to alleviate the obesity and dyslipidemia, but not the insulin resistance risk factors for T2D [17] induced by long-term (12 mo) HFHSD feeding in male Wistar rats. Induction of T2D by the HFHSD (Table 2) in the DC rats lead to significant increase in their BMI, AC:TC ratio, dyslipidemia, hyperglycemia, hyperinsulinemia and insulin resistance score (Figures 1-4). The HFHSD also decreased their RPW (%) and its content of islets of Langerhans (Figure 2) relative to the control NC rats consuming the normal chow diet (Table 1).

Rodent diets high in sucrose and fats increase BMI of Wistar rat [13,14]. On Days 60 and 120, we found that quercetin administered at 50 mg.kg⁻¹ bw.day⁻¹ normalized (*P*>0.05) BMI and the AC:TC ratio of the QT rats relative to the NC rats (Figures 1A and 1B). Consistent with previous findings, administration of quercetin decreases the body weight and adiposity in rats [18] and decreases liver and visceral fat in C57BL/6J mice via inhibiting adipogenesis and activating fatty acid β-oxidation in the mitochondria [19]. Promotion of energy expenditure by quercetin is mediated via upregulation of adiponectin gene expression (Authors' manuscript accepted for publication).

Consistent with previous report [20], induction of T2D by HFHS diet in our rats was accompanied by significant dyslipidemia (Figures 3A-3C). Curiously enough, under quercetin effect, the QT rats demonstrated normal plasma TAG, LDL-cholesterol and total cholesterol concentrations compared to the normal control NC rats on Day 120. The anti-dyslipidemic effects of quercetin are well documented in mice [9] and male Wistar rats [21]. Quercetin alleviates dyslipidemia via induction of the insulin-independent AMP-protein kinase and glucagon-like peptide-1 (GLP-1) promoting GLUT-4 gene expression. As a result, glucose uptake by myocytes is significantly enhanced increasing the energy expenditure. Thus, the carbon source for hepatic lipogenesis decreases [22]. Additionally, quercetin also promotes cholesterol-to-bile conversion [12] to lower hypercholesterolemia.

Here, we show for the first time that the hyperglycemia correlated significantly positive with plasma TAG, but not with plasma cholesterol concentrations in the diabetic DC rats (Figure 3A and Table 5). This correlation implies that plasma TAG is a predictor of T2D-associated dyslipidemia in male Wistar rats (Table 5).

Consisting with previous findings [9,11,12,23], we observed that quercetin administration attenuated the concentration of the inflammatory marker CRP in plasma of the QT rats on Day 120. Qurecetin mediates its anti-inflammatory property via down-regulation gene expression of glycoprotein (gp91phox) component of NADPH oxidase in hepatocytes, and decrease of plasma 8-isoprostane, a mediator and a marker of oxidative stress in rodents [9].

During evaluation of emerging antidiabetic drug, its effect on pancreatic mass is seriously considered [24]. Illustrated in Figures 2A and 2B, we noted significant decrease of the RPW (%) and number of islets of Langerhans in the pancreas of diabetic DC rats (Days 0, 60 and 120) and in QT rats (Day 0) as evidence of pancreatic tissue alteration induced by HFHSD and T2D. In contrasts, quercetin normalized RPW (%) and enhanced number of islet of Langerhans in the QT rats (Figures 2A and 2B) lending support to previous findings *in vitro* in INS-1E β-cell line [25] and *in vivo* in rats [26,27] and mice [28], that quercetin prevents pancreatic tissue injury induced by chemicals and proinflammatory cytokines insults.

In humans, the pancreatic weight and size correlate positively with BMI and body weight [29]. In our study, RPW (%) did not correlate with BMI, but correlated with AC:TC ratio and hyperglycemia in T2D male Wistar rats (Table 3).

One of the strengths of this study is its ability to determine preliminary data about the usefulness of the RPW (%) as marker of the obesity-related T2D induction. We clearly showed that while long-term HFHSD induced obesity-associated T2D and significantly decreases RPW (%) and number of islets of Langerhans, quercetin increases reverses this effect.

Additionally, because body weight does not increase under *ad libitum* feeding in all experimental rats [30] body weight parameter might not precisely predict obesity in rats. We found that the AC:TC ratio correlated positively with the hyperglycemia and negatively with RPW (%), suggesting that the abdominal circumference (visceral fats) component of the AC:TC adequately predicts obesity-associated T2D in rats (Table 3).

The significant (*P* ≤ 0.05) decrease of the RPW (%) and number of islets of Langerhans in the pancreas of diabetic DC rats fed the HFHSD on (Days 0, 60 and 120) and QT rats (Day 0) implies pancreatic tissue alteration. Chronic hyperglycemia in T2D induces glucotoxicity leading to β-cell mitochondrial damage, β-cell necroptosis [25,31] that could decrease the RPW. Our observation that quercetin normalized the RPW (%) and enhanced number of islet of Langerhans in the QT rats (Figure 2A and B) agrees with previous findings *in vitro* in INS-1E β-cell line [25] and *in vivo* in rats [25,26] and mice [30], which shows that quercetin prevent pancreatic tissue injury induced by chemicals and proinflammatory cytokines insults.

Thus, quercetin sufficiently normalized obesity, dyslipidemia and RPW, but failed to normalize the number of islets of Langerhans and insulin resistance in the QT rats. As a result, the hyperglycemia was not normalized.

In conclusion, quercetin cured the long-term obesity and dyslipidemia, which are long considered the underlying etiology of T2D in obese male Wistar rats. However, cure of obesity and dyslipidemia by quercetin did not lead to normalization of insulin resistance implying that other aberrant homeostatic alterations might have developed and blunted effect of quercetin in long-term T2D rats.

Acknowledgements

The authors thank the Faculty of Pharmacy, University of Khartoum for providing housing of the Wistar rats at their Restricted Animal Facility. Our appreciation is extended to Professor Hamid Suliman Abdulla, Faculty of Veterinary Medicine, University of Khartoum for assisting with the animal dissection. The authors also thank the Department of Statistics, University of Iowa, USA for helping with the statistical analysis.

References

1. World Health Organization (2016) "Fact sheet: Obesity and overweight".

2. Ouchi N, Parker JL, Lugus JJ, Walsh K (2011) Adipokines inflammation and metabolic disease. Nat Rev Immunol 11: 85-97.

3. Bingley PJ, Mahon JL, Gale EA (2007) Insulin resistance and progression to type 1 diabetes in the European Nicotinamide Diabetes Intervention Trial (ENDIT). Diabetes Care 31: 146-150.

4. Aguirre L, Arias N, Teresa M, Gracia A, Portillo MP (2011) Beneficial effects of quercetin on obesity and diabetes. Nutraceut J 4: 189-198.

5. Walle T, Otake Y, Walle UK, Wilson FA (2000) Quercetin glucosides are completely hydrolyzed in ileostomy patients before absorption. J Nutr 130: 2658-2661.

6. Cierniak A, Papiez M, Kapiszewska M (2004) Modulatory effect of quercetin on DNA damage, induced by etoposide in bone marrow cells and on changes in the activity of antioxidant enzymes in rats. Rocz Akad Med Bialymst 49: 167-169.

7. Ruiz MJ, Fernández M, Pico Y, Mañes J, Asensi M, et al. (2009) Dietary administration of high doses of pterostil to mice is not toxic. J Agric Food Chem 57: 3180-3186.

8. Alam M, Meerza D, Naseem I (2014) Protective effect of quercetin on hyperglycemia, oxidative stress and DNA damage in alloxan induced type 2 diabetic mice. Life Sci 109: 8-14.

9. Sun X, Yamasaki M, Katsube T, Shiwaku K (2015) Effects of quercetin derivatives from mulberry leaves: Improved gene expression related hepatic lipid and glucose metabolism in short-term high-fat fed mice. Nutr Res Pract 9: 137-143.

10. Kobori M, Masumoto S, Akimoto Y, Takahashi Y (2009) Dietary quercetin alleviates diabetic symptoms and reduces streptozotocin induced disturbance of hepatic gene expression in mice. Mol Nutr Food Res 53: 859-868.

11. Rivera L, Morón R, Sánchez M, Zarzuelo A, Galisteo M (2008) Quercetin ameliorates metabolic syndrome and improves the inflammatory status in obese Zucker rats. Obesity 16: 2081-2087.

12. Sekhon-Loodu S, Ziaullah Z, Rupasinghe P, Wang Y, Kulka M, et al. (2016) Novel quercetin-3-O-glucoside eicosapentenoic acid ester ameliorates inflammation and hyperlipidemia. Inflammopharmacology 23: 173-185.

13. Srinivasan K, Viswanad B, Asrat L, Kaul CL, Ramarao P (2005) Combination of high-fat diet-fed and low-dose streptozotocin-treated rat: A model for type 2 diabetes and pharmacological screening. Pharmacol Res 52: 313-320.

14. Novelli ELB, Diniz YS, Galhardi CM, Ebaid GMX, Rodrigues HG, et al. (2006) Anthropometrical parameters and markers of obesity in rats. Lab Anim 41: 111-119.

15. Mathews R, Hosker P, Rudenski S, Naylor A, Treacher DF, Turner RC (1985) Homeostasis model assessment: insulin resistance and β-cell function from fasting plasma glucose and insulin concentrations in man. Diabetologia 28: 412-419.

16. Carleton M, Drury R, Wallington A (1980) Carlton's histological technique (5th edn.) New York: Oxford University Press, pp: 173-174.

17. Forouzanfar MH, Afshin A, Alexander LT, Anderson HR, Bhutta ZA (2015) Global, regional and national comparative risk assessment of 79 behavioural, environmental and occupational, and metabolic risks or clusters of risks 1990-2015: a systematic analysis for the global burden of disease study 2015. Lancet 388: 1659-1724.

18. Lai Y, Yang J, Rayalam S, Della-Fera M, Ambati S, et al. (2011) Preventing bone loss and weight gain with combinations of vitamin D and phytochemicals. J Med Food 4: 1352-1362.

19. Koboro M, Masumoto S, Akimoto Y, Oike H (2011) Chronic dietary intake of quercetin alleviates hepatic fat accumulation associated with consumption of a Western-style diet in C57/BL6J mice. Mol Nutr Food Res 55: 530-540.

20. Torres-Villalobos G, Hamdan-Perez N, Tovar A, Ordaz-Nava G, Martínez-Benítez B, et al. (2015) Combined high-fat diet and sustained high sucrose consumption promotes NAFLD in a murine model. Ann Hepatol 14: 540-546.

21. Wein S, Behm N, Petersen RK, Kristiansen K, Wolffram S (2010) Quercetin enhances adiponectin secretion by a PPAR-γ independent mechanism. Eur J Pharm Sci 41: 16-22.

22. Eid H, Martineau L, Saleem A, Muhammad A, Vallerand D, et al. (2010) Stimulation of AMP-activated protein kinase and enhancement of basal glucose uptake in muscle cells by quercetin and quercetin glycosides, active principles of the antidiabetic medicinal plant Vaccinium vitis-idaea. Mol Nutr Food Res 54: 991-1003.

23. Stewart L, Soileau J, Ribnicky D, Wang Z, Raskin I, et al. (2008) Quercetin transiently increases energy expenditure, but persistently decreases circulating markers of inflammation in C57BL/6J mice fed a high-fat diet. Metabolism 57: S39-S46.

24. Vrang N, Jelsing J, Simonsen L, Jensen E, Thorup I, et al. (2012) The effects of 13 wk of liraglutide treatment on endocrine and exocrine pancreas in male and female ZDF rats: a quantitative and qualitative analysis revealing no evidence of drug-induced pancreatitis. Am J Physiol Endocrinol Metab 303: E253-E264.

25. Bhattacharya S, Oksbjerg N, Young J, Jeppesen P (2014) Caffeic acid, naringenin and quercetin enhance glucose stimulated insulin secretion and glucose sensitivity in INS-1E cells. Diabetes Obes Metab 16: 602-612.

26. Vessal M, Hemmati M, Vasei M (2003) Antidiabetic effects of quercetin in streptozocin-induced diabetic rats. Comp Biochem Physiol Part C: Toxicol Pharmacol 135: 357-364.

27. Youl EBG, Magous R, Cros G, Sejalon F, Virsolvy A (2010) Quercetin potentiates insulin secretion and protects INS-1 pancreatic β-cells against oxidative damage via the ERK1/2 pathway. British J Pharmac 161: 799-814.

28. Carvalho KM, Moris TC, de Melo TS, de Castro Brito GA, de Andrade GM, et al. (2010) The natural flavonoid quercetin ameliorates cerulein-induced acute pancreatitis in mice. Biol Pharmaceut Bull 33: 1534-1539.

29. Caglar V, Kkumral B, Uygur R, Alkoc O, Ozen O, et al. (2014) Study of volume, weight and size of normal pancreas, spleen and kidney in adults autopsies. Forensic Med Anat Res 2: 63-69.

30. Commerford S, Pagliassotti M, Melby C, Wei Y, Gayles E, et al. (2000) Fat oxidation, lipolysis and free fatty acid cycling in obesity-prone and obesity-resistant rats. Am J Physiol Endocrinol Metab 279: 875-885.

31. Dai X, Ding Y, Zhang Z, Cai X, Li Y (2013) Quercetin and quercetin protect against cytokine induced injuries in RINm5F beta-cells via the mitochondrial pathway and NF-kappaB signaling. Int J Mol Med 31: 265-271.

19

Retrospective Review of Weight Gain with Atypical Antipsychotics at GMH and COCMHC

Kothari DJ and Tabor A

Griffin Memorial Hospital, Norman, Oklahoma, US

Abstract

Objectives: Anti-Psychotics are a group of medications that are used to treat schizophrenia group of conditions, Mania caused by Bipolar disorder, and other conditions that can cause visual or auditory hallucinations. These hallucinations cause an individual to lose balance with reality and force their inner well being to lose self-control. The purpose of this research design is to identify the relationship between the atypical anti-psychotics and their associations with weight gain. The design is set to distinguish which of the three drugs leads to more weight gain and diabetogenic complications and added side effects in the patients at Griffin Memorial Hospital and Central Oklahoma Community Mental Health Center from 1/1/2010 to 12/31/2013.

Methods: Data from 555 patients were analyzed using a one-way ANOVA from Excel and R-version 3.0.3 statistics. Data was statistically analyzed using p tests.

Results: All of the atypical antipsychotics (Quetiapine, Olanzapine, Clozapine) led to weight gain with Risperidone having a synergistic effect. Diabetes was associated with all of the drugs and Quetiapine showed more GI complications than the other drugs and combinations ($p > 0.05$).

Conclusion: Our study suggests that atypical antipsychotics that were studied were associated with weight gain. Our findings demonstrated that no one drug was overwhelmingly led to more weight gain than the other. Adding risperidone had a synergistic effect and further enhanced weight gain. If replicated, the data may lead to clarification of the results and concluded analysis of the pharmacologic treatment plans of patients at Griffin Memorial Hospital and Central Oklahoma Mental Health Center.

Keywords: Quetiapine; Risperidone; Olanzapine; Seroquel; Antipsychotics; Weight gain

Introduction

Recent advancement in psychopharmacology and the implementation of atypical antipsychotics has made it possible for patients to have a more broad-spectrum efficacy with minimal side effect profile [1,2]. Unlike typical antipsychotics, the newer atypical drugs decrease the positive, negative and cognitive symptoms in the schizophrenia group of conditions and extrapyramidal side effects that pose with the older generation medications [3]. Atypical antipsychotics although efficacious, have shown to cause side effects, such as weight gain, that can lead to overall detrimental health effects. Increased weight gain and obesity has led to an increase in metabolic and cardiovascular complications and an increase in psychotic flare-ups due to poor compliance due via patients' efforts to avoid weight gain [4].

The purpose of this study is to analyze weight gain in patients 50 to 70 years of age at Griffin Memorial Hospital in Oklahoma (GMH) and Central Oklahoma Community Mental Health Care (COCMHC) with the different antipsychotics they are prescribed. In addition, this follow-up review will allow us to better identify which single or combination of drugs pose the most amount of weight gain and side effect profile.

Mechanism of action of atypical antipsychotics

First (typical) and second (atypical) generation antipsychotics have a propensity to bind dopamine D2 receptors in the brain. Typical antipsychotics have a higher affinity for the D2 receptors than atypical antipsychotics and therefore cause more Extrapyramidal Symptoms (EPS) and elevated prolactin levels [5]. The atypical antipsychotics, which include olanzapine (Zyprexa), quetiapine (Seroquel), and clozapine (Clozaril), have a lower affinity for D2 receptors but higher affinity for serotonin 5-HT2_A, 5-HT2_C, 5-HT2_6, 5-HT_6, histamine H1, and alpha 1 receptors [6].

Atypical antipsychotics and weight gain have been studied on the basis of the receptors that these drugs target. According to various studies and articles, weight gain is directly correlated with histamine H1 and 5-HT2_C receptor antagonism [7-9]. Clozapine and olanzapine have the greatest antagonist effect and the most potential to cause weight gain. Quetiapine has a high affinity for H1 receptors but lower affinity for 5-HT2_C receptors and hypothetically causes less weight gain in comparison.

Methods

Participants: Participants were taken from the patient database at two adult mental health facilities, Griffin Memorial Hospital (GMH) and Central Oklahoma Community Mental Health Care (COCMHC). GMH also includes an inpatient and outpatient facility. To be included in our study, participants had to receive services for at least two months in either or both facilities, had to have an admission date between 1/1/2010 and 12/31/2013, and had to be between the ages of 50 and 70

---

*Corresponding author: Kothari DJ, Griffin Memorial Hospital, Norman, Oklahoma, US, E-mail: dhaiwatk@yahoo.com

at the time of admission. This was to eliminate potential illnesses that can interfere with our results, and negate any confounding variables. Patients were selected randomly to eliminate bias. A final study roster of participants (N=555) was obtained; participants were 60% female and 40% male with a mean age at admission of 56.44 years.

Data: A retrospective study design was used with data received from patient's previous charts. Pre-existing condition data for diabetes mellitus and hypertension were taken from admissions forms. Prescription drug use was charted for five drugs, including four atypical antipsychotics: quetiapine, olanzapine, clozapine, and risperidone and metformin, as a secondary measure for diabetes mellitus. Data on weight gain and GI complications (most notably for nausea, vomiting, diarrhea, irritable bowel syndrome, constipation, and esophageal reflux) were also collected. This study was approved by the Oklahoma Department of Mental Health and Substance Abuse Services Institutional Review Board.

Analyses: Frequencies were obtained for all prescription drug use categories. Each participant was placed into a single category based upon the specific combination of antipsychotics he or she took while receiving mental health services. For instance, all participants taking both quetiapine and olanzapine were categorized separately from those taking olanzapine and clozapine. Means, standard deviations, and 95% confidence intervals were obtained for weight gain in each category. Proportions of patients having GI complications were also calculated. A one-way, between-subjects ANOVA comparing weight gains among the different antipsychotic categories were also run. All statistics were run in R version 3.0.3.

Results and Discussions

Out of the 555 patients included in this follow-up review, those that encountered the greatest average weight gain, 24.24 pounds, took quetiapine, followed by olanzapine, with an average weight gain of 19.59 pounds. Clozapine demonstrated a 16-pound average weight gain; however, the patient sample was small and the chance of error is high. The combination of quetiapine and olanzapine seemed to have a synergistic effect, with an average weight gain of 28.33 pounds; there was no relationship between intake and weight gain over time for the patient's that took the quetiapine-olanzapine combination. However, individual intake of either medication demonstrated a relationship with weight gain and metabolic side effects. This high average standard of deviation between single drug and combination intake illustrates a variability that exists and may indicate an error of collecting or reporting weight for some patients. Studies have shown Clozaril to cause the greatest weight gain [9], but our review was limited to three patients and therefore inconclusive for patients at GMH and COCMHC.

Of the 555 patients that were studied, 369 patients were not on any of the three drugs that were studied. These patients were on different atypical antipsychotics, such as aripiprazole (Abilify), ziprasidone (Geodon), or risperidone (Risperdal), which have been shown to cause minimal weight gain in comparison to those studied [10,16,17]. However, the patient population studied showed an average weight gain of 20.84 pounds when using either of these drugs. Out of these three atypical antipsychotics that were not studied, it has been shown that risperidone tends to lead to higher weight gain than either aripiprazole or ziprasidone [11,16].

Of the 369 patients not on quetiapine, olanzapine or clozapine, 104 patients were on risperidone strictly taken from the COCMHC database. We randomly chose patients at COCMHC and compared those only on

Risperdal to those on Risperdal combined with the medication(s) of interest. Patients only on risperidone showed a mean weight gain of 22.12 pounds, while those not on quetiapine, olanzapine, clozapine or risperidone showed an average weight gain of 20.59 pounds. However caution must be taken when interpreting these data since significant variability in the measured weight is a potential source of error. Patients who had risperidone added to their quetiapine showed a 7.78 pound weight gain over a 2 months to a 4 years span, while patients for whom risperidone was added to olanzapine showed an average gain of 5.57 pounds. There were very few patients on clozapine; therefore, the data were inconclusive in showing a relationship with risperidone. Patients on combinations of quetiapine and olanzapine with added risperidone showed a decrease in weight gain compared to patients on quetiapine and olanzapine alone. This was again inconclusive because only 15 patients were on risperidone with quetiapine and olanzapine (Table 1). With an increase in weight, there comes an increased risk of abdominal fat deposition and an increased risk of diabetes and hypertension [12-14]. Patients with pre-existing diabetes and Metformin, and hypertension were taken into account. This helped us eliminate a potential confounding factor, diabetes, for weight gain [12]. Out of the 79 patients on quetiapine, 14 were on metformin (18%). Fourteen patients were on metformin that were also on olanzapine (23%) and 1 patient was on metformin that was on clozapine (33%). Although not every patient with weight gain was on metformin, patients that were excessively obese were on metformin.

Similarly we also focused on which of the three antipsychotics were most associated with gastrointestinal symptoms, such as nausea, vomiting, diarrhea, irritable bowel syndrome, constipation, and esophageal reflux. Gastrointestinal symptoms were noted most with patients taking quetiapine, with 37 out of 79 (47%) patients complaining and being treated for gastrointestinal symptoms. 44% of the patients on Olanzapine (27/62) had G.I. complaints, and were treated accordingly.

Conclusively, quetiapine showed more patients complain of weight gain than olanzapine. Clozapine has been noted to cause weight gain [15], but the evidence was inconclusive at GMH and COCMHC for patients between 50-70 (Table 2). The combination of quetiapine and olanzapine had a synergistic effect for increase in weight. Patients on all three drugs also showed an increase, but the data were inconclusive. Evidence showed that risperidone had a synergistic effect when added to quetiapine or olanzapine. There was not much difference in diabetes prevalence amongst the quetiapine or olanzapine users (Figure 1).

Conclusion

Weight gain is a serious problem in patients taking atypical antipsychotics [2,12]. Along with increased weight, we encountered that patients had an increase in the risk of cardiovascular and metabolic complications such as diabetes, hypertension, and gastrointestinal

Antipsychotic Category	M	SD	(N)
Quetiapine	24.24	17.81	79
Zyprexa	19.59	13.00	62
Clozapine	16.00	5.66	3
Quetiapine and olanzapine	28.33	22.72	28
Olanzapine and clozapine	19.00	a	7
Quetiapine, olanzapine and clozapine	19.25	13.15	6
Other antipsychotics	20.84	13.78	369

[a]One participant took book olanzapine and clozapine, preventing the calculation of a standard deviation

Table 1: Means and Standard Deviations for Weight Gain (pounds) by Antipsychotics Used.

Drug	Total Patients on Drug	Total Patients on Metformin	Total Patients with G.I. Complaints (Nausea, Vomiting, Diarrhea, Ibs, Gerd)
Quetiapine	79	14 (18%)	37 (47%)
Olanzapine	62	14 (22%)	27 (44%)
Clozapine	3	1 (33%)	1 (33%)
Quetiapine-Olanzapine	28	4 (14%)	12 (43%)
Quetiapine-Clozapine	1	--	1
Olanzapine-Clozapine	7	2 (28%)	1 (14%)
Quetiapine-Olanzapine-Clozapine	6	3 (50%)	2 (33%)
No drugs of interest, but are on other atypical antipsychotics	369	52 (14%)	100 (27%)

This table demonstrates the relationship between patients on one Anti-Psychotic or combination with Metformin. The last column is the GI side effects associated with single antipsychotic use compared to the anti-psychotic combination use.

Table 2: Effect of Metformin and G.I. complaints on Anti-Psychotics.

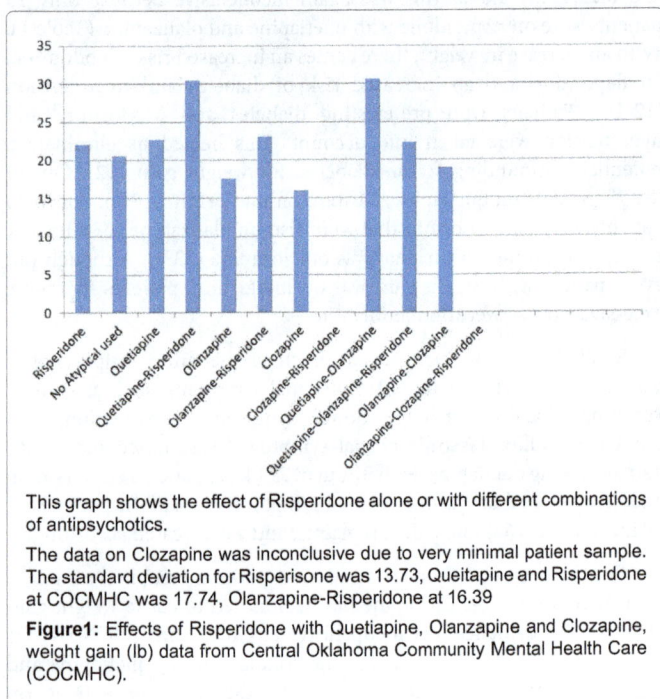

This graph shows the effect of Risperidone alone or with different combinations of antipsychotics.

The data on Clozapine was inconclusive due to very minimal patient sample. The standard deviation for Risperisone was 13.73, Queitapine and Risperidone at COCMHC was 17.74, Olanzapine-Risperidone at 16.39

Figure1: Effects of Risperidone with Quetiapine, Olanzapine and Clozapine, weight gain (lb) data from Central Oklahoma Community Mental Health Care (COCMHC).

manifestations. Although atypical antipsychotics are noted to cause weight gain, different drugs in the second-generation group can have different effects based on their affinity for histamine and serotonin receptors [6-9]. Our study was geared to identify all the atypical antipsychotic that cause more weight gain, what drugs are associated with more metformin intake, and which antipsychotic causes more common side effects such as gastrointestinal manifestations. Understanding that there may be errors in reporting or collecting data, we did manage to secure enough evidence to distinguish that both quetiapine and olanzapine caused weight gain in the patients of GMH and COCMHC. Adding risperidone had a synergistic effect and further enhanced weight gain. Evidently, there was not a great relationship of Metformin intake with any one or combination of anti-psychotics, it is still proved that chance of acquiring diabetes is more from the added weight gain. Studies have shown that diabetes complications have led to multiple cardiovascular manifestations, therefore, proper care needs to be take when on antipsychotics to eliminate the potential for such adverse reactions.

References

1. Das C, Mendez G, Jagasia S, Labbate LA (2012) Second Generation Antipsychotic use in Schizophreia and weight gain: A review and meta-analysis of behavioral and pharmacologic treatments. Ann Clin Psychiatry 24: 225-239.

2. Nasrallah H (2003) A review of the effect of atypical antipsychotics on weight. Psychoneuroendocrinology 28 Suppl 1: 83-96.

3. Javitt DC (1999) Treatment of negative and cognitive symptoms. Curr Psychiatry Rep 1: 25-30.

4. Weiner RL, Hunter GR, Heini AF, Goran MI, Sell SM (1998) The etiology of obesity: Relative contribution of metabolic factors, diet, and physical activity. Am J Med 105: 145-150.

5. Haase HJ, Janssen PAJ (1965) The Action of Neuroleptic drugs: A Psychiatric, neurologic and pharmacologic investigation. Chicago.

6. Meltzer HY (1999) The role of serotonin in antipsychotic drug action. Neuropsychopharmacology 21: 106S-115S.

7. Balt SL, Galloway GP, Baggott MJ, Schwartz Z, Mendelson J (2011) Mechanisms and genetics of antipsychotic-associated weight gain. Clin Pharmacol Ther 90: 179-183.

8. Nasrallah HA (2008) A typical antipsychotic-induced metabolic side effects: insights from receptor-binding profiles. Mol Psychiatry 13: 27-35.

9. Kannel WB, McGee DL (1979) Diabetes and cardiovascular disease. The Framingham study. JAMA 241: 2035-2038.

10. Gentile S (2009) A systematic review of quality of life and weight gain-related issues in patients treated for severe and persistent mental disorders: focus on aripiprazole. Neuropsychiatr Dis Treat 5: 117-125.

11. Claus A, Bollen J, De Cuyper H, Eneman M, Malfroid M (1992) Risperidone versus Haloperidol in the treatment of Schizophrenia inpatients: A multicenter double blind comparative study. Acta Psychiatr Scand 85: 295-305.

12. Haupt DW, Newcomer JW (2001) Hyperglycemia and antipsychotic medication. J Clin Psychiatry 62: 40-41.

13. Amdisen A (1964) Drug-produced obesity. Experiences with chlorpromazine, perphenazine and clopenthixol. Dan Med Bull 11: 182-189.

14. Citrome L, Jaffe A, Levine J, Allingham B, Robinson J et al. (2004) Antipsychotic medication treatment and new prescriptions for insulin and oral hypoglycemic. Eur Neuropharmacol.

15. Stanton JM (1995) Weight gain associated with neuroleptic medication: a review. Schizophr Bull 21: 463-472.

16. Csernansky JG, Mahmoud R, Brenner R; Risperidone-USA-79 Study Group (2002) A comparison of risperidone and haloperidol for the prevention of relapse in patients with schizophrenia. N Engl J Med 346: 16-22.

17. www.pfizer.com/hml/pi's/geodonpi.pdf

20

Sequence Symmetry Analysis and Disproportionality Analyses: What Percentage of Adverse Drug Reaction do they Signal?

Izyan A Wahab*, Nicole L Pratt, Lisa M Kalisch and Elizabeth E Roughead

School of Pharmacy and Medical Sciences, Quality Use of Medicines and Pharmacy Research Centre, Sansom Institute, University of South Australia, Adelaide, South Australia, Australia

Abstract

Background: Sequence Symmetry Analysis (SSA) is a method to detect Adverse Event (AE) signals using administrative claims data. Proportional Reporting Ratio (PRR), Reporting Odds Ratio (ROR) and Bayesian Confidence Propagation Neural Network (BCPNN) are methods to detect AE signals using spontaneous reporting data. The proportion of AEs detected by all four methods is unknown.

Objective: To determine sensitivity, specificity and predictive values of SSA, PRR, ROR and BCPNN for a set of medicine-AE pairs.

Methods: All AEs identified in published Randomised Controlled Trials (RCTs) and Product Information (PI) were extracted for 19 medicines. Gold standard positive AEs were events identified in powered RCTs and gold standard negative AEs were events not listed in the PI for that medicine or any other medicines in the class. SSA was performed for each medicine-AE pairs using Australian Goverrnment Department of Veterans Affairs' data, while the PRR, ROR and BCPNN, was calculated using the Food and Drug Administration Adverse Events Reporting System data.

Results: A total of 157 medicine-AE pairs (43 positive and 114 negative) were identified and tested. SSA, PRR, ROR and BCPNN had a sensitivity of 65%, 19%, 49% and 51% respectively. Specificities across all methods were similar; 89%-97%. Thirty percent of true positive pairs were detected by all methods. SSA detected an additional 35% different true positive pairs while PRR, ROR and BCPNN methods detected an additional 21% different true positive pairs.

Conclusions: Using the combination of signalling methods and data sources, more adverse drug reactions can be detected and could potentially strengthen the safety surveillance of post-marketing medicine.

Keywords: Sequence symmetry analysis; Disproportionality analysis; Adverse drug reaction detection

Introduction

Post-marketing surveillance systems rely on spontaneous reporting databases maintained by health regulators to identify safety issues arising from medicines once they are marketed. Quantitative safety signal detection methods such as Proportional Reporting ratio (PRR), Reporting Odds Ratio (ROR), Bayesian Confidence Propagation Neural Network (BCPNN), and empirical Bayesian technique are applied to spontaneous reporting data to identify safety signals [1-3]. These methods have been adopted as standard quantitative methods by many pharmaco-surveillance centres to screen for safety signals of medicines [2-5]. Studies have validated these methods and showed that the methods have low to moderate sensitivity to detect adverse drug reaction (ADR) signals, ranging between 28% to 56%, while the specificity of the methods ranged from 82% to 95% [6-8].

Voluntary reporting systems have contributed to early identification of previously unknown ADRs, such as flucoxacillin-induced hepatitis and cisapride-induced cardiac arrhythmia [9-11]. There are limitations associated with spontaneous reports such as under-reporting, uncertain quality of information in adverse event reports and inability to identify the incidence of adverse events in voluntary systems [12-13]. Administrative claims databases have the potential to complement spontaneous reports. The administrative claims data have wide population coverage and routine collection of data on exposures (prescription medicines) and outcomes (for an example hospitalisation diagnosis) and are usually stored electronically [14-16]. The advantages of claims data may enable detection of medicine adverse event signals because complete capture of exposures and outcomes can be investigated.

Sequence symmetry analysis (SSA) has been used in previous studies to investigate adverse events associated with medicines using administrative claims data [17-26]. A previous study showed SSA has moderate sensitivity (61%) and high specificity (94%) [27]. The aim of this study was to assess the extent of SSA method for ADR detection in administrative claims database compared to existing standard quantitative methods in spontaneous reporting databases (PRR, ROR and BCPNN) for the same set of medicine-adverse event pairs.

Methods

This study was approved by the Human Research Ethics Committee,

*Corresponding author: Izyan A Wahab, QUMPRC, Sansom Institute, School of Pharmacy and Medical Sciences, University of South Australia, GPO Box 2471, Adelaide 5001, South Australia, Australia,
E-mail: ayyiy001@mymail.unisa.edu.au

University of South Australia and the Department of Veterans' Affairs Research Ethics Committee.

Selection and identification of tested medicines and gold standard adverse events

The selection of medicine and adverse event have been reported elsewhere [27]. Adverse events were considered gold standard positive events if the event was statistically significant in adequately powered randomized clinical trials. Gold standard negative events were those not listed as an adverse event in the product information for the medicine or any other medicine in the class. One hundred and fifty seven medicine-adverse event pairs for 19 medicines were evaluated. The list of tested medicines-adverse event pairs can be found in Appendix A.

Study 1-ADR detection in spontaneous reporting database

Spontaneous reporting database: The United States Food and Drug Administration Adverse Events Reporting System (FAERS) database is a computerised spontaneous reporting database of medicines and adverse events that was used in this study [28]. The database is designed to support the FDA's post-marketing safety surveillance program for medicine and therapeutic products. In 2010, the majority of the reports (62%) were voluntarily reported by health professionals and consumers in the United States [29]. Other countries (32%) also contributed reports to the database [29]. All reported adverse events in the database are coded using a standardised, international terminology, MedDRA (Medical Dictionary for Regulatory Activities). Medicine names are coded using either generic names or trade names.

The FAERS raw data from 2004 and onwards were downloaded from the FDA website [30]. All reports received by the FDA between January 2004 until July 2010 was used in this analysis. Duplicate adverse event reports were excluded. Reports with missing information for adverse events or medicine name were also excluded. After excluding duplicates and cases with missing data, the total number of medicine-adverse event pairs for final analysis was 10,804,054. Because the FAERS data consist of reports around the world, all trade names of the tested medicines were identified using Martindale [31]. Extensive spelling checks for each medicine were applied. For the adverse events, all terms under the Preferred Term of MedDRA were searched. Keywords of the adverse events term were also used to identify the events in the database. The preferred terms used for adverse events are listed in Appendix B.

Identification of ADR in spontaneous reporting database: Three standard pharmaco-surveillance methods in spontaneous reporting databases; Proportional Reporting Ratio (PRR), Reporting Odds Ratio (ROR) and Bayesian Confidence Propagation Neural Network (BCPNN), were applied for each medicine-adverse event pairs in the FAERS database. These methods have been described in detail previously [1-3,5]. These methods are disproportionality analyses based on 2×2 tables as shown in Table 1. Table 2 shows the information used to support the calculation for all three methods. Signals are considered to be present when signal criteria for the three methods are met (Table 2). These signal criteria have been used by medicine regulatory agencies in the United Kingdom and European countries [2,3-5]. Counts of drug-event pairs were used as the unit of analysis in calculating the PRR and ROR statistics. For the BCPNN calculation, we used counts of reports

Medicines	Specific Adverse events	All other adverse events	Total
Specific medicine	A	B	A+B
All other medicines	C	D	C+D

Table 1: 2×2 table of the disproportionality analysis of PRR, ROR and BCPNN.

Method	Regulatory agencies	Information used	Criteria for signal detection
PRR	Australia, United Kingdom Medicines and Healthcare products Regulatory Agency (MHRA), Italian Regulatory Agency, European Medicine Agency.	[A/(A+B)]/[C/(C+D)]	PRR ≥ 2, A ≥ 3, x^2 ≥ 4
ROR	Netherlands Pharmacovigilance Foundation Lareb.	(A/B)/(C/D)	Lower limit of 95% CI ≥ 1
BCPNN	Uppsala Monitoring Centre (World Health Organization (WHO) Vigibase).	Log2 [p (x,y)/p(x)p(y)]	Lower limit of 95% CI>0

CI=Confidence interval; **A**=case reports of medicine associated with adverse events; x^2= chi-square; **p(x)**=probability of medicine 'x' reported on database, **p(y)**=probability of adverse event 'y' reported on the database, **p(x,y)**=probability of medicine 'x'- adverse event 'y' combination reported on the database

Table 2: Pharmaco-surveillance methods used by regulatory agencies, information used to generate signal and the threshold for ADR signal.

[1]. Sensitivity, specificity and predictive values were calculated based on the 2×2 table [32]. All analyses were carried out using SAS 9.2 (SAS Institute, Inc., Cary, NC, USA; www.sas.com).

Study 2-ADR detection in administrative claims database

Administrative claims database: Administrative claims data from the Australian Government Department of Veterans' Affairs (DVA) was used. The DVA database contains information on all medicines and healthcare utilisation by veterans for which DVA pays a subsidy. This includes data for all medicines dispensed on the Pharmaceutical Benefit Scheme (PBS) and Repatriation Pharmaceutical Benefits Scheme (RPBS) as well as hospitalisations, for a treatment population of 250,000 veterans [33]. Medicines are coded according to the World Health Organization (WHO) anatomical and therapeutic chemical (ATC) classification [34] and the Schedule of Pharmaceutical Benefits item codes [35]. Hospitalisations are coded according to the WHO international classification of disease, 10th revision (ICD-10) Australian modification [36].

Identification of ADR in administrative claims database: Sequence symmetry analysis (SSA) was undertaken for each medicine-adverse event pair within the DVA database. Prescription supply and hospitalisation records between 1 January 2000 and 31 December 2010 were used. SSA has been described in detail previously [24]. Briefly, sequence symmetry analysis determines asymmetry in the sequence of dispensing between medicine and indicator of adverse event within a given time window. The indicator of adverse event can be either a medicine used to treat the adverse event or hospitalisation that would describe the event. The indicators used for adverse events in this study are listed in Appendix C. The sequence ratio is robust to confounders that are stable over time. However, the SSA may be affected by prescribing or event trends overtime. To adjust for the trend, a null effect sequence ratio is calculated for prescription of investigated medicines dispensed within the time window limit before and after the indicator medicines dispensed based on the total exposed DVA population [24]. This ratio estimates the sequence ratio that might be expected due to the trends in medicine use under the assumption that the index medicine and the indicator are unrelated [24]. An adjusted sequence ratio (ASR) is obtained by dividing the crude sequence ratio by the null effect ratio [24] and 95% confidence intervals (CI) were calculated [37]. A signal is considered to be present when the lower limit of the 95% CI is one or more. Sensitivity, specificity and predictive values were calculated based on the 2×2 table [32]. All analyses were carried out using SAS 9.2 (SAS Institute, Inc., Cary, NC, USA; www.sas.com).

ADR detection in spontaneous reporting database and administrative claims database

Descriptive statistics were undertaken to compare detection of medicine-ADR pairs when using any of the four methods; PRR, ROR, BCPNN, and SSA.

Results

Study 1-ADR detection in spontaneous reporting database

Bayesian Confidence Propagation Neural Network (BCPNN) had higher sensitivity (51%) than PRR (19%) but similar to ROR (49%) (Table 3). Specificity, and predictive values across all disproportionality methods were similar (specificity: 89%-97%, positive predictive values: 65%-73%), negative predictive values: 76%-83% (Table 3)).

Study 2-ADR detection in administrative claims database

Sequence symmetry analysis (SSA) had 65% sensitivity and 90% specificity to detect ADRs (Table 3). Positive and negative predictive values were 72% and 87% respectively (Table 3).

Methods	Proportional reporting ratio (PRR)	Reporting odds ratio (ROR)	Bayesian Confidence Propagation Neural Network (BCPNN)	Sequence Symmetry Analysis (SSA)
Databases	FDA spontaneous reporting database	FDA spontaneous reporting database	FDA spontaneous reporting database	DVA administrative claims database
Signalling criteria	PRR ≥ 2, a ≥ 3, x^2 ≥ 4	Lower 95% CI ≥ 1	IC 95% CI>0	Lower 95% CI ≥ 1
Sensitivity (%)	19	49	51	65
Specificity (%)	97	92	89	90
Positive predictive value (%)	73	70	65	72
Negative prediciitive value (%)	76	83	83	87

Table 3: Sensitivity, specificity and predictive values results for SSA, PRR, ROR and BCPNN.

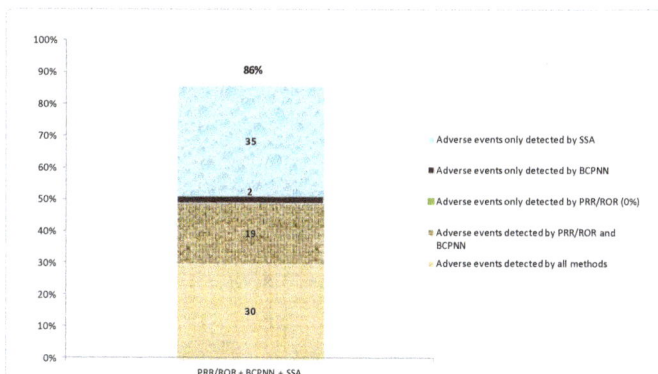

PRR: Proportional Reporting Ratio; ROR: Reporting Odds Ratio; BCPNN: Bayesian Confidence Propagation Neural Network; SSA: Sequence Symmetry Analysis

Figure 1: Combination of all signalling methods to detect true positive events.

ADR detection in spontaneous reporting database and administrative claims database

When using any of the four methods, 86% of true positive adverse events were detected (Figure 1). Thirty percent of true positive pairs were detected by all methods (PRR, ROR, BCPNN and SSA) (Figure 1). SSA detected an additional 35% true positive medicine-adverse event pairs that were not detected by other methods. PRR, ROR and BCPNN detected an additional 21% true positive association that were not detected by SSA.

Discussion

The findings of this study suggest that use of a combination signalling methods to detect adverse drug reactions (SSA in administrative claims database and PRR, ROR, BCPNN in spontaneous reporting database) is better than any of the four methods alone to detect adverse drug reactions. This study also has demonstrated that for a list of medicine-adverse event pairs, SSA has higher sensitivity compared to other signal detection algorithms using spontaneous reporting data (Table 1). Although the PRR had slightly higher specificity (97%) compared to SSA (90%), PRR had the lowest sensitivity (19%) to detect the tested medicine-adverse pairs. This study suggests that SSA is a potential complementary tool to enhance current pharmaco-surveillance methods used in spontaneous reporting database.

The sensitivity of PRR and ROR in this study (49%) is higher than that found in two previous studies that showed sensitivity ranged from 9.9% to 28% [8,38]. One reason for this may be the different gold standard medicine-adverse event pairs used in our study. Our study used only statistically significant adverse events from powered randomised controlled trials as gold standard positive events, while the previous studies used all adverse events listed in the product information. Adverse events listed in the product information may be based on case reports and causality not substantiated. The specificity for PRR and ROR in prior studies was similar to the specificity in our study [6,8,38]. The predictive values for the BCPNN in our study (PPV: 51%, NPV: 81%) were similar with a previous study that used Martindale and Physician Desk Reference as the gold standard reference to evaluate safety signal using spontaneous reporting database (PPV: 44%, NPV: 85%) (7)].

Our findings suggest in cases where an adverse event has a prescription treatment or hospital admission that could describe the event, symmetry analysis may be employed in the administrative claims data as a complementary tool to spontaneous reporting of adverse event system. As with PRR, ROR and BCPNN methods, signals detected by SSA should not replace expert clinical review. SSA uses only prescription dispensing records and hospitalisation admission data without consideration of a patient's clinical condition. Positive signals generated for a medicine do not provide causal evidence that the medicine induced the event. Any positive signals generated by SSA should be followed up with a thorough investigation.

The strength of this study was that we used only adverse events identified in powered randomised controlled trials (RCTs) as the gold standard for positive events. In the real world, the types of adverse events reported to spontaneous reporting database may be different from those identified in the RCTs. The adverse events identified in RCTs are generally common and expected due to the mechanism of action of the medicine, thus these adverse events maybe unlikely to be reported to the spontaneous reporting centres. In addition, the FDA has a requirement that serious adverse events are to be reported to the

FDA reporting website [39]. However, in this study we found about 50% of the adverse events identified in RCTs such as nausea and diarrhoea could be detected from the FDA spontaneous reporting database. Other studies have also found that non-serious adverse events are commonly reported to spontaneous reporting databases [40-42]. Similarly, in administrative claims data, medicines used to treat adverse events may not always be recorded. Patients could either discontinue the suspected medicine that caused the event or switch to another medicine without having to be treated or hospitalised. Medicines used to treat adverse events are sometimes available as over-the-counter (OTC) medicines in pharmacy without having a prescription, meaning that the supply is not be recorded in the administrative claims data. The omission of OTC medicines could result in an underestimation of the sensitivity of sequence symmetry method. In essence, both types of databases used in this study have limitations as a source of data to detect common adverse events. However, this study has demonstrated that SSA that uses health claims data, together with PRR, ROR and BCPNN that use spontaneous reporting data can enhance ADR signal detection.

Conclusions

This study has demonstrated that sequence symmetry analysis that uses prescription and hospitalisation claims data may be a complementary pharmaco-surveillance tool to enhance the current quantitative methods that use spontaneous reporting data in detecting safety signals of medicines.

Acknowledgement

The authors would like to thank the Australian Government Department of Veterans' Affairs for providing the data used in this study. No sources of funding were used in the preparation of this manuscript and the research. The authors have no conflicts of interest relevant to this study.

References

1. Gould AL (2003) Practical pharmacovigilance analysis strategies. Pharmacoepidemiol Drug Saf 12: 559-574.

2. Egberts AC, Meyboom RH, van Puijenbroek EP (2002) Use of measures of disproportionality in pharmacovigilance: three Dutch examples. Drug Saf 25: 453-458.

3. Evans SJ, Waller PC, Davis S (2001) Use of proportional reporting ratios (PRRs) for signal generation from spontaneous adverse drug reaction reports. Pharmacoepidemiol Drug Saf 10: 483-486.

4. Australia Government Department of Health and Ageing. Pharmacovigilance: Office of Product Review (2012).

5. Bate A, Lindquist M, Edwards IR, Olsson S, Orre R, et al. (1998) A Bayesian neural network method for adverse drug reaction signal generation. Eur J Clin Pharmacol 54: 315-321.

6. Lehman HP, Chen J, Gould AL, Kassekert R, Beninger PR, et al. (2007) An evaluation of computer-aided disproportionality analysis for post-marketing signal detection. Clin Pharmacol Ther 82: 173-180.

7. Lindquist M, Stahl M, Bate A, Edwards IR, Meyboom RH (2000) A retrospective evaluation of a data mining approach to aid finding new adverse drug reaction signals in the WHO international database. Drug Saf 23: 533-542.

8. Matsushita Y, Kuroda Y, Niwa S, Sonehara S, Hamada C, et al. (2007) Criteria revision and performance comparison of three methods of signal detection applied to the spontaneous reporting database of a pharmaceutical manufacturer. Drug Saf 30: 715-726.

9. Turner IB, Eckstein RP, Riley JW, Lunzer MR (1989) Prolonged hepatic cholestasis after flucloxacillin therapy. Med J Aust 151: 701-705.

10. Eckstein RP, Dowsett JF, Lunzer MR (1993) Flucloxacillin induced liver disease: histopathological findings at biopsy and autopsy. Pathology 25: 223-228.

11. Olsson S, Edwards IR (1992) Tachycardia during cisapride treatment. BMJ 305: 748-749.

12. Hazell L, Shakir SA (2006) Under-reporting of adverse drug reactions: a systematic review. Drug Saf 29: 385-396.

13. Alvarez-Requejo A, Carvajal A, Begaud B, Moride Y, Vega T, et al. (1998) Under-reporting of adverse drug reactions. Estimate based on a spontaneous reporting scheme and a sentinel system. Eur J Clin Pharmacol 54: 483-488.

14. Silverman SL (2009) From randomized controlled trials to observational studies. Am J Med 122: 114-120.

15. Berger ML, Mamdani M, Atkins D, Johnson ML (2009) Good research practices for comparative effectiveness research: Defining, reporting and interpreting nonrandomized studies of treatment effects using secondary data sources: The ISPOR good research practices for retrospective database analysis task force report - Part i. Value in Health 12: 1044-1052.

16. Schneeweiss S, Avorn J (2005) A review of uses of health care utilization databases for epidemiologic research on therapeutics. J Clin Epidemiol 58: 323-337.

17. Hallas J (1996) Evidence of depression provoked by cardiovascular medication: a prescription sequence symmetry analysis. Epidemiology 7: 478-484.

18. Hallas J, Bytzer P (1998) Screening for drug related dyspepsia: an analysis of prescription symmetry. Eur J Gastroenterol Hepatol 10: 27-32.

19. Bytzer P, Hallas J (2000) Drug-induced symptoms of functional dyspepsia and nausea. A symmetry analysis of one million prescriptions. Aliment Pharmacol Ther 14: 1479-1484.

20. Corrao G, Botteri E, Bagnardi V, Zambon A, Carobbio A, et al. (2005) Generating signals of drug-adverse effects from prescription databases and application to the risk of arrhythmia associated with antibacterials. Pharmacoepidemiol Drug Saf 14: 31-40.

21. Caughey GE, Roughead EE, Pratt N, Killer G, Gilbert AL (2011) Stroke risk and NSAIDs: an Australian population-based study. Med J Aust 195: 525-529.

22. Hersom K, Neary MP, Levaux HP, Klaskala W, Strauss JS (2003) Isotretinoin and antidepressant pharmacotherapy: a prescription sequence symmetry analysis. J Am Acad Dermatol 49: 424-432.

23. Lindberg G, Hallas J (1998) Cholesterol-lowering drugs and antidepressants- -a study of prescription symmetry. Pharmacoepidemiol Drug Saf 7: 399-402.

24. Tsiropoulos I, Andersen M, Hallas J (2009) Adverse events with use of antiepileptic drugs: a prescription and event symmetry analysis. Pharmacoepidemiol Drug Saf 18: 483-491.

25. Vegter S, de Jong-van den Berg LT (2010) Misdiagnosis and mistreatment of a common side-effect--angiotensin-converting enzyme inhibitor-induced cough. Br J Clin Pharmacol 69: 200-203.

26. Garrison SR, Dormuth CR, Morrow RL, Carney GA, Khan KM (2012) Nocturnal leg cramps and prescription use that precedes them: a sequence symmetry analysis. Arch Intern Med 172: 120-126.

27. Wahab IA, Pratt NL, Wiese MD, Kalisch LM, Roughead EE (2013) The validity of sequence symmetry analysis (SSA) for adverse drug reaction signal detection. Pharmacoepidemiol Drug Saf 22: 496-502.

28. United States Food and Drug Admistration. (2012) FDA Adverse Event Reporting System (FAERS).

29. United States Food and Drug Administration (2013) AERS Domestic and Foreign Reports by Year.

30. United States Food and Drug Administration (2013) The FDA Adverse Event Reporting System (FAERS): latest Quarterly Data files.

31. Medicines Complete. Martindale: The Complete Drug Reference 2013.

32. Altman DG, Bland JM (1994) Diagnostic tests. 1: Sensitivity and specificity. BMJ 308: 1552.

33. Australian Government Department of Veterans' Affairs. (2011) Treatment population statistics. Quarterly Report-March.

34. World Health Organization Collaborating Centre for Drug Statistics Methodology. (2011) Anatomical Therapeutic Chemical Code Classification/ Defined Daily Dose Index.

35. Australian Government, Department of Health and Ageing. Schedule of Pharmaceutical Benefits. PBS for health professional. 2011.

36. National Centre for Classification in Health. International statistical classification

of diseases and related health problems, Tenth Revision, Australian Modification (ICD-10-AM). National Centre for Classification in Health, Faculty of Health Sciences, University of Sydney 2004.

37. Rothman K (1986) Modern Epidemiology. Little Brown and Company: Boston, USA.

38. Choi NK, Chang Y, Kim JY, Choi YK, Park BJ (2011) Comparison and validation of data-mining indices for signal detection: using the Korean national health insurance claims database. Pharmacoepidemiol Drug Saf 20: 1278-1286.

39. United States Food and Drug Administration. (2012) Safety: Reporting Serious Problems to FDA.

40. Hornbuckle K, Wu HH, Fung MC (1999) Evaluation of spontaneous adverse event reports by primary reporter a 15-year review (1983 to 1997). Drug Information Journal 33: 1117-1124.

41. Gedde-Dahl A, Harg P, Stenberg-Nilsen H, Buajordet M, Granas AG, et al. (2007) Characteristics and quality of adverse drug reaction reports by pharmacists in Norway. Pharmacoepidemiol Drug Saf 16: 999-1005.

42. Thiessard F, Roux E, Miremont-Salame G, Fourrier-Reglat A, Haramburu F, et al. (2005) Trends in spontaneous adverse drug reaction reports to the French pharmacovigilance system (1986-2001). Drug Saf 28: 731-740.

21

Statins' Cardiovascular Benefits Outweigh their Diabetogenicity: A Direct Comparison between Number Needed to Treat and Number Needed to Harm

Shimoyama S*

Gastrointestinal Unit, Settlement Clinic, Towa, Adachi-ku, Tokyo, Japan

Abstract

Backgrounds: Although there are several metaanalyses showing that the risk of new onset diabetes mellitus (NODM) is more increased in statin or higher dose statin users than placebos or lower dose statin users, a small increase in the risk of NODM would be outweighed by the improved cardiovascular outcomes. However, these metaanalyses are accompanied by limitations of the inclusion of the studies with confounders. The aim of this study is to elucidate the risk-benefit balance by investigating the number needed to treat (NNT) and number needed to harm (NNH) in a simultaneous comparison according to the individual trial-based criteria of NODM and cardiovascular events.

Methods: A systematic review of the literature retrieves 6 randomized controlled trials (RCTs) comparing statins vs. placebos and 5 RCTs comparing higher vs. moderate doses of statin. Only RCTs which documented the number of patients who developed DM and who experienced cardiovascular events are included.

Results: NNH is consistently larger than NNT in trials of statin use vs. placebos, or in trials of higher vs. moderate dose. Furthermore, the benefit-risk ratios are consistently greater than 1 in most trial.

Conclusions: These results suggest that the absolute risk of NODM by statin is offset by the benefit for reducing cardiovascular events. The evaluation of an individual trial-based risk-benefit balance could resolve the limitations of previous studies as well as provide further reinforced evidence that the merit of statin use for the purpose of low-density lipoprotein cholesterol lowering outweighs the NODM risk.

Keywords: Statin; Diabetes mellitus; Risk-benefit balance; Number needed to treat; Number needed to harm

Introduction

Statins have now become the most widely prescribed drugs for lowering low-density lipoprotein cholesterol, which eventually achieves protective effects against cardiovascular events. Two metaanalyses recruiting only large-size randomized trials have convincingly demonstrated that statin therapy results in a substantial reduction of cardiovascular events regardless of the risk in such events, with a good safety profile [1,2]. However, several unintended, adverse events have been recently expressed [3]. Among them, new onset diabetes mellitus (NODM) has received considerable attention, because DM *per se* confers about a 2-fold excess risk for a wide range of vascular diseases [4], and cardiovascular diseases remain the chief cause of mortality among type 2 DM patients [5]. Therefore, statin use may lead to a dilemma that the beneficial effects of statins for the prevention of cardiovascular events would in turn be superseded by a NODM and a subsequent increase in the potential risks of cardiovascular events.

There is conflicting evidence from different statin trials concerning statin-induced NODM, and if it exists, its strength is a matter of debate. Several observation studies provided evidence of positive [6,7] and neutral [8] statin-DM association. Even in RCTs, the risk of NODM was reduced by 30% with pravastatin [9], was neutral with simvastatin [10], but was nonsignificantly increased by 15% with atorvastatin [11]. Against these backgrounds, several metaanalyses [12-19] have been conducted and have yielded possible evidence of a statin-DM association. However, such evidence –the increased likelihood of NODM in statin users than nonusers or in intensive rather than moderate dose users– does not indicate whether NODM is really harmful and consequently cancels any cardioprotective benefit of statin.

Furthermore, such evidence is based on the RCTs with substantial between-trial differences with regard to nonuniform criteria of NODM, varying numbers of components of metabolic syndrome, simultaneous analyses of primary and secondary prevention trials, and a wide range in age and male-to-female ratios of the participants. Such questions could be answered by carrying out simultaneous comparisons between diabetogenic risks and cardioprotective benefits under the individual trial-based diagnostic criteria of NODM and cardiovascular events in each cohort.

Accordingly, the present study considers the risk-benefit balance of statin use by focusing on a direct comparison between the number needed to treat (i.e., cardiovascular events) and the number needed to harm (i.e., statin-induced NODM) of statins in each trial. This systematic individual trial-based risk-benefit balanced analysis of the previous RCTs reduces currently raised background confounders and reinforces the opinion that the statin-induced NODM is outweighed by the reduction of cardiovascular events regardless of baseline cardiovascular event risk and statin dose.

*Corresponding author: Shimoyama S, Gastrointestinal Unit, Settlement Clinic, Towa, Adachi-ku, Tokyo, 120-0003, Japan, E-mail: shimoyama@apost.plala.or.jp

Methods

Data extraction

A computerized English literature search between 1992 and January 2015 was conducted in PubMed with "statin" and "diabetes" as keywords. As of January 2015, 4482 publications were initially extracted. Filters activated by "metaanalysis" or "systematic review" then retrieved 266 publications. Subsequently, those articles which were not apparently metaanalyses or systematic reviews from their titles/abstracts were excluded. Additional review articles that were considered pertinent were sought by manual search through reference lists in the retrieved publications. By these procedures, 24 metaanalyses and systematic review articles [12-35] were considered eligible sources of RCTs. Following a thorough review of the 73 RCTs included in these 24 metaanalyses and systematic reviews, 6 RCTs of statin use vs. placebos [10,11,36-39] and 5 RCTs of intensive vs. moderate doses of statin use (reviewed in ref.19) were finally judged as qualifying because of their reported actual number of NODM and cardiovascular events in the same cohort, in which participants were restricted to be without DM at the baseline.

NNT and NNH calculations

The number needed to treat (NNT) is defined as the number of patients needed to achieve one cardiovascular event prevention by statin use or intensive dose statin therapy. In the same sense, the number needed to harm (NNH) is defined as the number of patients needed by which one NODM patient appears. By definition, therefore, when NNH is larger than NNT, the cardiovascular benefit of statin treatment outweighs the diabetogenic harm. Actually, the absolute benefit gain is expressed by a difference of cardiovascular event rates between statin or intensive dose statin users and placebos or moderate dose statin users. The absolute risk increase is expressed by a difference of rate of NODM between the two groups. NNT or NNH is then respectively calculated by a reciprocal of the absolute benefit gain or a reciprocal of the absolute risk increase [40,41].

Benefit-risk ratio

In this study, cardiovascular event rates of reference and experimental arms are respectively expressed as p1 and p2. Similarly, rates of NODM in experimental and reference arms are respectively expressed as q1 and q2. Since NNT and NNH would be usable only when p1>p2 and q1>q2, the trials of p1<p2 and/or q1<q2, if any, could not be a subject of NNT and NNH calculations. This leads to a loss of information even in the valuable studies. To avoid this information loss, the benefit-risk ratio is calculated to evaluate benefit-risk balance. Where the benefit and risk ratios are respectively defined as p1/p2 and q1/q2, the benefit-risk ratio is then expressed by (p1/p2)/ (q1/q2). If this ratio is >1, then benefit outweighs the risk.

Results

The characteristics of the selected 11 RCTs are summarized in Tables 1,2. The trial design (primary or secondary prevention), definition of NODM, and predefined primary endpoint were different between trials.

Table 3 demonstrates each NNT, NNH, and benefit-risk ratio

Trial name (reference)	Trial design	Statin and doses(mg)	Number of patients		Male(%)/ Female(%)	Age (year)	Follow-up (year)	Definition	
			Total	non DM/DM				Endpoint	NODM
JUPITER [36]	1°	Ros20 vs. placebo	17802	17802/0	62/38	median 66	median 1.9	Nonfatal MI, nonfatal stroke, hospitalization for unstable angina, arterial revascularization, death from cardiovascular causes	Physician-reported
ASCOT-LLA [11]	1°+2°	Ato10 vs. placebo	10305	7773/2532	81/19	mean 63	median 3.3	Nonfatal MI and fatal CHD	Self-reported history and receiving any treatment
HPS [10]	2°	Sim40 vs. placebo	20536	14573/5963	75/25	more than 70	mean 5	Major vascular events (major coronary events, strokes, and revascularizations)	Initiation of oral hypoglycemic or insulin treatment, or specific report of new diabetes
GISSI-HF [37]	2°	Ros10 vs. placebo	4574	3378/1196	77/23	mean 68	median 3.9	Time to death or time to death or admission to hospital for cardiovascular reasons	NA
LIPID [38]	2°	Pra40 vs. placebo	9014	6997/2017†	83/17	median 62	mean 6.1	Nonfatal MI and fatal CHD	FBG>=7mmol/l or reported use of oral hypoglycemic or insulin treatment
AURORA [39]	2°	Ros10 vs. placebo	2773	2042/731	62/38	mean 64	mean 3.2	Time to major cardiovascular event (nonfatal MI, nonfatal stroke, death from cardiovascular causes)	NA

1°: primary prevention, 2°: secondary prevention, Ros: rosuvastatin, Ato: atorvastatin, Sim: simvastatin, Pra: pravastatin, PBO: placebo, NODM: new onset diabetes mellitus. MI: myocardial infarction, CHD: coronary heart disease, NA: not available, FBG: fasting blood glucose
†including impaired fasting glucose
Table 1: Study characteristics included in this study. Statins vs. placebos.

in each RCT comparing statin vs. placebos. Among them, p2>p1 and q2>q1 was respectively found in one [37] and two trials [38,39]. Therefore, the calculation of NNT and NNH was accurate in the other three RCTs [10,11,36]. The number needed to treat in order to prevent 1 primary endpoint was 18-83. The number needed to treat to cause 1 case of NODM was 165-213. Therefore, NNT was found to be consistently smaller than NNH across these three trials. Benefit-risk ratio was consistently greater than 1 except one trial [37]. This consistency was reserved both in primary and secondary prevention trials.

Table 4 demonstrates each NNT, NNH, and benefit-risk ratio in each intensive vs. moderate dose statin trial. Again, NNT was found to

be smaller than NNH in 4 of 5 trials and benefit-risk ratio was greater than 1 in 3 of 5 trials.

Discussion

This is the first report of a direct comparison between individual trial-based NNT and NNH under each diagnostic criterion of NODM and cardiovascular events. This analysis differs from the previous metaanalyses in that it simultaneously addresses two parameters (NNT and NNH) of clinical concern about the risk-benefit balance according to each diagnostic criterion of NODM and cardiovascular events. This approach elucidates that NNH is larger than NNT in statin users than placebos, or in population using intensive rather than moderate doses

Authors	Trial design	Statin and doses(mg)	Number of patients		Male(%)/ Female(%)	Age (year)	Follow-up (year)	Definition	
			Total	non DM/DM				primary endpoint	NODM
Cannon CP	2°	Ato80 vs. Sim40	4162	3428/734	78/22	mean 58	mean 2	Death from any cause, MI, unstable angina, revascularization, and stroke	NA
de Lemos JA	2°	Sim80 vs. Sim20	4497	3438/1059	76/24	median 61	up to 2	Cardiovascular death, nonfatal MI, admission for acute coronary syndrome, stroke	NA
LaRosa JC	2°	Ato80 vs. Ato20	10001	8500/1501	81/19	mean 61	median 4.9	Death from CHD, nonfatal MI, resuscitation after cardiac arrest, fatal or nonfatal stroke	NA
Pedersen TR	2°	Ato80 vs. Sim20	8888	7819/1069	81/19	mean 62	median 4.8	Coronary death, nonfatal MI, cardiac arrest with resuscitation	NA
Armitage J	2°	Sim80 vs. Sim20	12064	NA	83/17	mean 64	mean 6.7	Coronary death, MI, stroke, arterial revascularization	NA

2°: secondary prevention, Ato: atorvastatin, Sim: simvastatin, NODM: new onset diabetes mellitus. MI: myocardial infarction, CHD: coronary heart disease, NA: not available.

Table 2: Study characteristics included in this study. Intensive vs. moderate doses of statins. References are listed in a review article [19].

Trial name	Number of non DM patients at study entry		Number of patients with primary endpoint		Rates of primary endpoint		NNT	Number of patients with NODM		Rates of NODM		NNH	Benefit-risk ratio
	PBO	Statin	PBO	Statin	PBO (p1)	Statin (p2)	1/(p1-p2)	Statin	PBO	Statin (q1)	PBO (q2)	1/(q1-q2)	
JUPITER [36]	8901	8901	251	142	0.028	0.016	81.7	270	216	0.030	0.024	164.8	1.41
ASCOT-LLA [11]	3863	3910	108	62	0.028	0.016	82.6	154	134	0.039	0.035	212.9	1.55
HPS [10]	7282	7291	1837	1432	0.252	0.196	17.9	335	293	0.046	0.040	175.1	1.12
GISSI-HF [37]	1718	1660	919	908	0.535	0.547	NA	225	215	0.136	0.125	96.2	0.90
LIPID [38]	3501	3496	507	395	0.145	0.113	31.4	126	138	0.036	0.039	NA	1.40
AURORA [39]	1041	1001	272	261	0.261	0.261	1824.9	10	14	0.010	0.013	NA	1.35

PBO: placebo, NNT: number needed to treat, NNH: number needed to harm, NODM: new onset diabetes mellitus. Benefit-risk ratio is calculated by (p1/p2)/(q1/q2).

Table 3: NNT and NNH in trials of statin versus placebos.

Authors	Number of non DM patients at study entry		Number of patients with primary endpoint		Rates of primary endpoint		NNT	Number of patients with NODM		Rates of NODM		NNH	Benefit-risk ratio
	Moderate	Intensive	Moderate	Intensive	Moderate (p1)	Intensive (p2)	1/(p1-p2)	Intensive	Moderate	Intensive (q1)	Moderate (q2)	1/(q1-q2)	
Cannon CP	1688	1707	355	315	0.210	0.185	38.8	101	99	0.059	0.059	1927.4	1.13
de Lemos JA	1736	1768	234	212	0.135	0.120	67.2	65	47	0.037	0.027	103.2	0.83
LaRosa JC	3797	3798	830	647	0.219	0.170	20.7	418	358	0.110	0.094	63.4	1.10
Pedersen TR	3724	3737	917	776	0.246	0.208	25.9	240	209	0.064	0.056	123.5	1.04
Armitage J	5399	5398	1214	1184	0.225	0.219	181.3	625	587	0.116	0.109	141.6	0.96

PBO: placebo, NNT: number needed to treat, NNH: number needed to harm, NODM: new onset diabetes mellitus
Benefit-risk ratio is calculated by (p1/p2)/(q1/q2).

Table 4: NNT and NNH in trials of intensive vs. moderate doses of statin. References are listed in a review article [19].

of statin. In addition, benefit-risk ratio is mostly greater than 1 in both primary and secondary prevention trials or intensive dose statin use. These results suggest that the statins' advantage outweighs the statins' diabetogenicity regardless of statin dose and cardiovascular event risk at baseline.

Although there are many RCTs reporting statins' benefit for cardiovascular health, only 11 studies were considered pertinent in the present study. This is attributable to the fact that a NODM was not initially considered as a potential adverse event of statins, so that NODM was less likely to become a main topic and was not a primary endpoint. Therefore, many previous RCTs recruited patients both with and without DM at entry, and the incidence of a cardiovascular endpoint was analyzed in this mixed population with a different ability for glycemic control. In addition, even in the subanalysis studies, the information was very limited concerning the actual number of patients developing DM as well as with cardiovascular events among participants restricted to be without DM at entry. This may further make the selection of pertinent publications difficult for the purpose of carrying out a statin risk-benefit balance simultaneously.

Several confounders could be pointed out in previous observational studies and metaanalyses when considering the increased chance of statin-induced NODM than nonstatin users. First, the diagnostic criteria of NODM were different between studies, with some including an initiation of pharmacotherapy and some including personal or a physician report [12-14]. Second, patients carrying a higher number of risk factors for DM are more susceptible to statin-induced NODM than those carrying a smaller number of risk factors for DM [42-44]. This consideration is important since statin users may adopt a less healthy lifestyle than nonstatin users. Given that the risk factors of hyperlipidemia, such as increased body weight, excess calorie intake, less daily exercise habit, sedentary lifestyle, and further components of metabolic syndrome are equivalent to DM, statin may push predisposing individuals toward the development of DM or simply hasten the DM that would have developed anyway by these risk factors regardless of whether or not the person took statin. This context is relevant to the third confounder –a selection bias– in which choice and dose of statin may influence the statin-DM association [14,19]. Strong statin at higher doses may be more likely to be prescribed to those patients with severer metabolic syndrome. It is conceivable that patients with multiple components of metabolic syndromes are both at risk of developing DM [44] and liable to receive higher doses of statin. Fourth, participants in RCTs at different baseline cardiovascular risk –primary or secondary prevention trial– may also lead to a different risk-benefit outcome, because cardioprotective effects of statins are more prominent in secondary prevention than primary prevention. Fifth, the age of participants may also comprise a confounder. Statin appears to increase the risk of NODM in older patients [14]. The risk of DM by pravastatin was increased by 32% in PROSPER [14] in which the patients were aged 70-82 years, while it was decreased by 30% in WOSCOPS in which the mean age of participants was 55 years [9]. Finally, observational studies are unavoidably susceptible to detection bias. Statin users are more likely to have health concerns which lead to a doctor visit, subsequently having more frequent health checks and more chances to detect DM.

Against these backgrounds, several attempts have been made to explore the risk-benefit balance by comparing statin vs. placebo, intensive vs. moderate statin doses, and primary vs. secondary prevention. Cannon et al. estimated that the benefit of preventing total vascular events was 9 times higher than the risk of NODM [45].

Intensive dose statin documented a 16% absolute risk reduction of cardiovascular disease risk with a 12% absolute increase in DM risk [19]. In the primary prevention of statins, the magnitude of the increased risk of NODM is estimated to be 50 times smaller than the absolute cardiovascular benefit [2]. However, even these calculations still cannot avoid bias because they are based on metaanalyses in which the included RCTs have between-trial differences as mentioned above. Such limitations motivate the individual trial-based NNT and NNH comparison under the same diagnostic criteria of NODM and cardiovascular events in each cohort. The present study could resolve the aforementioned limitations of between-trial confounders, thereby providing evidence that statins' diabetogenicity can be canceled and outweighed by the more protective effects of cardiovascular events regardless of different baseline risks of cardiovascular events or statin dose.

Despite the strength, the relatively shorter observation period of the studies recruited in the present one could still render limitations. A glycemic disorder begins long before DM diagnosis [46], and type 2 DM requires a long latency period until cardiovascular events become manifest. In fact, major cardiovascular event rates cumulatively increased in proportion to the length of observation period [47,48]. On the other hand, the mean or median observation period of the studies in the present study is only between 1.9 and 6.1 years, suggesting that a firm conclusion concerning the statins' risk-benefit balance awaits further investigation. It should be noted that valsartan-induced DM occurs more frequently in the later period of its use [49]. Another limitation of concern is whether the present results, derived from studies in which most participants were Caucasians, could be extrapolated to Asian ethnicity. The increase of type 2 DM patients in Asian countries is an epidemic –the prevalence of type 2 DM has tripled or quintupled over the past 30 years in some Asian countries, a higher rate than in the USA where it doubled during the past 40 years. Since DM in Asian countries developed in a much shorter time, in a younger group, and in people with much lower BMI [50], further investigations are required concerning the NNT/NNH comparison in particular in Asian ethnicity.

As statins are consequently prescribed to the overwhelmingly majority of patients with hyperlipidemia, a specific investigation of the risk-benefit balance of statin treatment is merited and the present trial-based findings deserve clinical consideration. The present analyses add insight into the probable cardioprotective advantage of statins rather than their diabetogenic harm.

References

1. Baigent C, Keech A, Kearney PM, Blackwell L, Buck G, et al. (2005) Efficacy and safety of cholesterol-lowering treatment: prospective meta-analysis of data from 90,056 participants in 14 randomised trials of statins. Lancet 366: 1267-1278.

2. Cholesterol Treatment Trialists' (CTT) Collaborators, Mihaylova B, Emberson J, Blackwell L, Keech A, et al. (2012) The effects of lowering LDL cholesterol with statin therapy in people at low risk of vascular disease: meta-analysis of individual data from 27 randomised trials. Lancet 380: 581-590.

3. Macedo AF, Taylor FC, Casas JP, Adler A, Prieto-Merino D, et al. (2014) Unintended effects of statins from observational studies in the general population: systematic review and meta-analysis. BMC Med 12: 51.

4. Emerging Risk Factors Collaboration, Sarwar N, Gao P, Seshasai SR, Gobin R, Kaptoge S, et al. (2010) Diabetes mellitus, fasting blood glucose concentration, and risk of vascular disease: a collaborative meta-analysis of 102 prospective studies. Lancet 375: 2215-2222.

5. Emerging Risk Factors Collaboration, Seshasai SR, Kaptoge S, Thompson A, Di Angelantonio E, et al. (2011) Diabetes mellitus, fasting glucose, and risk of cause-specific death. N Engl J Med 364: 829-841.

6. Carter AA, Gomes T, Camacho X, Juurlink DN, Shah BR, et al (2013) Risk of incident diabetes among patients treated with statins: population based study. BMJ 346: f2610.

7. Dormuth CR, Filion KB, Paterson JM, James MT, Teare GF, et al. (2014) Higher potency statins and the risk of new diabetes: multicentre, observational study of administrative databases. BMJ 348: g3244.

8. Ko DT, Wijeysundera HC, Jackevicius CA, Yousef A, Wang J, et al. (2013) Diabetes mellitus and cardiovascular events in older patients with myocardial infarction prescribed intensive-dose and moderate-dose statins. Circ Cardiovasc Qual Outcomes 6: 315-322.

9. Freeman DJ, Norrie J, Sattar N, Neely RD, Cobbe SM, et al. (2001) Pravastatin and the development of diabetes mellitus: evidence for a protective treatment effect in the West of Scotland Coronary Prevention Study. Circulation 103: 357-362.

10. Collins R, Armitage J, Parish S, Sleigh P, Peto R, et al. (2003) Heart Protection Study Collaborative Group. MRC/BHF Heart Protection Study of cholesterol-lowering with simvastatin in 5963 people with diabetes: a randomised placebo-controlled trial. Lancet. 361: 2005-2016.

11. Sever PS, Dahlöf B, Poulter NR, Wedel H, Beevers G, et al. (2003) Prevention of coronary and stroke events with atorvastatin in hypertensive patients who have average or lower-than-average cholesterol concentrations, in the Anglo-Scandinavian Cardiac Outcomes Trial--Lipid Lowering Arm (ASCOT-LLA): a multicentre randomised controlled trial. Lancet. 361: 1149-1158.

12. Coleman CI, Reinhart K, Kluger J, White CM. (2008) The effect of statins on the development of new-onset type 2 diabetes: a meta-analysis of randomized controlled trials. Curr Med Res Opin 24: 1359-1362.

13. Rajpathak SN, Kumbhani DJ, Crandall J, Barzilai N, Alderman M, et al. (2009) Statin therapy and risk of developing type 2 diabetes: a meta-analysis. Diabetes Care 32: 1924-1929.

14. Sattar N, Preiss D, Murray HM, Welsh P, Buckley BM, et al. (2010) Statins and risk of incident diabetes: a collaborative meta-analysis of randomised statin trials. Lancet 375: 735-742.

15. Mills EJ, Wu P, Chong G, Ghement I, Singh S, et al. (2011) Efficacy and safety of statin treatment for cardiovascular disease: a network meta-analysis of 170,255 patients from 76 randomized trials. QJM 104: 109-124.

16. Naci H, Brugts J, Ades T (2013) Comparative tolerability and harms of individual statins: a study-level network meta-analysis of 246 955 participants from 135 randomized, controlled trials. Circ Cardiovasc Qual Outcomes 6: 390-399.

17. Taylor F, Huffman MD, Macedo AF, Moore TH, Burke M, et al. (2013) Statins for the primary prevention of cardiovascular disease. Cochrane Database Syst Rev 1: CD004816.

18. Navarese EP, Buffon A, Andreotti F, Kozinski M, Welton N, et al. (2013) Meta-analysis of impact of different types and doses of statins on new-onset diabetes mellitus. Am J Cardiol 111: 1123-1130.

19. Preiss D, Seshasai SR, Welsh P, Murphy SA, Ho JE, et al. (2011) Risk of incident diabetes with intensive-dose compared with moderate-dose statin therapy: a meta-analysis. JAMA 305: 2556-2564.

20. Ray KK, Seshasai SR, Erqou S, Sever P, Jukema JW, et al. (2010) Statins and all-cause mortality in high-risk primary prevention: a meta-analysis of 11 randomized controlled trials involving 65,229 participants. Arch Intern Med 170: 1024-1031.

21. 21. Naci H, Brugts JJ, Fleurence R, Tsoi B, Toor H, et al. (2013) Comparative benefits of statins in the primary and secondary prevention of major coronary events and all-cause mortality: a network meta-analysis of placebo-controlled and active-comparator trials. Eur J Prev Cardiol 20: 641-657.

22. Taylor F, Huffman MD, Macedo AF, Moore TH, Burke M, et al. (2013) Statins for the primary prevention of cardiovascular disease. Cochrane Database Syst Rev 1: CD004816.

23. Petretta M, Costanzo P, Perrone-Filardi P, Chiariello M (2010) Impact of gender in primary prevention of coronary heart disease with statin therapy: a meta-analysis. Int J Cardiol 138: 25-31.

24. Cholesterol Treatment Trialists' (CTT) Collaboration, Baigent C, Blackwell L, Emberson J, Holland LE, Reith C, et al. (2010) Efficacy and safety of more intensive lowering of LDL cholesterol: a meta-analysis of data from 170,000 participants in 26 randomised trials. Lancet 376: 1670-1681.

25. Brugts JJ, Yetgin T, Hoeks SE, Gotto AM, Shepherd J, et al. (2009) The benefits of statins in people without established cardiovascular disease but with cardiovascular risk factors: meta-analysis of randomised controlled trials. BMJ 338: b2376.

26. Cai R, Yuan Y, Zhou Y, Xia W, Wang P, et al. (2014) Lower intensified target LDL-c level of statin therapy results in a higher risk of incident diabetes: a meta-analysis. PLoS One 9: e104922.

27. Chang YH, Hsieh MC, Wang CY, Lin KC, Lee YJ (2013) Reassessing the benefits of statins in the prevention of cardiovascular disease in diabetic patients--a systematic review and meta-analysis. Rev Diabet Stud 10: 157-170.

28. Swerdlow DI, Preiss D, Kuchenbaecker KB, Holmes MV, Engmann JE, et al. (2015) HMG-coenzyme A reductase inhibition, type 2 diabetes, and bodyweight: evidence from genetic analysis and randomised trials. Lancet 385: 351-361.

29. Tonelli M, Lloyd A, Clement F, Conly J, Husereau D, et al. Efficacy of statins for primary prevention in people at low cardiovascular risk: a meta-analysis. CMAJ 183: E1189-1202.

30. Mills EJ, Rachlis B, Wu P, Devereaux PJ, Arora P, et al. (2008) Primary prevention of cardiovascular mortality and events with statin treatments: a network meta-analysis involving more than 65,000 patients. J Am Coll Cardiol 52: 1769-1781.

31. Thavendiranathan P, Bagai A, Brookhart MA, Choudhry NK (2006) Primary prevention of cardiovascular diseases with statin therapy: a meta-analysis of randomized controlled trials. Arch Intern Med 166: 2307-2313.

32. Kostis WJ, Cheng JQ, Dobrzynski JM, Cabrera J, Kostis JB (2012) Meta-analysis of statin effects in women versus men. J Am Coll Cardiol 59: 572-582.

33. Gould AL, Davies GM, Alemao E, Yin DD, Cook JR (2007) Cholesterol reduction yields clinical benefits: meta-analysis including recent trials. Clin Ther 29: 778-794.

34. Gould AL, Rossouw JE, Santanello NC, Heyse JF, Furberg CD (1998) Cholesterol reduction yields clinical benefit: impact of statin trials. Circulation 97: 946-952.

35. Gould AL, Rossouw JE, Santanello NC, Heyse JF, Furberg CD (1995) Cholesterol reduction yields clinical benefit. A new look at old data. Circulation 91: 2274-2282.

36. Ridker PM, Danielson E, Fonseca FA, Genest J, Gotto AM Jr, et al. (2008) Rosuvastatin to prevent vascular events in men and women with elevated C-reactive protein. N Engl J Med 359: 2195-2207.

37. Gissi-HF Investigators, Tavazzi L, Maggioni AP, Marchioli R, Barlera S, Franzosi MG, et al. (2008) Effect of rosuvastatin in patients with chronic heart failure (the GISSI-HF trial): a randomised, double-blind, placebo-controlled trial. Lancet 372: 1231-1239.

38. Keech A, Colquhoun D, Best J, Kirby A, Simes RJ, et al. (2003) Secondary prevention of cardiovascular events with long-term pravastatin in patients with diabetes or impaired fasting glucose: results from the LIPID trial. Diabetes Care 26: 2713-2721.

39. Fellström BC, Jardine AG, Schmieder RE, Holdaas H, Bannister K, et al. (2009) Rosuvastatin and cardiovascular events in patients undergoing hemodialysis. N Engl J Med 360: 1395-1407.

40. Mancini GB, Schulzer M (1999) Reporting risks and benefits of therapy by use of the concepts of unqualified success and unmitigated failure: applications to highly cited trials in cardiovascular medicine. Circulation 99: 377-383.

41. Schulzer M, Mancini GB (1996) 'Unqualified success' and 'unmitigated failure': number-needed-to-treat-related concepts for assessing treatment efficacy in the presence of treatment-induced adverse events. Int J Epidemiol 25: 704-712.

42. Waters DD, Ho JE, Boekholdt SM, DeMicco DA, Kastelein JJ, et al. (2013) Cardiovascular event reduction versus new-onset diabetes during atorvastatin therapy: effect of baseline risk factors for diabetes. J Am Coll Cardiol 61: 148-152.

43. Sattar N, McConnachie A, Shaper AG, Blauw GJ, Buckley BM, et al. (2008) Can metabolic syndrome usefully predict cardiovascular disease and diabetes? Outcome data from two prospective studies. Lancet 371: 1927-1935.

44. Ridker PM, Pradhan A, MacFadyen JG, Libby P, Glynn RJ (2012) Cardiovascular benefits and diabetes risks of statin therapy in primary prevention: an analysis from the JUPITER trial. Lancet 380: 565-571.

45. Cannon CP (2010) Balancing the benefits of statins versus a new risk-diabetes. Lancet 375: 700-701.

46. Tabák AG, Jokela M, Akbaraly TN, Brunner EJ, Kivimäki M, et al. (2009) Trajectories of glycaemia, insulin sensitivity, and insulin secretion before diagnosis of type 2 diabetes: an analysis from the Whitehall II study. Lancet 373: 2215-2221.

47. Tominaga M, Eguchi H, Manaka H, Igarashi K, Kato T, et al. (1999) Impaired glucose tolerance is a risk factor for cardiovascular disease, but not impaired fasting glucose. The Funagata Diabetes Study. Diabetes Care 22: 920-924.

48. Oizumi T, Daimon M, Jimbu Y, Wada K, Kameda W, et al. (2008) Impaired glucose tolerance is a risk factor for stroke in a Japanese sample--the Funagata study. Metabolism 57: 333-338.

49. Aksnes TA, Kjeldsen SE, Rostrup M, Omvik P, Hua TA, et al. (2007) Impact of new-onset diabetes mellitus on cardiac outcomes in the Valsartan Antihypertensive Long-term Use Evaluation (VALUE) trial population. Hypertension 50: 467-473.

50. Yoon KH, Lee JH, Kim JW, Cho JH, Choi YH, et al. (2006) Epidemic obesity and type 2 diabetes in Asia. Lancet 368: 1681-1688.

22

Subjectively Perceived Side-Effects of Anti-Epileptic Drugs in Chronic Refractory Epilepsy

IJff DM[1,2]*, Kinderen RJ[1,3], Vader CI[1], Majoie MHJM[1,2] and Aldenkamp AP[1,2,4-6]

[1]Epilepsy Center Kempenhaeghe, Heeze, The Netherlands
[2]MHENS School of Mental Health & Neuroscience, Maastricht University, Maastricht, The Netherlands
[3]CAPHRI School for Public Health and Primary Care, Maastricht University, Maastricht, The Netherlands
[4]Department of Neurology, Maastricht University Medical Center, Maastricht, The Netherlands
[5]Department of neurology, Gent University Hospital, Belgium
[6]Faculty of Electrical Engineering, University of Technology, Eindhoven, The Netherlands

Abstract

Purpose: Antiepileptic drugs (AEDs) can cause side-effects. Patient-reported side-effects due to this type of medication are very common, but thus far only investigated in community based populations. We investigated the subjectively perceived side-effects of anti-epileptic drug treatment in patients with refractory epilepsy.

Methods: A non-selected group, of patients visiting the outpatient department between September 2011 and November 2011 was invited to complete a questionnaire only if they had experienced side-effects of their AED treatment during last year. The questionnaire, the SIDAED, assessed four different categories; cognition, mood, cosmetics and general health. Subgroup analyses were based on their medication use: mono- or polytherapy, older and newer AEDs and AEDs with a high or a low risk for cognitive and behavioral/mood side-effects.

Results: In total, 203 patients or their relatives completed the questionnaire. Mean age of the patients was 37 years (2-81). Most reported complaints (85%) were about their general health followed by cognition, mood and cosmetics. Subgroup analyses showed no differences between patients using monotherapy or polytherapy. Also, no differences were found between patients using older AEDs or newer drugs. Patients using AEDs with a high risk for side-effects did complain more about their mood but not about their cognition. Regression analysis showed that using a high risk AED for behavioral side-effects contributed significantly to the total experienced side-effects.

Conclusion: In conclusion, our study illustrates that patients are a reliable respondent to indicate side-effects despite of their refractory epilepsy. Particularly, mood complaints due to antiepileptic drugs (such as levetiracetam) are correctly noticed.

Keywords: Antiepileptic drugs; Epilepsy; Side-effects

Introduction

The best possible outcome of antiepileptic drug (AED) treatment is to achieve complete seizure freedom without adverse events. However, AEDs are frequently accompanied by a variety of side-effects. The prevalence of AED-related subjective complaints in routine clinical practice in a community-based population was almost 60% [1]. The two domains which yielded the highest prevalence of complaints are general CNS-related complaints (68%) and cognitive complaints (62%). The most frequently reported complaints within the general CNS-related domain are fatigue and tiredness. Memory problems and concentration difficulties are most frequently reported within the cognitive domain. Mood and behavioral complaints such as agitation or irritability and depression are reported less frequently (22%). Another study reported a prevalence of 67% of moderate to severe subjective complaints of patients who were considered to be well-controlled (defined as unchanged medication for the last six months) [2]. Cognitive complaints were reported most frequently. Furthermore, patients on polytherapy reported more side-effects than patients on monotherapy [1-3].

The new antiepileptic drugs such as lamotrigine (LTG), levetiracetam (LEV), oxcarbazepine (OXC), gabapentin (GBP), pregabalin (PGB) and lacosamide (LCS) seem to be similar to the older compounds in efficacy, but superior in tolerability [4]. Cognitive complaints, related to confirmed cognitive dysfunction has been reported with almost all the older drugs and especially for phenobarbital (PB), phenytoin (PHT) and vigabatrin (VGB) [4,5]. Some newer AEDs such as topiramate

(TPM) and zonisamide (ZNS) are also known to cause significant cognitive side-effects: both have diffuse cognitive effects, as well as specific effects on language and memory [5-9]. This concurs with the patient-reported cognitive side-effects that are more common with TPM, followed by ZNS and phenytoin (PHT) and are least likely to be reported with GBP, valproate (VPA), LTG and carbamazepine (CBZ) [10,11]. Furthermore, the newer anti-epileptic drug LEV is known for its high-risk to cause mood effects [12,13]. Mood side-effects are therefore most common in patients-reports with (LEV) [14,15]. The subjective reports about these drugs seem to be by and large equivalent to measured cognitive effects of these AEDs [16,17].

Negative consequences of the antiepileptic drugs necessitate interventions ranging from minor interventions such as drug switches to very expensive hospitalization. It is estimated that side-effects due to antiepileptic drugs have a major impact on health care costs which

*Corresponding author: IJff DM, Epilepsy center Kempenhaeghe, Department of Behavioral Sciences, The Netherlands;
E-mail: ijffd@kempenhaeghe.nl

can be as high as €20.751 (US \$26.675) per patient per year [18]. It is desirable to reduce these costs to a level as low as possible. Earlier studies already showed that side-effects are more important for patients than efficacy in long-term treatment and that long-term retention time is mainly based on subjectively perceived side-effects [19]. Previous research showed also that subjectively perceived side-effects about cognitive functions are used as a sensitive screening instrument for clinical practice which can help to identify who is at risk and needs further referral for neuropsychological assessment while keeping the burden on financial and time resources to a minimum [20]. This allows screening at an early stage and minimizes the use of expensive assessment facilities.

In addition to the community-based studies from our group [1,2,21], we attempted to investigate the impact of subjective complaints in a hospital-based study, in patients with chronic refractory epilepsy. In the community based studies most patients were in remission or they had only infrequent seizures and most were on low dose monotherapy. In the patient population of a tertiary referral center most patients have frequent seizures, are afraid of status epilepticus, and often use high dosing polytherapy. Within this study we also focused on subgroup comparisons. Firstly, a combination of AEDs can produce negative interactions which can lead to side-effects. Separate subgroup analyses were, therefore, performed to check for differences between patients on monotherapy or polytherapy. Secondly, as side-effects of AEDs are claimed to have less effects in the newer generation of AEDs, differences between the newer and older generation of AEDs were compared. Thirdly, some drugs are known to have a higher risk for side-effects than others. Therefore a high-risk group was compared with a low-risk group.

Methods

Procedure

All epilepsy patients using antiepileptic drugs, who visited our tertiary epilepsy center Kempenhaeghe, Heeze, The Netherlands, between September 2011 and November 2011, received a patient information letter by mail including an invitation to complete a questionnaire [18]. Patients were invited to complete the questionnaire only when they had experienced side-effects of the AEDs during the previous 12 months. The questionnaire could either be completed digitally via the internet or on paper. For young children and patients with severe mental retardation, proxy measures were used. All participants (patients, parents or caregivers) gave their informed consent.

Questionnaire

The questionnaire was specifically developed for this study and was subdivided into five different categories of commonly reported side-effects. The side effects of AED treatment questionnaire (SIDAED) [2], developed by our group, was used as the basis for the questionnaire. The original 10 side-effect categories of the SIDAED were compressed into four categories in order to focus on the most commonly reported side-effects. The categories used in this study were: cognition, cosmetic, mood and general health (i.e., general CNS, vision, headache, gastrointestinal, sexuality/menses complaints).

Subgroup and statistical analysis

The subgroup analyses were performed using independent t-tests with SPSS version 21.0, Chicago, IL, USA. A p-value of ≤0.05 was considered significant. Linear regression analysis was used to evaluate the impact of the treatment factors (mono vs. polytherapy, old vs. new AEDs and cognitive/behavioral high vs. low risk AEDs) on the total number of complaints.

Results

Demographic and clinical characteristics

In total, 1386 epilepsy patients received the request to complete a questionnaire. In total, 210 patients completed the questionnaire. Although we asked patients only to fill out the questionnaire when they had experienced any side-effect during the previous 12 months, seven patients returned the forms reporting no side-effects. These patients were excluded from the analysis, yielding a total of 203 patients reporting side-effects (14.6%).

Main characteristics of the 203 patients are shown in Table 1. Mean age was 37 years, with a range from 2 to 81 years. Most patients were treated with polytherapy (range 2-6 AEDs). Most patients used LTG as AED during the last 12 months, followed by LEV, CBZ, VPA and CLB. OXC, TPM, PHT, PGB, GBP, LCS, PB and ethosuximide (ESX) were used less frequently. AEDs that were only used by one patient were primidone, ZNS, VGB and acetazolamide. These drugs were grouped as 'other drugs' (3.0%). Most of the patients were treated with a combination of an older (such as CBZ, VPA, PB, PHT, ETX or benzodiazepines) and a newer (such as LTG, LEV, OXC, GBP, PGB, LCS, TPM) anti-epileptic drug during the last 12 months. Table 2 shows that in monotherapy LTG, VPA, CBZ and LEV are mostly used and OXC and TPM are used less frequently.

Based on the literature [16,17,22], we grouped PB, PHT, TPM, ZNS, and VGB as drugs with a high risk for side-effects. The other AEDs are grouped as AEDs with a low risk for side-effects except LEV which is known for its behavioral effect but has no cognitive side-effects [23]. Therefore, this drug is only added in the behavioral high risk group and not in the cognitive high risk group. During the last 12 months 16% of the patients used at least one of the cognitive high risk drugs and 46.8% of the patients used at least one of the behavioral high risk AEDs.

Type of side-effects

The largest group of patients (38%, n = 78) reported problems in three of the five categories, 24% (n = 49) reported to have side-effects in two of the categories, 23% (n = 47) reported side-effects in four of the categories, 12% (n = 24) reported problems in one of the five categories and five patients (3%) reported to have problems in all categories (Figure 1). Most of the patients (85%) had experienced some kind of general health side-effect due to AEDs during the last 12 months, such as sleep problems and fatigue, motor and balance problems, headache and dizziness (Table 3). Cognitive side-effects were the second most commonly reported problem among the patients (77%). Most described cognitive complaint was memory problems and to a lesser extent concentration problems, language difficulties, mental slowing and problems with information processing. Behavioral side-effects were reported in 69% of the patients. Most commonly described mood complaint was a depressive mood, irritable and angry or agitated behavior. Cosmetic side-effects such as skin rash, weight problems and gum problems occurred in 42% of the patients and 7% reported other side-effects that could not be classified. Only in the cosmetic category of the questionnaire there was a significant difference between males and females. More females reported cosmetic problems during the last 12 months (t = -2.229, p = 0.027). Only in the mood category, there was a significant negative correlation found for age (r = -0.141, p = 0.044); the younger the patients, the more mood complaints were reported.

Subgroup analyses

No differences were found between the mono- and the polytherapy group; patients on polytherapy did not report more side-effects than patients on monotherapy (Table 4). For the comparison between the

	N	%
Age mean (range)	37 (2 – 81)	
Gender		
Male	101	49.8
Female	102	50.2
Mono vs. polytherapy		
Monotherapy	67	33.0
Polytherapy	136	67.0
Number of different AEDs per patient		
Two	71	35.0
Three	40	19.7
Four or more	25	12.3
AED use during the last 12 months		
LTG	77	37.9
LEV	68	33.5
CBZ	68	33.5
VPA	65	32.0
CLB	50	24.6
Other BZP	15	7.4
OXC	27	13.3
TPM	15	7.4
PHT	10	4.9
PGB	11	5.4
GBP	8	3.9
LCS	7	3.4
PB	7	3.4
ESX	6	3.0
Other AEDs	5	2.5
Old versus new AEDs		
Old AEDs	48	23.6
New AEDs	54	26.6
Combination of old and new AEDs	101	49.8
Low risk versus high risk AEDs		
Cognitive low risk AEDs	170	83.7
Cognitive high risk AEDs	33	16.3
Behavioral low risk AEDs	108	53.2
Behavioral high risk AEDs	95	46.8

Table 1: Demographic and clinical characteristics (N=203).

	N	%
LTG	14	20.9
VPA	13	19.4
CBZ	13	19.4
LEV	12	17.9
OXC	6	9.0
TPM	4	6.0
CLB	3	4.5
PHT	1	1.5
Other BZP	1	1.5

LTG: Lamotrigine; VPA: Valproate; CBZ: Carbamazepine; LEV: Levetiracetam; OXC: Oxcarbazepine; TPM: Topiramate; CLB: Clobazam; PHT: Phenytoin; BZP: Benzodiazepines
Table 2: AED use in monotherapy patients.

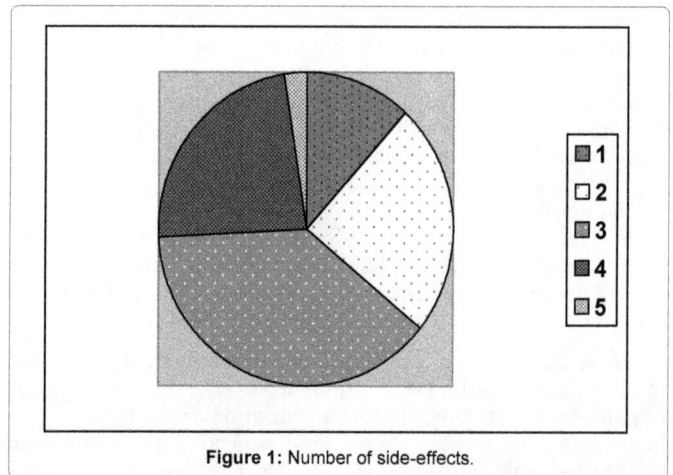

Figure 1: Number of side-effects.

older and the newer AEDs, patients who used a combination of these medication regimens were not taken into account. There were also no differences between the old and new AEDs; patients who used older AEDs did not experience more side-effects than patients who were treated with newer AEDs. Furthermore, there were also no differences between the cognitive risk groups; the cognitive high risk group did not report more side-effects than the cognitive low risk group. However, there was a significant difference between the behavioral risk groups for the mood complaints (t = -2.776, p = 0.006) and total number of complaints (t = -2.221, p = 0.027); patients from the behavioral high risk group did have significantly more problems than patients from the behavioral low risk group, especially concerning their mood.

Linear regression analysis

Thus far each comparison was made independently from the other treatment regimen. However, subgroup divisions are correlated. Therefore, regression analysis was performed with total number of complaints as dependent variable and 1) mono vs. polytherapy, 2) old vs. new AED, 3) cognitive high vs. low risk AED and 4) behavioral high vs. low risk AED as predictors. A backward procedure was used. Although both the cognitive and behavioral high vs. low risk AEDs contributed significantly (F-value: 3.044, p = 0.05), the procedure identified a one-factor solution as the strongest predictor of the total complaints: a behavioral high risk AED (F-value: 4.932, p = 0.027). The total percentage of explained variance was 2.4%.

Discussion

This study compared subjective reported side-effects among different AED treatments in a population referred to a tertiary epilepsy center. No more than 15% of the patients who visited the outpatient clinic reported to have side-effects. It is unlikely that this is due to the absence of side-effects. Rather this percentage reflects the weight the patients with chronic refractory epilepsy attribute to side-effects. Side-effects are commonly reported in community based studies in which the majority of the patients are in remission. In our population, much more importance is probably attributed to the seizures and, hence, the importance of the efficacy of the drugs.

Of the patients who did report side-effects, most had experienced some complaints in their general health, cognition or mood due to their AEDs during the last 12 months. Cosmetic side-effects occurred in a minority of the patients; more in females than males which is consistent with previous literature [24]. In our specific population, polytherapy did not induce more complaints than monotherapy. This

	N	%	Type of complaints	% [*]
General health complaints	172	84.7	Fatigue and sleep problems	62
			Motor and balance problems	29
			Headache	24
			Dizziness	23
			Gastrointestinal problems	14
			Nausea	13
Cognitive complaints	157	77.3	Memory problems	73
			Concentration problems	29
			Language difficulties	25
			Mental slowing	13
Mood complaints	139	68.5	Depressive mood	37
			Irritable and angry behavior	36
			Agitated behavior	20
			Mood sings	16
			Aggressive behavior	13
			Anxious behavior	5
Cosmetic complaints	86	42.4	Skin rash	45
			Weigh problems	44
			Problems with gums	26
			Hair loss	15
			Itch	4
			Shaking hands	4

[*] Patients can have problems in more than one area.

Table 3: Type of side-effect and complaints.

Type of side-effect	mono vs. poly	Old vs. new	Cognitive low risk vs. high risk	Behavioral low risk vs. high risk
Cognition	0.772	0.699	0.492	0.235
Mood	0.549	1.000	0.305	0.006[*]
General health	0.466	0.955	0.614	0.843
Cosmetic	0.309	0.962	0.696	0.620
Total	0.248	0.991	0.925	0.027[*]

[*] $p \leq 0.05$

Table 4: p-Values for the different subgroup analyses.

is inconsistent with previous literature who did report more side-effects [1-3] and a lower quality of life [25] for polytherapy. This probably again illustrates a different efficacy/tolerability attribution in our patient group compared to studies in the community. Furthermore, the generation of the AEDs (older versus newer) was not relevant. The newer AEDs have been thought to have decreased the incidence of certain side-effects such as cosmetic side-effects when compared with older antiepileptic medication [24,26]. However, previous research showed that there was no difference between patients using newer versus classic AEDs in their quality of life [25]. Moreover, patients with a high-risk AED for cognitive side-effects did not complain more about their cognitive functions than patients with a cognitive low-risk AED. However, when LEV was added to this high risk AED group, patients with a high risk AED for behavioral side-effects did complain more about their mood than patients with a behavioral low-risk AED. As shown in our regression analysis, using a high risk AED for behavioral

side-effects contributed significantly to the total experienced side-effects. Note however that the percentage explained variance is low, indicating that the complaints are also related to other factors, in this group probably the epilepsy. The mood complaints of patients using LEV treatment were an essential factor in our study and are in line with a number of studies and meta-analyses [27-30]. LEV had an adverse event profile within the range of the other older drugs like PHT but with a different profile; self-reported anger and hostility were particularly frequent [13,15].

The primary limitation of our study stem from self-reporting. The side-effects were subjectively reported. Our study therefore critically relied on the validity and reliability of subjective self-report as no formal neuropsychological testing was used. Nevertheless, this is a naturalistic situation and the assessment of possible side-effects of AEDs in routine daily care of patients with epilepsy is based on these same self-reports which can be used as a sensitive screening instrument [20].

In conclusion, our study illustrates that patients are a reliable respondent to indicate side-effects despite of their refractory epilepsy. Particularly, mood complaints due to antiepileptic drugs (such as LEV) are correctly noticed.

Acknowledgements

This study is part of a PhD project which is funded by the Netherlands Organization for Health Research and Development (ZonMw), grant application number 171002204. This study has been approved by the ethics committee of the Epilepsy Center Kempenhaeghe.

References

1. Carpay JA, Aldenkamp AP, Donselaar van CA (2005) Complaints associated with the use of antiepileptic drugs: results from a community-based study. Seizure 14: 198-206.

2. Uijl SG, Uiterwaal CS, Aldenkamp AP, Carpay JA, Doelman JC, et al. (2006) A cross-sectional study of subjective complaints in patients with epilepsy who seem to be well-controlled with anti-epileptic drugs. Seizure 15: 242-248.

3. Andrew A, Milinis K, Baker G, Wieshmann U (2012) Self-reported adverse effects of mono and polytherapy for epilepsy. Seizure 21: 610-613.

4. Beghi E (2004) Efficacy and tolerability of the new antiepileptic drugs: comparison of two recent guidelines. Lancet Neurol 3: 618-621.

5. Aldenkamp AP (2001) Effects of anti-epileptic drugs on cognition. Epilepsia 42: 46-49.

6. Bootsma HPR, Coolen F, Aldenkamp AP, Arends J, Diepman L, et al. (2004) Topiramate in clinical practice: long-term experience in patients with refractory epilepsy referred to a tertiary epilepsy center. Epilepsy Behav 5: 380-387.

7. Bootsma HPR, Aldenkamp AP, Diepman L, Hulsman J, Lambrechts D, et al. (2006) The effect of antiepileptic drugs on cognition: patient perceived cognitive problems of topiramate versus levetiracetam in clinical practice. Epilepsia 47: 24-27.

8. Bootsma HPR, Ricker L, Diepman L, Gehring J, Hulsman J, et al. (2008) Long-term effects of levetiractetam and topiramate in clinical practice: a head to head comparison. Seizure 17: 19-26.

9. Park SP, Hwang YH, Lee HW, Suh CK, Kwon SH, et al. (2008) Long-term cognitive and mood effects of zonisamide monotherapy in epilepsy patients. Epilepsy Behav 12: 102-108.

10. Arif H, Buchsbaum R, Weintraub D, Pierro J, Resor Jr SR, et al. (2009) Patient-reported cognitive side effects of antiepileptic drugs: Predictors and comparison of all commonly used antiepileptic drugs. Epilepsy Behav 14: 202-209.

11. Tatum WO, French JA, Faught E, Morris GL, Liporace J, et al. (2001) Post marketing experience with topiramate and cognition. Epilepsia 42: 1134-1140.

12. Bootsma HPR, Ricker L, Diepman L, Gehring J, Hulsman J, et al. (2007) Levetiracetam in clinical practice: long-term experience in patients with refractory epilepsy referred to a tertiary epilepsy center. Epilepsy Behav 10: 296-303.

13. Wieshmann UC, Baker GA (2013) Self-reported feelings of anger and aggression towards others in patients on levetiracetam: data from the UK antiepileptic drug register. BMJ Open 3: e002564.

14. Weintraub D, Buchsbau R, Resor Jr SR, Hirsch LJ (2007) Psychiatric and behavioral side effects of the newer antiepileptic drugs in adults with epilepsy. Epilepsy Behav 10: 105-110.

15. Wieshmann UC, Tan GM, Baker G (2011) Self-reported symptoms in patients on antiepileptic drugs in monotherapy. Acta Neurol Scand 124: 355-358.

16. IJff DM, Aldenkamp AP (2012) Comorbidities of treatment with antiepileptic drugs. In: M Duchowny, JH Cross, A Arzimanoglou, eds. Pediatric epilepsy. New York: McGraw-Hill Professional 424-436.

17. IJff DM, Aldenkamp AP (2013) Cognitive side effects of antiepileptic drugs in children. In: Dulac, Lassonde, Sarnat, eds. Handbook of Clinical Neurology: Pediatric Neurology. New York: Elsevier 738-749.

18. Kinderen de RJA, Evers SMAA, Rinkins R, Postulart D, Vader CI, et al. (2014) Side-effects of antiepileptic drugs: the economic burden. Seizure 23: 184-190.

19. Bootsma HP, Ricker L, Hekster YA, Hulsman J, Lambrechts D, et al. (2009) The impact of side effects on long-term retention in three new antiepileptic drugs. Seizure 18: 327-331.

20. Aldenkamp AP, van Meel HF, Baker GA, Brooks J, Hendriks MPH (2002) The A-B neuropsychological assessment schedule (ABNAS): the relationship between patient-perceived drug related cognitive impairment and results of neuropsychological tests. Seizure 11: 231-237.

21. Uijl SG, Uiterwaal CS, Aldenkamp AP, Carpay JA, Doelman JC, et al. (2009) Adjustment of treatment increases quality of life in patients with epilepsy: a randomized controlled pragmatic trial. Eur J Neurol 16: 1173-1177.

22. Loring DW, Marino S, Meador KJ (2007) Neuropsychological and behavioral effects of antiepilepsy drugs. Neuropsychol Rev 28: 413-425.

23. Mbizvo GK, Dixon P, Hutton JL, Marson AG (2012) Levetiracetam add-on for drug-resistant focal epilepsy: an updated Cochrane Review. Cochrane Database Syst Rev 19: CD001901.

24. Chen B, Choi H, Hirsch LJ, Moeller J, Jayed A, et al. (2015) Cosmetic side effects of antiepileptic drugs in adults with epilepsy. Epilepsy Behav 42: 129-137.

25. Haag A, Strzelczyk A, Bauer S, Kühne S, Hamer HM, et al. (2010) Quality of life and employment status are correlated with antiepileptic monotherapy versus polytherapy and not with use of "newer" versus "classic" drugs: results of the "Compliant 2006" survey in 907 patients. Epilepsy Behav 19: 618-622.

26. Talati R, Scholle JM, Phung OJ, Baker WL, Baker EL, et al. (2011) Effectiveness and safety of antiepileptic medications in patients with epilepsy. Rockville (MD): Agency for Healthcare Research and Quality, US.

27. Cramer JA, De Rue K, Devinsky O, Edrick P, Trimble MR (2003) A systematic review of the behavioral effects of levetiracetam in adults with epilepsy, cognitive disorders, or anxiety disorder during clinical trials. Epilepsy Behav 4: 124-132.

28. Dinkelacker V, Dietl T, Widman G, Lengler U, Elger CE (2003) Aggressive behavior of epilepsy patients in the course of levetiracetam add-on therapy: report of 33 mild to severe cases. Epilepsy Behav 4: 537-547.

29. Mula M, Trimble MR, Yuen A, Liu RS, Sander JW (2003) Psychiatric adverse events during levetiracetam therapy. Neurology 61: 704-706.

30. Weintraub D, Buchsbaum R, Resor SR Jr, Hirsch LJ. (2007) Psychiatric and behavioral side effects of the newer antiepileptic drugs in adults with epilepsy. Epilepsy Behav. 10: 105-110.

23

Synthesis and Biological Activities of 2-Carboxyphenyloxamoylamino Acids, their Salts with 2-ethoxy-6,9-Diaminoacridine and D-glucosamine

Khaldoon AL-Rahawi[1]*, Ali AL-Kaf[2], Shada Yassin[2], Sameh EL-Nabtity[3], Kotb EL-Sayed[4] and Napila AL-Shoba[2]

[1]*Department of Medicinal chemistry, Faculty of Pharmacy, Sana'a University, Sana'a, 14288, Yemen*
[2]*Department of Medicinal chemistry, Faculty of Pharmacy, Sana'a University, Yemen*
[3]*Department of Pharmacology, Faculty of Veterinary Medicine, Zagazig University, Egypt*
[4]*Department of Biochemistry and Molecular Biology, Faculty of Pharmacy, Helwan University, Egypt*

Abstract

As a result of this work, 17 new compounds were obtained. This group of compounds (2-carboxyphenyloxamoylamino acids) alone or with biologically active base showed diverse biological activity-Anti-inflammatory, antimicrobial and hepatoprotective activity- which can be used in medicine after further investigations.

Keywords: Synthesis; 2-carboxyphenyloxamoylamino acids; Salts of rivanol and D-glucosamine; Antimicrobial; Anti-inflammatory; Hepatoprotective activity

Introduction

N-acylamino acid derivatives are of significant interest due to their biological activities [1-4]. Our research in the chemistry and biological activity of oxamoylamino acids and their salts with biologically active base resulted in establishment of two methods for their synthesis one of which gave optically active compounds [5]. It was also found that, a representative of this chemical group possesses divers biological activities, including antioxidants, hepatoprotective, immunosuppressant, anti-inflammatory, antimicrobial, diuretic, hypoglycemic and antimalarial activities [5-9]. In continuation of research in this field we arrived to synthesize new derivatives of phenyloxamoylaminoacid (2-carboxyphenyloxamoylamino acid), and to obtaining their salts with biologically active base and to study the biological activities of the obtained compounds.

Experimental

Chemistry

The UV-spectra were measured on a UV-160 IPC (SHIMADZU) spectrophotometer using samples (10^{-4} mol) dissolved in ethanol. The IR spectra were obtained on a IR-FTIR-8300 (SHIMADZU) spectrophotometer in tablets of potassium bromide, at the range of 4000-400 cm^{-1}. The HNMR- spectra were recorded on spectrophotometer «Varian Mercury-VX-200 (200 MHz)», using DMSO-d_6 as solvent and TMS as the internal standard [1]. The ionization constants for acids 1-5 were determined by potentiometric titration in 50% aqueous dioxane. The measurements were performed on FTI-6 UNIVERSAL DIGITAL pH-meter (ENGLAND). The melting temperatures were determined on melting point apparatus SMP3 (England). The purity of the targeted products was checked by TLC on Silufon 0,25 mm silica gel 60 F_{254} (Merk, Germany).

I. I 2-Carboxyphenyloxamoylglycine (1)

11.53 g (0.05 mol) of ethyl ester of 2-Carboxyphenyloxamic acid in 50 ml absolute methanol was added to 3.53 g (0.05 mol) glycine in 15 mL methanolic solution of sodium methoxide, sodium methoxide solution, was obtained from 0.1 g atom sodium metal and 15 ml absolute methanol. The reaction mixture keeps standing to neutral pH, as detected by universal indicator. The formed precipitate dissolved in minimum volume of water and acidified with H:Cl to pH 2 with 1:1

HCl. The resulting precipitate was filtered, dried and crystallized from ethanol. Similarly compounds 2-5 were obtained. UV λ_{max} nm(log ε): 208 (4.17), 231 (4.19), 268 (3.88), 307 (3.83); IR (KBr, cm⁻¹): 3415,3377γNH; 2949-2650γOH(COOH); 1730γCO(COOH); 1680γCO; 1517CONH; 1600 γC=C; ¹HNMR (DMSO-d_6, δ): 3.88-4.20d (2H, CH_2); 7.10-7.34t (1H,$_{arom}$.); 7.54-7.69t (1H,$_{arom}$.) 7.9-8.2d (1H,$_{arom}$.); 8.51-8.75d (1H,$_{arom}$.) 9.11-9.35t (1H, $NHCH_2$); 12.42-12.65s (1H, NHCO).

II. 2-Carboxyphenyloxamoyl-β-alanine (2)

UV λmax nm(log ε): 208 (4.12), 231 (4.15), 268 (3.82), 307 (3.78); IR (KBr, cm⁻¹): 3300,3215 γNH; 2959-2528γOH (COOH); 1720 γCO(COOH); 1678 γCO; 1514 CONH; 1587 γC=C; 1HNMR (DMSO-d_6, δ): 1.24-1.49t (2H,CH_2COOH); 4.22-4.40m (2H, NHCH2CH2); 7.10-7.35t (1H,arom.); 7.40-7.65t (1H,arom.); 7.93-8.09d (1H,$_{arom}$.); 8.50-8.75d (1H,$_{arom}$.) 8.85-9.10-t (1H, $NHCH_2$) ; 12.33-12.57s (1H, NHCO).

III. 2-Carboxyphenyloxamoyl-α-alanine (3)

UV λ_{max} nm(log ε): 208(4.19), 231(4.22), 268(3.89), 307(3.85); IR (KBr, cm⁻¹): 3342,3400γNH; 2971-2771γOH (COOH); 1700 γCO(COOH);1670γCO;1514CONH;1585γC=C;1HNMR (DMSO-d6, δ): 1.25-1.51d(3H,CH_3); 4.22-4.45m(1H ,CH);7.10-7.33t(1H,$_{arom}$.); 7.42-7.65t(1H,$_{arom}$.) 7.90-8.15d(1H,$_{arom}$.); 8.50-8.75d(1H,$_{arom}$.) 9.00-9.25-d(1H, $NHCH_2$); 12.40-12.63s(1H, NHCO).

IV. 2-Carboxyphenyloxamoyl-γ-aminobutyric acid (4)

UV λ_{max} nm(log ε): 210(4.26), 231(4.33), 267(4.01), 307(3.95); IR (KBr, cm⁻¹): 3346,3323 γNH; 2961-2532γOH (COOH); 1720 γCO(COOH);1674γCO; 1516CONH; 1570 γC=C; ¹HNMR (DMSO-d_6, δ): 1.55-1.80p(2H,βCH_2); 2.05-2.29t(2H, αCH_2) ; 3.10-3.25t (2HγCH2);

*Corresponding author: Khaldoon AL-Rahawi, Medicinal Chemistry Department, Faculty of Pharmacy, Sana'a University, Sana'a, 14288, Yemen, E-mail: alrahawi_65@yahoo.com

7.10-7.34t (1H,$_{arom}$.); 7.54-7.78t (1H,$_{arom}$,); 7.95-8.19d (1H,$_{arom}$.); 8.55-8.79d (1H,$_{arom}$.); 9.0-9.24t (1H, NHCH$_2$); 12.42-12.65s (1H, NHCO).

V. 2-Carboxyphenyloxamoylserine (5)

UV λ$_{max}$ nm(log ε): 210(4.21); 228(4.25), 268(4.01), 307(3.82); IR (KBr, cm^{-1}): 3446γOHass. 3360,3280 γNH; 2900-2638γOH(COOH); 1700 γCO(COOH); 1685γCO; 1517 CONH; 1590γC=C; ^{1}HNMR (DMSO-d$_6$, δ): 3.72-3.94d (2H,CH$_2$OH); 4.19-4.40q (1H,CH); 5.00-5.21s (1H,OH); 7.10-7.32t (1H,$_{arom}$.); 7.55-7.78t (1H,$_{arom}$.); 7.93-8.15d (1H, $_{arom}$.); 8.50-8.71d (1H,$_{arom}$.); 8.80-9.05t (1H, NHCH); 12.40-12.55 (1H, NHCO).

VI. 2-Ethoxy-6,9-diaminoacridinium 2-carboxyphenyloxamoylglycinate (6)

To an ethanolic solution of 0.266 g (0.001 mol) of 2-Carboxyphenyloxamoylglycine, an ethanolic solution of 0.252 g (0.001 mol) 2-ethoxy-6,9-diaminoacridinium base was added. The mixture allowed to stand to neutral pH, as detected by universal indicator. The formed precipitate (salt) was filtered, washed with diethyl ether and dried. Salt 7-10 were obtained similarly.

VII. 2-Ethoxy-6, 9-diaminoacridinium 2-carboxyphenyloxamoyloxalate (16)

The equivalent mole of an ethanolic solution of 2-ethoxy-6,9-diaminoacridine and 2-carboxyphenyloxamic acid were mixed together and the reaction mixture allowed to stand to pH neural. The formed precipitate, was filtered, washed with diethyl ether and dried. C$_{24}$H$_{22}$N$_4$O$_6$, Yield, 3.88 g (85%); mp., 250°C.

VIII. 2-D-(+)-glucosamonium 2-carboxyphenyloxamoylglycinate (11)

0.862 g (0.004 mole) of D(+)-glucosaminium chloride was dissolved by heating in potassium hydroxide solution, obtained from 0.224 g (0.004 mol) of potassium hydroxide and 10 mL 50% aqueous ethanol. The precipitate of potassium chloride was filtered, then the filtrate was added to a solution of 1.064 g (0.004 mol) of 2-carboxyphenylglycine in 15 mL ethanol. The reaction mixture was allowed to stand for one night. The formed precipitate (salt) was filtered, washed with diethyl ether and dried. Other salts (12-15) were similarly obtained.

IX. 2-D-(+)-glucosamonium 2-carboxyphenyloxaminate (17)

0.862 g (0.004 mol) of D(+)-glucosaminium chloride was dissolved by heating in potassium hydroxide solution, obtained from 0.224 g (0.004 mol) of potassium hydroxide and 10 mL 50% aqueous ethanol. The precipitate of potassium chloride was filtered, then the filtrate was added to a solution of 1.5 g (0.004 mol) of 2-carboxyphenylxamic acid in 15 mL ethanol. The reaction mixture was allowed to stand for one night. The formed precipitate (salt) was filtered, washed with diethyl ether and dried. C$_{15}$H$_{20}$N$_2$O$_{10}$, Yield, 1.3 g (84%); mp., 160°C.

Biological activity assays

Antimicrobial activity

i. Agar well diffusion bioassay: Six of new compounds 6-10,16 in DMF (Table 3) were tested for their in vitro antimicrobial action against five microorganisms (i.e. S.aureus ATCC 25923, B.subtilis ATCC 6633, E.coli ATCC 2592, P. aeruginosa ATCC-9027, Candida albicans ATCC -885-653), following agar well-diffusion method, [10] and using the antiseptic rivanol as standard drug. Microbial growth was determined by measuring the diameter of inhibition zone in mm. DMF alone showed no inhibition zone.

ii. Dilution method: The minimal inhibitory concentrations of synthesized compounds 6-10, 16 were determined by the tube dilution method [11].

Anti-inflammatory activity: Animals were obtained from Animal house, Faculty of Science, Sana'a University, Yemen. Male Swiss albino mice weighing 25-30 g were used. All animal experiments were performed according to the ethical guidelines suggested by the Institutional animal ethics committee (IAEC).

Carrageenan-induced paw edema in mice was used as an acute inflammatory model as described by Winter et al. [12]. 50 µL of a 1% carrageenan solution was injected subcutaneously into the sub plantar surface of the right hind paws of the mice using a 25-gauge needle. Seventy two mice were used and were divided into 8 groups (n=9 in each group) as follows: Group I served as control (vehicle treated) and received normal saline (0.3 ml/kg i.p intraperitoneal) only, Group II served as a positive control and received diclofenac sodium (10 mg/kg i.p), Groups (III-VIII) served as test groups and received 10 mg/kg i.p., of compounds (ii,1-5) one hour before carrageenan injection. The differences in weight between right and left hind paws represent the amount of edema developed in the right hind paw [13].

Edema was calculated using the following formula;

$$EWD=EW_R-EW_L$$

Where; EWD=Edema weight difference between right and left hind paw.

EW$_R$=Edema weight of right hind paw (test). EW$_L$=Edema weight of left hind paw (control). Percentage Inhibition of Edema (PI) was calculated from equation:

$$PI=\frac{EW_C-EW_T}{EW_C}\times100$$

Where; EW$_C$=Edema Weight difference of Control animal's paw, and EW$_T$=Edema Weight difference of test animal's paw.

i. Statistical analysis

All results were expressed as the arithmetic mean ± SE. Differences between groups were evaluated by analysis of variance (ANOVA) complemented by Student's t-test. A difference was considered significant at P value less than 0.05.

Hepatoprotective activity: This study was performed to assess the hepatoprotective activity of the synthesized salts 2-D-(+)-glucosamonium-2-carboxyphenyloxamoylamino acids (compounds 11-15,17) in rats against carbon tetrachloride (CCl$_4$) as hepatotoxin using silymarin as standard hepatoprotective.

a) Animals: Fifty four male albino rats weighing 175- 225 g. maintained under good husbandry conditions (Temp. 23 ± 2°C. relative humidity 55 ± 10% and 12 h light dark cycle) were used for all studies. Animals were allowed to take standard laboratory feed and tap water. Ethical committee in accordance with animal experimentation and care has approved all animal procedures.

b) Evaluation of hepatoprotective activity: Fifty four male albino rats were divided into nine equal groups; control, silymarin, carbon tetrachloride (CCl$_4$) and test groups.

Group (1) The rats of control group received three doses of 5% acacia mucilage each (1 ml/Kg, per oral) at 12 h intervals (0 h, 12 h and 24 h).

Group (2) The rats of silymarine group received three doses of silymarine (25 mg /kg) at 0 h, 12 h and 24 h. CCl_4 (1.25 ml /kg i.p) was administered 30 min. after the first dose of silymarine.

Group (3) The rats of CCl_4 group received three doses of vehicle at 12 h intervals and a single dose of CCl_4 (1.25 ml/kg i.p) diluted in liquid paraffin (1:1) 30 min after the administration of the first dose of vehicle .

Group (4, 5, 6, 7, 8 and 9) were given the first dose of the tested compounds at a dose of (25 mg/kg p.o) in acacia mucilage at 0 h. which was followed by a dose of CCl_4 (1.25 ml/kg p.o) after 30 min., while at 12 h and 24 h the second and third dose of the test compounds (25 mg/ kg p.o) were administered.

After 36 h of administration of CCl_4 blood was collected and serum was separated and used for determination of biochemical tests.

c) **Measurement of biochemical parameters:** Liver function was investigated by estimation of alanine aminotransferase ALT [14], aspartate aminotransferase AST [14], and alkaline phosphatase ALP [15], Serum total protein T.P. was determined according to Henry 1964 [16], serum albumin was measured according to Doumas and Biggs, 1976 [17], Serum total bilirubin T.B. and serum direct bilirubin D.B. were determined according to Walters and Gerarde [18].

d) **Statistical analysis:** All results were expressed as the arithmetic mean ± SE. Differences between groups were evaluated by analysis of variance (ANOVA) complemented by Student's t-test. A difference was considered significant at P value less than 0.05.

Results and Discussion

Chemistry

The synthesis of 2-carboxyphenyloxamoylamino acids 1-5 was performed by acylation of ethyl ester of 2-carboxyphenyloxamic acid, compound i [19], with amino acids in the presence of sodium methoxide and absolute methanol as shown in the scheme 1.

Generally, the 2-carboxyphenyloxamoylaminoacids 1-5 (Table 1)

Com.	X	Yield, %	M.p.,C0	Empirical formula	*R$_f$	pK$_a$ I	pK$_a$ II
1	CH_2	67	228-230	$C_{11}H_{10}N_2O_6$	0.89	5.2	6.1
2	CH_2CH_2	54	238-240	$C_{12}H_{12}N_2O_6$	0.80	5.3	6.0
3	$CHCH_3$	56	233-235	$C_{12}H_{12}N_2O_6$	0.81	5.3	6.3
4	$CH_2CH_2CH_2$	81	221-223	$C_{13}H_{14}N_2O_6$	0.89	5.5	6.7
5	$CHCH_2OH$	58	195-197	$C_{12}H_{12}N_2O_7$	0.75	4.5	6.0

*The TLC systems: n-butanol-acetic acid-water (4:1:1)

Table 1: Physical Constants of 2-Carboxyphenyloxamoylamino acid (1-5).

Compd.	X	Yields,%	mp., C0	Empirical formula
6	CH_2	80	251-253	$C_{26}H_{25}N_5O_7$
7	CH_2CH_2	81	268-270	$C_{27}H_{27}N_5O_7$
8	CH_2CH_3	81	193-195	$C_{27}H_{27}N_5O_7$
9	$CH_2CH_2CH_2$	81	258-260	$C_{28}H_{29}N_5O_7$
10	$CHCH_2OH$	81	196-198	$C_{27}H_{27}N_5O_8$
11	CH_2	52	155 dec.	$C_{18}H_{25}O_{11}N_3$
12	CH_2CH_2	98	180 dec.	$C_{19}H_{27}O_{11}N_3$
13	CH_2CH_3	87	115 dec.	$C_{19}H_{27}O_{11}N_3$
14	$CH_2CH_2CH_2$	65	185 dec.	$C_{20}H_{29}O_{11}N_3$
15	$CHCH_2OH$	20	117-119	$C_{19}H_{27}O_{12}N_3$

Table 2: Physical Constants of salts (6-10) and salts (11-15).

are pale yellow crystalline substances, soluble in hot water, ethanol, alkaline solution and insoluble in most organic solvents. The purity and identity of the synthesized compounds were checked by using thin layer chromatography eluted with two systems of solvents (Table 1). Since the obtained substances (1-5) are acids the ionization constants (pKa) were measured (Table 1), the obtained results confirm that the synthesized compounds are dibasic acids. The values corresponded to high acidity (pKa I) belong to the aliphatic carboxylic group's ionization.

The proposed structures of compounds 1-5 were confirmed by the UV, IR and 1H NMR spectroscopic data.

The UV spectra of compounds (1-5) contain four absorption bands at 208-210, 228-231, 267-268 and 307 nm. The first three bands originates from π-π*-electronic transition of benzene ring. The 307 nm band originate from n-π*-electronic transition characteristic for N-acylanthranilic acid derivatives [20].

In accordance with the number and position of proton's signal, the result of ^{1}HNMR spectra of 2-carboxyphenyloxamoylamino acids 1-5 corresponds with the proposed structures. It should be noted that proton's signal of Ar-NHCO of compounds 1-5 is shifted from high field 10.24-10.90 ppm (signals characterized for other substituted phenyloxamoylamino acids) to low field 12.33-12.65 due to the effect of hydrogen bonding between the amide's hydrogen and ortho-carboxylic group [6,8,21].

Based on the synthesized acids 1-5, salts with the base of rivanol 6-10 and D-glucosamine 11-15 were obtained.

The obtained salts 6-10 (Table 2) are yellow crystalline substances, soluble in hot water and insoluble in most organic solvents.

UV spectra of salts 6-10 are attributed to the absorption of cation and are definitely identical to the ethacridine lactate's spectrum. This is the evidence that the salts were formed at ring's nitrogen atom. The IR spectra of salts 6-10 and 16 exhibit stretching absorption bands of the initial acids without the stretching absorption band of CO (COOH), the absence of this band in the salts may be due to the resonance effect between C-O bonds [22]. Furthermore, they exhibit absorption bands

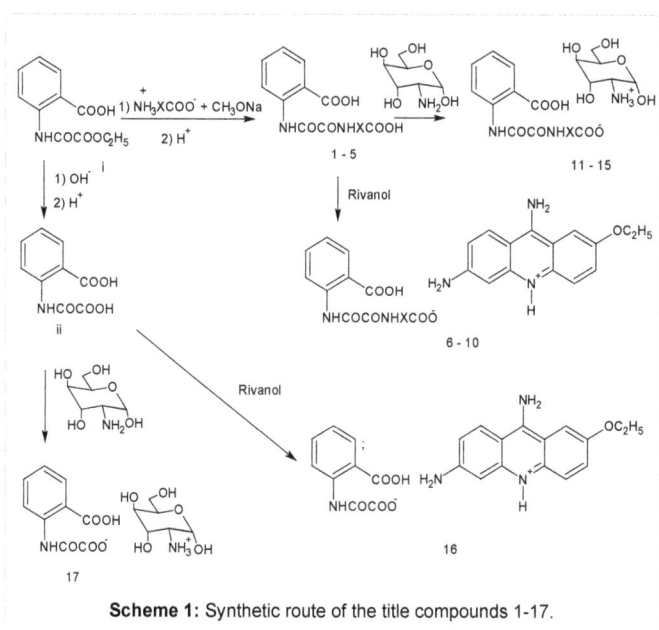

Scheme 1: Synthetic route of the title compounds 1-17.

belonging to the acridine's rings (1491-1500 см⁻¹; 1446-1455 см1; 1370-1395 см⁻¹).

The obtained salts 11-15 (Table 2) appeared as white crystalline substances, readily soluble in water with the formation of neutral solution. Adding mineral acid into the solutions of the obtained salts leads to formation of the precipitate of initial compounds 2-carboxy-phenyloxamoylaminoacids 1-5.

The UV spectra of the salts 11-15 and 17 were determined by anions and were found to be almost similar to the spectra of acids 1-5. The IR spectra of compounds 11-15 and 17 contain broad absorption bands due to the stretching vibration of associated NH and OH groups in the of region of 3430-3251 см⁻¹, CO amid I in the region of 1680-1660 см⁻¹ and groups of stretching absorption bands in the region of 3000-2810 см⁻¹, arising from symmetrical and asymmetrical stretching in the ammonium groups. Moreover, the hydrocarbon ring of D-(+)-glucosamine exists in pyranose form and shows two bands in IR spectrum; asymmetric at 925-910 cm⁻¹ and symmetric at 775-765 cm⁻¹ due to the pyranose vibration.

To study the effect of the amino acids residues upon the biological activity, the salts 16,17, which don't contain amino acids fragments, were obtained.

The obtained salt 16 is a yellow crystalline substances, soluble in hot water, insoluble in most organic solvents. The obtained salt 17 is a white crystalline substance, soluble in water and insoluble in most organic solvents. The UV and IR spectra of compound 16 and 17 were almost identical to the UV and IR spectra of compounds 6-10 and compounds 11-15, respectively.

Antimicrobial activity

Well diffusion method: From the data presented in table 3, in general it may be seen that compound 10 possesses strong activity (33 mm) against S.aureus when compared to rivanol, whereas compounds 8,10 possess strong activity (29.5 mm, 32 mm, respectively) against.

B.subtilis. Compound 10 possesses strong activity (32 mm) against *E. coli* in comparison with rivanol. Compounds 10, 16 possess strong activity (25.5 mm, 24.5 mm respectively) against P.aeruginosa. Compounds 8, 10 possess strong activity (33 mm, 32 mm) against C. albicans in comparison with rivanol.

From the presented results it was found that combination of acids with rivanol have clear effect on the antimicrobial activity of rivanol especially in compound 10 (2-ethoxy-6, 9-diaminoacridinum-2-

carboxyphenyloxamoylserinate), which showed stronger antimicrobial activity than rivanol against all test microorganisms.

Dilution method: From the data presented in table 3 it is clear that compound 8 possesses strong activity against B.subtilis, (MIC 6.25 µg/ml) and against E.coli (MIC 50 µg/ml) when compared with rivanol. Compound 10 possesses strong activity against B.subtilis (MIC 3.25 µg/ml), E.coli (MIC 1.55 µg/ml), and against C.albicans (MIC 12.5 µg/ml) as compared to standard rivanol.

The obtained results confirmed that only the combination of 2-carboxyphenyloxamoyl serine with rivanol has strengthened the antimicrobial activity of the later. Herewith, the most active one is compound 10 (2-ethoxy-6, 9-diaminoacridinum-2-carboxyphenyloxamoyl serinate).

Anti-inflammatory activity

Result of investigation (Table 4) showed that compounds ii, 3, 4 treated group possess higher % of inhibition of paw volume (61.1, 64.2, 77.8, respectively) than the standard drug, diclofenac (58.8). The best anti-inflammatory activity was exhibited by compound 4 (2-carboxyphenyloxamoyl-γ-aminobutyric acid), which superior to the reference drug, Diclofenac sodium in 35%.

Previously, we synthesized 3,4-dimethylphenyloxamoylamino acids and investigated their anti-inflammatory activity. In present study, it was found that introduction of carboxylic group to ortho position instead of the 3,4-dimethyl-groups, increases the anti-inflammatory activity when compared to Diclofenac sodium. This result is predictable, because insertion of COOH group, produces the known anti-inflammatory chemical group, N-substituted anthranilic acid derivatives [23,24].

Hepatoprotective activity

As is shown in table 5, CCl_4 elicited a significant increase in the activities of serum ALT, AST, ALP which may be attributed to cellular leakage and loss of functional integrity of cell membrane of hepatocytes [25].

Rats in CCl_4 group evoked a significant decrease in serum total proteins and albumin. This decline is due to disruption and disassociation of polyribosomes from endoplasmic reticulum following CCl_4 adminstration [26]. A similar significant decrease in serum total proteins was noted by Achliya et al. [27] and Shanmugasundaram [28]. They attributed these results to depression of liver ability to synthesize the proteins due to CCl_4–induced hepatic damage.

Rats in CCl_4 group showed significant increase in serum total and

Compd	S.aureus	B.subtilis	E.coli	P.aeruginosa	C.albicans
Rivanol	22.5 ± 0.17	24.5 ± 0.12	26 ± 0.12	19.5 ± 0.12	30 ± 0.07
	<50	<50	<50	<50	50 ± 0.06
6	12.5 ± 0.09	18.5 ± 0.15	14 ± 0.13	16.5 ± 0.08	19.5 ± 0.08
	<50	<50	<50	<50	<50
7	12 ± 0.07	19.5 ± 0.33	14 ± 0.29	12.5 ± 0.17	18.5 ± 0.13
	<50	<50	<50	<50	<50
8	21 ± 0.02	29.5 ± 0.29	26 ± 0.18	19.5 ± 0.07	33 ± 0.07
	<50	6.25 ± 0.17	50 ± 0.04	<50	50 ± 0.12
9	17.5 ± 0.12	23 ± 0.07	14 ± 0.16	16 ± 0.18	24.5 ± 0.05
	<50	<50	<50	<50	50 ± 0.08
10	33 ± 0.03	32 ± 0.03	32 ± 0.13	25.5 ± 0.17	32 ± 0.06
	<50	3.25 ± 0.06	1.55 ± 0.05	<50	12.5 ± 0.13
16	14.5 ± 0.17	19.5 ± 0.77	<50	24.5 ± 0.08	17 ± 0.11

Table 3: Antimicrobial activity of compounds 6-10,16 [inhibition zone (in mm)/ minimum inhibitory concentration (µg/ml)].

NO.	Group Name (n=9)	EWD (M+Se)	PI (%)
I	Control (0.9% NaCl)	750.9 ± 0.47	- - -
II	Diclofenac	319.4 ± 0.32 ∗ ∗ ∗; N.S.	58.8
III	ii	292.0 ± 0.29 ∗ ∗ ∗; N.S.	61.1
IV	1	311.1 ± 0.75 ∗ ∗ ∗; N.S.	58.6
V	2	416.8 ± 0.56 ∗ ∗; N.S.	44.5
VI	3	268.8 ± 0.37 ∗ ∗ ∗; N.S.	64.2
VII	4	166.7 ± 0.49 ∗ ∗ ∗; N.S.	77.8
VIII	5	544.4 ± 0.47 ∗; N.S.	27.5

The statistical data were expressed as M ± SE. M, mean; SE, standard error; n, number of rats; ∗ or ★=P<0.05; ∗∗ or ★★=p<0.01; ∗∗∗ or ★★★=p<0.001; ∗compare between different groups and control group while ★ compare between different groups and diclofenac group.

Table 4: The anti-inflammatory effects of compounds ii, 1-5 comparing with Diclofenac.

Synthesis and Biological Activities of 2-Carboxyphenyloxamoylamino Acids, their Salts...

127

№	AST U/L	ALT U/L	A.P. U/L	Alb g/dl	T.P. g/dl	T.B mg/dl	D.B mg/dl
Gp$_1$ Control	86.00^d ± 1.14	66.83 ± 0.60	19.40^e ± 0.46	4.17^a ± 0.03	6.97^a ± 0.04	0.45^f ± 0.02	0.14^d ± 0.001
Gp$_2$ Sily +CCL$_4$	77.17^d ± 13.64	93.83^{ab} ± 15.72	18.58^e ± 0.39	3.95^b ± 0.04	6.87^a ± 0.03	0.53^{ef} ± 0.03	0.15^d ± 0.004
Gp$_3$ CCL$_4$	119.83^a ±16.14	105.00^a ± 2.22	38.42^a ± 0.74	2.97^e ± 0.042	5.98^b ± 0.05	1.14^a ± 0.06	0.42^a ± 0.006
Gp$_4$ 1+CCL$_4$	95.80^{bcd} ± 1.66	74.80^{cd} ± 1.77	21.90^d ± 0.33	3.60^c ± 0.03	6.92^a ± 0.04	0.57^{de} ± 0.01	0.15^d ± 0.009
Gp$_5$ 2+CCL$_4$	89.60^{cd} ± 0.51	67.67^d ± 0.71	20.00^e ± 0.71	4.14^a ± 0.05	7.04^a ± 0.05	0.45^f ± 0.03	0.14^d ± 0.002
Gp$_6$ 3+CCL$_4$	113.67^{ab} ± 1.76	90.50^{abc} ± 0.92	25.80^c ± 0.37	3.32^d ± 0.04	6.64^a ± 0.05	0.72^c ± 0.04	0.23^c ± 0.01
Gp$_7$ 4+CCL$_4$	96.00^{bcd} ± 1.37	82.83^{bcd} ± 1.82	29.17^b ± 0.31	3.30^d ± 0.03	6.48^a ± 0.11	0.63^{cd} ± 0.01	0.16^d ± 0.01
Gp$_8$ 5+CCL$_4$	112.50^{abc} ± 1.12	100.33^a ± 1.05	27.17^c ± 0.48	3.25^d ± 0.03	6.41^a ± 0.11	0.86^b ± 0.02	0.35^b ± 0.02
Gp$_9$ 6+CCL$_4$	102.00^{abc} ± 1.41	104.17^a ± 1.54	29.00^b ± 0.37	3.34^d ± 0.02	6.38^a ± 0.05	0.61^{de} ± 0.01	0.15^d ± 0.009

Means within the same column having different alphabetical superscript letters are significantly different (P<0.01)

Table 5: Effects of the test compounds (11-15,17) on various biochemical parameters in rats with carbon tetrachloride induced hepatotoxicity.

direct bilirubin levels. Similar effects were bosomed by Nevin and Vijayammal [29]. They evaluated the toxic effect of CCl$_4$ on the liver and found that CCl$_4$ administered rats showed an elevation in serum bilirubin.

The test compounds 11-15 and 17 elicited a significant reduction in the levels of AST, ALT towards the normal value which is an indication of regeneration process.

Reduction of ALP levels with concurrent depletion of raised bilirubin level suggests the stability of the biliary function during injury with CCl$_4$.

The protein and albumin levels were also raised, suggesting stability of endoplasmic reticulum leading to protein synthesis.

The data presented in table 5, showed that the rank order of potency was silymarin >compd 12 >compd 11, compd13 >compd14 >compd 17 and compd 15, this promising hepatoprotection activity of the tested compounds may be due to their antioxidant and free radical scavenging properties.

From the obtained result it was established that not only glucosamine salt of 3,4-dimethylphenyloxamoylamino acids [5], and 4-bromophenyloxamoylamino acid [30], possess hepatoprotective properties, but also glucosamine salt of 2-carboxyphenyloxamoylamino acids. This effect may be due to the glucosamine as hepatoprotective [31], and antioxidant [32], or to the combination of glucosamine and substituted phenyloxamoylamino acids in one molecule as salts [5,30].

Further study should be done to clarify the biological rule of each molecule and to study relationship between the D-glucosamine, amino acid moiety, the substituent on the aromatic ring and the hepatoprotective property.

Conclusion

1. Seventeen new compounds were synthesized, their structures were established by using different physico-chemical methods.

2. TThe results of biological study clearly demonstrated that some compounds of 2-carboxyphenyloxamoylamino acids, their salts with rivanol and D-glucosamine possess strong anti-inflammatory, antimicrobial and hepatoprotective activities.

References

1. Moise M, Sunel V, Profire L, Popa M, Desbrieres J, et al. (2009) Synthesis and biological activity of some new 1,3,4-thiadiazole and 1,2,4-triazole compounds containing a phenylalanine moiety. Molecules 14: 2621-2631.

2. Kumar HV, Gnanendra CR, Naik N, Bulg (2009) Chem cammun 41: 72-79.

3. El-Sharief AM, Amma YA, Zahran MA, El-Gaby MS (2001) Aminoacids in the Synthesis of Heterocyclic Systems: The Synthesis of Triazinoquinazolinones,

Triazepinoquinazolinones and Triazocinoquinazolinones of Potential Biological Interest. Molecules 6: 267-278.

4. Connor M, Vaughan CW, Vandenberg RJ (2010) N-acyl amino acids and N-acyl neurotransmitter conjugates: neuromodulators and probes for new drug targets. Br J Pharmacol 160: 1857-1871.

5. Alrahawi Kh, Petyunin GP, Maloshtan LN (2008) J Org Pharm Chem 23: 53-58.

6. Alrahawi Kh, Petyunin GP, Diki IL (2008) Farm Zh 2: 73-76.

7. Alrahawi Kh, Petyunin GP, Diki IL (2008) Farm Zh 5: 62-66.

8. Alrahawi Kh, Al-kaf A, Yem (2007) J Med Sci 3: 32-36.

9. Al-rahawi KM, Al-haj M, Petyunina VN, Al-daidamoni G (2010) Actual issues Pharm Med Sci 4: 4-7.

10. Perez C, Paul M, Bazerque P (1990) An antibiotic assay by the agar–well diffusion method. Acta Biol Med Exp 15: 113–115.

11. Murray PR (1998) Manual of clinical microbiology, Editor in chief, ASM Press, Washington.

12. WINTER CA, RISLEY EA, NUSS GW (1962) Carrageenin-induced edema in hind paw of the rat as an assay for antiiflammatory drugs. Proc Soc Exp Biol Med 111: 544-547.

13. Gerner P, Mujtaba M, Sinnott CJ, Wang GK (2011) Anesthesiology 94: 611-617.

14. Tietz NW (2001) Fundamentals of clinical chemistry, Saunders, W.B., Philadelphia.

15. Belfield A, Goldberg DM (1971) Revised assay for serum phenyl phosphatase activity using 4-amino-antipyrine. Enzyme 12: 561-573.

16. Henry RJ (1964) Clinical chemistry, Harper & Row publishers, New York.

17. Doumas BT, Biggs HG (1976) Standard methods of clinical chemistry, Academic Press N. Y., Massachusetts, USA.

18. Walters MI, Gerarde HW (1970) Michrochem J 15: 229- 231.

19. Wallach O, West P (1887) Ann Chem 184: 57-59.

20. Petyunin GP, Chobenko AV (1987) Synthesis, chemistry and anti-inflammatory activity of oxamoylaminobenzoic acids and their derivatives, KhMAPE, Ukraine.

21. Silverstein RM, Clayton G (1991) Spectrometric Identification of Org Compounds, John Wiley, New York.

22. Bellamy LJ (1975) The infra-red spectra of complex molecules, Chapman and Hall London.

23. Wilson CO, Delgado JN (2004) Textbook of Organic Medicinal and Pharmaceutical Chemistry, John Block; John Beale; Lippincott Williams & Wilkins, Philadelphia.

24. Sharma S, Srivastava VK, Kumar A (2002) Newer N-substituted anthranilic acid derivatives as potent anti-inflammatory agents. Eur J Med Chem 37: 689-697.

25. Mukherjee PK (2003) Plant products with hypocholesterolemic potentials. Adv Food Nutr Res 47: 277-338.

26. Clawson GA (1989) Mechanisms of carbon tetrachloride hepatotoxicity. Pathol Immunopathol Res 8: 104-112.

27. Achliya GS, Wadodkar SG, Dorle AK (2004) Evaluation of hepatoprotective

effect of Amalkadi Ghrita against carbon tetrachloride-induced hepatic damage in rats. J Ethnopharmacol 90: 229-232.

28. Shanmugasundaram P, Venkataraman S (2006) Hepatoprotective and antioxidant effects of Hygrophila auriculata (K. Schum) Heine Acanthaceae root extract. J Ethnopharmacol 104: 124-128.

29. Nevin KG, Vijayammal PL (2005) Effect of Aerva lanata against hepatotoxicity of carbon tetrachloride in rats. Environ Toxicol Pharmacol 20: 471-477.

30. Petyunin GP, Karashok UV (1990) Synthesis and biological activity of oxamoyl derivatives of aminopropionic acid, KhMAPE, Ukraine.

31. Sal'nikova SI, Drogovoz SM, Zupanets IA (1990) Farmakol Toksikol 53: 32-35.

32. Yan Y, Wanshun L, Baoqin H, Changhong W, Chenwei F, et al. (2007) The antioxidative and immunostimulating properties of D-glucosamine. Int Immunopharmacol 7: 29-35.

24

The Effects of Obesity on the Comparative Effectiveness of Linezolid and Vancomycin in Suspected Methicillin-Resistant Staphylococcus aureus Pneumonia

Caffrey AR[1*], Noh E[2], Morrill HJ[2] and LaPlante KL[3]

[1]Infectious Diseases Research Program, Veterans Affairs Medical Center, Providence, Rhode Island, USA
[2]Department of Pharmacy Practice, College of Pharmacy, University of Rhode Island, Kingston, Rhode Island, USA
[3]Division of Infectious Diseases, Warren Alpert Medical School of Brown University, Providence, Rhode Island, USA

Abstract

Background: Methicillin-Resistant Staphylococcus aureus (MRSA) has become a leading cause of pneumonia in the United States and there is limited data on treatment outcomes in obese patients. We evaluated the effectiveness of linezolid compared to vancomycin for the treatment of MRSA pneumonia in a national cohort of obese Veterans.

Methods: This retrospective cohort study included obese patients (body mass index ≥ 30) admitted to Veterans Affairs hospitals with MRSA-positive respiratory cultures and clinical signs of infection between 2002 and 2012. Patients initiating treatment with either vancomycin or linezolid, but not both, were selected for inclusion. Propensity matching and adjustment of Cox proportional hazards regression models quantified the effect of linezolid compared with vancomycin on time to hospital discharge, intensive care unit discharge, 30-day mortality, inpatient mortality, therapy discontinuation, therapy change, 30-day readmission, and 30-day MRSA reinfection. We performed sensitivity analyses by vancomycin Minimum Inhibitory Concentrations (MICs) and true trough levels.

Results: We identified 101 linezolid and 2,565 vancomycin patients. Balance in baseline characteristics between the treatment groups was achieved within propensity score quintiles and between propensity matched pairs (76 pairs). No significant differences were observed for the outcomes assessed. Among patients with vancomycin MICs of ≤ 1 µg/mL, the linezolid group had a significantly lower mortality rate, increased length of hospital stay, and longer therapy duration. There were no differences between the linezolid and vancomycin MICs of ≥ 1.5 µg/mL groups. Clinical outcomes among those with vancomycin trough concentrations of 15-20 mg/L were similar to patients treated with linezolid.

Conclusions: In our real-world comparative effectiveness study among obese patients with suspected MRSA pneumonia, linezolid was associated with a significantly lower mortality rate as compared to the vancomycin-treated patients with lower vancomycin MICs. Further studies are needed to determine whether this beneficial effect is observed in other study populations.

Keywords: Comparative effectiveness; Linezolid; Methicillin-resistant *Staphylococcus aureus* (MRSA) Pneumonia; Obesity; Vancomycin

Abbreviations: BAL: Bronchoalveolar Lavage; BMI: Body Mass Index; CI : Confidence Interval; HR: Hazard Ratio; ICD-9-CM: International Classification of Diseases, 9th Revision, Clinical Modification; ICU: Intensive Care Unit; MIC: Minimum Inhibitory Concentrations; MRSA: Methicillin-Resistant *Staphylococcus aureus*; US: United State

Introduction

Methicillin-Resistant *Staphylococcus aureus* (MRSA) is one of the most prevalent, pathogenic antimicrobial-resistant organisms, causing invasive infections worldwide [1]. MRSA has become a leading cause of pneumonia in both healthcare and community settings [2,3]. Furthermore, approximately 69% of adults in the United States (US) are either overweight or obese [4], which is concerning as obesity is an independent risk factor for developing pneumonia [5,6].

Limited treatment options exist for patients with MRSA pneumonia, and for many years, vancomycin, a glycopeptide antibiotic that inhibits Gram-positive bacterial cell wall synthesis by binding a D-alanyl-D-alanine cell wall precursor that is essential for peptidoglycan cross-linking, has served as the standard of care [7-9]. However, over time, clinical outcomes among vancomycin-treated patients with MRSA pneumonia have worsened [10]. In addition, the use of the vancomycin in MRSA pneumonia has been questioned due to poor penetration into alveolar fluid and the emergence of bacteria with decreased vancomycin susceptibility [2,7,10]. These limitations have prompted the need for additional therapeutic options. Linezolid, an oxazolidinone antibiotic that inhibits protein synthesis at the 50S ribosome, is recommended for the treatment of pneumonia caused by *Staphylococcus aureus* (methicillin-susceptible and resistant strains) bacteria [11]. While linezolid has been shown to achieve high lung concentrations, there is limited evidence to support clinical superiority over vancomycin [10,12-15]. Moreover, the optimal treatment in obese patients is largely unknown.

*Corresponding author: Caffrey AR, College of Pharmacy, University of Rhode Island, 7 Greenhouse Road, Kingston, Rhode Island, USA, E-mail: Aisling.Caffrey@uri.edu

Obesity is associated with an increased risk of pneumonia [5,6]. Decreased immunity, a higher risk of aspiration, reduced lung volume, and an altered ventilation pattern, impact pneumonia risk in obese patients [5,6]. Furthermore, obesity itself is an independent predictor of antibiotic treatment failure [16]. To date, there is no published research comparing linezolid and vancomycin in obese patients with MRSA pneumonia in the real-world clinical setting. Due to the increasing complexity of treating MRSA pneumonia, controversial superiority data, and the scarcity of data in the obese, we sought to evaluate the effectiveness of linezolid therapy compared to vancomycin for the treatment of suspected MRSA pneumonia in a national cohort of obese Veterans.

Materials and Methods

Data sources

The Veterans Health Administration has utilized an electronic medical record system since 1999 [17]. Our study included national standardized databases capturing patient care including International Classification of Diseases, 9th Revision, Clinical Modification (ICD-9-CM) diagnostic and procedure codes, microbiology results, pharmacy records for prescriptions and barcode administration, laboratory results, vital status, and vital signs.

Study population

We conducted a national retrospective cohort study quantifying the effectiveness of linezolid compared to vancomycin among obese patients with suspected MRSA pneumonia. We identified hospital in patients with positive MRSA cultures from a pulmonary site between January 1, 2002 and December 1, 2012. Patients exposed to at least 1 day of therapy with linezolid (intravenous or oral) or vancomycin (intravenous only) were selected for inclusion. Next we identified all obese patients with a body mass index (BMI) ≥ 30 [18]. BMI calculations were based on the most recent height and weight measurements within a year of treatment initiation. Additionally, we included patients initiating linezolid or vancomycin therapy within a window of 3 days prior to culture through 4 days after culture with an absence of linezolid or vancomycin therapy in the 7 days prior to treatment initiation.

Of the patients with culture-positive MRSA treated with either linezolid or vancomycin, an additional inclusion criterion included clinical signs of infection based on the presence of a chest x-ray, or a fever, or an elevated white blood cell count [3,19]. Each clinical sign was assessed between the admission date and treatment initiation date. Fever was defined as a temperature ≥ 100.4°F. An elevated white blood cell count was defined as ≥10,000/mm³. We excluded patients who died or were discharged within 2 days of treatment initiation and patients exposed to more than 2 consecutive days of other antibiotic therapy with activity against MRSA (clindamycin, daptomycin, doxycycline, linezolid, minocycline, tigecycline, trimethoprim/sulfamethoxazole, vancomycin) in the 3 days prior to or during treatment with linezolid or vancomycin. Only the first admission within the study period meeting all inclusion and exclusion criteria was included. The purpose of the exclusion criteria were three-fold, to identify patients: (1) with clinical signs of infection in addition to a positive culture, (2) who were still in the hospital the day after treatment initiation, and (3) treated with monotherapy.

Outcomes

The primary outcome of interest was time to hospital discharge.

Therapy initiation was used to define the index date of treatment. Time calculations were made from the index date to the event date for each endpoint. The secondary endpoints of interest included time to Intensive Care Unit (ICU) discharge, 30-day mortality, inpatient mortality, therapy discontinuation, therapy change, 30-day readmission, and 30-day MRSA reinfection. For hospital discharge, patients who died during the admission were censored on their date of death. Transfer out of an ICU was assessed among patients initiating linezolid or vancomycin therapy in the ICU.

Antimicrobial drug exposures with activity against MRSA were assessed for each patient during the admission. These exposures were classified into dichotomous variables based on the class of the antimicrobial agent and by the duration of receipt of agents in each class. Therapy change was defined as discontinuation of linezolid or vancomycin and initiation of another agent with anti-MRSA activity. As such, therapy change could have included switching from linezolid to vancomycin, switching from vancomycin to linezolid, or switching from either linezolid or vancomycin to another anti-MRSA antibiotic (listed above). Switching an antibiotic (i.e. linezolid) from an intravenous to an oral route was not considered a therapy change. Clinical rationale for therapy change, such as de-escalation resulting from clinical improvement or change in therapy as a result of failure was not ascertained. For 30-day readmission to a VA medical unit and 30-day MRSA reinfection, patients who died after discharge were censored on their date of death. The end of the follow-up period was December 31, 2012.

Statistical analysis

To assess baseline differences between the two study groups, we utilized a Fisher's exact or χ^2 test for categorical data. For continuous variables of interest, we used a t-test for normally distributed data and the non-parametric Wilcoxon Rank Sum test was used otherwise. We employed propensity score methods, where the predicted probability of treatment with linezolid was derived from an unconditional logistic regression model using a manual backward, non–computer-generated, elimination approach [20-22]. Propensity score stratification and matching within propensity score calipers were implemented, related assumptions were assessed, and subsequent covariate balance was reviewed [20,21].

In the second stage of modeling, we used Cox proportional hazards regression models to quantify the effect of linezolid treatment in obese patients with MRSA pneumonia compared to vancomycin on the aforementioned outcomes. We further evaluated Cox proportional hazards model assumptions, including that of proportionality, with formal tests and graphical displays [23]. If the confidence interval of the hazard ratio included one, then the clinical outcome occurred at comparable rates in both the linezolid and vancomycin groups. A hazard ratio greater than one indicated an increased probability of the event occurring sooner in the linezolid group compared to the reference vancomycin group. In terms of the study outcomes, a hazard ratio greater than one would represent a higher mortality rate, decreased length of stay, or a higher readmission rate among patients treated with linezolid. Alternatively, a hazard ratio less than one would mean time to mortality was lower and length of stay was higher in the linezolid group as compared to vancomycin.

We conducted subgroup analyses among patients with morbid obesity (BMI ≥ 40) and with positive Bronchoalveolar Lavage (BAL) cultures. Additionally, we assessed the study outcomes among a restricted study population of those with a pneumonia-related diagnosis code present during the hospital admission (ICD-9-CM codes 003.22, 020.3, 020.4, 020.5, 021.2, 022.1, 031.0, 039.1, 052.1, 055.1, 073.0, 083.0, 112.4, 114.0, 114.4, 114.5, 115.05, 115.15, 115.95, 130.4, 136.3, 480-486, 513.0, 517.1) [24].

We also performed several sensitivity analyses. First, we assessed linezolid effectiveness as compared to patients with vancomycin minimum inhibitory concentrations (MICs) of ≤ 1 µg/mL and those with vancomycin MICs of ≥ 1.5 µg/mL. Second, we assessed linezolid effectiveness as compared to patients with true vancomycin trough concentrations of 15-20 mg/L and no evidence of acute kidney injury (defined as an increase in serum creatinine of 0.3 mg/dL or 50% prior to starting vancomycin) [25]. True vancomycin troughs were defined as levels obtained at steady state, with at least 3 vancomycin doses before the level, that were taken less than 2 hours before the next vancomycin dose or within 2 hours of the average interval between the two prior vancomycin doses [25]. Only the first trough level after the third vancomycin dose which met our steady state definition was assessed. We did not assess change in vancomycin dosing based on trough results. All analyses were performed using SAS (SAS Institute Inc., Cary, NC, Version 9.3).

Results

We identified 2,666 obese patients with suspected MRSA pneumonia who met our inclusion and exclusion criteria (Figure 1). There were 2,565 (96.2%) patients in the vancomycin group and 101 (3.8%) in the linezolid group. Among those treated with linezolid, approximately 91% (n=92) were dosed twice daily. The mean patient age at the time of culture collection was 66 years for linezolid and 68 years for vancomycin (Table 1). Several statistically significant differences in the frequency of current comorbidities, present during the suspected MRSA pneumonia admission, were observed, including chronic ulcer, dialysis, rheumatoid arthritis, and cerebrovascular disease. Medical histories in the year prior to the suspected MRSA pneumonia hospitalization, including pneumonia, osteomyelitis, and allergy to vancomycin, differed significantly between the treatment groups. Patients in the linezolid group had higher utilization of linezolid in the 90 days prior to the suspected MRSA pneumonia hospitalization (Table 2). Furthermore, surgical procedures in the previous 90 days and MRSA bronchial culture sites were more common in the linezolid group compared to the vancomycin group.

Though differences in baseline variables were observed between the treatment groups, balance was achieved within propensity score quintiles and between propensity matched pairs (linezolid=76, vancomycin=76). In propensity score quintile adjustment, quintile I served as the reference. Propensity score matching was achieved within 0.001 caliper. The propensity score model can be found in the footnote of Table 3. This model demonstrated excellent discrimination between the treatment groups (C-statistic 0.84) [22].

The median time to discharge was 15 days (interquartile range [IQR] 7-30) among linezolid-treated patients versus 12 days (IQR 7-23) in vancomycin-treated patients. Time to discharge was significantly longer in the linezolid group compared to the vancomycin group in the unadjusted analysis (hazard ratio [HR] 0.76, 95% confidence interval [CI] 0.60-0.96) and non-significantly longer in propensity adjusted (HR 0.85, 95% CI 0.66-1.08) and propensity matched analyses (HR 0.96, 95% CI 0.56-1.65; Table 3). The inpatient mortality (28%) and 30-day mortality (28%) rates were high but similar between treatment groups among this obese cohort with positive MRSA pulmonary cultures. No significant differences were observed in unadjusted, adjusted, or

matched Cox proportional hazards models for time to ICU discharge, 30-day mortality, inpatient mortality, therapy discontinuation, therapy change, 30-day MRSA pneumonia reinfection, or 30-day readmission.

Results similar to the overall cohort were observed in subgroup analyses among morbidly obese patients (BMI ≥ 40; linezolid n=29, vancomycin n=562) and those with positive BAL cultures (linezolid n=13, vancomycin n=165). Time to hospital discharge in the morbidly obese was significantly longer in the linezolid group in the unadjusted (HR 0.50, 95% CI 0.32-0.79) and propensity adjusted (HR 0.51, 95% CI 0.32-0.81) analyses and non-significant in propensity matched analyses (HR 0.50, 95% CI 0.15-1.66). No significant differences were observed for the other outcomes or by BAL subgroup. Regarding the subgroup analysis among patients with a pneumonia diagnosis code (linezolid n=67, vancomycin n=1,612), patients treated with linezolid demonstrated a significantly lower rate of therapy discontinuation (propensity matched HR 0.42, 95% CI 0.20-0.87) compared to patients treated with vancomycin, indicating length of therapy was longer in the vancomycin group.

Among the vancomycin group, we identified 984 eligible patients (38%) for the sensitivity analyses evaluating effectiveness by vancomycin MICs. Of them, 85% (n=833) had vancomycin MICs ≤ 1 µg/mL, 1% (n=10) had a MIC=1.5 µg/mL, 14% (n=141) had a MIC=2 µg/mL, and no patients had MICs > 2 µg/mL. Patients on linezolid showed significantly lower rates of 30-day mortality (Table 4; propensity matched HR 0.35, 95% CI 0.14-0.90) and therapy discontinuation (propensity matched HR 0.49, 95% CI 0.27-0.87) than those with vancomycin MICs of ≤ 1 µg/mL, meaning linezolid patients had longer survival in the 30 days after discharge and a longer duration of therapy than vancomycin patients with MICs of ≤ 1 µg/mL. Time to hospital discharge was significantly longer in the linezolid group compared to the vancomycin group with MICs of ≤ 1 µg/mL (unadjusted HR 0.69, 95% CI 0.54-0.89; propensity adjusted HR 0.72, 95% CI 0.55-0.93; and propensity matched HR 0.52, 95% CI 0.29-0.93).

Only 12% (n=301) of vancomycin patients had accurately obtained through concentrations without evidence of acute kidney injury. In sensitivity analyses among these patients with vancomycin trough levels obtained at steady state, 19% (n=58) had therapeutic trough concentrations less than 10 mg/L, 29% (n=86) had 10-15 mg/L, 22% (n=66) had 15-20 mg/L, and 30% (n=91) had greater than or equal to 20 mg/L. All clinical outcomes were similar among linezolid patients as compared to vancomycin patients with vancomycin trough concentrations between 15-20 mg/L.

Discussion

To our knowledge, this is the first real-world comparative effectiveness study assessing linezolid and vancomycin for the treatment of suspected MRSA pneumonia in obese patients. Rates of hospital discharge, ICU discharge, 30-day mortality, inpatient mortality, therapy discontinuation, therapy change, 30-day MRSA pneumonia reinfection, and 30-day readmission did not differ significantly between linezolid and vancomycin in our study.

Our results agree with a recently published analysis of two linezolid clinical trials in which clinical success and microbiologic success were similar across all quartiles of weight in patients with nosocomial MRSA pneumonia [26]. This appears to be the only other study evaluating clinical outcomes among obese MRSA pneumonia patients treated with linezolid or vancomycin. Additionally, our findings are consistent with previous research comparing linezolid and vancomycin in non-obese

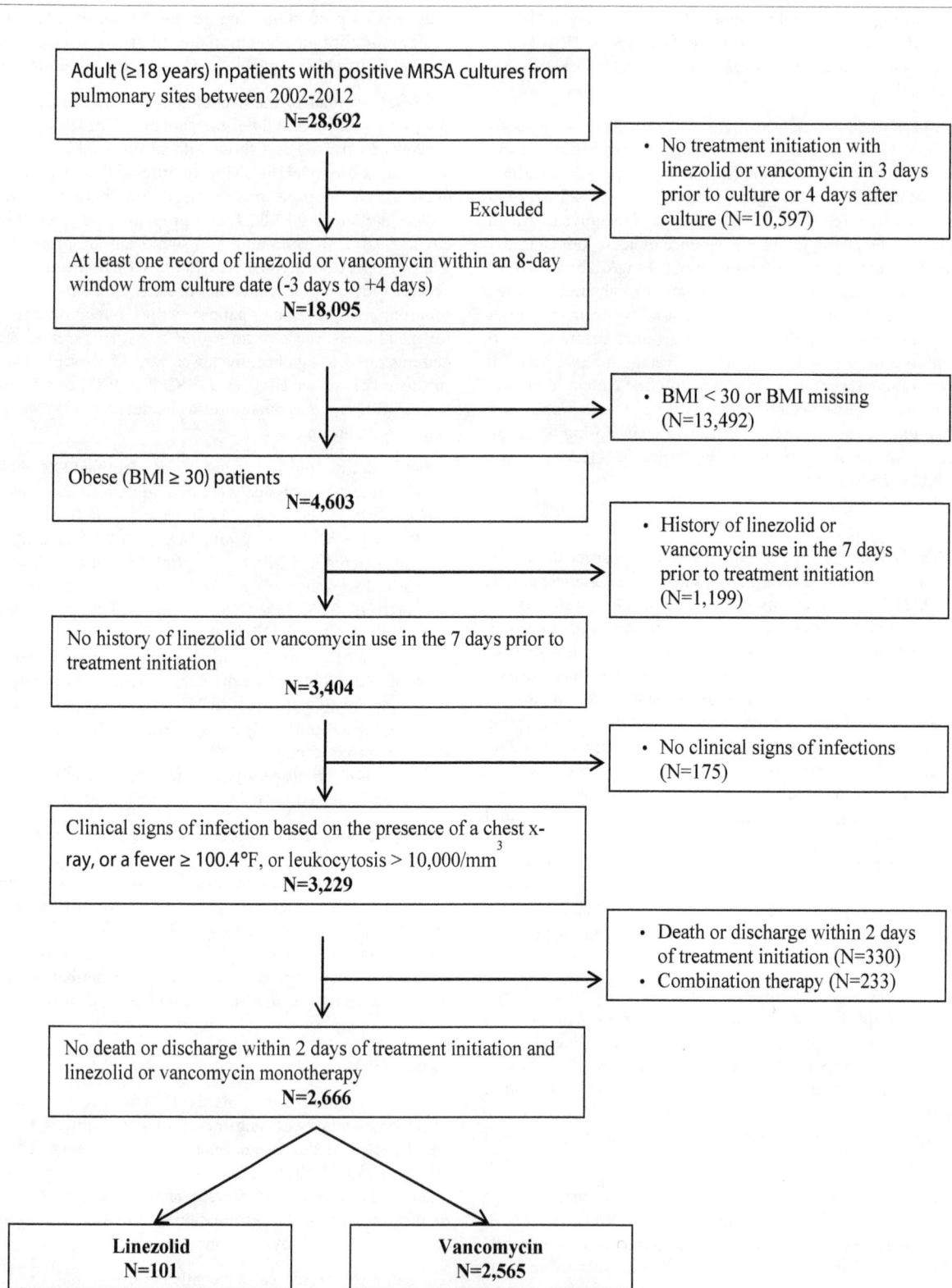

```
┌─────────────────────────────────────────────┐
│ Adult (≥18 years) inpatients with positive   │
│ MRSA cultures from pulmonary sites between    │
│ 2002-2012                                     │
│ N=28,692                                      │
└─────────────────────────────────────────────┘
```

Excluded

- No treatment initiation with linezolid or vancomycin in 3 days prior to culture or 4 days after culture (N=10,597)

At least one record of linezolid or vancomycin within an 8-day window from culture date (-3 days to +4 days)
N=18,095

- BMI < 30 or BMI missing (N=13,492)

Obese (BMI ≥ 30) patients
N=4,603

- History of linezolid or vancomycin use in the 7 days prior to treatment initiation (N=1,199)

No history of linezolid or vancomycin use in the 7 days prior to treatment initiation
N=3,404

- No clinical signs of infections (N=175)

Clinical signs of infection based on the presence of a chest x-ray, or a fever ≥ 100.4°F, or leukocytosis > $10,000/mm^3$
N=3,229

- Death or discharge within 2 days of treatment initiation (N=330)
- Combination therapy (N=233)

No death or discharge within 2 days of treatment initiation and linezolid or vancomycin monotherapy
N=2,666

Linezolid
N=101

Vancomycin
N=2,565

MRSA: Methicillin-Resistant *Staphylococcus*; BMI: Body Mass Index

Figure 1: Study Cohort Identification

Demographic characteristics	Linezolid N=101	Vancomycin N=2,565	P-value
Age (years)	66.2 ± 12.3	67.6 ± 11.2	0.22
Male	98 (97.0)	2,489 (97.0)	0.99
Body mass index			
30-35	63 (62.4)	1,652 (64.4)	0.15
35-40	9 (8.9)	351 (13.7)	
40+	29 (28.7)	562 (21.9)	
Current comorbid conditions[1]			
Charlson score	3.7 ± 2.7	3.6 ± 2.5	0.84
Elixhauser score	4.7 ± 2.5	4.3 ± 2.0	0.18
Chronic renal disease	34 (33.7)	718 (28.0)	0.21
Peripheral vascular disease	9 (8.9)	236 (9.2)	0.92
Cancer	17 (16.8)	487 (19.0)	0.59
Cerebrovascular disease	6 (5.9)	363 (14.2)	0.02*
Congestive heart failure	43 (42.6)	1,031 (40.2)	0.63
Diabetes	53 (52.5)	1,196 (46.6)	0.25
Rheumatoid arthritis	5 (5.0)	27 (1.1)	< 0.001*
Hypertension	53 (52.5)	1,532 (59.7)	0.15
Hypothyroidism	10 (9.9)	148 (5.8)	0.08
Coagulopathy	6 (5.9)	233 (9.1)	0.28
Fluid and electolyte disorder	45 (44.6)	986 (38.4)	0.22
Depression	25 (24.8)	365 (14.2)	0.003*
Other neurological disorders	22 (21.8)	440 (17.2)	0.23
Bactremia	11 (10.9)	419 (16.3)	0.14
Skin/subcutaneous infection	32 (31.7)	638 (24.9)	0.12
Chronic ulcer	26 (25.7)	424 (16.5)	0.02*
Dialysis	18 (17.8)	285 (11.1)	0.04*
Pneumonia	67 (66.3)	1,612 (62.9)	0.48
Culture-confirmed infections with			
Enterococcus	31 (30.7)	463 (18.1)	0.001*
VRE	20 (19.8)	218 (8.5)	< 0.001*
Psudomonas aeruginosa	31 (30.7)	508 (19.8)	0.008*
Concomitant[2] MRSA infection site			
Blood	12 (11.9)	359 (14.0)	0.55
Bone	5 (5.0)	25 (1.0)	0.002*
Nares	< 5 (<5.0)	112 (4.4)	1.00
Skin	20 (19.8)	404 (15.8)	0.27
Urine	9 (8.9)	183 (7.1)	0.50
Medical history[3]			
Previous Elixhauser score	5.4 ± 3.1	5.0 ± 3.0	0.24
Previous chronic renal disease	31 (30.7)	593 (23.1)	0.08
Previous diabetes	63 (62.4)	1,350 (52.6)	0.05*
Previous rheumatoid arthritis	5 (5.0)	56 (2.2)	0.07
Previous congestive heart failure	44 (43.6)	903 (35.2)	0.09
Previous hypothyroidism	16 (15.8)	248 (9.7)	0.04
Previous bactremia	7 (6.9)	115 (4.5)	0.25
Previous osteomyelitis	8 (7.9)	74 (2.9)	0.004*
Previous surgery/medical care complication	13 (12.9)	234 (9.1)	0.20
Previous allergy to vancomycin	9 (8.9)	14 (0.6)	< 0.001*
Previous pneumonia	32 (31.7)	598 (23.3)	0.05*
Previous culture-confirmed infections with			
Enterococcus	12 (11.9)	163 (6.4)	0.03*
VRE	6 (5.9)	48 (1.9)	0.004*

Data are mean ± standard deviation or number (%) of patients. MRSA: Methicillin-Resistant Staphylococcus aureus; VRE: Vancomycin-Resistant Enterococcus

1. Present during the MRSA pneumonia hospitalization.

2 Present between the MRSA pneumonia admission and the end of treatment

3. Present in the 1 year prior to the admission with a positive MRSA pulmonary culture.

* p<0.05

Table 1: Demographics and Comorbid Conditions by Treatment Group

Healthcare and antibiotic exposures	Linezolid N=101	Vancomycin N=2,565	P-value
Hospital unit at treatment initiation			
Intensive care	39 (38.6)	895 (34.9)	0.44
General medicine / Other	62 (61.4)	1,669 (65.1)	
Surgery during the current admission	46 (45.5)	1,039 (40.5)	0.31
MRSA culture site			
Bronchial	13 (12.9)	165 (6.4)	0.01*
Non-bronchial (i.e. lung)	88 (87.1)	2,400 (93.6)	
Year			
2002	5 (5.0)	112 (4.4)	
2003	5 (5.0)	238 (9.3)	
2004	10 (9.9)	271 (10.6)	
2005	8 (7.9)	258 (10.1)	
2006	5 (5.0)	247 (9.6)	0.15
2007	11 (10.9)	253 (9.9)	
2008	16 (15.8)	253 (9.9)	
2009	7 (6.9)	235 (9.2)	
2010	16 (15.8)	234 (9.1)	
2011	8 (7.9)	263 (10.2)	
2012	10 (9.9)	201 (7.8)	
Region of facility			
Northeast	14 (13.9)	434 (16.9)	
South	53 (52.5)	1,198 (46.7)	0.23
Midwest	24 (23.8)	515 (20.1)	
West	10 (9.9)	418 (16.3)	
Length of therapy (days)	8.3 ± 5.3	7.3 ± 5.9	0.08
Previous hospitalization, 90 days	38 (37.6)	991 (38.6)	0.84
Previous surgery, any, 90 days	22 (21.8)	324 (12.6)	0.01*
Previous nursing home stay, 90 days	7 (6.9)	166 (6.5)	0.85
Previous anti-MRSA antibiotic[1]			
Number of antibiotics	1.6 ± 0.6	1.3 ± 0.5	< 0.001*
Number of days with antibiotic use	13.3 ± 11.6	8.2 ± 9.4	0.01*
Linezolid	10 (9.9)	22 (0.9)	<0.001*
Vancomycin	18 (17.8)	300 (11.7)	0.06
Other antibiotics	9 (8.9)	120 (4.7)	0.05*

Data are mean ± standard deviation or number (%) of patients. MRSA: Methicillin-Resistant *Staphylococcus aureus*.
1. Present in the 90 days prior to the admission with a positive MRSA pulmonary culture.
* p<0.05

Table 2: Healthcare and Antibiotic Exposures and Hospitalization-Related Characteristics by Treatment Group

patients [15,27-30]. Two meta-analyses which compared vancomycin and linezolid for nosocomial pneumonia, found no differences in clinical and microbiologic outcomes or mortality [29,30]. While many trials have demonstrated equivalent efficacy between linezolid and vancomycin [12,14], a recent prospective, randomized, double-blind trial of MRSA pneumonia demonstrated higher clinical and microbiologic success rates with linezolid over vancomycin, however mortality was similar between the two groups [15]. Although several studies have shown benefits for linezolid treatment compared with vancomycin [10,15,31], their methodological and statistical limitations have been frequently debated in the literature [32-34].

There is conflicting evidence surrounding treatment outcomes with vancomycin at higher MICs. Some studies suggest patients with MRSA infections are more likely to experience clinical success with vancomycin if the vancomycin MIC is < 1 µg/mL as compared to patients with higher MICs [35,36]. In an observational study of 158 patients with hospital-acquired, ventilator-associated or healthcare-associated MRSA pneumonia, mortality increased as a function of the vancomycin MIC [37]. The overall all-cause 28-day mortality rate in these patients was 32.3%, with the majority of isolates having a vancomycin MIC $\geq$ 1.5 µg/mL (115/158, 72.8%) [37]. However, a recent meta-analysis examining the association between vancomycin MIC and mortality rates in patients with *Staphylococcus aureus* bacteremia demonstrated no significant differences in mortality between patients with lower-vancomycin MICs (< 1.5 µg/mL) and those with higher-MICs ($\geq$ 1.5 µg/mL) [38].

In our sensitivity analyses, we observed significant differences between treatment groups when restricting the vancomycin group to patients with lower MICs ($\leq$ 1 µg/mL). Linezolid was associated with a significantly lower discharge rate, representing an increased length of stay, a significantly decreased rate of therapy discontinuation, indicating longer therapy duration, and a significantly lower rate of 30-day mortality, representing greater survival, as compared to the vancomycin group with MICs of $\leq$ 1 µg/Ml. We believe this is the first study to demonstrate improved outcomes with linezolid in obese patients, as compared to those receiving vancomycin and infected with

Outcomes	No.of events/No.of patients		HR (95% CI)	Sooner outcomes in vancomycin ← → Sooner outcomes in linezolid
	Linezolid	Vancomycin		
Discharge				
Unadjusted	70/101	1,852/2,565	0.76 (0.60 - 0.96)	
Propensity Adjusted[1]	70/101	1,852/2,565	0.85 (0.66 - 1.08)	
Propensity Matched[2]	56/76	53/76	0.96 (0.56 - 1.65)	
ICU discharge				
Unadjusted	27/39	643/895	0.92 (0.62 - 1.35)	
Propensity Adjusted[1]	27/39	643/895	1.02 (0.68 - 1.53)	
Propensity Matched[2]	18/26	21/30	7.00 (0.86 - 56.9)	
30-day mortality				
Unadjusted	22/101	731/2,565	0.75 (0.49 - 1.15)	
Propensity Adjusted[1]	22/101	731/2,565	0.82 (0.53 - 1.27)	
Propensity Matched[2]	14/76	20/76	0.58 (0.28 - 1.22)	
Inpatient mortality				
Unadjusted	31/101	713/2,565	0.76 (0.53 - 1.08)	
Propensity Adjusted[1]	31/101	713/2,565	0.91 (0.63 - 1.33)	
Propensity Matched[2]	20/76	23/76	0.77 (0.34 - 1.75)	
Therapy discontinuation				
Unadjusted	74/101	1,903/2,565	0.93 (0.73 - 1.17)	
Propensity Adjusted[1]	74/101	1,903/2,565	0.93 (0.73 - 1.19)	
Propensity Matched[2]	56/76	56/76	0.62 (0.37 - 1.05)	
Therapy change				
Unadjusted	20/101	470/2,565	1.00 (0.64 - 1.56)	
Propensity Adjusted[1]	20/101	470/2,565	0.99 (0.62 - 1.58)	
Propensity Matched[2]	16/76	15/76	0.69 (0.30 - 1.62)	
30-day MRSA pneumonia reinfection				
Unadjusted	<5/70	26/1,852	1.01 (0.14 - 7.45)	
Propensity Adjusted[1]	<5/70	26/1,852	1.11 (0.14 - 8.81)	
Propensity Matched[2]	<5/56	<5/53	0.33 (0.04 - 3.21)	
30-day readmission				
Unadjusted	10/70	367/1,852	0.71 (0.38 - 1.34)	
Propensity Adjusted[1]	10/70	367/1,852	0.66 (0.35 - 1.26)	
Propensity Matched[2]	6/56	14/53	0.30 (0.08 - 1.09)	

HR (95% CI): 0, 1, 2 axis

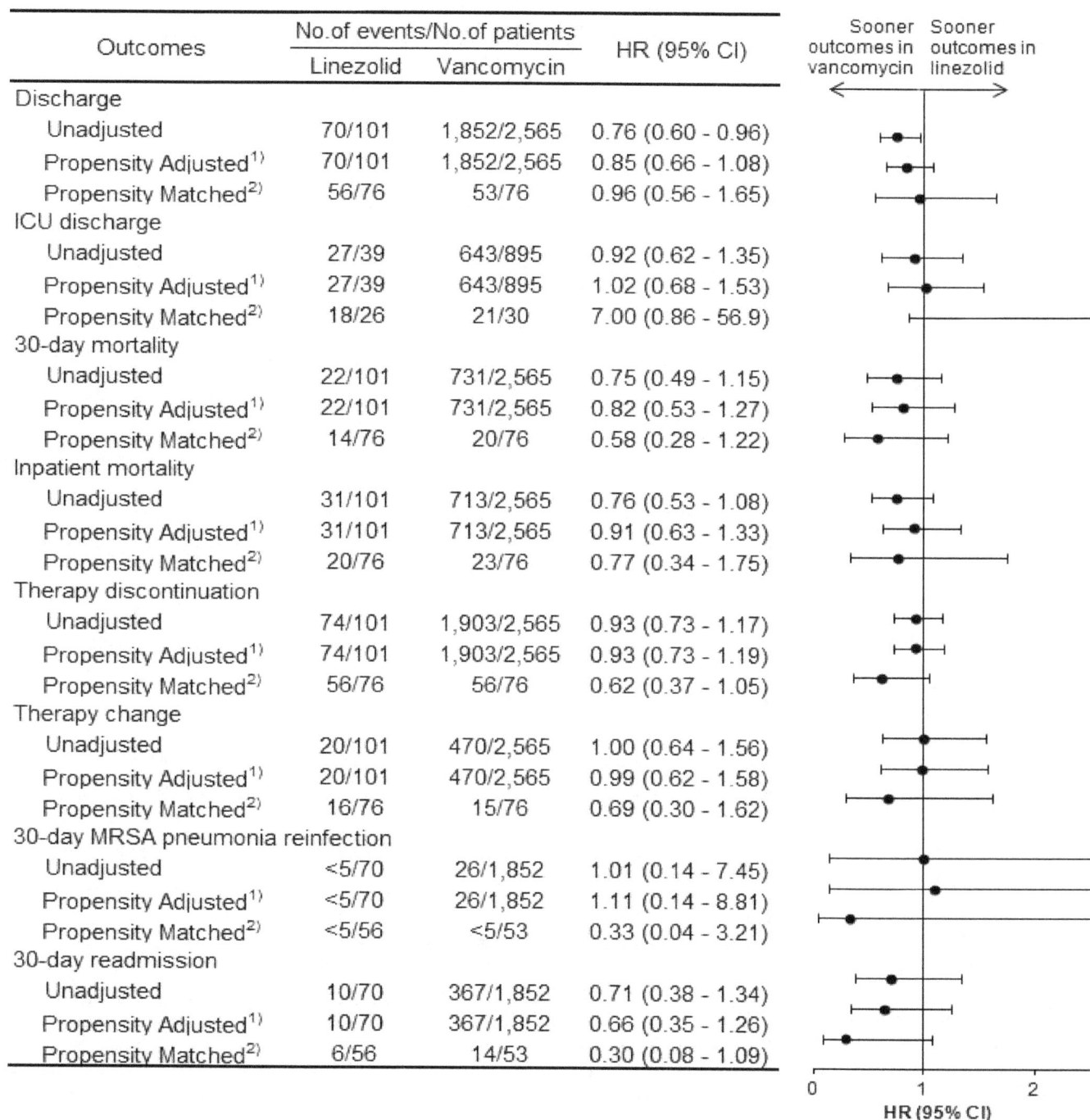

HR: Hazard Ratio; CI: Confidence Interval; ICU: Intensive Care Unit; MRSA: Methicillin-Resistant *Staphylococcus aureus*.
1. Adjusted by propensity score quintiles (reference quintile I).
2. Propensity score matched within 0.001 caliper.

The propensity score was derived from an unconditional logistic regression model controlling for age, body mass index, Elixhauser score, time to therapy initiation from culture date, year, region of facility, hospital unit at treatment initiation, culture site, history of MRSA infection, elevated white blood cell count, current diabetes complications, current myocardial infarction, current cerebrovascular disease, current rheumatoid arthritis, current hypertension, current other neurological disorders, current coagulopathy, current fluid and electrolyte disorder, current depression, current skin infection, current chronic ulcer, current bacteremia, current immune disorder, current dialysis, current VRE infection, current *Psudomonas aeroginosa* infection, concomitant MRSA infection in bone, history of chronic renal disease, history of diabetes, history of cancer, history of congestive heart failure, history of hypothyroidism, history of burn, history of pneumonia, history of bacteremia, history of osteomyelitis, history of neutropenia, history of VRE infection, history of allergy to vancomycin, nursing home stay in previous 30 days, surgery in previous 90 days, linezolid in previous 90 days, trimethoprim/sulfamethoxazole in previous 90 days, daptomycin in previous 90 days, number of antibiotic used in previous 90 days (C-statistic 0.84).

Table 3: Outcomes in Overall Cohort: Linezolid Compared with Vancomycin

Subgroups	Outcomes	No. of events/No. of patients		HR (95% CI)	Sooner outcomes in vancomycin / Sooner outcomes in linezolid
		Linezolid	Vancomycin		
Morbidly obese (BMI ≥ 40)	Discharge				
	Unadjusted	20/29	421/562	0.50 (0.32 - 0.79)	
	Propensity Adjusted[1]	20/29	421/562	0.51 (0.32 - 0.81)	
	Propensity Matched[2]	12/17	12/17	0.50 (0.15 - 1.66)	
ICD-9-CM pneumonia diagnosis	Therapy discontinuation				
	Unadjusted	47/67	1,188/1,612	0.89 (0.67 - 1.19)	
	Propensity Adjusted[1]	47/67	1,188/1,612	0.85 (0.63 - 1.15)	
	Propensity Matched[2]	32/48	34/48	0.42 (0.20 - 0.87)	
MIC ≤1.0 µg/mL	Discharge				
	Unadjusted	70/101	623/833	0.69 (0.54 - 0.89)	
	Propensity Adjusted[1]	70/101	623/833	0.72 (0.55 - 0.93)	
	Propensity Matched[2]	47/62	43/62	0.52 (0.29 - 0.93)	
	30-day mortality				
	Unadjusted	22/101	221/833	0.82 (0.53 - 1.27)	
	Propensity Adjusted[1]	22/101	221/833	0.56 (0.48 - 1.21)	
	Propensity Matched[2]	9/62	18/62	0.35 (0.14 - 0.90)	
	Therapy discontinuation				
	Unadjusted	74/101	589/833	0.97 (0.76 - 1.23)	
	Propensity Adjusted[1]	74/101	589/833	0.97 (0.74 - 1.26)	
	Propensity Matched[2]	46/62	49/62	0.49 (0.27 - 0.87)	

HR: Hazard Ratio; CI: Confidence Interval; BMI: Body Mass Index; ICD-9-CM: International Classification of Diseases, 9th Revision, Clinical Modification; MIC: Minimum Inhibitory Concentration.
1. Adjusted by propensity score quintiles (reference quintile I).
2. Propensity score matched within 0.001 caliper.

Table 4: Subgroup and Sensitivity Analyses: Linezolid Compared with Vancomycin

low MIC strains. On the contrary, there were no significant differences in clinical outcomes between treatment groups when restricting the vancomycin group to those with vancomycin MICs of ≥ 1.5 µg/mL. Since this was a national study, MIC testing systems varied by facility and MIC testing methodology was not specified in the data.

Appropriate dosing of antibiotics in obese patients is extremely difficult and may result in underdosing [9,39]. Furthermore, 28% of our cohort had a diagnosis of chronic renal disease during the admission, which further complicates appropriate dosing in the obese population. Obese patients treated with vancomycin may be less likely to achieve optimal dosing, which puts patients at risk for poor outcomes [40], even if they had a favorable vancomycin susceptibility.

Vancomycin trough concentrations of 15-20 mg/L are recommended for severe infections, including MRSA pneumonia, in order to improve penetration, increase the probability of optimal serum vancomycin concentrations, and improve clinical outcomes [25]. However the optimal trough in obese patients is largely unknown. Among patients with true vancomycin trough concentrations, only 22% (n=66) were in therapeutic range. All clinical outcomes were similar in patients with vancomycin trough levels of 15-20 mg/L compared to patients receiving linezolid. Although we found no significant

differences between linezolid and vancomycin, the relatively small number of patients with true trough levels of 15-20 mg/L may have affected our ability to detect differences between the treatment groups.

There is always the potential for observational studies to be impacted by bias and residual confounding. To address these potential limitations, we took steps in the design and analytic phases to minimize bias. To capture potential confounders, we assessed a variety of patient data, including pharmacy data, microbiology data, and records of inpatient and outpatient care. To address the impact of confounding by indication, we utilized propensity score methods in the analytic phase [20,21,41]. Although balance was achieved within propensity score quintiles and between propensity matched pairs, there is the potential for residual confounding by unobserved covariates. Additionally, due to the relatively small sample size after matching propensity scores, we may have been unable to detect small differences in clinical outcomes between the two treatment groups.

Though we sought to develop accurate definitions for exposures, outcomes, and known potential confounders, misclassification bias may have impacted our study results. Our definition of suspected MRSA pneumonia may not have captured all MRSA pneumonia infections. Previous research has shown that as many as 30% of patients never have cultures taken [27]. In addition, we included patients with positive MRSA respiratory cultures from both sputum and BAL. The sensitivity of culture-positive isolates from non-bronchoscopic lung lavage for confirming ventilator-associated pneumonia is reported to be 72% with a Positive Predictive Value (PPV) of 14%, while the sensitivity of BAL for confirming pneumonia is 89% with a PPV of 33% [42]. Since our cohort definition for suspected MRSA pneumonia was based on culture confirmation and the presence of clinical signs of infection, we performed a subgroup analysis restricting the cohort to patients with a pneumonia diagnosis code in addition to a positive culture from a respiratory culture site and clinical signs of infection. This subgroup analysis demonstrated consistent results with those of the overall cohort.

Lastly, our study findings were further impacted by the limited generalizability of the VA population to the general US population. However, the Veterans Health Administration is the largest integrated healthcare system in the US. Due to the implementation of electronic medical records in 1999, large standardized databases, unique in size and content, include a wealth of information not available from other national data sources, including barcode medication administration, microbiology, and lab chemistry data [43].

Conclusions

We evaluated the effectiveness of linezolid therapy compared to vancomycin in obese patients with culture-confirmed MRSA from a pulmonary site and found no significant differences in clinical outcomes between the two treatment groups. In sensitivity analyses, however, we found that linezolid was associated with a significantly higher survival rate compared to vancomycin patients with lower MICs (≤ 1 µg/mL). Based on our review of the literature, this is the first study to demonstrate improved survival with linezolid as compared to vancomycin among obese patients with suspected MRSA pneumonia infected with low vancomycin MICs. As such, further studies are needed to determine whether this beneficial effect is observed in other study populations and to determine the clinical implications of this finding.

Acknowledgement

This work was supported, in part, by an Advancing Science through Pfizer Initiated Research (ASPIRE) grant from Pfizer Inc.

References

1. Diekema DJ, Climo M (2008) Preventing MRSA infections: finding it is not enough. JAMA 299: 1190-1192.

2. Kollef MH, Shorr A, Tabak YP, Gupta V, Liu LZ, et al. (2005) Epidemiology and outcomes of health-care-associated pneumonia: results from a large US database of culture-positive pneumonia. Chest 128: 3854-3862.

3. Mandell LA, Wunderink RG, Anzueto A, Bartlett JG, Campbell GD, et al. (2007) Infectious Diseases Society of America/American Thoracic Society consensus guidelines on the management of community-acquired pneumonia in adults. Clin Infect Dis 44 (Suppl 2): S27-72.

4. Flegal KM, Carroll MD, Kit BK, Ogden CL (2012) Prevalence of obesity and trends in the distribution of body mass index among US adults, 1999-2010. JAMA 307: 491-497.

5. Kornum JB, Nørgaard M, Dethlefsen C, Due KM, Thomsen RW, et al. (2010) Obesity and risk of subsequent hospitalisation with pneumonia. Eur Respir J 36: 1330-1336.

6. Hingston CD, Holmes TW, Saayman AG, Wise MP (2011) Obesity and risk of pneumonia in patients with influenza. Eur Respir J 37: 1299.

7. Lodise TP Jr, McKinnon PS (2007) Burden of methicillin-resistant Staphylococcus aureus: focus on clinical and economic outcomes. Pharmacotherapy 27: 1001-1012.

8. Sakoulas G, Moellering RC Jr (2008) Increasing antibiotic resistance among methicillin-resistant Staphylococcus aureus strains. Clin Infect Dis 46 Suppl 5: S360-367.

9. Grace E (2012) Altered vancomycin pharmacokinetics in obese and morbidly obese patients: what we have learned over the past 30 years. J Antimicrob Chemother 67: 1305-1310.

10. Kollef MH, Rello J, Cammarata SK, Croos-Dabrera RV, Wunderink RG (2004) Clinical cure and survival in Gram-positive ventilator-associated pneumonia: retrospective analysis of two double-blind studies comparing linezolid with vancomycin. Intensive Care Med 30: 388-394.

11. Liu C, Bayer A, Cosgrove SE, Daum RS, Fridkin SK, et al. (2011) Clinical Practice Guidelines by the Infectious Diseases Society of America for the Treatment of Methicillin-Resistant Staphylococcus aureus Infections in Adults and Children. Clin Infect Dis 52: e18-55.

12. Kohno S, Yamaguchi K, Aikawa N, Sumiyama Y, Odagiri S, et al. (2007) Linezolid versus vancomycin for the treatment of infections caused by methicillin-resistant Staphylococcus aureus in Japan. J Antimicrob Chemother 60: 1361-1369.

13. Stein GE, Wells EM (2010) The importance of tissue penetration in achieving successful antimicrobial treatment of nosocomial pneumonia and complicated skin and soft-tissue infections caused by methicillin-resistant Staphylococcus aureus: vancomycin and linezolid. Curr Med Res Opin 26: 571-588.

14. Stevens DL, Herr D, Lampiris H, Hunt JL, Batts DH, et al. (2002) Linezolid versus vancomycin for the treatment of methicillin-resistant Staphylococcus aureus infections. Clin Infect Dis 34: 1481-1490.

15. Wunderink RG, Niederman MS, Kollef MH, Shorr AF, Kunkel MJ, et al. (2012) Linezolid in methicillin-resistant Staphylococcus aureus nosocomial pneumonia: a randomized, controlled study. Clin Infect Dis 54: 621-629.

16. Longo C, Bartlett G, Macgibbon B, Mayo N, Rosenberg E, et al. (2013) The effect of obesity on antibiotic treatment failure: a historical cohort study. Pharmacoepidemiol Drug Saf 22: 970-976.

17. http://www.hsrd.research.va.gov/for_researchers/cyber_seminars/archives/751-notes

18. (1998) Clinical Guidelines on the Identification, Evaluation, and Treatment of Overweight and Obesity in Adults--The Evidence Report. National Institutes of Health. Obes Res 6 Suppl 2: 51S-209S.

19. American Thoracic Society; Infectious Diseases Society of America (2005) Guidelines for the management of adults with hospital-acquired, ventilator-associated, and healthcare-associated pneumonia. Am J Respir Crit Care Med 171: 388-416.

20. D'Agostino RB Jr (1998) Propensity score methods for bias reduction in the comparison of a treatment to a non-randomized control group. Stat Med 17: 2265-2281.

21. Rubin DB (1997) Estimating causal effects from large data sets using propensity scores. Ann Intern Med 127: 757-763.

22. Hosmer DW and Lemeshow S (2000) Applied Logistic Regression (2nd ed), Hohn Wiley & Sons, Inc., New York.

23. Hosmer DW and Lemeshow S (1999) Applied Survival Analysis: Regression Modeling of Time to Event Data. John Wiley & Sons Inc, New York.

24. Katz LS, Bolen CR, Harcourt BH, Schmink S, Wang X, et al. (2009) Meningococcus genome informatics platform: a system for analyzing multilocus sequence typing data. Nucleic Acids Res 37: W606-611.

25. Rybak MJ, Lomaestro BM, Rotschafer JC, Moellering RC, Craig WA, et al. (2009) Vancomycin Therapeutic Guidelines: A Summary of Consensus Recommendations from the Infectious Diseases Society of America, the American Society of Health-System Pharmacists, and the Society of Infectious Diseases Pharmacists. Clin Infect Dis 49: 325-327.

26. Puzniak LA, Morrow LE, Huang DB, Barreto JN (2013) Impact of weight on treatment efficacy and safety in complicated skin and skin structure infections and nosocomial pneumonia caused by methicillin-resistant Staphylococcus aureus. Clin Ther 35: 1557-1570.

27. Caffrey AR, Morrill HJ, Puzniak LA, Laplante KL (2014) Comparative effectiveness of linezolid and vancomycin among a national veterans affairs cohort with methicillin-resistant Staphylococcus aureus pneumonia. Pharmacotherapy 34: 473-480.

28. Caffrey AR, Quilliam BJ, LaPlante KL (2010) Comparative effectiveness of linezolid and vancomycin among a national cohort of patients infected with methicillin-resistant Staphylococcus aureus. Antimicrob Agents Chemother 54: 4394-4344.

29. Kalil AC, Murthy MH, Hermsen ED, Neto FK, Sun J, et al. (2010) Linezolid versus vancomycin or teicoplanin for nosocomial pneumonia: a systematic review and meta-analysis. Crit Care Med 38: 1802-1808.

30. Walkey AJ, O'Donnell MR, Wiener RS (2011) Linezolid vs glycopeptide antibiotics for the treatment of suspected methicillin-resistant Staphylococcus aureus nosocomial pneumonia: a meta-analysis of randomized controlled trials. Chest 139: 1148-1155.

31. Wunderink RG, Rello J, Cammarata SK, Croos-Dabrera RV, Kollef MH (2003) Linezolid vs vancomycin: analysis of two double-blind studies of patients with methicillin-resistant Staphylococcus aureus nosocomial pneumonia. Chest 124: 1789-1797.

32. Lahey T (2012) Questionable superiority of linezolid for methicillin-resistant Staphylococcus aureus nosocomial pneumonia: watch where you step. Clin Infect Dis 55: 159-160.

33. Torres A (2012) Antibiotic treatment against methicillin-resistant Staphylococcus aureus hospital- and ventilator-acquired pneumonia: a step forward but the battle continues. Clin Infect Dis 54: 630-632.

34. Wolff M, Mourvillier B (2012) Linezolid for the treatment of nosocomial pneumonia due to methicillin-resistant Staphylococcus aureus. Clin Infect Dis 55: 160-161.

35. van Hal SJ, Lodise TP, Paterson DL (2012) The clinical significance of vancomycin minimum inhibitory concentration in Staphylococcus aureus infections: a systematic review and meta-analysis. Clin Infect Dis 54: 755-771.

36. Lodise TP, Graves J, Evans A, Graffunder E, Helmecke M, et al. (2008) Relationship between vancomycin MIC and failure among patients with methicillin-resistant Staphylococcus aureus bacteremia treated with vancomycin. Antimicrob Agents Chemother 52: 3315-3320.

37. Haque NZ, Zuniga LC, Peyrani P, Reyes K, Lamerato L, et al. (2010) Relationship of vancomycin minimum inhibitory concentration to mortality in patients with methicillin-resistant Staphylococcus aureus hospital-acquired, ventilator-associated, or health-care-associated pneumonia. Chest 138: 1356-1362.

38. Kalil AC, Van Schooneveld TC1, Fey PD2, Rupp ME1 (2014) Association between vancomycin minimum inhibitory concentration and mortality among patients with Staphylococcus aureus bloodstream infections: a systematic review and meta-analysis. JAMA 312: 1552-1564.

39. Leong JV, Boro MS, Winter M (2011) Determining vancomycin clearance in an overweight and obese population. Am J Health Syst Pharm 68: 599-603.

40. Kullar R, Davis SL, Levine DP, Rybak MJ (2011) Impact of vancomycin exposure on outcomes in patients with methicillin-resistant Staphylococcus aureus bacteremia: support for consensus guidelines suggested targets. Clin Infect Dis 52: 975-981.

41. Johnson ML, Crown W, Martin BC, Dormuth CR, Siebert U (2009) Good research practices for comparative effectiveness research: analytic methods to improve causal inference from nonrandomized studies of treatment effects using secondary data sources: the ISPOR Good Research Practices for Retrospective Database Analysis Task Force Report--Part III. Value Health 12: 1062-1073.

42. Flanagan PG, Findlay GP, Magee JT, Ionescu A, Barnes RA, et al. (2000) The diagnosis of ventilator-associated pneumonia using non-bronchoscopic, non-directed lung lavages. Intensive Care Med 26: 20-30.

43. Brown SH, Lincoln MJ, Groen PJ, Kolodner RM (2003) VistA--U.S. Department of Veterans Affairs national-scale HIS. Int J Med Inform 69: 135-156.

25

The Potential Effect of L-arginine on Mice Placenta

Mohanad A Al-Bayati[1]*, Marawan A Ahmad[1] and Wael Khamas[2]

[1]University of Baghdad, Collage of Veterinary Medicine, Department of Physiology and Pharmacology, Iraq
[2]Western University of Health Science, College of Veterinary Medicine, Pomona, CA, USA

Summary

L-arginine-nitric oxide pathway has emerged as novel regulators of several vital roles in the reproductive function which comprise pregnancy events, such as placental development. This study was done to pharmacologically enhance the performance of female reproductive system by using L-arginine powder as forerunner of nitric oxide. The study protocol consists of total number of 96 pregnant mice divided equally into two main groups (48 animals per group) and handled as follows: 1st Control group given normal saline orally daily and 2nd L-arginine dosed group 200 mg/kg BW 20% orally daily, both groups were randomly divided into four subgroup according to dosed period of pregnancy term, the dosed periods were 1-15 days, 7-15 days, 7-21 days and 15-21 days.

Several parameters were evaluated and displayed the following results: L-arginine concentration in uterine tissue was elevated in association with increased body, uterine, placenta and fetus weights. That presumably was controlled by an increase food and water intakes. Hormonal levels (estrogen and progesterone) mainly at 7-21 days and 15-21 days of gestation dosed periods. Those results showed histological and stereological profile which illustrated the activity and enlargement of placental layers acquaintance with increasing blood vessels (angiogenesis and vasodilation) and vascular density (%) especially in 7-21 and 15-21 of dosed gestation periods led to an increase placental volume and geometric parameters (cm), weight (gm) and proportional thickness (cm), vascular density, and blood vessels. Fetal traits parameters, displayed significant statistical values of fetuses and weights in all gestation periods expressed at 15-21 days as the best results. Also, increases other parameters: blood volume, steriometry values, histological assessments and alkaline phosphatase and lactogens values. The endpoints of this study presented the L-arginine donated NO which was capable of increasing remodeling blood supply and improvement of some reproductive phenotypic properties of animal models and significant number of fetuses viability.

Introduction

L-arginine was an essential amino acid found in proteins of the animal body and different sources of foods. L-arginine derived nitric oxide converted by catalyzed enzymes nitric oxide synthase. L-arginine had emerged as an important intracellular and intercellular messenger (Nitric oxide-cGMP) controlling many physiological processes [1].

L-arginine and derived nitric oxide plays important roles in numerous biochemical reactions in the body including ammonia detoxification by formation of urea, hormonal stimulation such as pituitary stimulus lead to release of growth hormone and pancreatic release of glucagon and insulin [2] and immune modulation in which it improved the immune status [3] in those suffering from sepsis, burn and trauma [4]. L-arginine donated nitric oxide was indisputable that such a polyvalent molecule could play a decisive role in the male and female reproductive system. Nitric oxide was first recognized in the reproductive system by [5]. Presently the L-arginine play an important role in male fertility which were provoke penile erectile [6-8], enhancement sperm motility [7,9,10] and also play positive position in sexual hormone regulation and ovarian function such as ovulation [11,12] . The role of NO in the uterus was suppression of myometrial contractility during pregnancy [13-17] in other explored extension held and fixed the facts participation of sexual and neuronal behaviors in reproductive fitness in L-arginine dosed mice [18].

Few ideas in the literature revealed the effect of L-arginine on placental efficiency and angiogenic process and therefore would lead to the placental growth and fetal development [6,19]. Therefore, if L-arginine was a potent vasodilator that gives a speculation lead to increase the weight of the fetus by placental competence and fitness [6,20]. So L-arginine-NO was upset the perinatal mortality and superior numbers of live fetuses [6,13,21].

According to philosophies and speculation of literatures and thesis that donation the positive appearance on functional placenta functions and the fetus's fitness, which rendering this study and aimed to evaluation of functional morphometric and stereology profile alteration in mouse placenta subjected to and explored the best time of maximal beneficial effect.

Material and Methods

Animals

This experiment was carried out at the department of physiology, College of Veterinary Medicine, University of Baghdad. Healthy adult female mice were obtained from the animal house of the pharmacology censorship center, ministry of health, Baghdad-Iraq.

Virgin female mice (8-10 weeks) with weight range of 30-35 gram were used in this study. Induction of pregnancy after 2 weeks of acclimatization mated for 48 hours female to male ratio (2:1) then separated and examined to detect pregnancy by observing vaginal mucus seal and/or vaginal smear to ensure of positive mating. These

*Corresponding author: Mohanad A Al-Bayati, University of Baghdad, Collage of Veterinary Medicine, Department of Physiology and Pharmacology, Iraq,
E-mail: aumnmumu@yahoo.com

animals were kept under 20-25°C in an air-conditioned room and light/dark cycle of 12 hours daily.

Study protocol

Ninety six female mice were randomly divided into two main equal groups held as follows; Control and L-arginine treated group. Each group was divided into 4 subgroups according to L-arginine administration: 7-2 days; 7-15; 7-21 and 15-21 days of pregnancy.

The pregnant mice of the control subgroups were given normal saline orally 0.1 ml/10 g by modified stomach tube and sacrificed at the end of the dosed period. The L-arginine dosed subgroups were orally administrated at dose of 200 mg/kg BW/per day, the amount of dosed L-arginine was adjusted individually according to the body weight. Treated mice were sacrificed at the end of the experiment. Pregnant mice in each group were anesthetized using diethyl ether before being sacrificed the placentas were dissected and excised; fetuses were carried out and taken to record their parameters and blood samples were collected for analysis by direct cardiac puncture.

Experimental parameters: The reflection of loading dose of L-arginine on placental function and their shading of fet uses development, the parameter derived to assess placental changes are described.

Fetal and placental weights and geometric values: After sacrificed the pregnant mice the excised uterus was transferred to watch glass and dissected carefully to extract the fetuses and placentas by incising the uterine horn and then weighing the fetuses and placentas using electrical scale, the morphometric analysis of changes in placentas as well as geometrical distances were recorded using a vernier scale.

Umbilical cord length: The umbilical cord was dissected from the maternal tissue and placental and fetal parts were measured using a vernier scale.

Placental thickness, area and volume: The thickness of placenta was measured of the pregnant mice and the placenta was extracted.

After measuring the major and minor diameters to obtain the mean diameter, the surface area of the placenta was calculated (Placental surface area=PM 2/4), and the volume of the placenta (Volume=p/6M³), P: perimeter, M: mean diameter, finally, the ratio between both was calculated (Ratio=3/2M).

Blood collection for hormonal assays: Blood samples were obtained by cardiac puncture from each anesthetized animal by using disposable insulin syringes. Samples were centrifuged at 2500 rpm for 15 minutes and serum samples were stored in a freezer at -18 C° until use.

Placentas tissue histology

Sample collection for stereological assessment: The entire placentas were gently removed and cleaned from adherent attachment after severing the umbilical cords and expulsion the fetuses from it. They were placed in normal saline solution then fixed in Bouin's fluid. Tissues, after 20 hr. fixation were embedded in paraffin wax, serial sections (5 μm thick) mounted on glass slides and were stained with Heamatoxylin and Eosin [22]. Every five sections were examined to obtain an overall picture of the changes, if any.

Placental tissue stereometrical assessment: The nuclei of the giant cells from the placentas were assessed stereometrically by oculometer scale. The sections were examined with a light microscope attached

with fitted camera. Fifty nuclei per animal were measured [23].

o **Relative volume of the placental giant cells:** To assess the placental giant cells on a percent basis we used the technique of Chalkley [24] formula: Vv=(Pn+Pct)/Pt, Where Pn are the points counted in the nucleus of the structure, Pct are the points counted in the cytoplasm and Pt is the total points.

o **Absolute volume of the placental giant cells:** Absolute volume was calculated by the following formula: V=Vv. W/ Wv, Where Vv is the relative volume, W is the weight of the placenta, and Wv is the specific total mean weight per volume of the placental tissue.

o **Relative nuclear volume:** Relative nuclear volume was calculated by the following formula: Vvn=Pn/(Pn + Pct) . [2M/(2M+3t)], Where Pn and Pct are number of points falling on the cell nucleus and cytoplasm, respectively, M is the mean nuclear diameter, and t is the thickness of the histological section.

o **Relative cytoplasm volume:** Relative cytoplasm volume was calculated by the following formula: Vvcyt=1–Vvn, Where Vvn is the relative nuclear volume

o **Nucleus/cytoplasm ratio:** The nucleus/cytoplasm ratio was calculated by the following formula: N/C=Vvn/Vvcyt

o **Nucleus, Cytoplasm and mean giant cell volume:** The above parameters were calculated by the following formula: Vct=Vvn/N/C and Vcell=Vn + Vct, Where Vn is the nuclear volume and Vct is the cytoplasm volume.

o **Numerical density of giant cells:** The numerical density of giant cells was calculated by the following formula: Nv=(Vv/Vcell).

o **Number of giant cells per placenta:** The number of giant cells per placenta was calculated by following formula: Np=(Nv. W/v)

Body weight and uterine weight: The pregnant mice weight were daily recorded using sensitive scale starting first day till the last day of the treatment The uterus of each animal was isolated at the end of the experiment and weight was recorded.

Prolactin assay

Placental tissue preparation: The procedure for dissecting the placenta and its separation into junctional and labyrinth zones was similar to that previously described for the mouse with the aid of a dissecting microscope; 10-20 X magnification. The tissues were collected and washed with Hank's balanced salt solution without Ca^{2+} and Mg^{2+}.

The tissues were immediately frozen on solid CO_2 and stored frozen at 25°C until further processing for placental lactogen and alkaline phosphatase assays. The tissues were homogenized in a Brinkman polytron tissue homogenizer for 60 sec at a setting of 6-5 in a Tris-saline buffer (l0 mM-Tris, 150 mM-NaCl, 1 mM-phenylmethylsulphonyl fluoride, pH 8.2). Aliquants of the homogenates were precipitated with perchloric acid, centrifuged at 4000 g. Supernatants from the centrifugation were used for assessment of placental lactogen and alkaline phosphatase activities.

Placental Lactogen assays and measurement: Placental lactogen was measured with a modification of the procedure described by

Shiuetai. Briefly, the prolactin receptor source was mammary gland membranes isolated from the lactating rabbit. Ovine prolactin (NIAMDD-OPRL-15) was used for radio-iodination and as a reference standard for the radio receptor assay. Radio iodination was accomplished with the solid-phase reagent 'Iodo-Gen' as described by Markwell and Fox. The radio iodinated hormone was purified by gel filtration on Sephadex G-100. The specific activity of the radio-iodinated ovine prolactin ranged from 55 to 95 pCi^g. The buffer for the radioreceptor assay was 25 mM-Tris-HCl, pH 7.6, containing 10 mM-CaCl$_2$ and 0.5% bovine serum albumin. The remainder of the procedure was similar to the method developed by Shiuetai. The sensitivity of the assay ranged from 0.1 to 0.2 ng/tube and within- and between assay coefficients of variation were 7% and 11%, respectively.

Alkaline phosphatase assay

Alkaline phosphatase activity was determined as previously described by Lowry. The procedure measures the cleavage of P-nitrophenyl phosphate to P-nitrophenol in a 1 M-2-amino-2-methyl-l propanol buffers at pH 10.3. Aliquants of the placental homogenates were appropriately diluted with phosphate-buffered saline. 50-µl sample was added to tubes placed in an ice bath, followed by the addition of 200 µ 8 mM-disodium p-nitrophenyl phosphate, 1 M-2-amino-2-methyl-l-propanol, pH 10.3. The reaction vessels were then incubated for 30 min at 37°C. The reaction was stopped by placing the tubes in an ice bath and adding 750 µ 0.25 N-NaOH. Samples were then read by spectrophotometry at 410 nm. A standard curve of P-nitrophenol from 1 to 50 nmol was generated. Results were expressed in nanomoles of P-nitrophenol released per mg protein per min or per placenta per min. The within- and between-assay coefficients of variations were 5% and 10%, respectively.

Results and Discussion

The effect of L-arginine on placental weight

The L-arginine treatment caused significant (P<0.05) increase of placental weight of treated groups in periods 1-15, 7-15, 15-21 and 7-21 days of pregnancy as compared with the control groups (Table 1). Also, the 15-21 days of treatment was significantly higher (P<0.05) than other periods of the treatment groups. Furthermore, the high value of placental weight in L-arginine treated group might be due to increase of the umbilical blood flow velocity and decreased the umbilical cord length by the role of L-arginine-NO system induced to the vasodilation this might coincides with our results that showed in Table 8 due to nitric oxide of maternal circulation and that might be cross the nitric oxide to the placenta and dilate the placental villous vasculature with increased number of villous vessels [25], dilating lumens and thinner muscular appearance of vessel walls [26]. Also this result was agreement with Myatt et al. [27] they attributed the dilatation of placental villous

Gestation periods[3] (days)	L-arginine treated groups		Control groups[2]	
1-15	0.109 ± 0.015	Aa	0.103 ± 0.040	Aa
7-15	0.117 ± 0.020	Aa	0.104 ± 0.022	Ab
7-21	0.133 ± 0.011	Ba	0.116 ± 0.028	Ab
15-21	0.187 ± 0.029	Ba	0.141 ± 0.031	Bb

[1]L-arginine 200 mg/Kg BW, daily, orally, 2%; [2]Control normal saline treatment; [3]Gestation periods; Time of loading daily dose of drugs (L-arginine and normal saline); [4]N 12 pregnant mice; Capital letters denoted significant (p<0.05) differences among gestations periods; Small letters denoted significant (p<0.05) differences among L-arginine and control groups

Table 1: Effect of L-arginine[1] loading dose on means placental weights g at in different gestation periods of pregnant mice[4].

Gestation periods[3] (days)	L-arginine treated groups		Control groups[2]	
1-15	1.25 ± 0.601	Aa	0.93 ± 0.111	Ab
7-15	1.01 ± 0.144	Ba	0.86 ± 0.048	Ab
7-21	0.94 ± 0.085	Ba	0.20 ± 0.012	Bb
15-21	0.53 ± 0.079	Ca	0.11 ± 0.010	Bb

[1]L-arginine 200 mg/Kg BW, daily, orally, 2%; [2]Control normal saline treatment; [3]Gestation periods; Time of loading daily dose of drugs (L-arginine and normal saline); [4]N 12 pregnant mice; Capital letters denoted significant (p<0.05) differences among gestations periods; Small letters denoted significant (p<0.05) differences among L-arginine and control groups

Table 2: Effect of L-arginine[1] loading dose on means umbilical cord length cm at different gestation periods of pregnant mice[4].

Gestation periods[3] days	L-arginine treated groups		Control groups[2]	
1-15	0.23 ± 0.034	Aa	0.14 ± 0.028	Ab
7-15	0.20 ± 0.064	Aa	0.12 ± 0.041	Ab
7-21	0.11 ± 0.005	Ba	0.08 ± 0.073	Bb
15-21	0.09 ± 0.011	Ba	0.06 ± 0.055	Bb

[1]L-arginine 200 mg/Kg BW, daily, orally, 2%; [2]Control normal saline treatment; [3]Gestation periods; Time of loading daily dose of drugs (L-arginine and normal saline); [4]N 12 pregnant mice; Capital letters denoted significant (p<0.05) differences among gestations periods; Small letters denoted significant (p<0.05) differences among L-arginine and control groups

Table 3: Effect of L-arginine[1] loading dose on means thickness of placenta cm at different gestation periods of pregnant mice[4].

Gestation period[3] (days)	L-arginine treated groups		Control groups[2]	
1-15	0.31 ± 0.007	Aa	0.24 ± 0.049	Ab
7-15	0.40 ± 0.001	Ba	0.31 ± 0.019	Bb
7-21	1.02 ± 0.266	Ca	0.41 ± 0.053	Cb
15-21	1.31 ± 0.113	Da	0.64 ± 0.012	Db

[1]L-arginine 200 mg/Kg BW, daily, orally, 2%; [2]Control normal saline treatment; [3]Gestation periods; Time of loading daily dose of drugs (L-arginine and normal saline); [4]N 12 pregnant mice; Capital etiters denoted significant (p<0.05) differences among gestations periods; Small etiters denoted significant (p<0.05) differences among L-arginine and control groups

Table 4: Effect of L-arginine[1] loading dose on means fetal weight gm at different gestation periods of pregnant mice[4].

vasculature due to the nitric oxide found in the endothelium of the umbilical, chorionic plate and stem villous vessels appears to contribute the maintenance of basal vascular tone and to attenuate the action of vasoconstrictors such as endothelin (ET-1) and thromboxane [28].

The placental weight increase may be attributed to the high level of L-arginine during gestation period 7-21 as compared with other treated groups and also with control groups suggested these changes might be due to enhanced placental angiogenesis through their donation of L-arginine and growth during this period, thereby promoting an optimal intrauterine environment throughout pregnancy [29]. The dramatically increase placental blood flow and blood volume (Tables 2, 5 and 6) increased the nutrients that transfer from maternal to the placental blood and then enter to the fetus. Subsequently increased the placental and fetal weight [30]. That explains the superior results of L-arginine at period 15-21 days as compared with control group in period.

Others attributed superior placental weight at gestation period 7-21 and 15-21 day due to enlarged placental volume at same period gestation time (Table 6) that through maximized placental transport capacity in late periods of gestation. That occurs presumably under provocation effect of L-arginine nitric oxide by encouragement to rise

Gestation periods[3] (days)	Control groups[2]	L-arginine treated groups
1-15	0.102 ± 0.028 Aa	0.184 ± 0.008 Ab
7-15	0.164 ± 0.011 Ba	0.193 ± 0.010 Bb
7-21	0.169 ± 0.025 BCa	0.222 ± 0.022 Cb
15-21	0.138 ± 0.016 Ca	0.179 ± 0.010 Db

[1]L-arginine 200 mg/Kg BW, daily, orally, 2%; [2]Control normal saline treatment; [3]Gestation periods; Time of loading daily dose of drugs (L-arginine and normal saline); [4]N 12 pregnant mice; Capital letters denoted significant (p<0.05) differences among gestations periods; Small letters denoted significant (p<0.05) differences among L-arginine and control groups

Table 5: Effect of L-arginine[1] loading dose on blood volume gm at different gestation periods of pregnant mice[4].

Gestation periods[3] (days)	L-arginine treated groups	Control groups[2]
1-15	0.71 ± 0.059 Aa	0.32 ± 0.061 Ba
7-15	1.23 ± 0.206 Ab	0.37 ± 0.010 Ba
7-21	1.5 2 ± 0.175 Ac	0.90 ± 0.043 Bb
15-21	1.58 ± 0.222 Ac	0.96 ± 0.197 Bb

[1]L-arginine 200 mg/Kg BW, daily, orally, 2%; [2]Control normal saline treatment; [3]Gestation periods; Time of loading daily dose of drugs (L-arginine and normal saline); [4]N 12 pregnant mice; Capital letters denoted significant (p<0.05) differences among gestations periods; Small letters denoted significant (p<0.05) differences among L-arginine and control groups

Table 6: Effect of L-arginine[1] loading dose on placental volume cm at different gestation periods of pregnant mice[4].

Gestation Periods[3] days	L-arginine treated groups	Control groups[2]
1-15	0.59 ± 0.044 Aa	0.20 ± 0.005 Ab
7-15	1.32 ± 0.201 Ba	0.33 ± 0.039 Bb
7-21	1.90 ± 0.115 Ca	0.40 ± 0.079 CBb
15-21	2.17 ± 0.265 Da	0.67 ± 0.022 Db

[1]L-arginine 200 mg/Kg BW, daily, orally, 2%; [2]Control normal saline treatment; [3]Gestation periods; Time of loading daily dose of drugs (L-arginine and normal saline); [4]N 12 pregnant mice; Capital etiters denoted significant (p<0.05) differences among gestations periods; Small letters denoted significant (p<0.05) differences among L-arginine and control groups

Table 7: Effect of L-arginine[1] loading dose on placental surface area cm at different gestation periods of pregnant mice[4].

of extraction rate for both oxygen and substances per unit of uterine blood or umbilical blood from the arterio-venous concentration difference [30].

De Boo et al. [31], Reynolds et al. [32] Faber and Thornburg [33] and Meschia [34] reported results that L-arginine derived NO into animal during 7-21 days and 15-21 days periods of gestation increased protein accretion, this presumably led to increase the placental weight and also fetal weight.

Furthermore, L-arginine-NO pathway transport against the concentration gradient (active transport), in which they activate carrier proteins in microvilli of the placental membrane led to partially factor promoted increasing placental weight, That speculated by Logic et al. [35] for amino acids turnovers and exogenous transport.

So, the placental weight showed at the gestation periods 1-15 and 7-15 appeared lesser than other L-arginine treated groups due to placental thickness at this periods was greater and lesser its permeability to cross high amounts of nutrients and oxygen and also level of L-arginine less than other periods which coincides with our results that showed in Table 3. But in gestation periods 7-21 and 15-21 the placental weight increased more than other L-arginine treated groups and control groups attributed to the natural diminution of

placental thickness due to high level and important role of L-arginine-NO pathway in inducing vasodilatation led to augmentation of permeability with greater placental diffusion thus increased the nutrients and oxygen that cross into the placenta which were coincides with our results that showed in periods 7-21 days and 15-21 days of gestation, therefore led to increased placental weight [36-39].

The effect of L-arginine on fetal weight

The L-arginine treatment caused significant increase (P<0.05) of fetal weight of treated groups from period 1-15, 7-15, 7-21 and 15-21 days of pregnancy as compared with the control groups Table 4. Also the period of treatment 15-21 days is significant (P<0.05) increased as compared with other treatment periods.

The fetal weight increase presumably due to contribution of nitric oxide in placental vasculature [26], its important regulator of placental perfusion, Therefore enhanced fetal growth, this led to improve the fetal-maternal circulation by vasodilation, subsequently increased the volume and deceased viscosity of the blood in fetal-maternal circulation [40].

Furthermore, Lampariello et al. [41] attributed the fetal growth and increased birth weight of newborns might be due to the nitric oxide improve the utero-placental blood flow and thereby increase oxygen delivery to the fetus, also its effect on the pregnancy and neonatal by indirect influencing the utero-placental circulation. Thureen et al. [42] recorded the L-arginine had influenced mechanism of hyper synthesis and release of insulin from B cells aggregated pancreatic island that directed our attitude to direct attribution rise of fetal weight might be play the L-arginine essential role in the acceleration of fetal growth by stimulation of insulin secretion utilized circulating glucose.

In otherwise, administration of L-arginine increased the number of born alive or live litter birth weight in pregnant animal during the periods 7-15 days and 7-21 days of gestation, as reported previously [42], an increased in plasma concentrations of L-arginine likely resulted in enhancement of placental transport from mother to fetus. This would provide adequate amounts of L-arginine from the pregnant animal to their fetuses, thereby supporting their optimal metabolism and growth during the periods 7-15 days and 7-21 days of gestation of most rapid fetal growth as compared with other period in same group and also with control group. Indeed, results of a recent study showed that L-arginine infusion into animal during 7-21 days and 15-21 days periods of gestation increased protein accretion in fetus [31], therefore, increased the fetal weight.

Roberto et al. [43] and Salvemini et al. [44] attributed the decreased in the results of fetal weight in the early period (1-15) of gestation due to reduce corpus luteum (CL) number due to the nitric oxide caused upset of CL through exaggeration of the biochemical event derived prostaglandin F2α (PGF2α) synthesis by up regulating expression of cyclooxygenase enzyme that key enzyme for (PGF2α) synthesis which considered a luteolytic agent, therefore reduce CL number and thereby resulting impairs the progesterone production, also this lack of progesterone production reduce the availability of amino acids, subsequently reduce protein synthesis which important for fetal growth, also CL was the main source for progesterone required for establishment and maintenance of pregnancy and increased the fetal weight [45].

Furthermore, the administration of L-arginine and in control group but the L-arginine more pronounce accelerated fetal weight reception gain through certain 7-15 days and15-21 days periods of gestation, which coincides with the period of rapid fetal growth [46], thereby increased the weight in this periods. Previous reports had shown that uterine capacity starts to become limiting for embryonic survival at as early 1-15 days period of gestation, thereby affecting fetal growth [47] and leading to losses of viable fetuses. This was in agreement with the finding of this study that almost all born dead were fully formed. Administration of L-arginine reduced the number of dead born, probably due to an improved uterine environment capacity for fetal growth and development [48].

The effect of L-arginine on blood volume

The blood volume displayed significant increase in blood volume at all periods of gestation in L-arginine dosed groups as compared with control groups whereas the superior values occur in 15-21day of gestation in L-arginine dosed group showed in Table 5.

Dong and Yallamplalli [49] attributed increased blood volume might be induced vasodilation that regulates by intrinsic ability of L-arginine-nitric oxide system to regulate cytosolic [Ca++], that L-arginine-NO system activity indicated an upset in cytosolic [Ca++] enable reduction of contraction cellular events associated with restricted of their tonicity partially, the placental vasculature expressed NOS [50] that had been presence in stem villious of placenta modulated NO production and enhanced activity NO synthase by L-arginine substrate or under systematic loading L-arginine which led to play a local role in controlling of placental blood volume [51].

That demonstrated the sequel of NO vasodilator effect provoked blood outflow then blood flow by relaxation of the blood vessels wall [52]. In addition to previous studies which were in agreement with our results indicated that progesterone [6] might be regulates the c.GMP effectors system for relaxation of blood vessels, and then led to increase blood demand through enlarging the blood vessel capacity then blood volume [53].

Furthermore, attributed increase blood volume might be due to increase estrogen during early pregnancy that initiated a receptor-mediated event that activated NOS and probably (nNOS) [6,54] to produce NO this NO increased and persist smooth muscle cyclic guanosine monophosphate (c.GMP) which activated a c.GMP-dependent kinase that encouraged velocity of Ca++ activated K+ channel activity and decreased Ca++ inflow by voltage gated Ca++ channel, resulting in vasodilation and quiescence during pregnancy [50]. Thus, an increase of NO availability might be included as one of the mechanisms through which estrogen reduces arterial wall thickness and increases vessel distention ability.

The loading of L-arginine capable of elevating the NO levels in CNS and reproductive organs; placenta, that NO had triggered, regulator and demined of gonadotrophin releasing hormone (GnRH) that involvement the stimulation and regulation of Luteinizing hormone (LH) released production, these findings are supported by [55] and increased postpone CL-Progesterone functionally.

Furthermore, the anatomical localization of NO neurons in close proximity to GnRH neurons in hypothalamus these adjacent between neuron may be regulated physiologically and regulator manner of GnRH secretion that increase blood volume [56].

At the endpoint may give an impression to say increase blood content (volume) which produced raise in placental weight and volume, finally it is reflected to increase physiological demand of fetal growth and fetal vital processes.

The morphometric parameter of placenta

Placental volume and surface area: The L-arginine loading dose caused significant (P<0.05) increase of placental volume and surface area in treated groups at periods 1-15 days , 7-15 days, 7-21 days and 15-21days of pregnancy as compared with the control groups Tables 6 and 7. The group treatment at 15-2 days presented higher significant (P<0.05) of placental volume and surface area than other periods of L-arginine treated groups.

The increased of the placental volume which might be through the L-arginine-NO pathway enhance the intrauterine growth trophoblast cells and labyrinth zone volume due to excessive provocation and produced of NO in the placental stem villous that encouragement the micro blood vessels network vasodilation .

Furthermore, the placental volume and placental surface area increased might be due to the labyrinth zone encouragement in their density was considered principle site in hemotrophic exchange "nutrient, hormones, ions, waste and water" between maternal and fetal parts [57,58] associated directly with increase functionally placental fluids in their layers these give a true impression geometrically exaggerated in dimensional and out line, this results was coincided with histological appearance through hyperplasia and hypertrophy in placental zones with comparable with control showed increased patches and multiple area increased of giant cells.

In otherwise, the NO induced vasodilation that promote compensatory mechanism and utilized reserved blood volume to increase blood flow in the placental layers and also the NO play a key role in angiogenesis of placenta [19,29]. NO is a proangiogenic growth factors in the systemic circulation, rise NO production led to stimulate new vessels growth and thus increasing total vessel length and subsequently, augmentation of permeability with greater placental diffusion due to increased Labyrinth zone surface area and decreased inter-hemal membrane thickness with an increased diffusion capacity necessary for exponential growth of embryonic tissues thus increased the nutrients and oxygen that cross into the placenta [36-39] that led to increase in geometric and enlarged morphometric of placental volume and placental surface area.

Giles et al. [25] demonstrated and explained the relationship between placental enlargement and vasculogenic functional remodeling and histological convention as dramatic influenced by L-arginine-NO metabolic pathway and their sequel due to increase the number of villous vessels and dilated the placental villous vasculature led to the expansion of the fetal capillary volume continues until at least embryonic day 18.5, would need for continually greater volumes of fetal blood to exchange with the maternal circulation to obtain enough nutrient and oxygen for fetal growth then increased the blood flow in this vessels and subsequently increased the placental volume and surface area [26].

The placental volume and surface area results under L-arginine loading dose was coincided with Babaei et al. [59] suggestion could use for attribution the increased of placental volume might be due to L-arginine-NO pathway which had important role in vasculogenesis (formation of blood vessels from mesoderm precursor cells) and angiogenesis (creation of new vessels from a pre-existing blood supply) in the placental villi which led to develops the labyrinth layer that was critical for maternal-fetal exchange, subsequently increased the placental volume and surface area. Finally, the placental enlargement was positive directly proportional with increased fetal weight and increased survival of fetuses (viable fetus).

Histological assessment of placenta: In both control and L-arginine dosed groups the giant cells and placental volumes were positivly increased parallel in period 15-21 days of gestation but the L-arginine dosed group showed superior values than control group that attributed to normally cessation and attained in placental volume at 16 days in control group [60] (Table 6) whereas, placental volume in L-arginine loading doses 15-21 day of gestation increase may be due to:

First, increase maximized stereological volume of giant cells of labyrinth zone (Table 7).

Second, increase giant cell volume (%) that provoked their endocrine releasing factor or hormones [61]. These promotion effects and locally control of labyrinth and junctional zones caused differentiation of trophoblast glycogen cell which finally increased volume indirectly [61].

Third, L-arginine-NO system facilitated migration of trophoblast cell to the maternal deciduas layer to differentiation to trophblast glycogen and that supply a spare weight and volume of placenta maximized function activity and apparent morphometrical enlargement (Figure 1).

Furthermore, these suggestions were encouraged by stereological profile by increased geometrical value of nucleo-cytoplasmic volumes; relative nuclear volume %, relative cytoplasm volume (%), cytoplasm volume (mm³), nuclear volume (μm³) and mean cell volume (μm³)) and decrease nucleus/cytoplasm ratio due to hyper functional activity of storage form and synthesis of cytoplasm.

Finally, increased endocrine function and extended the main location of nutrients and gaseous area through increased labyrinth and junction zones in volume which were play a key role in maternal-fetal transference that underlies fetal growth and weights (Table 5).

Furthermore, surface area and thickness also correlated with capillary length and diameter and volume in the same period 15-21 due to increased capillary length and important factor merged with labyrinth inter-hemal membrane that coincided with the results. The blood volume increased under the facts of increases capillary density according to primary function of L-arginine-nitric oxide system.

The endpoint was improved placental development and reduce shortcomes occur in the cessation of development occur between 15-18 days of pregnancy [60] and undergo the preceded and succeeded by relatively quiescence periods primary that may be caused L-arginine

Parameters steriometry	Control groups[2]	L-arginine treated groups
Relative volume of giant cells (%)	1.66 ± 0.21 a	1.85 ± 0.13 b
Absolute volume of giant cells (mm³)	2.27 ± 0.39 a	3.06 ± 0.21 b
Relative nuclear volume (%)	15.49 ± 1.95 a	16.01±1.04 b
Relative cytoplasm volume (%)	84.51 ± 5.01 a	85.99 ± 3.28 b
Nucleus/cytoplasm ratio	0.1819 ± 0.0096 a	0.1462 ± 0.0065 b
Cytoplasm volume (mm³)	15037.59 ± 48.91 a	16333.71 ± 33.33 b
Nuclear volume (μm³)	3512.19 ± 26.43 a	3905.72 ± 14.60 b
Mean cell volume (μm³)	22306.47 ± 11.92 a	41397.51 ± 12.85 b
Numerical density (n/mm³)	0.000074± 0.0086 a	0.000044± 0.0055 b
Number of giant cells/placenta	0.000095± 0.0095 a	0.000066± 0.0072 b

[1]L-arginine 200 mg/Kg BW, daily, orally, 2%; [2]Control normal saline treatment; [3]Gestation periods; Time of loading daily dose of drugs (L-arginine and normal saline); [4]N 12 pregnant mice; Capital letters denoted significant (p<0.05) differences among gestations periods; Small letters denoted significant (p<0.05) differences among L-arginine and control groups

Table 8: Effect of L-arginine[1] loading dose on placental steriometry cm at gestation periods (15-21)[3] of pregnant mice[4].

remodeling the discounting changes in maternal blood pressure and hence blood flow. The volume of maternal blood that may be through flow the placenta in the 17 days of pregnancy were is maximized in L-arginine treated group faster than in control group in 15-17 day.

In 17 days of pregnancy this is suggesting that maternal blood space develop more in L-arginine dosed group and sufficient at this stage with satisfactory and necessary maternal blood flow through term. On the other hand, the placental-fetal capillary may be increased in L-arginine dosed group extensively in 18 day of pregnancy than control [48] and extend their function to determine their need as controversy in control suggesting a call for greater fetal blood to exchange with the maternal circulation in order prepare enough nutrient and gaseous agents for fetal growth, that's taking into account the fetal weight [48]. The L-arginine-nitric oxide behaves as an angiogenic factor which acts either elongation and /or branching capillary network. In Figure 2, the control group manifested that thin barrier minimized the diffusion distance and maximized the area of passive exchange L-arginine treated group had a wide barrier proportional with a large surface area in physiologically maximized the diffusion distance and minimized area of passive exchange which play selective barrier not chance passive exchange according the gradient [36,37], in the contrast to compensate reduction of diffusion capacity by increased vasodilation and angiogenic process to overlap the increased, thickness of placenta which is necessary for exponential growth of embryonic tissues which may be harmonic alteration between thickness and vasodilation in L-arginine treated group is a more critical determinant of diffusion capacity of placenta [36,37]. That is interesting finding which might be explained by the difference in growth pattern of the fetus and placenta.

Whereas in control group, the decreased in fetal and placental growth in other periods presumably due to the fact that the fetus is small and therefore as a little total volume and reduction capillary with suggesting the inter-hemal membrane and capillary volume is triggered first in this period but not fully working in the control group. In L-arginine treated group, the total capillary network developed showed in well rather than control and inter-hemal membrane remained thick in control group at first due to narrow capillary and volume this would perturb diffusion of substances to the fetus. That's highly density of enlarged fetal capillary in L-arginine treated group enlarged capillary volume for compensation of inter-hemal membrane thickness to accumulate more molecular weight selection agent processes for fetal growth demand which play a supersized roles and expected a

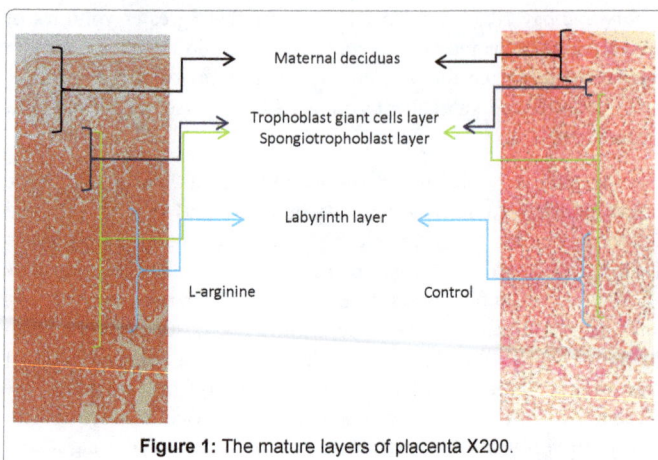

Figure 1: The mature layers of placenta X200.

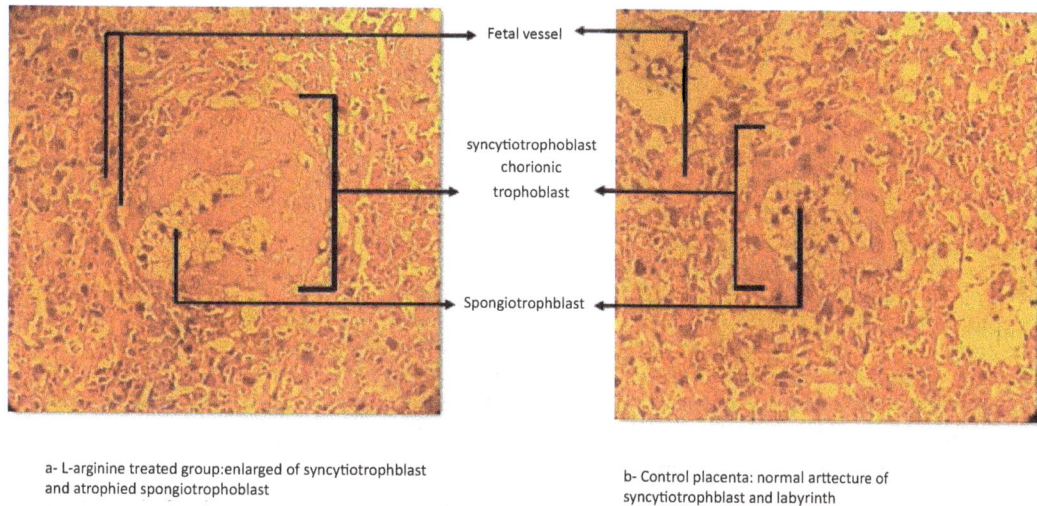

a- L-arginine treated group:enlarged of syncytiotrophblast and atrophied spongiotrophoblast

b- Control placenta: normal arttecture of syncytiotrophblast and labyrinth

Figure 2: Syncytiotrophoblast unit.

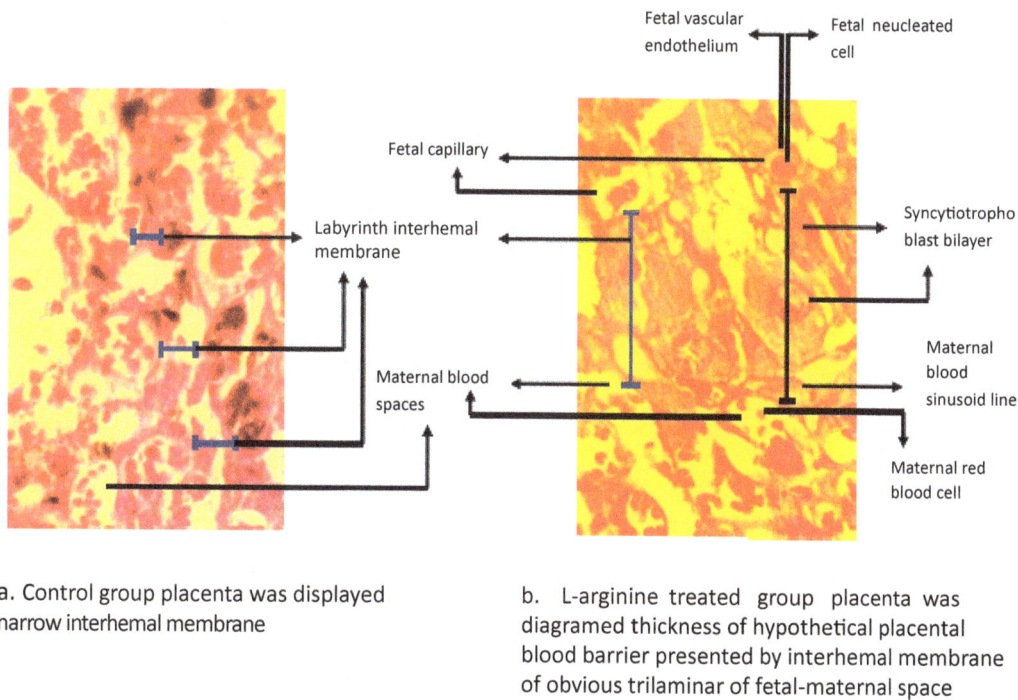

a. Control group placenta was displayed narrow interhemal membrane

b. L-arginine treated group placenta was diagramed thickness of hypothetical placental blood barrier presented by interhemal membrane of obvious trilaminar of fetal-maternal space

Figure 3: Cross-section of the maternal – fetal functional i X1025.

greater balance between placental supply and fetal requirements for exaggerated effect needed to fluctuation in local nutrition and reduced placental oxidative stress and prevent hypoxia-reoxygenatal type energy by direct chelating or indirect fating neutralization.

Placental Steriometry parameters: In a histological study of the placenta of mice treated with the L-arginine, cytometry of the giant trophoblastic cells showed that the placentas from the treated group was more positively changed, also in terms of cell volume. Thus, the relative volume, absolute volume, numerical density and total number of giant cells were significantly (P<0.05) superior in the placenta of this group than in control placenta showed in Table 8.

In rodents, giant cells differentiate by endo-reduplication and their functions are endocrine secretion and invasion of the maternal deciduas. These cells are a private source of placental lactogens I and II (PL-I and PL-II) and in the second trimester of pregnancy they likewise synthesize numerous prolactin-like proteins and a different of placental lactogen I (PL-IV) [62]. PL-I, PL-II and PL-IV also served on the fetus. Faria et al. [61] established the cellular derivation of placental lactogen I and the PL-I to PL-II transition at the end of the first half of pregnancy, with these cells starting to express PL-II thereafter.

The changes provoked by the L-arginine are trophoblastic cells and the difference in behavior observed among the cell populations of different placental regions may affect intra-uterine development, probably by efficient production of hormones such as placental lactogen, which acts to motivate a fetal development hormone.

Zybina and Zybina, [63] demonstrated that rat and mouse giant cells have 4c-8c ploidy on the 12th day of pregnancy, whereas on the 13th-14th day ploidy is 8c-16c this increase in ploidy may be important for trophoblast differentiation, allowing invasion of the deciduas. Therefore, L-arginine-NO may play a positive profile to increase ploidy presumably reach to 32-64 ploidy which promote secretory process and increase hormone like protein.

Keighren and West [64,65] did not observe higher order polyploidy in giant cells of the trophoblast of the mouse placenta suggesting that these may be polytene and not polyploidy cells. At a given stage of differentiation, giant cells divide into numerous nuclear fragments forming multinucleated cells that swiftly degenerate into nuclear fragments with 1 to 32c ploidy. Those seen in Figure 3 different multinucleated cells as same area of trophoblastic giant cell that may be L-arginine slowed degeneration of multinucleated cell by promoting anti free radical an ions and engorgement metabolic process to provoked cell long life. So L-arginine could act in promotion of cell cyclic in anaphase sensation telophase.

Furthermore, several areas occupancy were extended and differentiated large zoon of giant cells and given an impression darkely stained and hypertrophy to hyper functional activity for hormonal synthesis.

This result was coincided with hormonal level estimated and displayed higher levels of placental lactogens and alkaline phosphatase activity.

References

1. Moncada S, Palmer RM, Higgs EA (1991) Nitric oxide: physiology, pathophysiology, and pharmacology. Pharmacol Rev 43: 109-142.

2. McCann SM, Rettori V (1996) The role of nitric oxide in reproduction. Proc Soc Exp Biol Med 211: 7-15.

3. Lin PH, Johnson CK, Pullium JK, Bush RL, Conklin BS, et al. (2003) L-arginine improves endothelial vasoreactivity and reduces thrombogenicity after thrombolysis in experimental deep venous thrombosis. J Vasc Surg 38: 1396-1403.

4. Yallampalli C, Garfield RE, Byam-Smith M (1993) Nitric oxide inhibits uterine contractility during pregnancy but not during delivery. Endocrinology 133: 1899-1902.

5. Ignarro LJ, Bush PA, Buga GM, Wood KS, Fukuto JM, et al. (1990) Nitric oxide and cyclic GMP formation upon electrical field stimulation cause relaxation of corpus cavernosum smooth muscle. Biochem Biophys Res Commun 170: 843-850.

6. Bayaty MA, Tahan FJ, Hasan HF (2012) Influence of Protein Extract of Helianthus annuus L-seeds on blood volume of Reproductive organs in pregnant mice. JPCS 6: 02.

7. Al-Shaty ER (2007) Study The Effect of L.arginine Injection on Reproductive Efficiency of Local Iraqi Buck out of breeding season.

8. Anderson E, Wagner G (1995) Physiology of penile erection. Physiol Rev 75: 191-236.

9. Shaheed AS (2010) The Effect of Adding Different Concentrations of L.arginine on Poor Motility of Bull Semen in Vitro in Different Months. MSc Thesis, University of Baghdad, College of Veterinary Medicine. J Vet Med A Physiol Pathol Clin Med 4: 130-135.

10. Aydin S, Inci O, Alagöl B (1995) The role of arginine, indomethacin and kallikrein in the treatment of oligoasthenospermia. Int Urol Nephrol 27: 199-202.

11. Mahdi, Ferial Majed (2008) Some Reproductive Effect of Nitric oxide Precursor L-arginine and antagonist L.NAME in Female Mice. MSc. thesis Pharmacology and Toxicology, College of Veterinary Medicine, University of Baghdad.

12. Bonello N, McKie K, Jasper M, Andrew L, Ross N, et al. (1996) Inhibition of nitric oxide: effects on interleukin-1 beta-enhanced ovulation rate, steroid hormones, and ovarian leukocyte distribution at ovulation in the rat. Biol Reprod 54: 436-445.

13. Shakir IM (2009) The Effect of L.arginine on Uterine Muscle Contraction of Pregnant Mice. MSc Thesis, University of Baghdad, College of Veterinary Medicine.

14. Kuenzli KA, Bradley ME, Buxton IL (1996) Cyclic GMP-independent effects of nitric oxide on guinea-pig uterine contractility. Br J Pharmacol 119: 737-743.

15. Bradley KK, Buxton IL, Barber JE, McGaw T, Bradley ME (1998) Nitric oxide relaxes human myometrium by a cGMP-independent mechanism. Am J Physiol 275: C1668-1673.

16. Buxton IL, Kaiser RA, Malmquist NA, Tichenor S (2001) NO-induced relaxation of labouring and non-labouring human myometrium is not mediated by cyclic GMP. Br J Pharmacol 134: 206-214.

17. Radomski MW, Palmer RM, Moncada S (1990) An L-arginine/nitric oxide pathway present in human platelets regulates aggregation. Proc Natl Acad Sci U S A 87: 5193-5197.

18. Askar SJ (2012) The Neurobehavioral Effect of L.arginine and its Antagonist L.Name and Methylene Blue in mice. MSc Thesis, University of Baghdad, College of Veterinary Medicine.

19. Wu G, Bazer FW, Cudd TA, Meininger CJ, Spencer TE (2004) Maternal nutrition and fetal development. J Nutr 134: 2169-2172.

20. Vane JR, Botting RM (1991) Endothelium-derived vasoactive factors and the control of the circulation. Semin Perinatol 15: 4-10.

21. Greenberg SS, Lancaster JR, Xie J, Sarphie TG, Zhao X, et al. (1997) Effects of NO synthase inhibitors, arginine-deficient diet, and amiloride in pregnant rats. Am J Physiol 273: R1031-1045.

22. Bancroft J, Marilyn G (2008) Theory and Practice of histological techniques, 6th edition, Churchill Livingstone, Elsevier.

23. Sala MA, Komesu MC, Lopes RA, Maia Campos G (1994) Karyometric study of basal cell carcinoma. Braz Dent J 5: 11-14.

24. Chalkley HW (1943) method for the quantitative morphologic analysis of tissues. J Natl cancer Institute Bethesda 4: 47-53.

25. Giles WB, Trudinger BJ, Baird PJ (1985) Fetal umbilical artery flow velocity waveforms and placental resistance: pathological correlation. Br J Obstet Gynaecol 92: 31–38.

26. Giles W, O'Callaghan S, Boura A, Walters W (1992) Reduction in human fetal umbilical-placental vascular resistance by glyceryl trinitrate. Lancet 340: 856.

27. Myatt L, Brockman DE, Eis AL, Pollock JS (1993) Immunohistochemical localization of nitric oxide synthase in the human placenta. Placenta 14: 487-495.

28. Myatt L, Brewer AS, Langdon G, Brockman DE (1992) Attenuation of the vasoconstrictor effects of thromboxane and endothelin by nitric oxide in the human fetal-placental circulation. Am J Obstet Gynecol 166: 224-230.

29. Reynolds LP, Redmer DA (2001) Angiogenesis in the placenta. Biol Reprod 64: 1033-1040.

30. Myatt L, Brewer A, Brockman DE (1991) The action of nitric oxide in the perfused human fetal-placental circulation. Am J Obstet Gynecol 164: 687-692.

31. de Boo HA, van Zijl PL, Smith DE, Kulik W, Lafeber HN, et al. (2005) Arginine and mixed amino acids increase protein accretion in the growth-restricted and normal ovine fetus by different mechanisms. Pediatr Res 58: 270-277.

32. Reynolds LP, Ferrell CL, Robertson DA, Ford SP (1986) Metabolism of the gravid uterus, foetus and uteroplacenta at several stages of gestation in cows. J Agric Sci (Camb) 106: 437–444.

33. Faber JJ, Thornburg KL (1983) Placental Physiology. Structure and Function of Fetomaternal Exchange. Raven Press, New York.

34. Meschia G (1983) Circulation to female reproductive organs. In Handbook of Physiology, 2, 3: 241–269.

35. Logic H, Berk A, Zipursky SL, Matsudaira P, Baltimore D, et al. (2002) Transporte através das membrana. Biologia Celular e Molecular. 4 ed. Rio de Janeiro, Revinter, .578-585.

36. Guyton AC, Hall JE (2006) Tratado de fisiologia médica. 11 ed. Rio de Janeiro, Guanabara Koogan, 1264.

37. Rezende J (2005) Obstetrcia. 10 ed. Rio de Janeiro, Guanabara-Koogan1588.

38. Roby KF, Soares MJ (1993) Trophoblast cell differentiation and organization: role of fetal and ovarian signals. Placenta 14: 529-545.

39. Davies J, Glasser SR (1968) Histological and fine structural observations on the placenta of the rat. Acta Anat (Basel) 69: 542-608.

40. Neri I, Mazza V, Galassi MC, Volpe A, Facchinetti F (1996) Effects of L-arginine on utero-placental circulation in growth-retarded fetuses. Acta Obstet Gynecol Scand 75: 208-212.

41. Lampariello C, De Blasio A, Merenda A, Graziano E, Michalopoulou A, et al. (1997) [Use of arginine in intruterine growth retardation (IUGR). Authors' experience]. Minerva Ginecol 49: 577-581.

42. Thureen PJ, Baron KA, Fennessey PV, Hay WW Jr (2002) Ovine placental and fetal arginine metabolism at normal and increased maternal plasma arginine concentrations. Pediatr Res 51: 464-471.

43. Roberto da Costa RP, Costa AS, Korzekwa AJ, Platek R, Siemieniuch M, et al. (2008) Actions of a nitric oxide donor on prostaglandin production and angiogenic activity in the equine endometrium. Reprod Fertil Dev 20: 674-683.

44. Salvemini D, Misko TP, Masferrer JL, Seibert K, Currie MG, et al. (1993) Nitric oxide activates cyclooxygenase enzymes. Proc Natl Acad Sci U S A 90: 7240-7244.

45. Bazer FW, Spencer TE, Johnson GA, Burghardt RC, Wu G (2009) Comparative aspects of implantation. Reproduction 138: 195-209.

46. McPherson RL, Ji F, Wu G, Blanton JR Jr, Kim SW (2004) Growth and compositional changes of fetal tissues in pigs. J Anim Sci 82: 2534-2540.

47. Pope WF (1994) Embryonic mortality in swine. In: Geisert RD, editor. Embryonic mortality in domestic species. Boca Raton (FL): CRC; 53–78.

48. Wu G, Bazer FW, Wallace JM, Spencer TE (2006) Board-invited review: intrauterine growth retardation: implications for the animal sciences. J Anim Sci 84: 2316-2337.

49. Dong YL, Yallampalli C (2000) Pregnancy and exogenous steroid treatments modulate the expression of relaxant EP(2) and contractile FP receptors in the rat uterus. Biol Reprod 62: 533-539.

50. Magness RR, Shaw CE, Phernetton TM, Zheng J, Bird IM (1997) Endothelial vasodilator production by uterine and systemic arteries. II. Pregnancy effects on NO synthase expression. Am J Physiol 272: H1730-1740.

51. Telfer JF, Lyall F, Norman JE, Cameron IT (1995) Identification of nitric oxide synthase in human uterus. Hum Reprod 10: 19-23.

52. Albrecht EW, Stegeman CA, Heeringa P, Henning RH, van Goor H (2003) Protective role of endothelial nitric oxide synthase. J Pathol 199: 8-17.

53. Izumi H, Yallampalli C, Garfield RE (1993) Gestational changes in L-arginine-induced relaxation of pregnant rat and human myometrial smooth muscle. Am J Obstet Gynecol 169: 1327-1337.

54. Salhab WA, Shaul PW, Cox BE, Rosenfeld CR (2000) Regulation of types I and III NOS in ovine uterine arteries by daily and acute estrogen exposure. Am J Physiol Heart Circ Physiol 278: H2134-2142.

55. Bhat GK, Mahesh VB, Lamar CA, Ping L, Ping K, et al. (1995) Histochemical localization of nitric oxide neurons in the hypothalamus: association with gonadotropine releasing hormone neurons and co-localisation with N-methyl-D-aspartate receptors. Neuroendocrinology 62:187-197.

56. Zackrisson U, Brannstrom M, Granberg S, Janson PO, Collins WP, et al. (1998) Acute effects of a transdermal nitric oxide donor on perifollicular and intrauterine blood flow. Ultrasound Obstet Gynecol 12: 50-55.

57. Georgiades P, Ferguson-Smith AC, Burton GJ (2002) Comparative developmental anatomy of the murine and human definitive placentae. Placenta 23: 3-19.

58. Mayhew TM, Ohadike C, Baker PN, Crocker IP, Mitchell C, et al. (2003) Stereological investigation of placental morphology in pregnancies complicated by pre-eclampsia with and without intrauterine growth restriction. Placenta 24: 219-226.

59. Babaei S, Stewart DJ (2002) Overexpression of endothelial NO synthase induces angiogenesis in a co-culture model. Cardiovasc Res 55: 190-200.

60. Adamson SL, Lu Y, Whiteley KJ, Holmyard D, Hemberger M, et al. (2002) Interactions between trophoblast cells and the maternal and fetal circulation in the mouse placenta. Dev Biol 250: 358-373.

61. Faria TN, Ogren L, Talamantes F, Linzer DI, Soares MJ (1991) Localization of placental lactogen-I in trophoblast giant cells of the mouse placenta. Biol Reprod 44: 327-331.

62. Soares MJ, Chapman BM, Rasmussen CA, Dai G, Kamei T, et al. (1996) Differentiation of trophoblast endocrine cells. Placenta 17: 277-289.

63. Zybina EV, Zybina TG (1996) Polytene chromosomes in mammalian cells. Int Rev Cytol 165: 53-119.

64. Keighren M, West JD (1993) Analysis of cell ploidy in histological sections of mouse tissues by DNA-DNA in situ hybridization with digoxigenin-labelled probes. Histochem J 25: 30-44.

65. Luna LG (1968) Manual of histological staining methods of armed forces institute of Pathology. 4th ed. Lange Medical Printer. UK; 65-78.

26

The Role of Transporters in the Pharmacokinetics of Antibiotics

Hua WJ* and Hua WX

Department of Pharmacy, The First Affiliated Hospital of Nanchang University, Nanchang, China

Abstract

Aims: Various transporters including efflux transporters and uptake transporters play an important role in the pharmacokinetics of drugs. At present, interestingly, more and more studies had found that numbers of antibiotics were the substrates of transporters, and these antibiotics were usually combined with other drugs to treat disease more effectively in clinic. Therefore, it is necessary to focus on the role of transporters in pharmacokinetics and drug-drug interactions of antibiotics.

Methods: This review summarized the findings of recent studies as well as information obtained from several databases (update to June 2012): ISI Web of Knowledge SM (ISI WoK), SciFinder (Caplus, Medline, Registry, Casreact, Chrmlist, Chemcasts) and PubMed (indexed for Medline).

Results: The present review will provides useful information for studying the role of transporters in pharmacokinetics and drug-drug interactions of antibiotics, and should be of help to those intending to further research on these topics.

Conclusions: The drug transporter plays a significant role in the pharmacokinetics and drug-drug interactions of antibiotics.

Keywords: Antibiotics; CYP; Drug transporters

Introduction

Various drug transporters, including efflux transporters and uptake transporters, are widely expressed in body and play an important role in the absorption, distribution, excretion and metabolism of drugs [1]. At present, more and more drugs, including antibiotics, have been found as the substrates of transporters. Most of the antibiotics are eliminated by kidney and or biliary excretion, and this process mainly depends on renal or biliary tubular secretion through the function of transporters. Therefore, transporters play an important role in the pharmacokinetics of antibiotics.

Antibiotics are widely applied in infected patients of China and some other drugs may be combined with antibiotics to treat disease more effectively. Because transporters are involved in secretion and reabsorption of antibiotics, we should recognize which antibiotics were the substrate of transporter and considered that drug-drug interaction may be occurred between antibiotics and other drugs by inhibiting or inducing the same drug transporters .This paper makes a review on the roles of drug transporters in the pharmacokinetics of antibiotics.

OATPs/Oatps and antibiotics

OATPs/Oatps are expressed in a wide range of tissues in the body and are responsible for the Na+-independent uptake of large amphipathic organic anions into cells [2]. This suggests that OATPs/Oatps may act as an important role in drugs pharmacokinetic. At present, some antibiotics are found as the substrates or inhibitors of OATPs/Oatps.

Fluoroquinolones and OATPs/Oatps

Fluoroquinolones are antimicrobial drugs that are widely used for the treatment of bacterial and fungal infections. Although has hydrophilic nature, most fluoroquinolones are absorbed efficiently from the small intestine and show relatively high bioavailability [3]. The reasons for this might be explained by an involvement of carrier-mediated transport of fluoroquinolones across intestinal epithelial cells [4]. By using Xenopus oocytes expressing OATP1A2 model, a study found that ciprofloxacin and levofloxacin can be transported by organic anion transporting polypeptide 1A2 (OATP1A2/SLCO1A2) [5]. Therefore, both ciprofloxacin and levofloxacin are the substrates of OATP1A2. In rats, a study furtherly found that Oatp1a5 is involved in the intestinal absorption of ciprooxacin and naringin inhibited the uptake with an IC50 value of 18 uM by Xenopus oocytes expressing Oatp1a5 [6]. However, other investigations have shown that naringin has a significant inhibitory effect not only on Oatps but also P-gp and Bcrp [7,8]. Therefore, Oatp1a5 is involved in the intestinal absorption of ciprofloxacin in rats, but other influx and/or efflux transporters cannot be excluded.

Macrolide antibiotics and OATPs/Oatps

A study showed that when co administered with rifamycin SV, an OATP inhibitor, the exposures of erythromycin and clarithromycin were reduced 65 and 45%, respectively, but rifamycin SV had no affect on the total blood clearance of these macrolides. The study also confirm that rifamycin SV did not cause induction of metabolizing enzymes and/ or transporters. Therefore, it suggests that the intestinal Oatps may be involved in the p.o. absorption of erythromycin and clarithromycin in the rat [9]. However, although the inhibition of OATP/Oatp-mediated transport by rifamycin SV is well documented, it is possible that the decreased oral exposure of the macrolides following co administration

*Corresponding author: Hua WJ, Department of Pharmacy, The First Affiliated Hospital of Nanchang University, Nanchang, China,
E-mail: wenjh866@163.com

of rifamycin SV is caused by inhibition of other members of the OATP/Oatp family or other non-Oatp uptake transporters involved in the intestinal absorption of the macrolides.

Therefore, further study should be explored to confirm that OATPs/Oatps be involved the transport of macrolide antibiotics. In fact, more studies were proved that macrolide antibiotics act as inhibitor of OATPs/Oatps.

For intance, by using HEK293 cells stably expressing the human uptake transporters OATP1B1 or OATP1B3, the study explored the influence of macrolide antibiotics on the OATP1B1-and OATP1B3-mediated uptake of organic anions and drugs, and demonstrated that the OATP1B1-and OATP1B3-mediated uptake of BSP and pravastatin can be inhibited by increasing concentrations of all macrolides except azithromycin [10]. The results were showed in Tables 1 and 2.

Furthermore, the study found that azithromycin and clarithromycin can inhibit the uptake of taurocholate in rat Oatp1a5-transfected Madin-Darby canine kidney (MDCK) cell [9]. The same result also be found in another study , which showed that azithromycin and clarithromycin were potent inhibitors of rat Oatp1a5-mediated taurocholate uptake with apparent inhibitor constant (Ki) values of 3.3 and 2.4 uM, respectively [11]. However, azithromycin and clarithromycin did not significantly inhibit OATP2B1 mediated uptake of estrone-3-sulfate, a prototypical substrate of OATP. Simultaneously, the study showed that no significant transport of azithromycin or clarithromycin was observed in direct uptake studies using COS cells transfected with OATP1A2 or human/rat OATP2B1/Oatp2b1 [11]. Therefore, macrolide may play different role in different OATPs/Oatps.

The influence of macrolide antibiotics on the pharmacokinetic of substrate of OATPs/Oatps was also found in a study. The study demonstrated that the macrolides clarithromycin and erythromycin significantly increase pravastatin plasma concentrations [12]. Although cytochrome P450 (CYP) 3A is mainly responsible for 3"-hydroxy pravastatin formation, there is no clinically important pharmacokinetic interaction of pravastatin with a number of common CYP3A inhibitors [13]. In fact, pravastatin is little metabolized by cytochrome P450 enzymes. Therefore, macrolides may act as the inhibitor of OATPs/Oatps that acted as main transporters in the hepatic uptake of pravastatin.

Rifampin and OATPs/Oatps

Rifampin, an antibiotic mainly used for the treatment of

Macrolide	OATP1B1 (IC50)	OATP1B3(IC50)
Telithromycin	121 ± 19 uM	11 ± 0.3 uM
Clarithromycin	96 ± 5 uM	32 ± 7 uM
Erythromycin	217 ±19 uM	34 ± 14 uM
Roxithromycin	153 ± 4 uM	37 ± 6 uM
Azithromycin	no inhibition	no inhibition

Table 1: The influence of macrolide antibiotics on the OATP1B1- and OATP1B3-mediated uptake of BSP [18].

Macrolide	OATP1B1	Macrolide	OATP1B3
Telithromycin (10 uM)	Moderate inhibition	Telithromycin (100 uM)	19%
Clarithromycin (10 uM)	64%	Clarithromycin (100 uM)	37%
Erythromycin (100 uM)	24%	Erythromycin (100 uM)	36%
Roxithromycin (10 uM)	65%	Roxithromycin (100 uM)	52%
Azithromycin	no inhibition	Azithromycin	no inhibition

Table 2: The influence of macrolide antibiotics on the OATP1B1- and OATP1B3-mediated uptake of pravastatin (the reduction of intracellular accumulation of pravastatin compared with the control experiments) [18].

tuberculosis, is an effective inhibitor of OATP [14]. We previously showed that concomitant dosing of rifamycin SV, a general OATPs/Oatps inhibitor [15], significantly reduced the oral area under the blood-concentration time curve (AUC) for azithromycin and clarithromycin in rats [16]. Simultaneously, rifampin also is a strong inducer of CYP3A4 and MDR1 expression by pregnane X receptor (PXR)-mediated pathways [17].

β-Lactam antibiotics and OATPs/Oatps

Most of the β-lactam antibiotics were taken up by hepatocytes via a common carrier-mediated transport mechanism. For instance, by using cell models of Xenopus laevis oocytes expressing organic anion transporting peptides (Oatp1, 2, and 4) , the study showed that nafcillin was transported by multiple Oatps with Km values of 4120 microM (Oatp1/Oatp1a1), 198 microM (Oatp2/Oatp1a4), and 1570 microM (Oatp4/Oatp1b2), and indicated that Oatp2 is the predominant contributor to the hepatic uptake of nafcillin. This study also found that cefadroxil, cefazolin, cefmetazole, cefoperazone, cefsulodin, and cephalexin, but not cefotaxime or ceftriaxone, were also the substrates of Oatp2 [18]. In another study, by using Xenopus oocytes and cultured cells expressing human OATPs, revealed that OATP1B3 and OATP1B1 transported nafcillin with Km values of 74 microM and 11 mM, respectively, and suggested that OATP1B3 contributes mainly to nafcillin uptake and OATP1B1 contributes moderately [19]. Furthermore, the study also found that all the tested β-lactam antibiotics were transported by OATP1B3, while OATP1B1 transported cefazolin, cefditoren and cefoperazon, but not cefmetazole, cefadroxil or cephalexin.Compared with OATP1B3, OATP1B1showed limited activity for the transport of β-lactam antibiotics. The study showed that the contributions of OATP1B1 and OATP1B3 to the overall uptake of nafcillin in human hepatocytes were determined to 20.5% and 53.3%. The rank orders of affinity (Km) and particularly uptake clearance obtained as V_{max}/km, were similar for OATP1B3 and Oatp1a4, which indicates a functional correlation between human OATP1B3 and rat Oatp1a4 and suggests that Oatp1a4 plays a major role in the hepatic uptake of nafcillin in rats. This result is the same as former [19].

Ciprofloxacin, a drug of fluoroquinolones, was also found may be the substrate of oatp. The study showed that the Oatp1a5-mediated uptake of ciprofloxacin was saturable with a Km value of 140 mM, and naringin inhibited the uptake with an IC50 value of 18 uM by Xenopus oocytes expressing Oatp1a5. Naringin reduced the permeation of ciprofloxacin from the mucosal-to-serosal side, with an IC50 value of 7.5 uM by the Using-type chamber method. The estimated IC50 values were comparable to that of Oatp1a5. These dates suggest that Oatp1a5 is partially responsible for the intestinal absorption of ciprofloxacin [20]. However, recent investigations have shown that naringin has a significant inhibitory effect not only on Oatp1a5 but also P-gp and Bcrp. The present study demonstrates that Oatp1a5 is involved in the intestinal absorption of ciprofloxacin in rats, although other influx and/or efflux transporters cannot be excluded [21].

BCRP/Bcrp and antibiotics

Breast cancer resistance protein (BCRP/ABCG2), one important member of the ABC family of transporters, is apically expressed and mediates the active and outward transport of a range of anticancer drugs, dietary compounds, food carcinogens, and antibiotics. BCRP/Bcrp is found not only in tumor cells but also in a variety of normal tissues such as intestine, liver, brain, and mammary gland. Several in vivo and in vitro studies indicated that BCRP/Bcrp mediates the excretion of antibiotics.

BCRP/Bcrp and fluoroquinolone antibiotics

A study has demonstrated that ciprofloxacin is likely to be a substrate for BCRP in human intestinal cells (Caco-2), as indicated by sensitivity to Ko143 (BCRP inhibitor) inhibition. It is possible that BCRP is the predominant transporter responsible for ciprofloxacin secretion in both rat and human intestine [22]. But, other transport pathway cannot be excluded. Furthermore, by using the polarized canine kidney cell line MDCK-II and its subclones transduced with murine Bcrp1 and human BCRP cDNAs to test the possible role of murine Bcrp1 and human BCRP in the in vitro transport of ciprofloxacin, ofloxacin, and norfloxacin, the results showed that ciprofloxacin, ofloxacin, and norfloxacin were efficiently transported by murine Bcrp1 and moderately transported by human BCRP in the cell lines used [23]. Furthermore, this study also found that Bcrp1 play an important role in rat. The plasma concentration of ciprofloxacin was more than 2-fold increased in Bcrp1_/_ compared with wild-type mice (1.77 ± 0.73 versus 0.85 ± 0.39 ug/ml, $p<0.01$) 15 min after oral administration. At the same time, to test whether Bcrp1 plays a role in the secretion of fluoroquinolones into milk, ciprofloxacin (10 mg/kg) was administered i.v. to lactating Bcrp1_/_ and wild-type females, and 10 min after administration, milk and blood were collected. The result showed that the concentration of ciprofloxacin was 2-fold lower in the milk of Bcrp1_/_ mice (2.19 ± 0.13 vs. 4.44 ± 0.84 ug/ml, $p<0.01$). Ciprofloxacin appears to be actively transported into the milk of mice by Bcrp1 [23].

Plasma and bile concentrations of fluoroquinolones were determined in wild-type and Bcrp (_/_) mice after i.v. bolus injection. The cumulative biliary excretion of fluoroquinolones was significantly reduced in Bcrp (_/_) mice, resulting in a reduction of the biliary excretion clearances to 86, 50, 40, and 16 of the control values, for ciprofloxacin, grepafloxacin, ofloxacin, and ulifloxacin, respectively [24]. This study also showed that, in Madin-Darby canine kidney II cells expressing human BCRP or mouse Bcrp, the basal-to-apical transport of grepafloxacin and ulifloxacin was greater than that of the mock control, which was inhibited by a BCRP inhibitor(Ko143) [24]. Therefore, BCRP/Bcrp play a significant role in the biliary excretion of fluoroquinolones.

β-lactam antibiotics and BCRP/Bcrp

By using membrane vesicles of Sf9 cells transfected with Bcrp, an uptake study revealed that the uptake of cefoperazone, cefbuperazone, cefpiramide, cefotetan, ceftriaxone, cefotiam, cefamandole, and cefazolin by rBcrp-expressing vesicles was significantly higher than that by control vesicles, which suggests that all these compounds all are substrates of rBcrp. Whether the same result has in hBCRP is not explored in this study. Simultaneously, it is not exclude that other transporters are involved the efflux transporting of these β-lactam antibiotics [25].

Other transporters (P-gp and MRP) and antibiotics

ATP dependent efflux transporter P-glycoprotein (P-gp, MDR1) and multidrug resistance associated protein (MRP) also play an important role in the pharmacokinetics of antibiotics.

Fluoroquinolone and P-gp and MRP

MDCKII-MDR1 was employed as an in vitro model to evaluate the effects of antiretrovirals, azole antifungals, macrolide, and fluroquinolone antibiotics on efflux transporters. These in vitro studies indicate that grepafloxacin, levofloxacin, and sparfloxacin are potent inhibitors of P-gp-mediated efflux of 14C erythromycin and (3) H cyclosporine [26].

Gatifloxacin (2.5 mM) also raised the uptake of [14C] erythromycin by 1.6-fold and 1.7-fold in MDCKII-MDR1 cells and MDCK-MRP2 cells, respectively, suggests that this fluoroquinolone is a potent inhibitor of P-gp and MRP2 [27].

A studies also demonstrated that gemifloxacin is effluxed by both P-gp and MRP2. This compound inhibited both P-gp and MRP2 mediated efflux of [14C] erythromycin in a dose dependent manner with IC50 values of 123 ± 2 µM and 16 ± 2 µM, respectively [28]. The P-gp inhibitors PSC833 and GF120918 and the MRP-inhibitor MK571 partially decreased the secretion of Danofloxacin-Mesylate (DM) and increased its absorption rate in Caco-2 cells .Therefore, DM is a substrate for the efflux transporters P-gp and MRP29 [29].

Macrolide Antibiotics and P-gp and MRP

Azithromycin is a substrate for P-gp, the product of the ABCB1 (ATP-binding cassette B1) gene [30] A number of Single Nucleotide Polymorphisms (SNPs) have been identified in ABCB1 gene between individuals and ethnic groups [31]. Three of the most frequently occurring SNPs within ABCB1 include C1236T in exon 12, G2677T/A in exon 21 and C3435T in exon 26 [32]. Azithromycin pharmacokinetics may be influenced by particular polymorphisms of the ABCB1 gene. Cmax was significantly lower among individuals with 2677TT/3435TT genotype (468.0 ± 173.4 ng • h/ml) than those with 2677GG/3435CC (911.2 ± 396.4 ng • h/ml, $p=0.013$). However, the t_{max} value was higher among subjects with 2677TT/3435TT (2.0 ± 0.5 h) than those with 2677GT/3435CT (1.6 ± 0.3 h) or 2677GG/3435CC (1.4 ± 0.4 h) genotypes ($p=0.068$ and $p=0.026$, respectively). Furthermore, the AUC_{0-24} tended to be higher among subjects with 2677GG/3435CC than those with 2677GT/3435CT or 2677TT/3435TT genotypes (5000.2 ± 1610.0 vs. 4558.0 ± 805.0 vs. 4131.0 ± 995.1 ng/ml) [33]. Therefore, polymorphisms of the ABCB1 gene have significantly effect on the pharmacokinetics of azithromycin.

Bidirectional transport studies were conducted using our Caco-2 subclone with high P-gp expression (CLEFF9).Clarithromycin and roxithromycin are likely to exhibit drug interactions with digoxin via inhibition of efflux mechanisms, but azithromycin appears to have little influence on P-gp–mediated digoxin absorption or excretion and would be the safest macrolide to use concurrently with oral digoxin. As well, the study found that erythromycin had no effect on the transport of digoxin [34].

Mrp2 acted as a major canalicular transport protein responsible for spiramycin biliary excretion Mrp2-knockout mice was also confirmed. The study found that approximately 8-fold decrease in the recovery of spiramycin in the bile of Mrp2-knockout mice [35].

β-Lactam antibiotics and MRP

A study found that the uptake of cephalosporins by rMrp2- and hMRP2-expressing vesicles was also examined, and uptake of cefoperazone, cefbuperazone, cefpiramide, and ceftriaxone was significantly higher than that in control vesicles. Uptake of cefotetane and cefotiam was also significantly higher in hMRP2-expressing vesicles than that in control vesicles. This means that β-lactam antibiotics were the substrates of Mrp and MRP. Because most β-Lactam antibiotics are mainly excreted by kidney, therefore, MRP may act as one of efflux transporter in kidney tubules membranes. Simultaneously, possible involvement of other transporters on kidney tubules membranes, such as P-glycoprotein and/or bile salt export pump, should also be considered for the kidney excretion of all the cephalosporins [36].

Conclusion

In clinic, patients are usually treated by multiple drugs. Therefore, it is necessary to pay close attention to drug-drug interactions when these drugs are combined to treat the diseases. At present, more and more antibiotics agents are found as the substrates of transporters. There may be potential drug-drug interactions based on transporters binding site competition. Therefore, further study should be explored when these antibiotic agents are combined with other drugs to treat diseases.

Acknowledgement

This study was supported by the National Natural Science Foundation of China (8202583), Education Department Fund of Jiangxi Province (GJJ12145) and Research Fund Project of Traditional Chinese Medicine of the Health Department of Jiangxi Province (2012A137).

References

1. Coves-Orts FJ, Borrás-Blasco J, Navarro-Ruiz A, Murcia-López A, Palacios-Ortega F (2005) Acute seizures due to a probable interaction between valproic acid and meropenem. Ann Pharmacother 39: 533-537.

2. Wen JH, Wu W, Yang D, Guo LY, Xu WW, et al. (2013) The role of OATPs in pharmacokinetics and drug-drug interaction of cardiovascular agents. Drugs Fut 38: 257-262.

3. Wolfson JS, Hooper DC (1989) Fluoroquinolone antimicrobial agents. Clin Microbiol Rev 2: 378-424.

4. Arakawa H, ShirasakaY, Haga M, Nakanishia T, Tamai I (2012) Active intestinal absorption of fluoroquinolone antibacterial agent ciprofloxacin by organic anion transporting polypeptide, Oatp1a5. Biopharmaceutics and drug disposition 33: 332-341.

5. Maeda T, Takahashi K, Ohtsu N, Oguma T, Ohnishi T, et al. (2007) Identification of influx transporter for the quinolone antibacterial agent levofloxacin. See comment in PubMed Commons below Mol Pharm 4: 85-94.

6. Shirasaka Y, Li Y, Shibue Y, Kuraoka E, Spahn-Langguth H, et al. (2009) Concentration-dependent effect of naringin on intestinal absorption of beta(1)-adrenoceptor antagonist talinolol mediated by p-glycoprotein and organic anion transporting polypeptide (Oatp). Pharm Res 26: 560-567.

7. Shirasaka Y, Suzuki K, Nakanishi T, Tamai I (2011) Differential effect of grapefruit juice on intestinal absorption of statins due to inhibition of organic anion transporting polypeptide and/or P-glycoprotein. J Pharm Sci 100: 3843-3853.

8. Dresser GK, Bailey DG, Leake BF, Schwarz UI, Dawson PA, et al. (2002) Fruit juices inhibit organic anion transporting polypeptide-mediated drug uptake to decrease the oral availability of fexofenadine. Clin Pharmacol Ther 71: 11-20.

9. Garver E, Hugger ED, Shearn SP, Rao A, Dawson PA, et al. (2008) Involvement of intestinal uptake transporters in the absorption of azithromycin and clarithromycin in the rat. Drug Metab Dispos 36: 2492-2498.

10. Seithel A, Eberl S, Singer K, Auge D, Heinkele G, et al. (2007) The influence of macrolide antibiotics on the uptake of organic anions and drugs mediated by OATP1B1 and OATP1B3. Drug Metab Dispos 35: 779-786.

11. Lan T, Rao A, Haywood J, Davis CB, Han C, et al. (2009) Interaction of macrolide antibiotics with intestinally expressed human and rat organic anion-transporting polypeptides. Drug Metab Dispos 37: 2375-2382.

12. Jacobson TA (2004) Comparative pharmacokinetic interaction profiles of pravastatin, simvastatin, and atorvastatin when coadministered with cytochrome P450 inhibitors. Am J Cardiol 94: 1140-1146.

13. Lee CK, Choi JS, Choi DH (2012) Effects of pravastatin on the pharmacokinetic parameters of nimodipine after oral and intravenous administration in rats: possible role of CYP3A4 inhibition by pravastatin. Indian J Pharmacol 44: 624-628.

14. Niemi M, Backman JT, Fromm MF, Neuvonen PJ, Kivistö KT (2003) Pharmacokinetic interactions with rifampicin: clinical relevance. Clin Pharmacokinet 42: 819-850.

15. Vavricka SR, Van Montfoort J, Ha HR, Meier PJ, Fattinger K (2002) Interactions of rifamycin SV and rifampicin with organic anion uptake systems of human liver. Hepatology 36: 164-172.

16. Garver E, Hugger ED, Shearn SP, Rao A, Dawson PA, et al. (2008) Involvement of intestinal uptake transporters in the absorption of azithromycin and clarithromycin in the rat. Drug Metab Dispos 36: 2492-2498.

17. Liu CL, Lim YP, Hu ML (2012) Fucoxanthin attenuates rifampin-induced cytochrome P450 3A4 (CYP3A4) and multiple drug resistance 1 (MDR1) gene expression through pregnane X receptor (PXR)-mediated pathways in human hepatoma HepG2 and colon adenocarcinoma LS174T cells. Mar Drugs 10:242-257.

18. Nakakariya M, Shimada T, Irokawa M, Koibuchi H, Iwanaga T, et al. (2008) Predominant contribution of rat organic anion transporting polypeptide-2 (Oatp2) to hepatic uptake of beta-lactam antibiotics. Pharm Res 25: 578-585.

19. Nakakariya M, Shimada T, Irokawa M, Maeda T, Tamai I (2008) Identification and species similarity of OATP transporters responsible for hepatic uptake of beta-lactam antibiotics. Drug Metab Pharmacokinet 23: 347-355.

20. Arakawa H, Shirasaka Y, Haga M, Nakanishi T, Tamai I (2012) Active intestinal absorption of fluoroquinolone antibacterial agent ciprofloxacin by organic anion transporting polypeptide, Oatp1a5. Biopharm Drug Dispos 33: 332-341.

21. Shirasaka Y, Suzuki K, Nakanishi T, Tamai I (2011) Differential effect of grapefruit juice on intestinal absorption of statins due to inhibition of organic anion transporting polypeptide and/or P-glycoprotein. J Pharm Sci 100: 3843-3853.

22. Haslam IS, Wright JA, O'Reilly DA, Sherlock DJ, Coleman T, et al. (2011) Intestinal ciprofloxacin efflux: the role of breast cancer resistance protein (ABCG2). Drug Metab Dispos 39: 2321-2328.

23. Merino G, Alvarez AI, Pulido MM, Molina AJ, Schinkel AH, et al. (2006) Breast cancer resistance protein (BCRP/ABCG2) transports fluoroquinolone antibiotics and affects their oral availability, pharmacokinetics, and milk secretion. Drug Metab Dispos 4: 690-695.

24. Ando T, Kusuhara H, Merino G, Alvarez AI, Schinkel AH, et al. (2007) Involvement of breast cancer resistance protein (ABCG2) in the biliary excretion mechanism of fluoroquinolones. Drug Metab Dispos 35: 1873-1879.

25. 25. Kato Y, Takahara S, Kato S, Kubo Y, Sai Y, et al. (2008) Involvement of Multidrug Resistance-Associated Protein 2 (Abcc2) in Molecular Weight-Dependent Biliary Excretion of B-Lactam Antibiotics. Drug Metab Dispos 36:1088-1096.

26. Pal D, Mitra AK (2006) MDR- and CYP3A4-mediated drug-drug interactions. J Neuroimmune Pharmacol 1: 323-339.

27. Kwatra D, Vadlapatla RK, Vadlapudi AD, Pal D, Mitra AK (2010) Interaction of gatifloxacin with efflux transporters: a possible mechanism for drug resistance. Int J Pharm 395: 114-121.

28. Vadlapatla RK, Vadlapudi AD, Kwatra D, Pal D, Mitra AK (2011) Differential effect of P-gp and MRP2 on cellular translocation of gemifloxacin. Int J Pharm 420: 26-33.

29. Schrickx JA, Fink-Gremmels J (2007) Danofloxacin-mesylate is a substrate for ATP-dependent efflux transporters. Br J Pharmacol 150: 463-469.

30. Sugie M, Asakura E, Zhao YL, Torita S, Nadai M, et al. (2004) Possible involvement of the drug transporters P glycoprotein and multidrug resistance-associated protein Mrp2 in disposition of azithromycin. Antimicrob Agents Chemother 48: 809-814.

31. Marzolini C, Paus E, Buclin T, Kim RB (2004) Polymorphisms in human MDR1 (P-glycoprotein): recent advances and clinical relevance. Clin Pharmacol Ther 75: 13-33.

32. Bosch TM, Meijerman I, Beijnen JH, Schellens JH (2006) Genetic polymorphisms of drug-metabolising enzymes and drug transporters in the chemotherapeutic treatment of cancer. Clin Pharmacokinet 45: 253-285.

33. He XJ, Zhao LM, Qiu F, Sun YX, Li-Ling J (2009) Influence of ABCB1 gene polymorphisms on the pharmacokinetics of azithromycin among healthy Chinese Han ethnic subjects. Pharmacol Rep 61:843-850.

34. Hughes J, Crowe A (2010) Inhibition of P-glycoprotein-mediated efflux of digoxin and its metabolites by macrolide antibiotics. J Pharmacol Sci 113: 315-324.

27

The SULPYCO Method Using Sulpiride Integrated with an Atypical Adjuvant Therapy for Treating Depressive Syndrome: An Observational Study

Amgad M. Rabie*

Pharmaceutical Organic Chemistry Department, Faculty of Pharmacy, Mansoura University, Mansoura, Dakahlia Governorate, Egypt

Abstract

In this observational study, we studied the effects of a new drug combination on depression. Patients were analyzed before and after antidepressant treatment using the Hamilton rating scale for depression (HAMD). One group of patients was treated with the new integrated medicine consisting of two separate subcutaneous injections of a low dose (20 mg) of sulpiride and a 2.2 ml complex homeopathic solution based on the Krebs cycle elements; each injection was administered once daily. Another group of patients was treated with conventional therapy of 20 mg sulpiride only. The third group was treated with only the homeopathic solution. The differences in the HAMD scores were evaluated before and after 3 months of treatment in these three groups of patients. The HAMD score showed a statistically significant decrease in the group treated with combined sulpiride and homeopathy. This observation suggests that a low parenteral dose (20 mg) of sulpiride, when administered subcutaneously with a complex homeopathic remedy, may give better therapeutic results for mild and moderate depression than either sulpiride or complex homeopathy alone.

Keywords: Allohomeo; Depression; Homeopathy; Sulpiride

Introduction

Sulpiride is an atypical antipsychotic drug used mainly for the treatment of psychosis and depression [1]. At doses of over 600 mg daily, it predominantly acts as a selective antagonist of the dopamine D2 and D3 receptors. At doses of 600-1600 mg, sulpiride is mildly sedating and antipsychotic. At low doses (100-200 mg daily), its prominent feature is antagonistic action against presynaptic inhibitory dopamine receptors, which accounts for some antidepressant activity and a stimulating effect. It also alleviates vertigo. The oral bioavailability of sulpiride is only 25-35% [2].

In Croatia, parenteral sulpiride is available at a dose of 100 mg per vial. Oral sulpiride is available in a 50-mg tablet dose. When used for depression, this drug is usually administered orally at a 3×50 mg daily dose [3].

This observational study analyzed patient records after treatment in order to determine whether the therapeutic action of sulpiride given parenterally by subcutaneous injection would improve if it were combined with a liquid homeopathic complex remedy based on Krebs cycle elements suitable for parenteral use. The remedy was a commercial preparation produced and sold by the German company Heel, called Coenzyme Compositum, which is available in 2.2-ml vials and is sold as an over-the-counter drug.

Material and Methods

Preparation of the combined drug

A dose of 0.4 ml (20 mg) of an isotonic solution of sulpiride was combined in two separate syringes with 2.2 ml of an isotonic solution of mixed homeopathic substances. The dose of sulpiride was measured using a micropipette. These two injections (one with sulpiride and the other with the homeopathic remedy) were given simultaneously in the waist region using a 23 G (0.6×25) needle, once daily at 10 AM.

Homeopathic substances contained in this complex parenteral isotonic preparation were mainly compounds involved in the Krebs cycle as well as some herbal homeopathic remedies, and they were all present in equal volume:

1. Intermediates: Citric acid (D8), cis-aconitic acid (D8), alpha ketoglutaric acid (D8), succinic acid (D10), fumaric acid (D8), DL malic acid (D8), sodium diethyloxalateoacetate (D6), sodium pyruvate (D8), and barium oxalosuccinate (D10)

2. Vitamins, Nucleosides, and their Biosynthetic Intermediates: Coenzyme A (D8), nicotinamide adenine dinucleotide (NAD) (D8), adenosine triphosphate (ATP) (D10), ascorbic acid (D6), thiamine hydrochloride (D6), sodium riboflavin phosphate (D6), pyridoxine hydrochloride (D6), nicotinamide (D6), cysteine (D6), and DL-alpha-lipoic acid (D6)

3. Minerals: Magnesium orotate (D6), cerium oxalate (D8), and manganese phosphate (D6)

4. Herbal Extracts: Pulsatilla (D6) and Beta vulgaris (D4)

5. Miscellaneous Ingredients: Sulfur (D10) and Hepar sulfuris (D10).

The letter "D" in parentheses stands for "decimal dilution", whereas the numbers that follow the "D" represent the number of (decimal) dilution procedures repeated according to basic homeopathy principles [4]. In this manner, "D" means that the corresponding solution of a given active homeopathic ingredient (drug) is obtained by decimal dilution of the starting mother solution. According to the German Homeopathic Pharmacopoeia published by Driehsen [5], a solution of six (6) repeated decimal dilutions in a predefined diluent-water or

***Corresponding author:** Amgad M. Rabie, M.Sc., Pharm. Sci. Pharmaceutical Organic Chemistry Department, Faculty of Pharmacy, Mansoura University, Mansoura, Dakahlia Governorate, Egypt, E-mail: amgadpharmacist1@yahoo.com

aqueous ethanol, e.g., 1 ml of mother solution, is diluted with 9 ml of diluent to give D1; this D1 solution (1 ml) is subsequently diluted with 9 ml of diluent, giving a D2 solution, etc.

After the present study, sulpiride and the complex homeopathic remedy were integrated to create a new drug, which was patented and was approved as new and inventive according to an international evaluation. Its commercial name is SULPYCO.

Treatment with sulpiride alone

In a 5-ml syringe, 0.4 ml (20 mg) of isotonic sulpiride solution was combined with 2.2 ml of isotonic NaCl solution. The quantity of sulpiride was measured using a micropipette.

This injection was given simultaneously in the waist region using a 23 G (0.6×25) needle, once daily at 10 AM.

Treatment with only the complex homeopathic solution

One syringe with 2.2 ml of an isotonic solution of mixed homeopathic substances in relatively equal amounts was used.

Homeopathic substances present in this complex parenteral isotonic preparation were mainly Krebs cycle compounds as well as some herbal homeopathic remedies, all in equal volume:

1. Intermediates: Citric acid (D8), cis-aconitic acid (D8), alpha ketoglutaric acid (D8), succinic acid (D10), fumaric acid (D8), DL malic acid (D8), sodium diethyloxalateoacetate (D6), sodium pyruvate (D8), barium oxalosuccinate (D10).

2. Vitamins, Nucleosides, and Their Biosynthesis Intermediates: Coenzyme A (D8), nicotinamide adenine dinucleotide (NAD) (D8), adenosine triphosphate (ATP) (D10), ascorbic acid (D6), thiamine hydrochloride (D6), sodium riboflavin phosphate (D6), pyridoxine hydrochloride (D6), nicotinamide (D6), cysteine (D6), DL-alpha-lipoic acid (D6).

3. Minerals: Magnesium orotate (D6), cerium oxalate (D8), manganese phosphate (D6).

4. Herbal Extracts: Pulsatilla (D6) and Beta vulgaris (D4).

5. Miscellaneous Ingredients: Sulfur (D10) and Hepar sulfuris (D10).

This injection was given in the waist region using a 23 G (0.6×25) needle, once daily at 10 AM. This group was treated in the period before the first and second groups were treated.

Patient groups

The subjects of this study were 67 women, 44–80 years of age, who were suffering from depressive syndrome. One day prior to the experiment (day 0), all patients were tested using a 17-item version of the Hamilton rating scale for depression (HAMD test). These patients came to my clinic for antidepressant treatment. Because I run a private integrated medicine clinic, they had the choice of combined treatment or only conventional or homeopathic treatment. After the treatment was completed, we analyzed the patients' HAMD scores and compared them to scores taken before the treatment, and we noticed some significant differences. These are the three patients groups that were studied:

1. The first group (N=35) received one dose of the combined drug (sulpiride and complex homeopathy) as two separate injections daily in the morning for 3 months.

2. The second group (N=32) received one dose of the single drug (sulpiride only) daily in the morning for 3 months.

3. The third group (N=15) received one dose of the complex homeopathy remedy as one injection daily in the morning for 3 months, but during an earlier period. At the beginning of this study, the HAMD scores in the third group were determined before and after treatment, so the data were used for statistical analysis.

The HAMD test is generally accepted as the gold standard for quantifying severity of depression symptoms such as low mood, anxiety, agitation, insomnia, and weight loss. It was performed on day 90 of taking the injections. For the 17-item version of the HAMD test, scores can range from 0 to 54. In relation to depression, scores between 0 and 6 indicate normal personality; 7–17, mild depression; 18–24, moderate depression; >24, severe depression.

Results

• The average HMD score in the three groups prior to the study was 20.2 ± 7.1.

• In the second group, the HAMD score was 18.8 ± 9.2 before the study and 17.3 ± 8.8 after the study (Table 1).

• In the first group, the HAMD score was 21.3 ± 5.0 before the study and 8.8 ± 4.1 after the study (Table 1).

• In the third group, the HAMD score was 20.7 ± 4 before the study and 19.4 ± 4.5 after the study.

The results in table 1 were subjected to a paired t-test. The results of the paired t-test, performed with the Analyse-it version 2.21 software, are shown in table 2.

The results from the HAMD test strongly suggest that the combined therapy has a strong antidepressant activity (Table 2). The HAMD mean score decreased by 12.5 points in the first group and were far better than the results of treatment with sulpiride only and complex homeopathy.

No side effects, such as sedation, constipation, dryness of the mouth, or prolactinogenic activity, were observed.

Discussion

Sulpiride is an atypical antipsychotic drug used mainly to treat psychosis and depression. For productive psychosis, high doses of more than 600 mg daily are used. It can be administered orally or parenterally.

	Group	HAMD
	Before the study	
1	Second group/Third group	18.9 ± 9.2/20.7 ± 4.6
2	First group	21.3 ± 5.0
	After	
3	Second group/Third group	17.3 ± 8.8/19.4 ± 4.5
4	First group	8.8 ± 4.1

Table 1: Mean HAMD score before and after therapy.

Paired t-test parameters	Second group	First group	Third group
Mean difference	1.6	12.5	1.7
95% confidence interval (CI)	0.9–2.2	10.9–14.2	0.9–2.1
Standard error (SE)	0.31	0.81	0.32
t-statistic	4.97	15.47	5.0
Degrees of freedom (DF)	31	34	31
2-tailed p value	<0.0001	<0.0001	<0.0001

Table 2: Paired t-test results for the first and second groups.

For psychosis with negative symptoms, long-term treatment uses moderate doses (approximately 600 mg daily). Depression and vertigo are treated with low to moderate doses (100–200 mg daily) [1-3].

Sulpiride is absorbed slowly from the gastrointestinal tract. Its oral bioavailability is only 25–35%, with marked individual differences. The peak plasma concentration is reached 4.5 h after oral dosing. The usual half-life is 6-8 h. Ninety-two percent (92%) is excreted unchanged in the urine. Sulpiride is usually given in 2 or 3 divided doses [3].

Sulpiride is a selective antagonist of the dopamine D_2 and D_3 receptors. This action predominates at doses exceeding 600 mg daily. At low doses (in particular, 50–200 mg daily), its prominent feature is antagonistic action against presynaptic inhibitory dopamine receptors, which accounts for some antidepressant activity and a stimulating effect. Therefore, at these doses, it is used as a second-line antidepressant. Additionally, it alleviates vertigo [1-3]. For depression, sulpiride is given orally, at 100–200 mg daily, divided into 3 doses.

If 20 mg of sulpiride is given subcutaneously, one part of the drug is lost in the process of injection: according to my rough estimation, only about 17.5 mg reaches subcutaneous tissue because the process of injection results in some loss. Therefore, the overall amount of sulpiride in blood after subcutaneous injection with 20 mg is less than 17.5 mg. In the case of a 150-mg daily dose (which is the average dose prescribed for sulpiride to treat depression), 37.5 to 52.5 mg of the drug would be present in the blood at approximately 4.5 h after oral dosing [2]. In this study, I explored whether sulpiride given subcutaneously at a low dose (20 mg) would act better if combined with the complex homeopathic remedy than with isotonic NaCl solution.

Sulpiride was administered at a 20 mg dose, combined either with a complex homeopathic/isopathic remedy mainly based on diluted and potentized Krebs cycle elements or with isotonic NaCl solution. Homeopathized (potentized) Krebs cycle components act as nonspecific metabolism activators (Witt et al. [6], according to the Reckeweg theory of isopathy and homotoxicology).

According to integrative medicine principles, we combine paradigmatically different therapeutic actions in time and space in order to possibly magnify therapeutic potential in a given patient. This is achieved by means of "synergy", which is defined as "a cooperative action of discrete agencies such that the total effect is greater than the sum of the two effects that act independently" [7].

We therefore followed the principle of integrative medicine to combine sulpiride and a complex homeopathic remedy. Two paradigmatically different substances were used together in order to multiply the therapeutic potential. We can define a "paradigm" as "a mental model, a way of seeing, a filter for one's perceptions, a frame of reference, a framework of thought or belief through which one's world or reality is interpreted, an example used to define a phenomenon, and a commonly held belief among a group of people such as scientists of a given discipline" [8]. Thomas Kuhn, a philosopher of science, says that a paradigm is a constellation of concepts, values, perceptions and practices shared by a (scientific) community that forms a particular vision of reality that is the basis of the way a (scientific) community organizes itself [8].

Conventional medicine is mainly based on a biochemical paradigm, so drugs are perceived as acting by interacting with receptors on cells. Health and disease are perceived as purely biochemical processes [9]. Although medicine strongly holds for a biochemical paradigm of biological processes, we are now in a process of revising the past

century's biochemical concept. Therefore, major biological processes can also be electromagnetic in nature. Thus, we come to the concept of energy medicine, where illness is regarded also and at the same time as a disturbance in energy fields and can be addressed via interventions into those energies and energy fields [9]. The paradigm shift, as a change from one way to another, is not a transformative revolution but a sort of gradual metamorphosis driven by agents of small bits of slow change [8], and integrative medicine is surely one of those small bits.

Consequently, sulpiride acts at a biochemical level or paradigm, while homeopathic medicines surely do not, since the quantity of diluted matter is so small that it cannot satisfy the receptor theory in a biochemical paradigm [10,11]. There are disputes about the efficiency of homeopathic medicine. Although many suppose that homeopathy works on a placebo principle, others hold a different opinion [12-14]. Nevertheless, even though we do not fully understand how homeopathy works, it is usually perceived as being energetically programmed water interacting with water in the body, which affects cells on an energetic (quantum field) level [13]. This is the proposed mechanism of action for high dilutions/potencies, which integrate global dynamics also by electromagnetic regulation.

Another model emerging from the nonlinear complex systems theory has been proposed for low potencies [7]. A quantum and nonlinear physical model for homeopathy may work in concordance as well, so at the same time both mechanisms of action may be in play.

The findings of the present study indicate that sulpiride at a low dose, given subcutaneously in combination with a complex homeopathic remedy, acts better than sulpiride with isotonic NaCl solution does.

My opinion is that the body exists on different levels or in different paradigms that are mutually related concurrently. Therefore, we cannot say definitively that the body is just a machine or just a computer or just a quantum operator. It is all of these at the same time. For example, if a bone is fractured, it should first be treated mechanically, i.e., operated on with osteosynthesis (mechanical paradigm). In order for it to be healed, growing processes (biochemical paradigm) should be applied. If we apply magnetic therapy to a fracture site, it can grow even faster (energetic paradigm), so by combining mechanical, biochemical and energetic processes, we may achieve positive synergy and multiply the healing potential. Thus, we see that the body is a complex system, which means at least two things:

1. It is a system composed of interconnected parts that, as a whole, exhibits one or more properties that are not obvious from the properties of the individual parts; the whole is more than merely the sum of its parts.

2. It is also a network of heterogeneous components that interact nonlinearly. In a linear system, an effect is always directly proportional to cause, whereas in a complex system, a small perturbation may cause a large effect (the butterfly effect), a proportional effect, or even no effect at all. Here, we come to the principle of the chaos theory [7].

In the context of this study, I speculate that a homeopathic remedy can make a small change in cellular energy production so that sulpiride can perform better and at a smaller dose. The foremost problem with sulpiride in low doses is a strong stimulation of prolactin secretion; whether this may contribute to the development of breast cancer in women is currently not known, but in this study, no milk production or breast stimulation was observed.

Whether such combined allohomeo (R) therapy is really a therapeutic possibility needs to be investigated in further studies, and it will have paramount significance. It would enable us to reduce the dose of chemical drugs, thereby helping to avoid drug side effects while still achieving the desired therapeutic effect.

Conclusion

This study confirms that sulpiride at a low dose (20 mg) taken parenterally has a significantly better effect on depression if combined with a complex homeopathic/isopathic remedy based on Krebs cycle components than if combined with an isotonic solution of NaCl. It also presupposes that homeopathy does not work on the placebo system. Further experiments are necessary to determine whether this speculation is valid.

References

1. Komossa K, Depping AM, Gaudchau A, Kissling W, Leucht S (2010) Second-generation antipsychotics for major depressive disorder and dysthymia. Cochrane Database Syst Rev 12: CD008121.

2. Martí Massó JF, Ruiz-Martínez J, Bergareche A, López de Munain A (2011) Parkinsonism induced by sulpiride and veralipride: two different stories. Med Clin (Barc) 137: 473-474.

3. Jo SH, Lee SY (2010) Response of i(kr) and HERG currents to the antipsychotics tiapride and sulpiride. Korean J Physiol Pharmacol 14: 305-310.

4. Weingarther O (2007) The nature of the active ingredient in ultramolecular dilutions. Homeopathy 96: 220-226.

5. Driehsen W (2003) German Homeopathic Pharmacopoeia, (5thedn), Gauteng, South Africa, Medpharm, November 3, 2003.

6. Witt CM, Bluth M, Albrecht H, Weisshuhn TE, Baumgartner S, et al. (2007) The in vitro evidence for an effect of high homeopathic potencies-a systematic review of the literature. Complement Ther Med 15: 128-138.

7. Rocha LM (1999) Complex Systems Modeling: Using Metaphors From Nature in Simulation and Scientific Models. BITS: Computer and Communications News. Computing, Information, and Communications Division. Los Alamos National Laboratory. November 1999.

8. Kuhn TS (1965) The structure of Scientific Revolutions, (2ndedn) University of Chicago Press, Chicago, IL,U.S.A.

9. Becker RO (2004) Exploring new horizons in electromedicine. J Altern Complement Med 10: 17-18.

10. Taylor MA, Reilly D, Llewellyn-Jones RH, McSharry C, Aitchison TC (2000) Randomised controlled trial of homoeopathy versus placebo in perennial allergic rhinitis with overview of four trial series. BMJ 321: 471-476.

11. Bell IR, Lewis DA 2nd, Brooks AJ, Schwartz GE, Lewis SE, et al. (2004) Improved clinical status in fibromyalgia patients treated with individualized homeopathic remedies versus placebo. Rheumatology (Oxford) 43: 577-582.

12. Linde K, Clausius N, Ramirez G, Melchart D, Eitel F, et al. (1997) Are the clinical effects of homeopathy placebo effects? A meta-analysis of placebo-controlled trials. Lancet 350: 834-843.

13. Vickers AJ, Smith C (2009) Homeopathic Oscillococcinum for preventing and treating influenza and influenza-like syndromes. Cochrane Database Syst Rev CD001957.

14. Lüdtke R, Rutten AL (2008) The conclusions on the effectiveness of homeopathy highly depend on the set of analyzed trials. J Clin Epidemiol 61: 1197-1204.

28

Trainees' Attitudes and Preferences towards the Use of Over the Counter Analgesics in Patients with Chronic Liver Disease

Nguyen D, Banerjee N, Abdelaziz D and Lewis JH*

Division of Gastroenterology, Hepatology Section, Department of Medicine, Georgetown University Medical Center, Washington, USA

Abstract

Background: The use of certain medications in patients with chronic liver disease and cirrhosis remains controversial. No formal evidence-based guidelines have been published regarding the use of acetaminophen or non-steroidal anti-inflammatory drugs in patients in this setting. As a result, whether or not to prescribe these medications and at what dosages in patients with chronic liver disease or cirrhosis is often met with much consternation.

Objective: We assessed the prescribing preferences of senior medical students, internal medicine residents, and gastroenterology fellows for using NSAIDs and acetaminophen in patients with chronic liver disease (CLD), including those with cirrhosis.

Methods: A 21-question web-based survey was distributed to several major teaching hospitals in Washington, DC. An online survey software (Survey Monkey) was used to collect and analyze responses.

Results: A total of 543 trainees were sent the survey with 174 (32%) responding. The majority of respondents who were willing to use acetaminophen recommended a daily dose of 2 gms or less regardless of their level of training. Internal medicine residents and senior medical students tended to recommend against acetaminophen at any dose in favor of NSAIDs in decompensated cirrhotics. All trainee levels showed a diminishing preference towards using a therapeutic dose of 4 gms acetaminophen per day as a function of CLD severity.

Conclusions: There is a wide divide at the trainee level regarding the usage and dosing for acetaminophen in patients with chronic liver disease. Additional education on the safe use of NSAIDs and acetaminophen in CLD and cirrhosis needs to begin in medical school. Senior students in particular voiced the need for controlled prospective studies in order to develop evidence-based guidelines to determine the appropriate indications for use of NSAIDs and acetaminophen along the spectrum of hepatic impairment in chronic liver disease.

Keywords: Cirrhosis; Physician prescribing patterns; Acetaminophen; Academic training; NSAIDS

Introduction

Objective

The safe use of medications in patients with Chronic Liver Disease (CLD) and cirrhosis remains clinically challenging [1]. Increasing degrees of hepatic impairment may alter the disposition and effects of many drugs through changes in pharmacokinetics and end-organ response. The greater the degree of liver dysfunction, the higher the potential for impaired drug metabolism with the risk of adverse hepatic and other drug effects [1-3]. This may be especially true when it comes to the use of OTC prescription analgesics.

Intentional Acetaminophen (APAP) overdose is the most common cause of acute liver failure in the United States [4], and as a result, the drug is often perceived by many patients and clinicians alike as being too dangerous to use in patients with any form of chronic liver disease, especially cirrhosis, even when therapeutic doses are taken [1,5-7]. While a number of authors have suggested that 2-3 gm/day of APAP given for short durations is safe in patients with cirrhosis [1,5,7-9], this recommendation is largely based on anecdotal clinical experience and expert opinion. As a result, many clinicians still suggest that their chronic liver disease patients, especially those with cirrhosis, not use APAP in any dose or under any circumstances [1,10].

Nonsteroidal Anti-Inflammatory Drugs (NSAIDs) as a group carry a class warning about the possibility of hepatic injury, raising the possibility of acute on chronic injury developing in a cirrhotic patient [11]. However, a more likely concern with NSAID use in cirrhosis is renal impairment [12], in particular precipitating hepatorenal syndrome—a frequently fatal complication of advanced liver disease [13]. Therefore, it is usually recommended that NSAIDs be avoided in cirrhosis, especially those with ascites [14]. NSAIDs can also cause mucosal bleeding or worsen acute bleeding in patients at increased risk of bleeding as a result of the thrombocytopenia and coagulopathy associated with advanced liver disease [1,15,16]. This risk may even be greater in patients with portal hypertension–related complications, such as esophageal or gastric varices, portal hypertensive gastropathy, or Gastric Antral Vacular Ectasias (GAVE) [15,17].

The work of a limited number of investigators has helped to clarify the usage patterns of Over the Counter Analgesics (OTCAs) including APAP and various NSAIDs with respect to their safety in cirrhosis. Khalid et al. [18] found that among non-cirrhotic patients

***Corresponding author:** Lewis JH, Division of Gastroenterology, Hepatology Section, Department of Medicine, Georgetown University Medical Center, Washington, USA, E-mail: lewisjh@gunet.georgetown.edu

in their subspecialty liver clinic, 70% used APAP or NSAIDs. In their patients with compensated cirrhosis, over half mentioned the use of over the counter analgesics, with 25% taking APAP and 31% receiving NSAIDs. Among those with advanced cirrhosis who were hospitalized for a number of common causes of hepatic decompensation, a lower percentage (35%) mentioned taking over the counter analgesics with 19% saying they used acetaminophen and 16% took NSAIDs [14]. Of importance was the fact that hospitalization rates were not increased among cirrhotics using these over the counter analgesics, as reported by Fenkel et al. [19].

In 2008, Rossi et al. studied physicians' attitudes regarding the use of over-the-counter nonprescription analgesics in CLD [10]. The results of their web-based questionnaire survey found that internists and family physicians were significantly more likely *not* to recommend the use of acetaminophen in patients with compensated cirrhosis compared to gastroenterologists, who felt that APAP would, in fact, be safe. In patients with decompensated cirrhosis, 95% of family physicians and 70% of internists would not recommend the use of acetaminophen compared to just 22% of gastroenterologists. Even among patients with mild chronic hepatitis without cirrhosis, 15 to 20% of general practitioners would not recommend APAP. In contrast, none of the gastroenterologists questioned in their survey would avoid APAP in that setting. Overall, non-gastroenterologists were more likely to recommend NSAIDs compared to gastroenterologists who were more likely to recommend the use of APAP [10]. Their survey, however, did not address the specific reasoning behind these recommendations, nor did it specify what daily APAP dose the physicians responding would recommend.

It is unclear whether or not medical students or physicians in training (medical residents or GI fellows) are aware of, or put any of these findings to use. We are also unaware of any information regarding trainees' reasoning for or against prescribing OTCAs in CLD patients, nor their familiarity with any APAP dosing recommendations. This study was designed to examine the preferences and perspectives of senior medical students (MS4), internal medicine residents (PGY I,II,III), and gastroenterology fellows, in order to identify their attitudes and prescribing habits for NSAIDs and APAP patients with CLD and cirrhosis.

Design

A 21-question web-based survey was designed and distributed via email. Included trainees were senior medical students, residents and GI fellows at several of the major teaching institutions in Washington, DC. These included Medstar Georgetown Hospital, Medstar Washington Hospital Center, and George Washington University Hospital. There were no specific exclusion criteria; the survey was not sent to anybody outside of the aforementioned training designations. The survey sought to determine what recommendations they would make regarding NSAID and APAP use in patients with chronic hepatitis without cirrhosis of any cause (group I), in compensated cirrhosis (group II), and in decompensated cirrhosis (group III). During 2012, the email was sent 6 separate times to maximize responses and all results were kept confidential. An online survey software (Survey Monkey) was

used to collect and analyze responses. The questionnaire can be found in the supplemental section as an attached PDF.

The study was submitted to and approved by the Georgetown Institutional Review Board prior to online distribution of the survey. No statistical analysis software was used.

Results

The survey was sent to a total of 543 trainees. A total of 177 responses were collected, accounting for a 33% overall response rate. The survey was answered by 72 senior medical students, 86 internal medicine residents (35 PGY-1, 23 PGY-2, 28 PGY-3), and 19 GI fellows (in all 3 years of training).

The respondents' preferences and recommendations for APAP and NSAID use based on the severity of the CLD and their level of training are summarized in Table 1. Overall, the willingness to use APAP decreased as liver disease severity increased; 62% of MS4s would recommend APAP use in chronic hepatitis patients, but this decreased to only 4% in decompensated cirrhotics. Similar trends were observed for the PGY1-3 medicine residents regarding recommendations for APAP use from CLD group I to III, from 74% to 19% in PGY1s, 57% to 14% in PGY2s and from 89% to 4% in PGY3s. GI fellows were the only group of trainees in which the majority continued to favor APAP use for every stage of liver disease, with only a small drop from 89% to 79% in the recommendation as CLD severity progressed from groups I to III. In comparison, this trend was reversed with NSAID use. Only 5% of GI fellows recommended NSAID use for any stage of CLD. In contrast, among the other trainees (medical students and internal medicine residents), the majority recommended NSAID usage in groups I and II. MS4s were most likely to recommend NSAID use for any stage of liver disease, with 96% recommending use in groups I and II and 58% recommending NSAID use in group III.

Trainees were also surveyed regarding the maximum daily APAP dose that they would recommend based on the severity of liver disease, with the results summarized in Table 2. The maximum therapeutic dose of 4 gm daily of APAP was recommended least often for any stage of chronic liver disease at every level of physician training. In contrast, a maximum daily dose of 2 gm APAP was most often recommended for any stage of chronic liver disease, although responses were not unanimous amongst the trainees. Those who most strongly favored the 2 gm maximum daily dose were the MS4s and GI fellows, with over 60% expressing that dose preference for any stage of CLD. PGY 1-3s were more hesitant about the safety of any daily dose, with a majority feeling that 2 gm per day of APAP was acceptable for groups I and II while no maximal daily dose was acceptable for group III.

Medical students and internal medicine and GI physician trainees were also surveyed as to why they would avoid NSAIDs and/or APAP in patients with CLD. As Table 3 shows, there was wide variability in the reasons cited to avoid NSAID use in this setting. One-third of MS4s, 44% of PGY1s, 80% of PGY2s, 25% of PGY3s, and 22% of GI fellows expressed concern that NSAIDs would increase the risk of gastric ulcers and/or would precipitate GI bleeding. The risk of renal

	MS4 N=72		PGY1 N=35		PGY2 N=23		PGY3 N= 28		GI Fellow N=19	
	APAP	NSAID	APAP	NSAID	APAP	NSAID	APAP	NSAID	APAP	NSAID
Group I	62%	96%	74%	61%	57%	71%	89%	85%	89%	5%
Group II	32%	96%	55%	56%	61%	57%	59%	69%	89%	5%
Group III	4%	58%	19%	25%	13%	29%	4%	27%	79%	5%

Table 1: Percentage of trainees by level of training who recommended APAP or NSAIDs (dose not specified) at varying levels of CLD.

	4 gms daily				
	MS4 N=72	PGY1 N=35	PGY2 N=23	PGY3 N=28	GI Fellow N=19
Group I	22%	23%	22%	22%	26%
Group II	8%	3%	9%	8%	0%
Group III	0%	0%	0%	4%	0%
	2 gms or less daily				
	MS4 N=72	PGY1 N=35	PGY2 N=23	PGY3 N=28	GI Fellow N=19
Group I	61%	45%	26%	48%	63%
Group II	62%	43%	52%	36%	84%
Group III	63%	24%	17%	4%	73%
	No daily dose is acceptable				
	MS4 N=72	PGY1 N=35	PGY2 N=23	PGY3 N=28	GI Fellow N=19
Group I	6%	26%	43%	11%	11%
Group II	15%	47%	39%	32%	11%
Group III	36%	76%	83%	92%	21%

Table 2: Percentage of trainees who recommended a specified daily dose of APAP at given stages of CLD.

	MS4 N=72	PGY-1 N=35	PGY-2 N=23	PGY-3 N=28	GI Fellow N=19
Risk of precipitating ulcers/GI bleeding	33%	44%	80%	25%	22%
Risk of renal failure	24%	33%	20%	25%	67%
Concern about worsening underlying liver disease	20%	11%	NS	50%	11%
Preference for APAP over NSAIDS	23%	12%	NS	NS	NS

Table 3: Primary reasons given for not wanting to use NSAIDs in patients with CLD.

	MS4 N=72	PGY-1 N=35	PGY-2 N=23	PGY-3 N=28	GI Fellow N=19
Concern of worsening underlying liver disease	33%	33%	100%	100%	100%
Concern of inadvertent overdose	31%	67%	NS	NS	NS
Lack of information regarding use of APAP in CLD patients	36%	NS	NS	NS	NS

Table 4: Primary reasons for not wanting to use of APAP in patients with CLD.

failure with NSAID use was the primary concern of 24% of MS4s, 33% of PGY1s, 20% of PGY2s, 25% of PGY3s, and 67% of GI fellows. Twenty percent of MS4s, 11% of PGY1s, 0% of PGY2s, 50% of PGY3s, and 11% of GI fellows felt that worsening of the underlying liver disease was the primary reason to avoid NSAIDs.

Specific reasons why trainees would not use APAP in CLD patients are shown in table 4. All of the PGY- 2 and 3 residents and GI fellows who did not recommend use of APAP in CLD patients were primarily concerned over worsening of underlying liver disease. Two thirds of PGY1 residents were concerned with the risk of an inadvertent overdose. MS4s were more split in their reasoning between a risk of worsening of the underlying disease, concern about an inadvertent overdose and the lack of formal guidelines on APAP use in CLD patients. No trainee groups avoided APAP due to a preference for using NSAIDs or narcotics.

Discussion

The results of this survey show that for every stage of CLD, senior level medical students favored the use of NSAIDs over APAP. Internal medicine residents also preferred NSAIDs over APAP in nearly every stage of CLD. In contrast, GI fellows overwhelmingly favored the use of APAP over NSAIDs at every stage of CLD. We did note, however,

that the willingness to prescribe either type of OTCA decreased as a function of CLD severity in most trainee groups. These findings among medical students and internal medicine residents are very similar to previously published studies [10]. The reasons given by the trainees, who were worried about using APAP, primarily reflected their concerns about worsening the underlying liver disease, precipitating an inadvertent overdose, and the lack of evidence-based information on which to justify clinical decisions.

Our study indicates that a significant variability exists among health care providers and physicians in training regarding their recommendations on the use of OTCAs, and affords an opportunity for physician and patient education on medication use in CLD. Non-specialty trainees (senior medical students and IM residents) were much more willing to use NSAIDs at all levels of CLD as compared with GI fellows- a trend not seen between general practitioners and GI specialists. However, the trend towards avoiding NSAID use in Group III cirrhotics held is similar to results from Rossi et al. [10].

The recommendations for using APAP differed significantly among practicing physicians in the study by Rossi et al for all levels of CLD severity [10]. APAP was deemed safe for use by 100%, 95%, and 80% of gastroenterologists for patients in groups I, II, III respectively. In contrast, APAP use was deemed suitable for CLD groups I, II, III by 85-90%, 50-80%, and 10-30% of general internists (GIMs) and family practitioners (FPs) respectively. The gastroenterologists' recommendations for APAP use were similar to those of the GI fellows in our survey for all levels of CLD. While the recommendations for APAP use varied among senior level medical students and residents and among practicing FPs/GIMs, the overall trend of using APAP less in patients with more advanced stages of CLD (group III) was confirmed in both studies. GI fellows and practicing gastroenterologists were both more likely to recommend APAP over NSAIDs at the most advanced stages of CLD (groups II, and III).

Although no formal evidence-based guidelines have been published regarding the use of APAP or NSAIDs in patients with CLD or cirrhosis, expert opinion suggests that a daily dose of 2-3gm or less of APAP is safe for short term use in patients with CLD including cirrhosis[1,5-10]. While APAP remains the single leading cause of acute liver failure in the US, the UK and other westernized countries, the majority of instances involve an intentional overdose [4,20]. In contrast, the vast majority of APAP users take the drug safely and without incident [21]. Although it has been demonstrated that doses of 4 grams daily over the course of 2 weeks given to healthy volunteers can lead to marked, but clinically silent, elevations in ALT and AST in more than 40% of subjects [22], other groups have not shown significant ALT elevations with doses up to 8 grams daily when used for shorter periods [23,24], including in patients who have recently used alcohol [25]. The issue of "therapeutic misadventure", a termed coined by Maddrey and Zimmerman in the mid-1990s [26], is still a cautionary tale, in that unsuspecting chronic alcohol users (which can include cirrhotics), may experience an inadvertent overdose from APAP (in doses far lower than the traditional 10 grams implicated in most intentional overdoses) leading to acute on chronic liver failure. However, such reports remain relatively anecdotal and limited in number compared to the billions of doses taken annually [21,27], and no instances of acute liver failure were seen with daily doses less than 2.5 gm [26]. Moreover, the toxic-metabolic premises upon which the alcohol-acetaminophen interaction was based (i.e. increased formation of NAPQI by CYP2E1 induction, and glutathione depletion by alcohol), have been challenged [25,28]. Unfortunately, there are no long-term prospective studies looking at APAP use in cirrhotics.

In contrast to the concerns about using APAP in patients with CLD, most lay persons and many physicians consider NSAIDs to be a safer analgesic option. However, owing to their inhibition of prostaglandin synthesis, NSAIDs are generally not recommended for use in cirrhosis due to the risk of precipitating GI bleeding and renal failure [1,12-17]. Patients with cirrhosis have increased synthesis of renal prostaglandins to counteract the renin-angiotensin-aldosterone and sympathetic systems that reduce perfusion to the kidneys [14]. Circulating renal prostaglandins help to maintain and regulate renal hemodynamics, glomerular filtration and the renal handling of sodium and water. In addition, NSAIDs are largely protein bound and metabolized by CYP P450 enzymes and thus increased serum levels can be anticipated in cirrhosis [29]. The inhibition of prostaglandin synthesis leads to a profound decrease in renal perfusion, reduction in GFR, impairment in water clearance, and marked sodium retention. Moreover, NSAIDs have deleterious effects on platelets that can increase the risk of GI hemorrhage [30]. In addition, ibuprofen has been associated with exacerbating chronic hepatitis C, suggesting it might not be safe in this setting [31], although others have challenged this notion [32]. Although celecoxib may not impair platelet or renal function in cirrhosis to the extent of non-selective NSAIDs, its long-term safety in cirrhosis remains to be established [33].

In general, the majority of physician trainees in our survey believed that a daily APAP dose of 2 gm or less was safe for some CLD patients, regardless of their level of training. However, for patients with decompensated cirrhosis, a majority of IM residents felt that no daily dose of APAP was safe. Moreover, all trainee levels showed a diminished preference for a full dose of 4gms per day as a function of CLD severity. When offered a range of APAP doses, most trainees in our survey had the strongest preference for using a daily dose of 2gms or less in patients with chronic hepatitis or stable cirrhosis. For decompensated cirrhosis, the majority of trainees felt that no daily dose was acceptable.

In 2011, in an effort to help encourage and ensure appropriate acetaminophen use, the maker of Extra Strength TYLENOL' implemented new dosing instructions that lowered the maximum daily dose for single-ingredient Extra Strength TYLENOL' products sold in the U.S. from 8 pills per day (4,000 mg) to 6 pills per day (3,000 mg). The dosing interval has also changed from 2 pills every 4-6 hours to 2 pills every 6 hours [34]. Although these recommendations were for the general population at large, with no specific guidelines offered for patients with CLD, there is evidence to suggest that APAP taken at therapeutic doses may be safe in patients with CLD. Fenkel et al. demonstrated that "non-excessive" doses of OTCAs (NSAIDs and/or APAP) in patients with cirrhosis were not associated with an increased rate of hospitalization for liver related events [19]. The non-excessive dosage referred to in the study were listed as being less than the maximally recommended dose in the package label, although actual dosages in the study were not reported. Khalid et al found that reduced doses of APAP were not associated with acute hepatic decomposition, even among patients with recent alcohol ingestion [18].

In examining the reasons for why trainees would avoid using NSAIDs or APAP in CLD patients, their responses were found to be variable. The majority of MS4s and IM residents were concerned about NSAIDs causing ulcers or GI bleeding in patients with CLD, whereas GI fellows were more concerned about NSAIDs precipitating renal failure in these patients. The study by Rossi et al. [10] did not address the specific reasoning behind the practitioners' recommendations for or against NSAID use in CLD patients, and thus no direct comparison

can be made with our respondents. However, most senior level medical residents and GI fellows were concerned that APAP could worsen the underlying liver disease. Of note, senior medical students were the only group to suggest that the lack of evidence-based literature on the subject was the main reasoning behind their avoidance of APAP.

An interesting observation highlighted by the results of our survey, and also found by Rossi et al. [10], is why a preference for NSAIDs over APAP in CLD patients still exists. Given that NSAID-induced GI and renal toxicity and idiosyncratic hepatotoxicity have been well characterized in the literature, coupled with the evidence that APAP at low or therapeutic doses is generally safe in CLD patients, some might find it surprising that both primary care practitioners and non-GI trainees consistently chose NSAIDs over APAP at all levels of CLD severity. Based on the responses provided by our survey, it seems that while senior medical students and internal medicine residents are aware of the GI toxicity of NSAIDs, they appear to be less concerned with the risk of renal failure compared to GI fellows. It is possible that the often dramatic events surrounding acute liver failure associated with APAP outweighs the concern for NSAID-associated GI toxicity among non-GI physicians. While one might surmise that the absolute risk of renal failure might be a stronger reason to change their preference, at what level of training and how this information should this is introduced has not been studied. Nevertheless, it appears that given the responses to our survey, both trainees and general medical practitioners have an incomplete understanding of the potential for NSAID and APAP to cause toxicity in CLD patients.

Regarding information given to patients about using OTCAs, only about half of the patients included in the survey by Fenkel et al. ever reported having received medical advice on OTCA use by pharmacists or physicians [19]. The reluctance of trainees responding to our survey to use APAP at any dose in decompensated cirrhosis implies that further evidenced-based recommendations are needed for this patient population. Longer-term prospective studies examining the safety of APAP in CLD patients would bolster and extend recommendations that are currently based largely on expert opinion.

Conclusion

Our results show that there exists a divide, even at the training level, among IM residents and those specifically training to become gastroenterologists with respect to selecting OTCAs for use in patients with CLD. We also observed a preference for recommending that APAP be used in lieu of NSAIDs in CLD patients of any stage among trainees in GI fellowships. Senior medical students and internal medicine residents were more likely to recommend NSAIDs over APAP for CLD patients, with a majority still preferring NSAID use, even in patients with decompensated cirrhosis. Our survey results also found a variable response to what trainees consider to be the maximum daily safe dose of APAP for the various stages of CLD and the reasons why some trainees felt that NSAIDs should be avoided. Although 2 gm per day of APAP was the most agreed upon dose, this is an indication that additional education is needed beginning in medical school. Prospective studies would be welcomed to help determine a safe dose of APAP and duration of treatment in CLD patients.

References

1. Lewis JH, Stine JG (2013) Review article: prescribing medications in patients with cirrhosis-a practical guide. Aliment Pharmacol Ther 37: 1132-1156.

2. Delcò F, Tchambaz L, Schlienger R, Drewe J, Krähenbühl S (2005) Dose adjustment in patients with liver disease. Drug Saf 28: 529-545.

3. Verbeeck RK (2008) Pharmacokinetics and dosage adjustment in patients with hepatic dysfunction. Eur J Clin Pharmacol 64: 1147-1161.

4. Lee WM (2013) Drug-induced acute liver failure. Clin Liver Dis 17: 575-586.

5. Benson GD, Koff RS, Tolman KG (2005) The therapeutic use of acetaminophen in patients with liver disease. Am J Ther 12: 133-141.

6. Murphy EJ (2005) Acute pain management pharmacology for the patient with concurrent renal or hepatic disease. Anesthesia Intensive Care 33: 311-322.

7. Gupta NK, Lewis JH (2008) Review article:The use of potentially hepatotoxic drugs in patients with liver disease. Aliment Pharmacol Ther 28: 1021-1041.

8. Chandok N, Watt KD (2010) Pain management in the cirrhotic patient: the clinical challenge. Mayo Clin Proc 85: 451-458.

9. Lucena MI, Andrade RJ, Tognoni G, Hidalgo R, Sanchez de la Cuesta F, et al. (2003) Drug use for non-hepatic associated conditions in patients with liver cirrhosis. Eur J Clin Pharmacol 59: 71-76.

10. Rossi S, Assis DN, Awsare M, Brunner M, Skole K, et al. (2008) Use of over-the-counter analgesics in patients with chronic liver disease: physicians' recommendations. Drug Saf 31: 261-270.

11. Lewis JH (1998) NSAID-induced hepatotoxicity. Clin Liver Dis 2: 543-561.

12. Brater DC, Anderson SA, Brown-Cartwright D, Toto RD (1986) Effects of nonsteroidal antiinflammatory drugs on renal function in patients with renal insufficiency and in cirrhotics. Am J Kidney Dis 8: 351-355.

13. Salerno F, Gerbes A, Gines P, Wong F, Arroyo V (2007) Diagnosis, prevention and treatment of hepatorenal syndrome in cirrhosis. Gut 56: 1310-1318.

14. Laffi G, La Villa G, Pinzani M, Marra F, Gentilini P (1997) Arachidonic acid derivatives and renal function in liver cirrhosis. Semin Nephrol 17: 530-548.

15. Lee YC, Chang CH, Lin JW, Chen HC, Lin MS, et al. (2012) Non-steroidal anti-inflammatory drugs use and risk of upper gastrointestinal adverse events in cirrhotic patients. Liver Int 32: 859-866.

16. Castro-Fernandez M, Sanchez-Munoz D, Galan-Jurado MV, Larraona JL, Suárez E, et al. (2006) Influence of nonsteroidal antiinflammatory drugs in gastrointestinal bleeding due to gastroduodenal ulcers or erosions in patients with liver cirrhosis. Gastroenterol Hepatol 29: 11-14.

17. Deledinghen V, Heresbach D, Fourdan O, Bernard P, Liebaert-Bories M, et al. (1999) Anti-inflammatory drugs and variceal bleeding: a case-control study. Gut 44: 270-273.

18. Khalid SK, Lane J, Navarro V, Garcia-Tsao G (2009) Use of over-the-counter analgesics is not associated with acute decompensation in patients with cirrhosis. Clin Gastroenterol and Hepatol 7: 994-999.

19. Fenkel JM, Coron RN, Daskalakis C, Vega M, Rossi S, et al. (2010) Over-the-counter analgesics in cirrhotic patients: a case-control study examining the risk of hospitalization for liver-associated events. Scand J Gastroenterol 45: 1101-1109.

20. Prescott LF (2000) Therapeutic misadventure with paracetamol: fact or fiction? Am J Ther 7: 99-114.

21. Jones A (2002) Over-the-counter analgesics: a toxicology perspective. Am J Ther 9: 245-257.

22. Watkins PB, Kaplowitz N, Slattery JT, Colonese CR, Colucci SV, et al. (2006) Aminotransferase elevations in healthy adults receiving 4 grams of acetaminophen daily: a randomized controlled trial. JAMA 296: 87-93.

23. Temple AR, Lynch JM, Vena J, Auiler JF, Gelotte CK, et al. (2007) Aminotransferase activities in healthy subjects receiving three-day dosing of 4, 6, or 8 grams per day of acetaminophen. Clin Toxicol (Phila) 45: 36-44.

24. Heard KJ, Green JL, Dart RC (2010) Serum alanine aminotransferase elevation during 10 days of acetaminophen use in nondrinkers. Pharmacotherapy 30: 818-822.

25. Rumack B, Heard K, Green J, Albert D, Bartelson BB, et al. (2012) The effect of acetaminophen on serum alanine aminotransferase activity in subjects who consume ethanol: a systematic review and meta-analysis of published randomized, controlled trials. Pharmacotherapy 32: 784-91.

26. Zimmerman HJ, Maddrey WC (1995) Acetaminophen (paracetamol) hepatotoxicity with regular intake of alcohol: analysis of instances of therapeutic misadventure. Hepatology 22: 767-773.

27. Dart RC, Green JL, Kuffner EK, Heard K, Sproule B, et al. (2010) The effects of paracetamol (acetaminophen) on hepatic tests in patients who chronically abuse alcohol-a randomized study. Aliment Pharmacol Ther 32: 478-486.

28. Rumack BH (2004) Acetaminophen misconceptions. Hepatology 40:10-15.

29. Bosilkovska M, Walder B, Besson M, Daali Y, Desmeules J (2012) Analgesics in patients with hepatic impairment: pharmacology and clinical implications. Drugs 72:1645-1669.

30. Schafer AI (1995) Effects of nonsteroidal antiinflammatory drugs on platelet function and systemic hemostasis. J Clin Pharmacol 35: 209-219.

31. Riley TR 3rd, Smith JP (1998) Ibuprofen-induced hepatotoxicity in patients with chronic hepatitis C: a case series. Am J Gastroenterol 93: 1563-1565.

32. Andrade RJ, Lucena MI, Garcia-Cortes M, García-Ruiz E, Fernández-Bonilla E, et al. (2002) Chronic hepatitis C, ibuprofen, and liver damage. Am J Gastroenterol 97: 1854-1855.

33. Claria J, Kent JD, Lopez-Parra M, Escolar G, Ruiz-Del-Arbol L, et al. (2005) Effects of celecoxib and naproxen on renal function in nonazotemic patients with cirrhosis and ascites. Hepatology 41: 579-587.

34. McNEIL-PPC (2013) Acetaminophen Dosage for Adults.

29

Treatment of Hepatitis C with First Generation Protease Inhibitors

Marcos Cardoso Rios*, Evelyne de Andrade Mota, Layana Tyara Sandes Fraga, Saulo Makerran Loureiro, Tereza Virgínia Silva Bezerra Nascimento, Ângelo Roberto Antoniolli, Divaldo Pereira de Lyra-Junior and Alex Franca

Universidade Federal de Sergipe, São Cristovão, Sergipe, Brazil

Abstract

Recent changes in the treatment of hepatitis C have increased the demands for medical care and pharmacovigilance. The aim of this study was to evaluate the epidemiological profile, drug therapy, and response to treatment of chronic hepatitis C patients treated with interferon plus ribavirin in combination with Telaprevir (TVR) or Boceprevir (BOC), in an outpatient hospital in Northeast Brazil. A retrospective review of patient records archived at the Hepatology Unit of the University Hospital of the Federal University of Sergipe was conducted. A total of 48 treatments were analyzed, with TVR (35) being the most used antiviral drug. The overall Sustained Virologic Response (SVR) rate after a 48-week treatment course was 61.5% among patients who received TVR and 50% among patients who received BOC. However, the SVR rate was lower when intention-to-treat was considered, decreasing to 22.8% for TVR treatment, and 15.4% for BOC treatment. Cirrhosis was one of the main characteristics of patients with suspension of treatment due to adverse reactions associated with TVR use. During combination drug treatment, adverse reactions caused by the different drugs are cumulative, creating a scenario that is difficult to control. These findings indicate the need for multidisciplinary care, and for review of therapeutic indications or even evaluating the anticipation of treatment of chronic carriers of hepatitis C, in order to achieve better results. The availability of new direct antiviral drugs will negate the need for a therapy associated with significant adverse reactions and low therapeutic response.

Keywords: Hepatitis C; Pharmacotherapy; Drug Safety; Protease inhibitors; Telaprevir; Boceprevir

Introduction

The treatment of hepatitis C has advanced considerably in recent decades. The discovery of Protease Inhibitors (PIs), the first Direct Acting Antivirals (DAAs), was promising as these drugs were able to dramatically decrease the Viral Load (VL) [1,2]. In 2011, the first generation of DAAs, Telaprevir (TVR) and Boceprevir (BOC), was released for use against infection with Hepatitis C Virus (HCV) genotype 1, and triple therapy was subsequently considered the standard therapy [3,4]. In Brazil, the Ministry of Health began to provide these drugs in 2012 for patients with advanced fibrosis (F3 and F4) and/or for patients not responding to previous treatment [5].

The proposed treatment includes the elimination of the virus and a decrease in the progression of liver disease. The inclusion of PIs in association with Pegylated Interferon (PEG-IFN) and Ribavirin (RBV) increased the Sustained Virologic Response (SVR) rate, defined as the absence of detectable viral RNA in serum 3–6 months after the end of therapy; SVR is the best indicator of effective treatment [6,7]. The SVR to triple therapy can reach up to 83%, higher than the SVR to drug regimens with PEG-IFN and RBV [8]. In addition, triple therapy has been very effective in both treatment-naïve patients and in treatment-experienced patients, including the null response [9,10].

Treatment of hepatitis C is associated with increased medical demands due to increased costs and adverse reactions [8,11]. According to Kiser et al. [12], the correct use of TVR and BOC requires careful observation because there is clinical evidence of adverse reactions and more frequent drug interactions. Moreover, the long period of treatment and the negative experience associated with pharmacotherapy may contribute to an adverse clinical outcome [13-15].

Surveillance measures are essential for the collection and detection of data on adverse effects of drugs and for developing protocols for guidance on the use of medicines, risk minimization and prevention of adverse reactions [16]. Moreover, the use of PIs in Brazil is recent and there are not many studies evaluating the reactions of these drugs in our country. In the state of Sergipe, for example, to date there are no studies assessing the impact of implementation of these technologies?

The aim of this study was to evaluate the epidemiological profile, drug therapy, and response to treatment of patients with chronic hepatitis C treated with interferon plus ribavirin and TVR or BOC in an outpatient hospital in northeastern Brazil.

Material and Methods

A cross-sectional review was conducted of the medical records of all hepatitis C patients treated with BOC or TVR in combination with the alfa peginterferon 2a or 2b and ribavirin, between January 2013 and October 2015, as part of the Hepatology Service at the University Hospital of Sergipe in Northeast Brazil. The work was approved by the Research Ethics Committee of the Federal University of Sergipe. The study population included outpatients with chronic hepatitis C, regardless of sex or race, commencing treatment with triple therapy during the study period.

To characterize drug therapy, the following data were collected: Genotype, histologic evaluation (based on METAVIR classification), medical condition, and duration of treatment, antiviral drugs administered, and changes during drug therapy, adverse reactions,

*Corresponding author: Marcos Cardoso Rios, Universidade Federal de Sergipe, São Cristovão, Sergipe, Brazil, E-mail: mcrios_farma@yahoo.com.br

and medication used to treat adverse reactions. Antiviral therapy was assigned in accordance with the Clinical Protocols and Therapeutic Guidelines for viral hepatitis C and co-infections, issued by the Brazilian Ministry of Health. The medications administered were classified according to the Brazilian Common Denomination.

Patients with hepatitis B and HIV infection were excluded from the treatment response analysis. Patient response to antiviral treatment was categorized according to the Ministry of Health protocol [4,5]: RVR response; Extended Rapid Virologic Response (eRVR); virologic response at the End of Treatment (ETR); SVR; viral breakthrough. The evolution of the VL and manifestation of adverse reactions were monitored at weeks 4, 8, 12, 24 and 48 of treatment.

By intention-to-treat, all patients who started treatment were considered. Completion of treatment excluded patients who did not complete the proposed treatment. SVR and medication type were analyzed using the Chi-square test and Fisher's exact test (GraphPad Prism version 5'). The 95% confidence interval was calculated and a value of p<0.05 was considered significant. Following analysis, the results were expressed as text, graphics, and tables, using Microsoft Excel 2010.

Results

Records from 57 patients with clinical indication for triple-drug treatment with first generation PIs for treatment of chronic hepatitis C genotype 1, between January 2013 and October 2015, were selected from the archives of the Hepatology and Liver Diseases Sector. Six patients were excluded because they did not use the PIs: 2 used a single dose of PEG-IFN and ribavirin, 2 did not present VL decline >1 log after lead-in, 1 developed descompensated cirrhosis during the double-drug treatment, and one evaded treatment after the third week of treatment. For 3 further patients, no information was recorded regarding the reason for premature interruption of therapy.

According to the METAVIR classification, 15 patients presented with F4 fibrosis (31.9%), diagnosed by hepatic biopsy (8) and non-invasive methods, as elastography (7) (Table 1). One transplanted patient presented with F1 fibrosis.

The degree of fibrosis in patients receiving treatment for chronic hepatitis C, and treated with different PIs, is presented on Figures 1 and 2. A survey of the pharmacotherapeutic profile showed that 37.5% (18/48) of the patients were hepatitis C treatment-naive. The remaining 61.7% (30/48) did not respond to previous therapy with PEG-IFN+RBV, of which 46.6% (14/30) were relapsing, 6.6% (2/30) experienced virological breakthrough, 23.4% (7/30) were partial responders, and 23.4% (7/30) were null responders.

The TVR treatment was suspended in 48.6% of patients (17/35), 18% (3/17) did not complete the first 4 weeks of treatment, 2 patients (12%; 2/17) suspended treatment on week 10, and 2 (12%; 2/17) suspended treatment between week 12 and 24. Treatment suspension (53%; 9/17) was the main adverse reactions, and was more common in patients with advanced fibrosis (89%; 8/9). The reasons for treatment suspension included virological breakthrough (35.3%; 6/17), observed on week 4 (1/6), 12 (2/6) and 24 (3/6); and non-response (partial and null) (11.7%; 2/17).

For patient's treatment with BOC, treatment suspension occurred in 54% (7/13) of patients, due to the following: the presence of one or more reactions adverse (71.4%; 5/7), which was more common in cirrhotic patients (60%; 3/5); virological breakthrough in 1 case (14.3%) and failure to respond to treatment in 1 patient (14.3%). Virological

Variables	Patients selected for antiviral treatment		
	All patients	BOC	TVR
Patient number (n/%)	48	13/48 (27.1)	35/48 (72.9)
Mean Age ± SD (years)	55.2 ± 16	-	-
Gender (n/%)			
Male	36/48 (75)	9/36 (25)	27/36 (75)
Female	12/48 (25)	3/12 (25)	9/12 (75)
HCV genotype (n/%)			
1A	20/48 (40,4)	10 (50)	10 (50)
1B	25/48 (51,1)	3 (12)	25 (88)
1 not specified	3/48 (8,5)	-	3 (100)
Treatment experienced (n/%)			
Yes	30/48 (62,5)	-	-
No	18/48 (37,5)	-	-
Fibrosis stage (n/%)			
F1	5/48 (10.4)	2/5 (40)	3/5 (60)
F2	13/48 (27.1)	5/13 (38.4)	8 (61.6)
F3	15/48 (31.25)	4/15 (26.6)	11 (73.4)
F4	15/48 (31.25)	2/15 (13.3)	13/15 (86.7)
Viral charge	-	1.000.000 log 6.0	630.957 log 5.8

Table 1: Baseline characteristics of the study.

breakthrough occurred between week 24 and 48, and the reactions that determined treatment suspension were observed between week 4 and 12 (Table 2).

The association between SVR and lead-in was shown to be statistically significant for treatment with TVR (p=0.0238) and non-significant for BOC (p>0.05). The SVR and RVR associations were not significant for both drugs. The SVR for patients with different degrees of fibrosis and treatment conditions are presented in Figures 1 and 2.

Approximately 60 different types of reactions adverse were described, with a higher average frequency in patients using the IFN+RBV+BOC combination than in patients receiving the IFN+RBV+TVR combination. It should be noted that, because all patients received IFN+RBV+IP, the adverse reactions observed in the present study were associated with the triple-drug combination. Symptoms of depression, including irritability, insomnia, and despondency, which may be characteristic of the use of IFN, were therefore considered to be associated with the use of PIs (Figure 3). For patients receiving TVR, the following complaints were reported: weight loss (42.8%; 15/35), body itching (62.8%; 22/35), skin rash (32%; 11/35), anal discomfort and/or itching (28%; 10/35), and lower limb pain (23%; 8/35). For patients receiving BOC, the following complaints were reported: weight loss (46.1%; 5/13), body itching (38%; 5/13), and skin rash (15.4%; 2/13). These symptoms were prevalent in 46.1% (6/13) of patients treated with BOC, and 14.3% (5/35) of patients treated with TVR (Figure 3).

Discussion

A close association was observed between the predictive factors for response to treatment and the factors referred to in the literature as barriers to successful treatment. The higher prevalence of chronic hepatitis C observed for men, which was even higher than the reported hepatitis C prevalence for men in Brazil [5]; indicate a greater exposure of men to risk factors and an increased concern with their health. In addition, the prognosis of treatment outcome is worse for men than for women [17], making treatment more difficult. According to Poynard et al. [18], Tanaka et al. [19], Narciso-Schiavon et al. [20], women have not only fewer changes in liver biochemical tests, but also lower rates of fibrosis progression, and a lower risk of developing hepatocellular

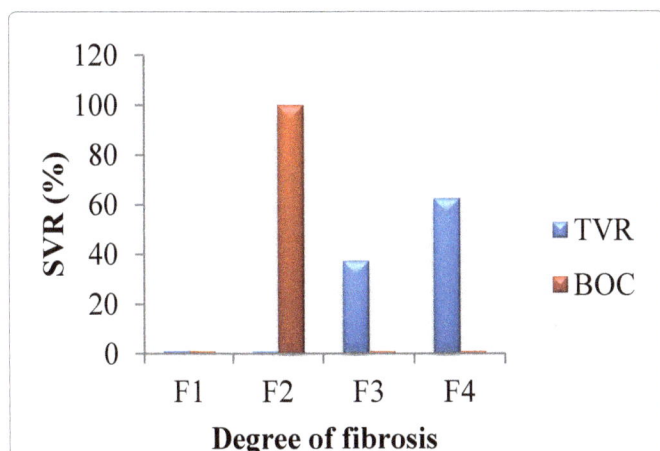

Figure 1: SVR for patients presenting different degree of fibrosis, and treated with TVR or BOC.

Variables	Patients selected for Antiviral Treatment		
	All patients	BOC	TVR
Effectiveness Variables			
Lead-in			
Patients number (n/%)	44/48 (91.6)	13/13 (100%)	31/35 (88.6)
Reduction of ≥1 log (n/%)	28/44 (64)	12/13 (90%)	16/27 (59.5)
Average log reduction (n/%)	-	2,9	1,9
RVR			
Rates (n/%)	32/48 (66.6)	5/13 (38.5)[1]	27/35 (77.1)[2]
SVR			
Related to Lead-in (n/%)	10/31 (32.25)	2/12 (16,6)	8/16 (50)
Related to RVR (n/%)	9/31 (29)	2/4 (50)	7/27 (25.9)
Global (n/%)	10/17 (58.8)	2/4 (50)	8/13 (61.5)
Intention-to-treat (n/%)	10/43 (23.25)	2/13 (15.4)	8/35 (22.8)
Other outcomes			
Breakthrough (n/%)	7/24 (29.2)	1/7 (14.3)	6/17 (35.3)
No answer (n/%)	3/24 (12.5)	1/7 (14.3)	2/17 (11.7)
Withdrawal due to adverse reactions (n/%)	14/24 (58.3)	5/7 (71.4)	9/17 (53)
Security variables			
Incidence of adverse reactions (n/ average per patient)	314/48 (6.5/ patient)	104/13 (8/ patient)	210/35 (6/ patient)
Anemia	28/48 (58.3)	8/13 (61.5)	20/35 (57.1)
Modification of dosage (n/%)	14/48 (29.2)	2/13 (15.4)	12/35 (34.3)
Use of erythropoietin (EPO) (n/%)	13/48 (27.1)	2/13 (15.4)	11/13 (84.6)
Use of packed red blood cells (n/%)	1/48 (2)	-	1/20 (5)
Leukopenia (n/%)	30/48 (62.5)	5/13 (38.5)	25/35 (72)
Neutropenia (n/%)	20/48 (41.6)	7/13 (54)	13/35 (13)
Use of Filgastrima (n/%)	15/33 (45.5)	5/15 (33,3)	10/15 (66,7)

Note: [1]Week 8 of BOC treatment; [2]Week 4 of TVR treatment

Table 2: Characteristics evaluated after the beginning of treatment.

carcinoma than men. It is believed that all of that is related to the protective effects of estrogen [21].

Regarding the election criteria adopted by the Brazilian guidelines, most patients presented advanced hepatic fibrosis (METAVIR F3 and F4), and hepatic fibrosis was detected in almost 71% of patients receiving TVR. These drugs were first available in 2013 to patient's monoinfected with genotype 1 and with advanced fibrosis (Metavir F3 and F4) or compensated hepatic cirrhosis (Child-Pugh ≤ 6) [6]. The

degree of liver fibrosis, particularly the presence of cirrhosis, is directly related to response to treatment [22]. Patients with F3 and, particularly, F4 fibrosis, usually present lower SVR rates. However, the success of treatment in these patients is essential to avoid complications, such as hepatocellular carcinoma, liver transplant, decompensation, and death [23].

The observed higher overall SVR rate in relapsing patients corroborates the findings by Mchutchison et al. [24] and Krawitt et al. [25], who observed that relapsing patients represented the group that best responded to retreatment. Null-responders are usually the most difficult group to retreat, because their VL never becomes negative, either during treatment or at the end of treatment [26]. The average pre-treatment VL (>600,000 IU/ml) observed in the present study was higher than the levels observed by McHutchison et al. [24] as good predictors of SVR. This may have contributed to the low response rate observed.

Out of the 64% (28/44) of patients presenting with VL decline ≥1 log during the lead-in period, only 35.7% (10/28) achieved SVR; none of the patients with no VL decline ≥1 log during the lead-in period achieved SVR. This is in accordance with previous reports. Despite being a good predictor of response to PI treatment [27-29], the lead-in SVR rates presented by this study were low and showed a significant association only for the treatments with TVR (p<0.05), in that the lead-in scheme is not mandatory. Nevertheless, SVR rates from the lead-in were low. According to Poordad [28], the lead-in is based upon the premise that if the viral load decreases in this 4-week period, relapse rates and treatment resistance may be reduced, while the no reduction of the viral load during this period requires more frequent viral load monitoring due to the increased risk of developing resistance.

Furthermore, in the lead-in period is possible to test adherence to pharmacotherapy and tolerance to peg IFN plus ribavirin before initiating the use of boceprevir, and patients who do not tolerate dual therapy should not be treated with the IP [28].

For patients treated with TVR, only 1 patient who achieved SVR (3.2%; 1/31) presented no prior positive RVR. For patients treated with BOC, all patients who achieved SVR previously, had a RVR. However, only a small proportion of patients who had a RVR achieved SVR, specifically, 26% (7/27) of patients treated with TVR, and 15.4% (2/13) treated with BOC. Although the RVR/SVR associations were not

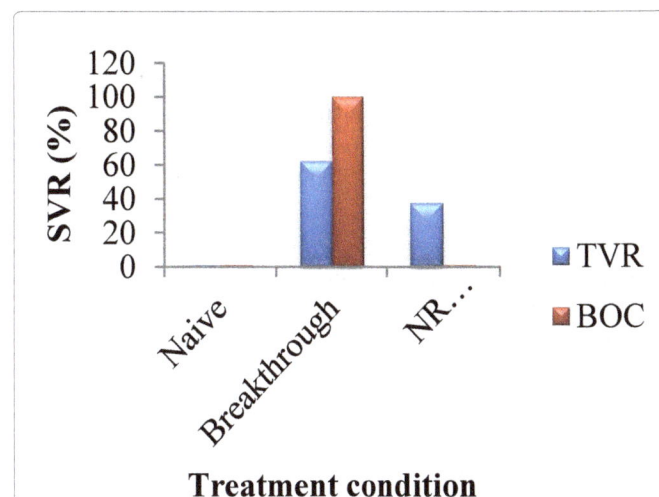

Figure 2: SVR in patients presenting different treatment condition, and treated with TVR or BOC.

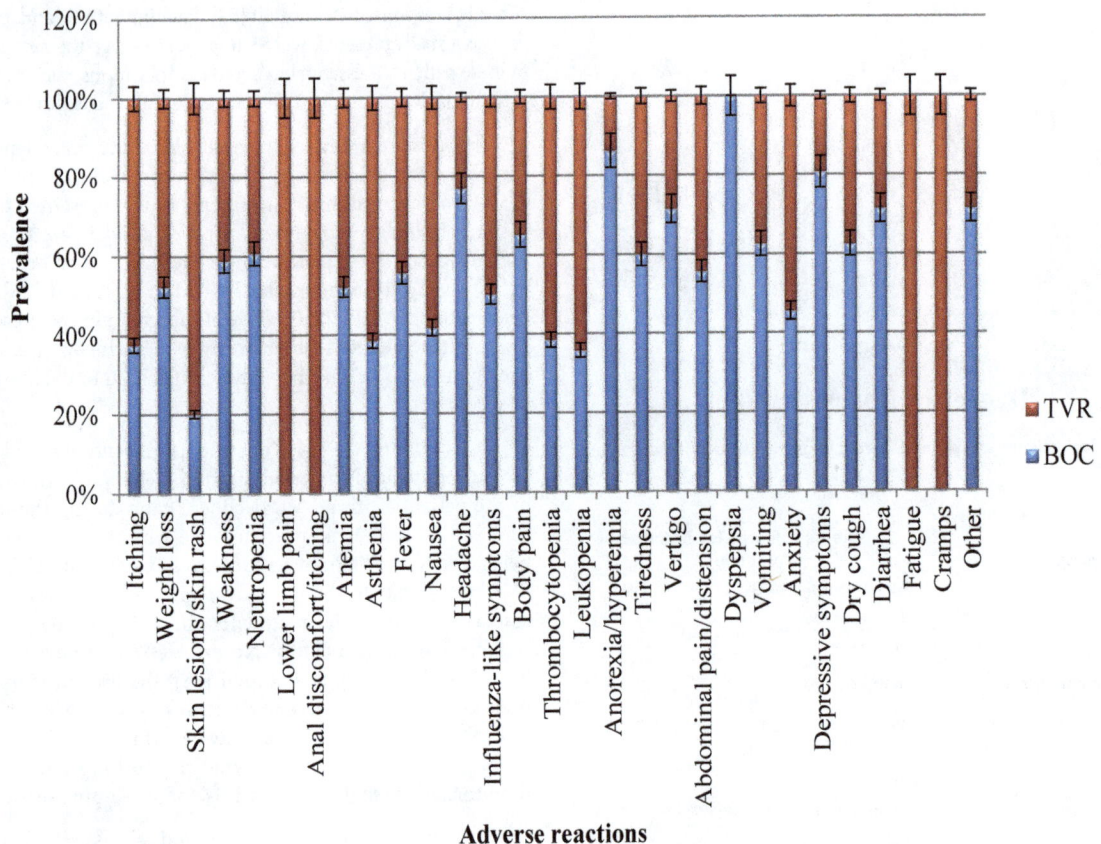

Figure 3: Frequency of the main adverse effects of triple therapy for hepatitis C.

significant in the present study, other studies highlight the predictive value of these variables [30,31].

As observed, patients that do not respond quickly to treatment (non-RVR) have decreased chances of achieving SVR. This indicates that the treatment for these patients should be reevaluated and, in selected cases, the period of treatment should be shortened to 24 weeks for TVR and 28 weeks for BOC, avoiding adverse reactions, for potentially curative treatments. The imposition of response-guided therapy (RGT) for the treatment with these drugs has already been highlighted in the literature, showing that it is possible to reduce the treatment time of certain patients within 24 weeks with peg IFN+RBV, without affecting SVR that is, in these cases the patient will not benefit from the 48-week treatment [28, 32]. In this way, RGT is essential to patient safety.

Adverse reactions were some of the causes for suspending treatment (24/48), and were slightly more frequent among cirrhotic patients [52.9% (9/17)] just as Vierling et al. [29]. The frequency of adverse reactions was considered serious in 41.4% (12/29) of patients with hepatic cirrhosis, and was even higher in the Model for End-stage Liver Disease (MELD) subgroup, when compared to patients without complications [33].

The main adverse reactions associated with treatment of the subjects were similar to those found in previous studies using PI [34]. However, the average frequency of side effects was higher than previously reported. Colombo et al. [35] described an average of two to

four adverse reactions experienced by patients receiving TVR, leading to suspension of treatment in 16% of cases. The average reported rate of treatment suspension due to adverse reactions during triple-drug therapy is 12.5% [24,27,31,36-37], lower than in the present study. However, Hezode et al. [38] highlighted the high incidence of adverse reactions associated with cirrhosis, including death and serious complications. The high incidence of adverse reactions observed in the present study were probably related to the severity of the hepatic disease, as most patients (62.5%; 30/48) presented with a high degree of fibrosis (F3, F4).

Anemia was more often prevalent with BOC than with TVR treatments, which is in agreement with the Comparative Assessment of Effectiveness of Antiviral Therapies in Hepatitis C (CMPASS) [39]. Anemia was the main adverse reaction associated with the use of BOC. However, the frequency of anemia in the present study was considerably higher than in previous studies and this is likely to be due to the higher proportion of cirrhotic patients. Hezode et al. [38] reported a frequency of anemia of approximately 50% for triple therapy with BOC, and 40% with TVR, lower than observed in the present study. The impact of anemia on SVR does not seem to be important in treatment-naive patients treated with TVR. However, it may have a negative impact in patients treated with BOC [38]. In the present study, no patients presenting with anemia during treatment with BOC achieved SVR.

The indication for EPO in patients treated with BOC was higher than in previous studies, with a reported variation of up to 46% [27-28,40]. This supports the conclusions of Hezode et al. [38] that the use of EPO does not seem to have a positive effect on SVR rates in studies with BOC. Blood transfusions were performed in 5% of patients, similar to previously reported rates (3-5%) [31-31,34,37]. It should be highlighted that in cirrhotic patients, in addition to the difficulty of managing anemia, the use of EPO (50.7%) and transfusions (12.1%) are more frequent [34]. Neutropenia occurrence was also higher than previously reported for both drug combinations. Although it is associated with the use of PEG-IFN [41], studies of treatments with BOC and TVR reported lower neutropenia values, approximately 25% for INF+RBV+BOC [40] and 37% for TVR [37].

The use of TVR caused anal discomfort and/or itching in 28% of patients, much higher than the 6% reported in the studies for drug approval [31,42]. In the present study, no association was observed between anal itching and BOC, in accordance with previous reports. The following adverse reactions were observed, with lower occurrence than previously reported: Dysgeusia [27-28,42], body itching in patients receiving TVR [31,42], skin lesions or rash [24,31,40], headaches [31,40], and depression and/or depressive symptoms [43]. It should be highlighted that the presence of neuropsychiatric symptoms is quite common during interferon treatment. Similar to in the present study, the psychiatric adverse reactions more often reported by patients are fatigue and sleep disturbance [43].

Because it is a combined drug treatment, the adverse reactions for each drug are cumulative and this is clinically challenging. Some of these reactions are quite significant, and may determine continuity of treatment, whereas others may affect the quality of life of patients. Fagundes et al. [44] reported that the transient decrease in quality of life in patients treated with TVR or BOC was higher than in patients treated with IFN+RBV double treatment. The authors highlighted that even subjective adverse reactions, such as fatigue, have a direct impact on patient quality of life, and decrease the chances of achieving SVR.

In addition to adverse reactions, the chances of achieving SVR may be lower in clinical practice and depend on several factors [45,46]. El-Zayadi [47], Loannou et al. [48] observed that a high percentage of patients with cirrhosis and comorbidities did not achieve SVR. Kim [49] suggested that medical conditions, such as diabetes, blood pressure, or thyroid diseases, should be optimized before commencing treatment. Namely, a careful selection of the individuals to be treated is crucial, particularly in patients presenting with advanced liver disease [50]. In a multidisciplinary context, studies have shown that the collaborative work of other professionals, such as the pharmacist, may prevent adverse reactions and improve the provision of adequate information associated with medications and pharmacotherapeutic management. Some of the pharmaceutical interventions still resulted in referral to other professionals (e.g., nutritionists, psychiatrists, dermatologists), which may have contributed to a higher SVR rate [51,52].

Differences in population characteristics may also account for the lower SVR rates observed among patients receiving BOC, compared to those of subjects involved in studies for drug registration. Sample selection is a weak point of randomized clinical assays, where samples are generally composed of white patients, presenting absent or minimal hepatic fibrosis, and include few null-responders to prior treatment. For example, in the REALIZE study [37], the percentage of white individuals was 93.5%. Fried et al. [17] indicated afro-descendant ethnicity as a predictor of bad prognosis. In ADVANCE [31], only 6% of patients were cirrhotic, comparable to the studies with BOC, where 11% of patients were METAVIR F3 or F4 [28] and 10% were cirrhotic [29]. These values were much higher in the present study (48%).

All these factors may have contributed to the different clinical outcomes observed in the large randomized studies used to define guidelines, and should be analyzed and considered in future drug therapy adjustments and individualization. The high incidence of adverse reactions and low SVR rate observed in the present study indicates that the processes of identification of the clinical indication for treatment and treatment monitoring should be reevaluated, particularly in eligible patients, and included in specific protocols.

Silva et al. [53] noted that, for non-urgent patients, it is prudent to wait for the inclusion of new treatment options into a single health system. Studies have shown that direct-acting antivirals have better cure rates, together with a reduction in the complexity of pharmacotherapy (e.g., reduction in the number of drugs, time of treatment, need for tests to monitor viral load, and incidence of adverse reactions) [54,55].

Although the results are expected, the data presented is relevant, and it does bring a great novelty to the evaluation of these treatments from the perspective of Brazil, thereby contributing to support and complement biomedical research and decisions in the field of hepatitis C drug policy.

Conclusion

The present results show that the treatment of chronic hepatitis C using triple therapy is not satisfactory, due to high rates of treatment suspension and several complications. These findings indicate the need for multidisciplinary care, and for review of therapeutic indications or even evaluating the anticipation of treatment of chronic carriers of hepatitis C, in order to achieve better results.

The availability of new direct antiviral drugs will negate the need for a therapy associated with significant adverse reactions and low therapeutic response.

Study limitations and future prospects

The study has some limitations, such as selection bias. This is not a prospective, randomized, controlled study, but a retrospective analysis of the results observed in the medical records of patients treated for hepatitis C. Single-centered research and the small sample size are also limiting. Therefore, loss of information wills likely results in extrapolation of data. However, this is a real life study that has allowed the evaluation of the use of medicines in various limiting conditions, such as biopsychosocial characteristics, encompassing all patients treated in the state, contributing to the medico-social and economic basis of regulatory activities and other decisions in the field of medication policy and treatment of hepatitis C.

Acknowledgements

The authors wish to acknowledge Fundação de Apoio à Pesquisa e Inovação Tecnológica do Estado de Sergipe (FAPITEC) for supporting funds- Grant Number 01920301343/2013-9.

References

1. Lin C, Kwoong AD, Perni RB (2006) Discovery and development of VX-950, a novel, covalent, and reversible inhibitor of hepatitis C virus NS3/4A serine protease. Infect. Disord. Drug Targets 6: 3-16.

2. Reesink HW, Zeuzem S, Weegink CJ, Forestier N, Vilet AV, et al. (2006) Rapid decline of viral RNA in hepatitis C patients treated with VX-950: a phase 1b, placebo-controlled, randomized study. Gastroenterology 13: 997-1002.

3. Ghany MG, Strader DB, Thomas DL, Seeff LB (2009) Diagnosis, Management, and Treatment of Hepatitis C: An Update. Hepatology 49:1335-1374.

4. Ghany MG, Nelson DR, Strader DB, Thomas DL, Seeff LB (2011) An update on treatment of genotype 1 chronic hepatitis C virus infection: 2011 practice guideline by the American Association for the Study of Liver Diseases. Hepatology 54: 1433-1444.

5. http://www.aids.gov.br/sites/default/files/anexos/publicacao/2012/51820/boletim_epidemiol_gico_hepatites_virais_2012_ve_12026.pdf

6. Brasil Ministério da Saúde (2013a) Secretaria de Vigilância em Saúde. Departamento de DST, Aids e Hepatites Virais. Suplemento 2 do Protocolo

Clínico e Diretrizes Terapêuticas (PCDT) para Hepatite Viral C e Coinfecções - genótipo 1 do HCV e fibrose avançada; Série A. Normas e Manuais Técnicos, Coordenação de Hepatites Virais - Brasília: Ministério da Saúde, p: 22.

7. Brasil Ministério da Saúde (2013b) Secretaria de Vigilância em Saúde. Protocolo Clínico e Diretrizes Terapêuticas para Hepatite Viral C e Coinfecções: manejo do paciente infectado cronicamente pelo genótipo 1 de HCV e fibrose avançada, Departamento de DST, Aids e Hepatites Virais - Brasília: Ministério da Saúde, p: 52.

8. Brasil Ministério da Saúde (2010) Secretaria de Vigilância em Saúde. Departamento de DST, Aids e Hepatites Virais. Relatório técnico do estudo de prevalência de base populacional das infecções pelos vírus das hepatites A, B e C nas capitais do Brasil: dados preliminares. Recife: Ministério da Saúde.

9. European Association for the Study of the Liver (EASL) (2014) Clinical Practice Guidelines: Management of hepatitis C virus infection. J Hepatol 60: 392-420.

10. Bersusa AAS, Bonfim JRA, Louvison MCP (2012) Inibidor de protease NS3/4 (boceprevir e telaprevir) associado aalfapeginterferona e ribavirina no tratamento de adultos com hepatite viral C crônica de genótipo 1. Parecertécnico-científico do Instituto de Saúde. São Paulo 14: 221-228.

11. Nogueira JBC, Sena LCS, Quintans JSS, Almeida JRGS, Franca AVC, et al. (2012) Side Effects of the Therapy With Peginterferon and Ribavirin in Chronic Hepatitis C: A Small Audit. J Pharm Pract 25: 85-88.

12. Kiser JJ, Burton JR Jr, Everson GT (2013) Drug-drug interactions during antiviral therapy for chronic hepatitis C. Nat. Rev. Gastroenterol. Hepatology 10: 596-606.

13. Brasil Ministério da Saúde (2011) Secretaria de Vigilância em Saúde. Boletim epidemiológico - hepatites virais. Ministério da Saúde. Departamento de DST, AIDS e hepatites virais. Ano II, n°1. Brasília: Ministério da Saúde.

14. McGowan CE, Fried MW (2012) Barriers to hepatitis C treatment. Liver Int 2: 151-156.

15. Garcia TJ, Lara PHS, Morimoto TP, Higasiaraguti M, Perejão AM, et al. (2012) Efeitos colaterais do tratamento da hepatite C no pólo aplicador do ABC. Rev Assoc Méd Brasil 58: 543-549.

16. Stenver DI (2008) Pharmacovigilance: What to do if you see an adverse reaction and the consequences. Eur J Radiol 66: 184-186.

17. Fried MW, Shiffman ML, Reddy RR, Smit C, Marinos C, et al. (2002) Peginterferon alfa-2a plus ribavirin for chronic hepatitis C virus infection. N Engl J Med 347: 975-982.

18. Poynard T, Ratziu V, Charlotte F, Goodman Z, McHutchison J, et al. (2001) Rates and risk factors of liver fibrosis progression in patients with chronic hepatitis C. J Hepatol 34: 730-739.

19. Tanaka J, Kumada H, Ikeda K, Chayama K, Mizui M, et al. (2003) Natural histories of hepatitis C virus infection in men and women simulated by the Markov model. J Med Virol 70: 378-386.

20. Narciso-Schiavon JL, Schiavon LL, Carvalho-Filho RJ, Freire FCF, Cardoso JR, et al. (2008) Anti-hepatitis C virus-positive blood donors: are women any different? Trans Med 18: 175-183.

21. Di Martino V, Rufat P, Boyer N, Renard P, Degos F, et al. (2001) The influence of human immunodeficiency virus coinfection on chronic hepatitis C in injection drug users: a long-term retrospective cohort study. Hepatology 34: 1193-1199.

22. Bruno S, Shiffman ML, Roberts SK, Gane EJ, Messinger D, et al. (2010) Efficacy and safety of peginterferon alfa-2a (40KD) plus ribavirin in hepatitis C patients with advanced fibrosis and cirrhosis. Hepatology 51: 388-397.

23. Morgan TR, Ghany MG, Kim HY, Snow KK, Schiffman ML, et al. (2010) Outcome of sustained virological responders with histological advanced chronic hepatitis C. Hepatology 52: 833-844.

24. McHutchison JG, Lawitz EJ, Shiffman ML, Muir AJ, Galler GW, et al. (2009) Peginterferon Alfa-2b or Alfa-2a with Ribavirin for Treatment of Hepatitis C Infection. N Engl J Med 362: 580-593.

25. Krawitt EL, Ashikaga T, Gordon SR, Ferrentino N, Ray MA, et al. (2005) New York New England Study Team. Peginterferon alpha-2b and ribavirin for treatment-refractory chronic hepatitis C. J Hepatol 43: 243-249.

26. Sociedade Brasileira de Infectologia (2008) I Consenso da Sociedade Brasileira de Infectologia para o Manuseio e Terapia da Hepatite C. Office Editora e Publicidade Ltda.

27. Bacon BR, Gordon S, Lawitz E, Marcellin P, Vierling JM, et al. (2011) Boceprevir for previously treated chronic HCV genotype 1 infection. N Engl J Med 364: 1207-1217.

28. Poordad F, McCone J, Bacon BR, Bruno S, Manns MP, et al. (2011) Boceprevir for untreated chronic HCV genotype 1 infection. N Engl J Med 364: 1195-1206.

29. Vierling JM, Zeuzem S, Poordad F, Bronowicki JP, Manns MP, et al. (2014) Safety and efficacy of boceprevir/peginterferon/ribavirin for HCV G1 compensated cirrhotics: Meta-analysis of 5 trials. J Hepatol 61: 200-209.

30. Harrington PR, Zeng W, Naeger LK (2012) Clinical relevance of detectable but not quantifiable hepatitis C virus RNA during boceprevir or telaprevir treatment. Hepatology 55: 1048-1057.

31. Jacobson IM, McHutchison JG, Dusheiko G, Di Bisceglie AM, Rajender K, et al. (2011) Telaprevir for previously untreated chronic hepatites C vírus infection. N Engl J Med 364: 2405-2416.

32. Sherman KE, Sulkowski MS, Zoulim F, Aberti A, Wei LJ, et al. (2011) Follow-up of SVR durability and viral resistance in patients with chronic hepatitis C treated with telaprevir-based regimens: Interim analysis of the EXTEND study. Hepatology 54: 1471.

33. Simmons B, Saleem J, Heath K, Cooke GS, Hill A (2015) Long-Term Treatment Outcomes of Patients Infected With Hepatitis C Virus: A Systematic Review and Meta-analysis of the Survival Benefit of Achieving a Sustained Virological Response. Clin Infect Dis 61: 730-740.

34. Hézode C (2012) Boceprevir and Telaprevir for the treatment of chronic hepatitis C: safety management in clinical practice. Liver Int 32: 32-38.

35. Colombo M, Strasser S, Moreno C, Abrao Ferreira P, Urbanek P, et al. (2014) Sustained virological response with telaprevir in 1078 patients with advanced hepatitis C: The international telaprevir access program. J Hepatol 61: 976-983.

36. McHutchison JG, Manns MP, Muir AJ, Terrault MD, Jacobson IM, et al. (2010) Telaprevir for previously treated chronic HCV infection. N Engl J Med 362: 1292-1303.

37. Zeuzem S, Andreone P, Stanislas P, Lawitz E, Diago M, et al. (2011) Telaprevir for retreatment of HCV infection. N Engl J Med 364: 2417-2428.

38. Hézode C, Fontaine H, Dorival C, Larrey D, Zoulim F, et al. (2013) Triple therapy in treatment-experience patients with HCV-cirrhosis in a multicenter cohort of the French. Early Access Programme. J Hepatol 59: 434-441.

39. Mauss S, Buti M, Ryder S, Isakov VA, Paraná R, et al. (2014) Virologic outcomes, adverse events, and health care costs associated with therapy of chronic HCV infection in clinical practice: results from the CMPASS study. Hepatology 1764: 1048A.

40. Manns M.P, Markova AA, Serrano BC, Cornberg M (2011) Phase III results of Boceprevir in treatment naïve patients with chronic hepatitis C genotype 1. Liver Int 32: 27-31.

41. Fried MW, Hadziyannis SJ (2004) Treatment of chronic hepatitis C infection with peg interferons plus ribavirin. Semin. Liver Dis 24: 47-54.

42. Kumada H, Toyota J, Okanoue T, Chayama, K, Tsoubouchi H, et al. (2012) Telaprevir with peginterferon and ribavirin for treatment-naive patients chronically infected with HCV of genotype 1 in Japn J Hepatol 56: 78-84.

43. Russo MW, Fried MW (2003) Side effects of therapy for chronic hepatitis C. Gastroenterology 124: 1711-1719.

44. Fagundes RN, Ferreira LEVV, Pace FHL (2015) Qualidade de vida relacionada à saúde em pacientes com hepatite C em terapia dupla e tripla. Rev Esc Enferm 49: 939-945.

45. Schott E, Schober A, Link R, Weber B, Rieke A, et al. (2014) Adverse events and co-medication: a comparison between dual and triple combination therapies in genotype 1 patients with chronic hepatitis C. BNG Study Group. J Hepatol 60: S313.

46. Strader DB, Wright T, Thomas DL, Seeff LB (2004) American Association for the Study of Liver Diseases. Diagnosis, management, and treatment of hepatitis C. Hepatology 39: 1147-1171.

47. El-Zayadi A (2009) Hepatitis C comorbidities affecting the course and response to therapy. World J Gastroenterol 15: 4993-4999.

48. Loannou GN, Beste LA, Gren PK (2014) Similar Effectiveness of Boceprevir and Telaprevir Treatment Regimens for Hepatitis C Virus Infection on the Basis of a Nationwide Study of Veterans. Clin Gastroenterol Hepatol 18: 1371-1380.

49. Kim AY (2013) Management algorithm for genotype 1 hepatitis C vírus. F1000 Prime Rep, pp: 5-24.

50. Maasoumy B, Port K, Markova AA, Serrano BC, Rogalska-Taranta M, et al. (2013). Eligibility and safety of triple therapy for hepatitis C: lessons learned from the first experience in a real world setting. PLoS ONE 8: 1-10.

51. Mohammad RA, Bulloch MN, Chan J, Deming P, Love B, et al. (2014) Provision of Clinical Pharmacist Services for Individuals With Chronic Hepatitis C Viral Infection. Pharmacotherapy 34: 1341-1354.

52. Rosa JA, Blatt CR, Bernardo NLMC, Silva R, Luiz MC, et al. (2010) Seguimento

farmacoterapêutico dos pacientes em tratamento da hepatite C crônica. Rev Bras Farm 91: 162-169.

53. Silva GF, Villela-Nogueira CA, Mello CEB, Soares EC, Coelho HS, et al. (2014) Peg interferon plus ribavirin and sustained virological response rate in HCV-related advanced fibrosis: a real life. Braz J Infect Dis 18: 48-52.

54. Londeix P, Forette C (2014) New treatments for hepatitis C virus. Strategies for achieving universal access. Medecins Du Monde.

55. Suthar AB, Harries AD (2015) A public health approach to hepatitis C control in low- and middle-income countries. PLoS Med 12: e1001795.

30

Trends in Antihypertensive Drug Use in Spanish Primary Health Care (1990-2012)

Cáceres MC[1], Moyano P[1], Fariñas H[1], Cobaleda J[1,2], Pijierro A[1], Dorado P[1]and LLerena A[1*]

[1]CICAB Clinical Research Centre, Extremadura University Hospital and Medical School, Badajoz, Spain
[2]Ciudad Jardin Primary Health Care Center.SES Servicio Extremeño de Salud, Badajoz, Spain

Abstract

Objective: This study aimed to describe the use of antihypertensive in Extremadura (Spain) from 1990 to 2012 and its economic impact.

Method: Information on antihypertensive drug (ATC C02, C03, C07, C08, C09) utilization was obtained from the community pharmacy sales figures reimbursed by the Health System of Extremadura (Spain). Data were expressed in Defined Daily Dose (DDD) and DDD per 1000 inhabitants per day (DHD).

Results: Antihypertensive consumption in Extremadura increased from 67.1 DHD in 1990 to 315.2 in 2012 (an increase of 3.7 times). Agents acting on the Renin-Angiotensin System (C09) are responsible for 75% of the total increase. Since 2007 the use of Angiotensin II antagonist increased over ACE inhibitors.

Conclusions: The consumption of antihypertensive drugs in Extremadura increased remarkably in the last 23 years. In the last years the use of angiotensin II antagonist drugs is having a significant economic impact.

Keywords: Antihypertensives; Drug use; Pharmacoepidemiology; Primary care

Introduction

Hypertension is currently considered a major public health problem because of its importance as a cardiovascular risk factor. Worldwide, high blood pressure is estimated to cause 7.5 million deaths, about 12.8% of the total of all annual deaths [1]. Blood pressure levels have been shown to be positively and progressively related to the risk for stroke and coronary heart disease [2]. In addition to coronary heart diseases and stroke, complications of high blood pressure include heart failure, peripheral vascular disease, renal impairment, retinal haemorrhage and visual impairment [3].

The 33.3% of adult population in Spain suffer from hypertension [4]. Moreover, 1 out of every 4 deaths and 1 out of every 2.5 deaths caused by cardiovascular disease is related to high blood pressure [5].

A great number of national and international guidelines for hypertension treatment have been published. The JNC 7 guideline recommended diuretics as first-line treatment in hypertension [6]. Therefore the current Guidelines advise that diuretics (including thiazides, chlorthalidone and indapamide), beta-blockers, calcium antagonists, Angiotensin-Converting Enzyme (ACE) inhibitors and angiotensin receptor blockers are all suitable for the initiation and maintenance of antihypertensive treatment, either as monotherapy or in some combinations [7].

The European guideline, on the other hand, suggests that unless a special indication exists, any of the five antihypertensive classes can be used as first-line treatment [8]. Although the number of prescriptions for Diuretics (Ds) and B-Blockers (BBs) is increasing, and for Calcium-Channel Blockers (CCBs) is decreasing, in most countries the most frequently antihypertensive classes prescribed are still Angiotensin-Converting Enzyme Inhibitors (ACEIs) or CCBs [9-15]. However, there is a considerable variation in the antihypertensive drug classes used in different countries [9-20].

The present study aimed to analyze the overall use and changes in the prescribing pattern of antihypertensive drugs by Family Medicine physicians in the Spanish region of Extremadura from 1990 to 2012, its compliance with guidelines, and its economic impact.

Method

In order to study the use of antihypertensive drugs in Extremadura, annual data from 1 January 1990 to 31 December 2012 about the prescribing of antihypertensive drugs were collected from the community pharmacy sales figures reimbursed by the Spanish Extremadura Health System (SES), which covers almost 100% of the Extremadura population (1.100.000 inhabitants).

All the antihypertensive drugs marketed in Spain and listed in the Anatomic Therapeutic Chemical (ATC) classification system were studied. The ATC studied groups studied are the followings: C02 [Antihypertensives]; C03 [Diuretics]; C07 [Beta blocking agents]; C08 [Calcium channel blockers]; C09 [Renin angiotensin system], including: C09A (Angiotensin-converting enzyme inhibitors (ACE inhibitors), C09B (ACE inhibitors, combinations), C09C (Angiotensin II antagonists), C09D (Angiotensin II antagonists, combinations).

Drug consumption figures were expressed as the number of Defined Daily Doses (DDD) per 1000 inhabitants per Day of Treatment (DHD), using the DDD values proposed by WHO [21].

Total costs were estimated by multiplying the number of sold

*Corresponding author: LLerena A, CICAB, Clinical Research Centre, Extremadura University Hospital and Medical School, Badajoz 06080, Spain, E-mail: allerena@unex.es

packages of each product by the price of each one. Cost per day was calculated by dividing the total cost by the total DDD consumed for the active ingredient or subgroup considered.

Study limitations: firstly, data were collected by auditing drug sales in all the pharmacies of Extremadura, which allowed us to estimate the prescription of antihypertensive drugs but not their real use; [22] second, the DDD methodology allows the possibility of analyzing trends of consumption over the years, but does not allow individual level analyses regarding the real DDD received by a patient daily.

Results

Antihypertensive consumption in Extremadura increased fivefold between 1990 and 2012 (Figure 1). It is estimated that in 1990 there were 73,781 people in treatment with an antihypertensive drug, increasing to 346,726 people in 2012.

Subgroup C09 (agents acting on the renin-angiotensin system) is responsible for 75% of the total increase (Figure 1).

Since 2007 the use of ARBs (C09C+C09D) increased over ACE inhibitors (C09A+C09B) (Figure 2).

The ranking of the most frequently prescribed renine-angyotensine drugs (C09) in the study period is shown in Table 1.

Total spending on antihypertensives (C02, C03, C07, C08 and C09)

1990		2000		2012	
Drug	%	Drug	%	Drug	%
Captopril	49.6	Enalapril	31.3	Enalapril	18.3
Enalapril	47.9	Candesartan	11.5	Candesartan	14.1
Captopril+diuretics	2.4	Ramipril	7.0	Ramipril	12.2
		Valsartan	6.6	Valsartan	8.2
		Olmesartan	5.3	Valsartan+diuretics	4.8

Table 1: Active ingredients most frequently prescribed in selected years, expressed in percentage of the total of the renin-angiotensin system drugs (C09). Combinations are fixed.

in 2012 was 42.5 million euros, of which 75.9% corresponds to the drug spending of the renin-angiotensin system (C09). Within this group, during the 2003-2012 spending on ACE inhibitors (C09A+C09B) decreased from 9.8 to 4.5 million euros, while in ARBs (C09C+C09D) increased from 22.1 to 27.0 million euros.

Discussion

There was an increase in the use of antihypertensive drugs in the study period, the same result was observed in similar studies performed in Spain [23-27]. This increase could be due to an increase in the number of people on antihypertensive treatment. It should be noted that antihypertensive drugs, except the C02 group, are not only used in hypertension, but also for treatment of other diseases such as diabetes, nephropathy, ischemic heart disease, peripheral arterial disease or stroke. Furthermore, the criteria for blood pressure control throughout the study period became more restrictive, considering as normal blood pressure values ever lower [6]. Therefore, it is increasingly common to find patients taking more than one drug, and also patients that at the beginning of the study period would be considered normotensive, at period end would not be [6]. Other possible causes for the increase in the prescription of antihypertensives may be the aging population, changes in lifestyle, a better knowledge of the condition by the population, the implementation of Health Programmes at Primary Care. Furthermore must be taking into account the important role that have the implementation on recent years of the ambulatory blood pressure monitoring and home blood pressure monitoring, these measures have facilitated the diagnosis and the management of hypertension, and have strengthened its prognostic value.

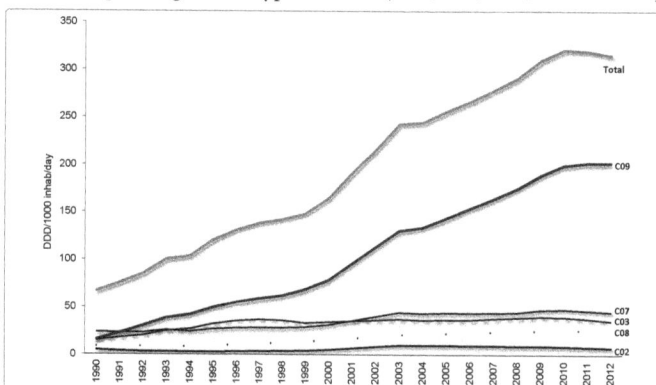

Figure 1: Antihypertensive drugs consumption in Extremadura, Spain (1990-2012).(C02 Antihypertensives; C03 Diuretics; C07 Beta-blockers; C08 Calcium channel blockers; C09 Agents acting on the renin-angiotensin system).

Study data shows that the total use of antihypertensives in Extremadura is higher than in other studies performed in Spain [25-27]. Extremadura is among the regions with higher rates of cardiovascular morbidity and mortality [28]and a high incidence of diabetic nephropathy and microalbuminuria [29,30] diseases that are related with the level of control of cardiovascular risk factors, particularly with high blood pressure. However, control of blood pressure in Extremadura is similar to the rest of Spain, 36.7% [31,32].

This rising use of antihypertensive over the past 20 years is not exclusive to Spain, also occurred in other European countries [33,34].

The increase in total use of antihypertensive drugs is mainly due to increased consumption of C09 group. The dramatic increase could be due to greater efficiency and tolerability of this group, although up today, clinical trials have failed to demonstrate greater efficacy and lower mortality of this group respect to others. Furthermore, it must be taken into account the possible influence of pharmaceutical companies. The C09 group is the most widely group used also in Europe, as it is shown in different European studies [33,34,38-40]. Within this group, the ACE inhibitors were the antihypertensive drugs most commonly used until 2007, at that moment they started to be replaced by ARBs. In a similar study published, in Murcia region the same fact is observed

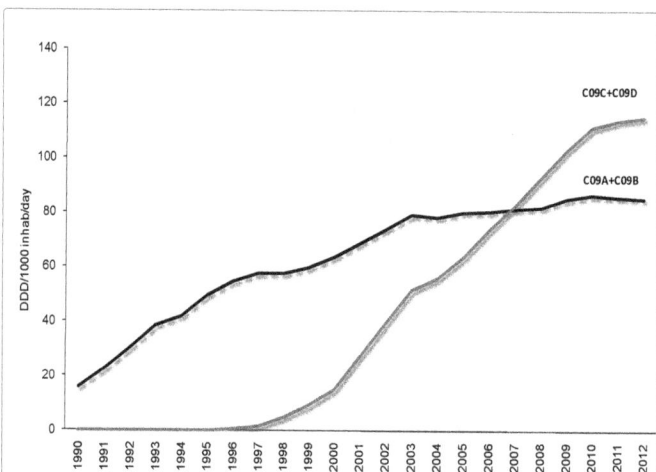

Figure 2: Angiotensin II antagonist (ARBs) and ACE inhibitors consumption in Extremadura, Spain (1990-2012).

since 2005 [27]. However Spanish data released shows that until 2006 the ACE inhibitors were the antihypertensive most prescribed [24].

Captopril was the active ingredient most widely used in 1990; from 1991 to the end of the study period, enalapril remained as the most active ingredient prescribed, even after the marketing of ACE inhibitor. This trend is also observed in other studies published [25,26]. Considering the causes of high consumption of enalapril, it should be noted that enalapril has a good tolerability and a long half-life which allows an adequate blood pressure control with a single daily dose; it is also worth noting that as its action mechanism was better known, enalapril began to be used in the treatment of other diseases such as heart failure in normotensive patients and the prevention of diabetic nephropathy in diabetic patients.

From the point of view of therapeutic recommendations, therapeutic guidelines agree on D_s as first line treatment followed by BB_s. Since the commercialization of ACE inhibitors and CCBs, they became part of the first-line treatment. Since 1997, the JNC VI, recommended by the first time ARBs only when the ACE inhibitor is not tolerated, but in 2003, both the JNC VII and the ESH-ESC 1, added ARBs as first-line treatment [6-8,35-37].

Despite all the measures that were taken in recent years to reduce drug spending, the significant increase in the use of antihypertensive drugs in the study period generated a major economic impact on the healthcare system, being due largely to the high cost of ARBs. This fact has been observed in other studies [24,27,33,40].

References

1. World Health Organization (2009) Global health risks: mortality and burden of disease attributable to selected major risks. Geneva, Switzerland.

2. Whitworth JA. World Health Organization, International Society of Hypertension Writing Group (2003) 2003 World Health Organization (WHO)/International Society of Hypertension (ISH) statement on management of hypertension. J Hypertens 21: 1983-1992.

3. Williams B, Poulter NR, Brown MJ, Davis M, McInnes GT, et al. (2004) British Hypertension Society guidelines for hypertension management 2004 (BHS-IV): summary.BMJ 328: 634-640.

4. Banegas JR, Graciani A, de la Cruz-Troca JJ, León-Muñoz LM, Guallar-Castillón P, et al. (2012) Achievement of cardiometabolic goals in aware hypertensive patients in Spain: a nationwide population-based study. Hypertension 60: 898-905.

5. Banegas Banegas JR, Rodríguez-Artalejo F, de la Cruz Troca JJ, de Andrés Manzano B, del Rey Calero J (1999) Hypertension-related mortality and arterial pressure in Spain. Med Clin (Barc) 112: 489-494.

6. Chobanian AV, Bakris GL, Black HR, Cushman WC, Green LA, et al. (2003) Seventh report of the Joint National Committee on Prevention, Detection, Evaluation, and Treatment of High Blood Pressure. Hypertension 42: 1206-1252.

7. Mancia G, Fagard R, Narkiewicz K, Redon J, Zanchetti A, et al. (2013) 2013 ESH/ESC Guidelines for the management of arterial hypertension: The Task Force for the management of arterial hypertension of the European Society of Hypertension (ESH) and of the European Society of Cardiology (ESC). J Hypertens 31:1281-357.

8. European Society of Hypertension-European Society of Cardiology Guidelines Committee (2003) 2003 European Society of Hypertension-European Society of Cardiology guidelines for the management of arterial hypertension. J Hypertens 21: 1011-1053.

9. Chamontin B, Poggi L, Lang T, Ménard J, Chevalier H, et al. (1998) Prevalence, treatment, and control of hypertension in the French population: data from a survey on high blood pressure in general practice, 1994. Am J Hypertens 11: 759-762.

10. Siegel D, Lopez J, Meier J, Cunningham F (2001) Changes in the pharmacologic treatment of hypertension in the Department of Veterans Affairs 1997–1999: decreased use of calcium antagonists and increased use of beta-blockers and thiazide diuretics. Am J Hypertens 14: 957-962.

11. Sturani A, Degli Esposti E, Serra M, Ruffo P, Valpiani G; PANDORA Study Group (2002) Assessment of antihypertensive drug use in primary care in Ravenna, Italy, based on data collected in the PANDORA project. Clin Ther 24: 249-259.

12. Esposti LD, Baio GL, Valpiani G, Buda S, Sturani A, et al. (2002) Cost allocation in antihypertensive drug therapies. Expert Rev Pharmacoecon Outcomes Res 2: 419-426.

13. Rotmensch HH, Mendelevitch L, Silverberg DS, Liron M (1996) Prescribing pattern of antihypertensive drugs in the community. J Hum Hypertens 10 Suppl 3: S169-172.

14. Siddiqui S, Ogbeide DO, Karim A, Al-Khalifa I (2001) Hypertension control in a community health centre at Riyadh, Saudi Arabia. Saudi Med J 22: 49-52.

15. Crucitti A, Cecchi E, Gensini GF, Simone I, Conti A, et al. (2000) Use of antihypertensive drugs in the Italian hospitals. GIFA group. Gruppo Italiano di Farmacoepidemiologia nell'Anziano. Pharmacol Res 41: 249-253.

16. Wallenius S, Kumpusalo E, Pärnänen H, Takala J (1998) Drug treatment for hypertension in Finnish primary health care. Eur J Clin Pharmacol 54: 793-799.

17. Walley T, Duggan AK, Haycox AR, Niziol CJ (2003) Treatment for newly diagnosed hypertension: patterns of prescribing and antihypertensive effectiveness in the UK. J R Soc Med 96: 525-531.

18. Gasse C, Stieber J, Döring A, Keil U, Hense HW (1999) Population trends in antihypertensive drug use: results from the MONICA Augsburg Project 1984 to 1995. J Clin Epidemiol 52: 695-703.

19. Al Khaja KA, Sequeira RP (2006) Pharmacoepidemiology of antihypertensive drugs in primary care setting of Bahrain between 1998 and 2000. Pharmacoepidemiol Drug Saf 15: 741-748.

20. Jassim al Khaja KA, Sequeira RP, Wahab AW, Mathur VS (2001) Antihypertensive drug prescription trends at the primary health care centres in Bahrain. Pharmacoepidemiol Drug Saf 10: 219-227.

21. Uchida N, Chong MY, Tan CH, Nagai H, Tanaka M, et al. (2007) International study on antidepressant prescription pattern at 20 teaching hospitals and major psychiatric institutions in East Asia: Analysis of 1898 cases from China, Japan, Korea, Singapore and Taiwan. Psychiatry Clin Neurosci 61: 522-528.

22. Jones G (2003) Prescribing and taking medicines. BMJ 327: 819.

23. Jabary NS, Herrero AM, Gonzalez JA (2000) The use of antihypertensive therapy in Spain (1986-1994). Am J Hypertens 13: 607-610.

24. García del Pozo J, Ramos Sevillano E, de Abajo FJ, Mateos Campos R (2004) Use of antihypertensive drugs in Spain (1995-2001). Rev Esp Cardiol 57: 241-249.

25. Prieto M, de Abajo FJ, Montero D, Martín-Serrano G, Madurga M, et al. (1998) Use of antihypertensive drugs in Spain, 1985-1995. Med Clin (Barc) 110: 247-253.

26. Montero D, García J, De Abajo FJ (2009) Use of Antihypertensive Drugs in Spain, 1992-2006. Essential Information System for Therapy and Health 1-14.

27. Ruiz JC, Ariza MA, Aguilera B, Leal M, Gómez R, et al. (2012) Analysis of the rational use of anti-hypertensives in the Murcia (Spain) region]. Aten Primaria 44: 272-279.

28. Comprehensive Plan for cardiovascular diseases of Extremadura. Merida: Junta de Extremadura (2007).

29. Robles NR, Cid MC, Roncero F, Pizarro JL, Sánchez-Casado E, et al. (1996) Incidence of diabetic nephropathy in the province of Badajoz along the period from 1990 to 1994. An Med Interna 13: 572-575.

30. Roberto Robles N, Velasco J, Mena C, Angulo E, Garrote T; MICREX Study (2006) Microalbuminuria in diabetic and hypertensive patients: a study of 979 patients. Med Clin (Barc) 127: 761-764.

31. Marcos G, Robles NR, Barroso S, Sánchez Muñoz-Torrero JF (2009) Blood pressure control in Extremadura control. Results from a study on Risk Control Factors in Extremadura (CHEST study). Hipertens Vasc Risk 26: 14-19.

32. Llisterri Caro JL, Rodríguez Roca GC, Alonso Moreno FJ, Banegas Banegas JR, González-Segura Alsina D, et al. (2008) Control of blood pressure in Spanish hypertensive population attended in primary health-care. PRESCAP 2006 Study. Med Clin (Barc) 130: 681-687.

33. Furtado C, Pinto M (2006) Anti-hypertensive drug utilization in Continental Portugal (1999-2004). Rev Port Cardiol 25: 273-292.

34. Rønning M, Sakshaug S, Strøm H, et al. (2009) Drug Consumption in Norway 2004-2008. Norwegian Institute of Public Health, Norway.

35. (1997) The sixth report of the Joint National Committee on prevention, detection, evaluation, and treatment of high blood pressure. Arch Intern Med 157: 2413-2446.

36. Mancia G, De Backer G, Dominiczak A, Cifkova R, Fagard R, et al. (2007) 2007 Guidelines for the Management of Arterial Hypertension: The Task Force for the Management of Arterial Hypertension of the European Society of Hypertension (ESH) and of the European Society of Cardiology (ESC). J Hypertens 25: 1105-1187.

37. Mancia G, Laurent S, Agabiti-Rosei E, Ambrosioni E, Burnier M, et al. (2009) Reappraisal of European guidelines on hypertension management: a European Society of Hypertension Task Force document. J Hypertens 27: 2121-2158.

38. Simó Miñana J (2012) Use of prescription drugs in Spain and Europe. Aten Primaria 44: 335-347.

39. Stolk P, Van Wijk BL, Leufkens HG, Heerdink ER (2006) Between-country variation in the utilization of antihypertensive agents: Guidelines and clinical practice. J Hum Hypertens 20: 917-922.

40. Vara L, Sangrador A, Muñoz P, Sanz S (2004) Use of antihypertensive agents in Cantabria, Spain [1995-2002]: discrepancy with the published evidence. Gac Sanit 18: 406-408.

31

Use of Psychotropics and Drug-Drug Interactions in Oncology: Reflections from a Study in a Portuguese Psycho-Oncology Unit

Oliveira L* and Santos Z

Department of Psychiatry, Psycho-Oncology Unit, Coimbra University Hospital Centre, Coimbra, Portugal

Abstract

Introduction: Psychopharmacological treatment is an important tool of the multidimensional approach in oncologic setting but cancer patient´s susceptibility to drug-drug interactions may pose them at risk.

Objective: To describe the use of psychotropics in patients referred to a psycho-oncology unit and to point out potential and clinical relevant drug-drug interactions in this context.

Methods: Descriptive study of a sample of patients referred for the first time to the Psycho-Oncology Unit of Coimbra University Hospital Centre, between April and December 2013. A retrospective collection of the socio-demographic, clinical and prescription data was made by consulting clinical processes.

Results: From the sample of 110 patients, 51,8% of the patients were already taking some psychotropic drug and 91,9% were on antineoplastic medication at the time of the psycho-oncology appointment. Among the psychotropic medication, almost all were benzodiazepines and antidepressants. Psychotropics can cause potential interactions with antineoplastic medication administered in cancer patients. Some pharmacological agents have more potential to cause drug-drug interactions.

Conclusions: Prescription of psychotropic medication by the oncological team is common and cancer patients usually take several drugs at the same time. This study outlines the importance of promoting scientific research on drug-drug interactions in psycho-oncology and a closer collaboration between oncology and psychiatry in order to reduce the risk of drug-drug Interactions, to increase its awareness and to adequately prescribe a psychopharmacologic treatment for each patient.

Keywords: Psychotropic drugs; Psycho-oncology; Drug-drug interactions; Antineoplastic agents

Abbreviations

ADs: Antidepressants; ANs: Antineoplastic Agents; APs: Antipsychotics; BDZ: Benzodiazepines; DDIs: Drug-Drug Interactions; NaSSA: Noradrenergic and Specific Serotonergic Antidepressants; SDRI: Selective Dopamine Reuptake Inhibitor; SSRIs: Selective Serotonin Reuptake Inhibitors; TMX: Tamoxifen

Introduction

Psychotropic medication represents a significant tool in the treatment of psychiatric symptoms or disorders cancer related that affects about half of the cancer patients [1]. Adjustment disorder and major depression are the most frequent in oncology. If undiagnosed and untreated, result in poor quality of life and worst cancer prognosis, which can contribute to exacerbate demoralization syndrome. Furthermore, 80% of the suicides in oncological population are committed by patients with depressive syndrome [2]. Pain, cognitive impairment and acute confusional states are common in advances states of the disease and also increase risk for suicide [3].

In the last decades, psychopharmacological treatment has been promoted in a multidisciplinary approach to cancer care in order to treat psychiatric disorders and improve cancer patients' quality of life [4]. Advances in psycho-oncology research have also shown the efficacy of psychotropic drugs as adjuvant treatment of cancer-related symptoms, such as pain, hot flushes, pruritus, nausea and vomiting, fatigue, and cognitive impairment [5]. The use of psychotropic medication in cancer patients has been studied in few oncological centres or services. In one of the first reports, data indicated that about half of patients were treated with psychotropic drugs. Hypnotics were the most frequently prescribed (48%), while antidepressants (ADs) were the least (1%) [6]. Another study reported that antipsychotic (61%) and hypnotics (56%) were the most prescribed drugs and ADs were used in only a minority (10%) [7]. The use of antipsychotics was a lot related to the management of physical symptoms like nausea and vomiting. A later study [8] investigated the use of psychotropic medication in patients referred to a psycho-oncology service and found that over half (55.5%) patients were already on psychotropic drugs at referral, mainly minor tranquilisers (51%) and antidepressants (24%); 22% were on more than one drug; 46% had been prescribed by the oncology team. A more recent study of cancer patients and matched-controls found that the prevalence of emotional distress was higher among cancer patients (15.6% versus 1.4%) and that the volume and duration of psychotropic drug prescriptions was correspondingly higher among cases than controls [9].

Cancer patients are likely to receive psychotropic agents but patients who concurrently receive psychotropic and antineoplastic agents are at high risk of drug–drug interactions (DDIs), which are thought to be

---

*Corresponding author: Oliveira L, Department of Psychiatry, Psycho-Oncology Unit, Coimbra University Hospital Centre, Coimbra, Portugal, E-mail: lucilia.guimaraes@gmail.com

the cause of approximately 20–30% of all adverse drug reactions [10]. In order to reduce the adverse outcomes of DDIs, potential interactions between anti-cancer drugs and ADs should be identified before these drugs are prescribed and administered in cancer patients.

To our knowledge, this study is the first that sets out to portray the practice in the psychotropic treatment of ambulatory patients referred to a psycho-oncology unit in a large cancer center in Portugal. Recognising the importance of psychopharmacological treatment in cancer patients but also cancer patient´s susceptibility to drug interactions, the aims of our study were to describe the use of psychotropic medication in patients referred to a psycho-oncology unit and to point out potential and clinical relevant drug-drug interactions in this clinical context.

Material and Methods

Patients referred for the first time to the psycho-oncology unit of the oncology day-hospital from Coimbra University Hospital Centre over a 9-month period, from of April to December 2013 were selected. This psycho-oncology unit only admitted cancer outpatients receiving oncological treatment at the oncology day-hospital and who were attending the oncology consultation at the moment of the psychiatric assessment. A descriptive and retrospective study was elaborated by consulting hospital records for each patient. Socio-demographic, clinical and therapeutic data were collected.

Results

A total of 110 oncological patients were referred to the psycho-oncology consultation during the 9-month period. Main demographic and clinical characteristics of the sample are shown in Table 1.

The most common causes for psychiatric assessment were addressed by the oncology team as 'depressive symptoms', 'anxiety', 'emotional problems' and 'insomnia'. In this sample, 51,8% of the patients were already taking some psychotropic medication at the time of the psycho-oncology appointment (Table 2). Drugs were most prescribed by the oncologist or another physician of the oncology team (80,6%). Among the psychotropic medication, almost all were anxiolytics (benzodiazepines) and/or ADs. With respect to the first class of the two pharmacological agents, short acting benzodiazepines (especially alprazolam and lorazepam) were the most prescribed; in the case of antidepressants, selective serotonin reuptake inhibitors (SSRIs), especially sertraline and paroxetine, were the most common physician's option. Following psychiatric assessment, the most common psychiatric diagnoses were adjustment disorder (58,6%) and depressive disorder (41,4%). In addition, some pharmacotherapeutic change occurred for the majority of patients, particularly with the introduction of an antidepressant, the increasing dosage of the antidepressant, drug discontinuation or the switch to a different pharmacological agent. Regarding oncological treatment, almost all patients (91,9%) were on chemotherapy cancer treatment and antineoplastic agents (ANs) used by the patients are listed on Table 3.

Discussion

The result that almost half patients referred to psycho-oncology unit had metastatic disease and received cancer diagnosis by one year is congruent to what has been reported by some studies. It seems that there is a tendency to prescribe psychotropic medications and/or refer patients to liaison psychiatry or psycho-oncology in the advanced phase or even palliative phase of cancer, as physical and psychological symptoms get worse and physicians feel they have no more to offer to their patients [11,12].

Psychiatric assessment was requested mainly because psychological distress and psychopathology was noted by physicians from the oncology team, which is a positive finding suggesting awareness about psychological/psychiatric morbidity. Our study found that more than half of patients were already taking some psychotropic medication at the psycho-oncology appointment, which is higher than the one found in other studies [6-8] and suggests that pharmacotherapy is being an increasingly intervention tool.

After psychiatric assessment, increasing the dosage or switching to another drug where the most frequent changes. In fact, correct use of psychotropic medication demands a careful evaluation, particularly concerning patient´s physical condition, clinical and psychiatric symptoms, drug-drug interactions and side effects.

Antidepressants

In our work we found a quite higher percentage (59,6%) of antidepressant use compared to what was reported by previous studies [6-8]. This might be related to many factors: more awareness to psychological distress from the oncological team; the development of new classes of ADs with a better tolerability and safety profiles; increasing scientific evidence showing that ADs, irrespective of their class, are more effective than placebo in treating depression in cancer patients [13]. Also the fact that recent ADs with sedative and increasing appetite properties, like mirtazapine, are useful and adequate to manage the sleep disturbance and anorexia, which are common symptoms in cancer patients [14,15]. Somnolence, hyperphagia and weight gain side effects may be attributed in part to the antihistaminic activity of mirtazapine at low doses.

Number of patients, *n*	110
Gender (%)	
Female	59,1
Male	40,9
Age (years)	
Mean	54
Min-Max	23-82
Civil status (%)	
Single	13,6
Married	69,1
Widow	11,8
Divorced	5,5
Cancer type (%)	
Gastro-intestinal	24,5
Breast	20,9
Lung	17,3
Hematological	12,7
Gynecological	8,2
Brain	4,5
Other	11,8
Clinical Stage (%)	
Advanced/metastatic	47,3
Local	52,7
Diagnosis date (%)	
>1 year	40,9
<1 year	59,1
Past psychiatric history (%)	
Yes	13,6
No	86,4

Table 1: Demographic and clinical characteristics of patients.

Patients taking psychotropics (%)	51,8
Anxiolytics (%)	90,5
Alprazolam	
Lorazepam	
Other	
Antidepressants (%)	59,6
SSRI	
NaSSA	
SDRI	
Other	
Antipsychotics (%)	8,2

Table 2: Psychotropic drugs before referral.

Alkylating agents	Cyclophosphamide, Procarbazine, Temozolomide
Antimetabolites	Capecitabine, Cytarabine, Fluorouracil, Methotrexate, Pemetrexed
Antimicrotubules	Docetaxel, Vinblastine, Vincristine
Hormone agonists/antagonists	Anastrozole, Cyproterone, Fulvestrant, Goserelin, Leuprolide, Octreotide, Tamoxifen
Platinum compounds	Cisplatin, Carboplatin, Oxaliplatin
Topoisomerase inhibitors	Doxorubicin, Epirubicin, Etoposide, Irinotecan
Tyrosine kinase inhibitors and monoclonal antibodies	Bevacizumab, Bortezomib, Erlotinib, Rituximab, Trastuzumab

Table 3: Antineoplastic agents used by the patients on chemotherapy treatment.

Psycho-oncology research indicates that ADs should be reserved for patients with clinical depression, moderate or severe in intensity, otherwise their use does not appear to have any significant benefit over placebo [16], and cancer patients with depressive-like symptoms as part of an adjustment disorder seem to respond weakly to ADs [17].

Among the new classes of ADs there are the serotonin reuptake inhibitors (SSRIs) (e.g., fluoxetine, paroxetine, sertraline, citalopram and escitalopram), selective serotonin and noradrenergic reuptake inhibitors (SNRIs) (e.g. venlafaxine, duloxetine), selective noradrenergic and dopamine reuptake inhibitors (NDRIs) (e.g., bupropion), and noradrenergic and specific serotonergic antidepressants (NaSSA) (e.g., mirtazapine). In our study the most prescribed ADs were sertraline, paroxetine and mirtazapine, which represent common psychopharmacologic options that have shown their efficacy in cancer patients, according to data of non-randomised controlled trials [18,19]. Although a better tolerability and safety profiles of these new classes of ADs might have contributed to their increasing prescription by non-psychiatrist in the last decades, the risk of inadequate or unnecessary ADs prescription should be take into account, especially in cases of high potential for drug interactions. Generally, anti-cancer drugs and ADs can interact through pharmacokinetic or pharmacodynamic mechanisms [10]. Pharmacokinetic interactions are mainly a result of inhibition or induction of the cytochrome P450 (CYP450) isozymes, since ADs are metabolized through the cytochrome P450 enzyme system (CYP450). Pharmacodynamic interactions occur when the concurrent use of two drugs results in an alteration of the therapeutic and/or toxic effects of either drug without altering their pharmacokinetics. These interactions can be additive, synergistic or antagonistic [10].

DDIs can result in clinically significant changes in pharmacokinetics and/or pharmacodynamics of antineoplastic agents (ANs) altering their therapeutic efficacy and toxicity. Both ADs and ANs have narrow therapeutic indices and consequently, small variations in their plasmatic concentrations may result in sub-therapeutic or toxic effects [20]. The literature is scarce on reviews or research addressing the drug interactions between ANs and ADs and their clinical consequences and the majority of information available comes from animal experiments or in vitro tests. The pharmacokinetic drug interactions with ADs are unlikely with busulfan, chlorambucil, estramustine, mechlorethamine, melphalan, temozolomide, 5-fluorouracil, gemcitabine, mercaptopurine, thioguanine, cisplatin, carboplatin, oxaliplatin, daunorubicin, doxorubicin, doxorubicin, epirubicin and vorinostat. Among the remaining ANs, the risk of loss of efficacy or increased toxicity, when coadministered with certain ADs, is a possibility [20]. Most of them are subjected to metabolization by CYP 450 3A4 should be used with caution concomitantly with inhibitors of this isoenzyme such as fluoxetine, sertraline, paroxetine and fluvoxamine. Fluvoxamine is a CYP3A4 inhibitor and therefore has many DDIs with ANs such as: doxorubicin and etoposide, both susceptible to pharmacokinetic interactions involving competitive CYP3A4 inhibition; cyclophosphamide and ifosfamide, both major substrates of CYP3A4; docetaxel and paclitaxel, both substrates of CYP3A4 and therefore, interactions that involve ADs which inhibit this isozyme [21]. Precautions should be employed when using irinotecan and ADs in colon cancer patients. Irinotecan has significant pharmacodynamic and pharmacokinetic interactions and drugs acting on the serotonergic system (e.g. desipramine, paroxetine, and sertraline) which are inhibitors of CYP2B6 may increase the levels/effects of irinotecan [22]. Cyclophosphamide and ifosfamide are inhibitors of CYP2B6, and can theoretically decrease the clearance of bupropion, a dopamine reuptake inhibitor which is a major substrate of the same isoenzyme. Co-administration of bupropion with these ACDs can potentially affect the clinical activity of bupropion [21]. Escitalopram, citalopram, venlafaxine, mirtazapine and milnacipram are ADs with minimal CYP 450 inhibitory potential and are therefore seems safer in these patients [20].

Tamoxifen (TMX) has been very studied for drug interactions with ADs and results point that drugs that inhibit CYP 2D6 can reduce the clinical benefit of TMX and SSRIs inhibit, to varying degrees, CYP 2D6 [20]. Certain SSRIs such as paroxetine and fluoxetine can interact most with TMX by strongly decreasing the levels of its active metabolites. Venlafaxine, mirtazapine, citalopram and escitalopram are small inhibitors of CYP 2D6, therefore being a safe choice when using TMX [20].

Benzodiazepines anxiolytics

The high rate of benzodiazepines (BDZ) anxiolytics use is similar to previous studies and it has been shown for many years to be useful for anxiety and emotional distress [23,24]. Most BDZ are metabolized by CYP P450 and possess potential for DDIs with other drugs. Alprazolam was one of the most frequent BDZ option in our study. It has significant potential for DDIs because cytochrome P450 3A (CYP 3A) metabolizes this drug, rendering sensitive to a wide array of CYP 3A inhibitors and inducers. Among CYP 3A inducers, there is dexamethasone, common in oncological practice. Because of the pharmacologic complexity of many cancer treatment regimens, anxiolytics with fewer interactions such as BDZ which are metabolized through glucuronidation (e.g., lorazepam, oxazepam) are preferable in this setting [25].

Midazolam has been used in the treatment of cancer related symptoms especially in the terminal phase of the disease, including extreme anxiety, pain, dyspnoea, nausea, restlessness, and agitated delirium. Tyrosine kinase inhibitors (e.g., erlotinib and gefitinib) have also been shown to interact with midazolam based on in vitro and substrate binding studies, possibly due to induction of CYP3A4 by the ANs [10]. Midazolam is a substrate of this isozyme, and pretreatment and co-administration with erlotinib was shown to decrease the total exposure to midazolam in a small open-label study of 16 cancer patients [10].

Antipsychotics

The use of antipsychotics (APs) in our sample was lower compared to the results obtained in the last decades, when typical antipsychotics, also called neuroleptics (e.g., haloperidol, prochlorperazine) have been used for the management of cancer-related symptoms (e.g., nausea and vomiting) for more than 30 years. Both haloperidol (a butyrophenone) and prochlorperazine (a phenothiazine) block D2 receptors found in the chemoreceptor trigger zone, but haloperidol is a more potent and pure D2 receptor blocker.

In more recent years, second generation antipsychotics (e.g., olanzapine, quetiapine, risperidone), also known as atypical APs, have been used in psycho-oncology in the treatment of delirium, as well as of medical symptoms and chemotherapy side effects in patients with cancer. APs are metabolized via the CYP450 system (especially CYP1A2, CYP2D6, and CYP3A4) with possible interaction with other medications that by inhibiting CYP450 enzymes or by inducing their activity may increase or reduce, respectively, plasma levels of APs. Concomitant administrations of antipsychotics in patients who are on anthracycline therapy (e.g., doxorubicin, epirubicin) may predispose them to increased risks of drug-induced QT prolongations and torsades. Antipsychotic related haematological disorders (neutropenia, aplastic anaemia, thrombocytopenia, and rarely agranulocytosis), observed with clozapine and some other atypical APs must be taken into account especially for myelo-suppressed patients [26].

Our study has several limitations, both the sample size and the unicentric methodology used compromises the external validity of the study. The use of descriptive statistical methods limits the projection of the conclusions. The discussion about DDIs in oncology did not intend to be exhaustive, but to point out potential DDIs that may be clinically important in cancer patients.

Conclusion

The use of psychotropic medication by oncologists in patients referred to psychiatric assessment is common. Psychopharmacological treatment represents some of the main challenges for the future of multicomponent interventions in psycho-oncology but cancer patients are a physically vulnerable population, usually, taking several drugs and, therefore, in particular risk of drug interactions.

This study outlines the importance of promoting scientific research on drug-drug interactions in psycho-oncology and a closer collaboration between oncology and psychiatry in order to reduce the risk of DDIs, to increase its awareness and to adequately prescribe a psychopharmacologic treatment for each patient.

References

1. Pasquini M, Biondi M, Costantini A, Cairoli F, Ferrarese G et al. (2006) Detection and treatment of depressive and anxiety disorders among cancer patients: Feasibility and preliminar findings from a Liason Service in an Oncology division. Depress Anxiety 23: 441-448.

2. Henriksson MM, Isometsa ET, Hietanen PS, Aroa HM, Lönnqvist JK (1995) Mental disorders in cancer suicides. Journal of Affective Disorders 36: 11-21.

3. Breitbart W, Gibson C, Abbey J (2006) Suicide in palliative care. Textbook of palliative medicine. London: Hodder Arnold 860-868.

4. Okamura M, Akizuki N, Nakano T, Shimizu K, Ito T, et al. (2008) Clinical experience of the use of a pharmacological treatment algorithm for major depressive disorder in patients with advanced cancer. Psychooncology 17: 154-160.

5. Thekdi SM, Irarrazaval ME, Dunn L, Luigi Grassi, Michelle Rib (2012) Psychopharmacological Interventions. Clinical Psycho-Oncology: An International Perspective. Wiley-Blackwell 109-126.

6. Derogatis LR, Feldstein M, Morrow G, Schmale A, Schmitt M, et al. (1979) A survey of psychotropic drug prescriptions in an oncology population. Cancer 44: 1919-1929.

7. Jaeger H, Morrow GR, Carpenter PJ, Brescia F (1985) A survey of psychotropic drug utilization by patients with advanced neoplastic disease. Gen Hosp Psychiatry 7: 353-360.

8. Cullivan R, Crown J, Walsh N (1998) The use of psychotropic medication in patients referred to a psycho-oncology service. Psychooncology 7: 301-306.

9. Desplenter F, Bond C, Watson M, Burton C, Murchie P, et al. (2012) Incidence and drug treatment of emotional distress after cancer diagnosis: A matched primary care case-control study. Br J Cancer 107: 1644 - 1651.

10. Yap KYL, Tay WL, Chui WK, Chan A (2011) Clinically relevant drug interactions between anticancer drugs and psychotropic agents. Eur J Cancer Care 20: 6-32.

11. Farriols C, Ferrández O, Planas J, Ortiz P, Mojal S, et al. (2012) Changes in the prescription of psychotropic drugs in the palliative care of advanced cancer patients over a seven-year period. J Pain Symptom Manage 43: 945-952.

12. Ng CG, Boks MP, Zainal NZ, Wit NJ (2011) The prevalence and pharmacotherapy of depression in cancer patients. J Affect Disord 131: 1-7.

13. Laoutidis ZG, Mathiak K (2013) Antidepressants in the treatment of depression/depressive symptoms in cancer patients: A systematic review and meta-analysis. BMC Psychiatry 13: 140.

14. Riechelmann RP, Burman D, Tannock IF (2010) Phase II trial of mirtazapine for cancer-related cachexia and anorexia. Am J Hosp Palliat Care 27: 106-10.

15. Savard J, Morin CM (2001) Insomnia in the context of cancer: A review of a neglected problem. J Clin Oncol 19: 895-908.

16. Stockler MR, O'Connell R, Nowak AK, Goldstein D, Turner J, et al. (2007) Zoloft's Effects on Symptoms and Survival Time Trial Group. Effect of sertraline on symptoms and survival in patients with advanced cancer, but without major depression: A placebo-controlled double-blind randomised trial. Lancet Oncol 8: 603-612.

17. Hart SL, Hoyt MA, Diefenbach M, Anderson DR, Kilbourn KM, et al. (2012) Meta-analysis of efficacy of interventions for elevated depressive symptoms in adults diagnosed with cancer. J Natl Cancer Inst 104: 990-1004.

18. Torta R, Siri I, Caldera P (2008) Sertraline effectiveness and safety in depressed oncological patients. Supportive Care in Cancer 16: 83-91.

19. Cankurtaran ES, Ozalp E, Soygur H, Akbiyik DI, Turhan L, et al. (2008) Mirtazapine improves sleep and lowers anxiety and depression in cancer patients: Superiority over imipramine. Supportive Care in Cancer 16: 1291-1298.

20. Miguel C, Albuquerque E (2011) Drug interaction in psycho-oncology: Antidepressants and antineoplastics. Pharmacology 88: 333-339.

21. Chan A, Rong DNT, Yap KYL (2012) Clinically relevant anticancer antidepressant drug interactions. Expert Opin Drug Metab Toxicol 8:173-199.

22. Di Paolo A, Bocci G, Polillo M, Del Re M, Di Desidero T, et al. (2012) Pharmacokinetic and pharmacogenetic predictive markers of irinotecan activity and toxicity. Curr Drug Metab 12: 932-943.

23. Tsavaris N, Kosmas C, Vadiaka M, Sougioultzis S, Kontos A, et al. (2001) Comparative study of tropisetron with the addition of dexamethasone or

alprazolam in breast cancer patients receiving adjuvant chemotherapy with CEF (cyclophosphamide, epirubicin and 5-fluorouracil). J Chemother 13: 641-647.

24. Roscoe JA, Morrow GR, Aapro MS, Molassiotis A, Olver I, et al. (2011) Anticipatory nausea and vomiting. Supportive Care in Cancer 19: 1533-1538.

25. Ilana M, William E (2010) Psychotropic Medication in Cancer Care. Oxford University Press.

26. Nooijen PM, Carvalho F, Flanagan RJ (2011) Haematological toxicity of clozapine and some other drugs used in psychiatry. Hum Psychopharmacol 26: 112-119.

32

A Review of Safety Data from Spontaneous Reports on Marketed Products Containing Tramadol and Celecoxib: A Vigibase Descriptive Analysis

Vaqué A[1], Sust M[2], Gascón N[3], Puyada A[4] and Videla S[5]*

[1]Drug Safety and Pharmacovigilance. Laboratorios del Dr. Esteve, Barcelona, Spain
[2]Clinical Investigation, Laboratorios del Dr. Esteve, Barcelona, Spain
[3]Drug Safety and Pharmacovigilance. Laboratorios del Dr. Esteve, Barcelona, Spain
[4]Clinical Investigation, Laboratorios del Dr. Esteve, Barcelona, Spain
[5]Clinical Investigation, Laboratorios del Dr. Esteve, Barcelona, Spain

Abstract

Background: The concomitant administration of opioids and non-steroidal anti-inflammatory drugs is used to manage pain in clinical practice, given their synergistic analgesic effect. Among their possible combinations, tramadol and celecoxib are routinely used. The aim of this study was to explore the safety profile of tramadol and celecoxib administered individually compared to their concomitant administration in clinical practice.

Methods: Retrospective analysis of adverse-drug-reactions from the safety database Vigibase, The WHO global individual case safety report database system.

A case was defined as an adverse-drug-reaction included in a report of Vigibase between January 2000 and March 2012. Three groups were studied: 'tramadol-no-celecoxib' (tramadol was only reported as suspected or interacting drug), 'celecoxib-no-tramadol' (celecoxib was only reported as suspected or interacting drug) and 'celecoxib+tramadol' (both drugs co-administered and reported as suspected or interacting drug). MedDRA dictionary was used to code adverse-drug-reactions. Reporting proportions were calculated as the number of adverse-drug-reactions of a given type divided by the overall total number of reported adverse-drug-reaction in each drug-group.

Results: Reporting proportions for global profile, and for each studied group of adverse-drug-reaction, were lower for the concomitant administration than for each individual drug, specifically for the drug (either tramadol or celecoxib) primary involved in the particular adverse-drug-reaction. Therefore, no safety signals were found for 'gastrointestinal bleeding' and 'gastrointestinal signs and symptoms'; 'cardiovascular' and 'cerebrovascular events' (related to 'ischemic and embolic-thrombotic events'); 'renal' and 'renovascular' events (including cardiac failure related events); neither for 'central nervous system' effects; neither for 'respiratory depression'; 'development of tolerance with repeated administration' (including abuse/dependence/withdrawal reported events); 'hepatic disorders (drug-related)'; 'skin events'; and neither for the most frequent preferred terms: 'nausea', 'vomiting', 'constipation', 'myocardial infarction' and 'hypertension'.

Conclusion: Based on reporting proportions, no trend was observed to an increased risk for any specific potential safety concern when both tramadol and celecoxib, are administered concomitantly.

Keywords: Tramadol and celecoxib concomitant administration; Safety profile; Adverse drug reaction

List of Abbreviations: ADR: Adverse Drug Reaction; CNS: Central Nervous System; GI: Gastrointestinal; HLGT: High Level Group Terms; HLT: High Level Terms; ICD: International Classification of Diseases; ICH: International Conference on Harmonisation; ICSR: Individual Case Safety Report; LLT: Lowest Level Terms; MedDRA: Medical Dictionary for Regulatory Activities; PT: Preferred Terms; PUB: GI Upper Bleeding; RP: Reporting Proportion; SMQ: Standardized MedDRA Queries; SOC: System Organ Classes; WHO: World Health Organization; WHO-ART: WHO Adverse Reaction Terminology; WHO-DD, WHO-DDE: WHO Drug Dictionaries and the medical terminologies

Introduction

Pain is the most common symptom for which patients seek medical attention. Currently, in developing countries in particular, a number of serious diseases can cause severe pain, but often little or no pain relief is available [1]. Strategies to address this unmet need include the concomitant administration of analgesic drugs. In fact, in clinical practice is a usual procedure to administer different painkillers at the same time to control the pain. This practice is based on the concept of multimodal analgesia, which is rapidly becoming the 'standard of care'.

Multimodal analgesia involves the use of different classes of analgesics and sometimes different sites of analgesic administration, with the ultimate goal of providing superior pain relief [2-4]. Among the different strategies in multimodal analgesia to manage the pain, the concomitant administration of opioids and non-steroidal anti-inflammatory drugs is one of the most used given their analgesic effect [5], being second step therapies in The WHO Pain Relief Ladder [6,7].

*Corresponding author: Videla S, Clinical Investigation, Laboratorios del Dr. Esteve, Barcelona, Spain, E-mail: svidela@esteve.es

The concomitant administration of tramadol and celecoxib is one of the approaches used in clinical practice (data from internal survey based on automated health care databases). Tramadol acts centrally as a weak μ-opioid receptor agonist and an inhibitor of the neuronal reuptake of norepinephrine and serotonin, and celecoxib as an inhibitor of the cyclo-oxygenase-2 enzyme. Currently, tramadol is indicated for the treatment of moderate to severe pain [8], and celecoxib for the relief of chronic inflammatory pain as of osteoarthritis, rheumatoid arthritis and ankylosing spondylitis [9].

Although, up to date, no detectable unexpected safety signals from the free concomitant administration of tramadol and celecoxib (neither in clinical trial data nor post-marketing surveillance data) has been identified; to our knowledge, specific epidemiological studies focused on the safety profile of this concomitant administration of analgesics are not available. An exploratory evaluation of the safety profile of concomitant free administration can be conducted in global safety databases, e.g., Vigibase from the World Health Organization (WHO). Global safety databases record Adverse Drug Reactions (ADR) in terms of Individual Case Safety Report (ICSR), format and content for the reporting of one or several suspected adverse reactions in relation to a medicinal product that occur in a single patient at a specific point of time.

Our hypothesis is that tramadol and celecoxib given concomitantly have a similar safety profile compared to the individual administration of both compounds (at similar doses). Therefore, the aim of this study was to explore the safety profile of tramadol and celecoxib administered individually compared to their free concomitant administration in clinical practice, based on the spontaneous ADR recorded in Vigibase, the WHO Global ICSR Database System.

Methods

Study design

This study was a retrospective analysis of ADRs from the global safety database Vigibase. This study was performed according to the stipulations of the Declaration of Helsinki and the level of protection of confidentiality concerning the protection of personal data as required by Spanish laws (LOPD 15/1999) was ensured.

Spontaneous adverse drug reactions

A case was defined as an ADR included in a report of Vigibase database in which product/s causality was defined as follows:

a) Group 'tramadol no celecoxib', a single drug reported: tramadol is reported as suspected or interacting drug and celecoxib is not present.

b) Group 'celecoxib no tramadol', a single drug reported: celecoxib is reported as suspected or interacting drug and tramadol is not present.

c) Group 'celecoxib+tramadol', both drugs concomitantly-administered (co-administered) and reported, including:

c.1) tramadol and celecoxib are both reported as suspected or interacting drugs,

c.2) tramadol is reported as suspected or interacting drug and celecoxib is reported as concomitant drug,

c.3) celecoxib is reported as suspected or interacting drug and tramadol is reported as concomitant drug.

The five above mentioned groups (a, b, c.1, c.2 and c.3) are mutually exclusive and do no overlap, i.e., no ADR is contained in more the one

group. Likewise, it is worth mentioning that cases in which tramadol and celecoxib are co-administered but both appear reported merely as concomitant drug were not included.

Vigibase

The main aim of the WHO International Drug Monitoring Programme, started in 1968, is to identify the earliest possible pharmacovigilance signals. The data held is collected from countries participating in the WHO Medicines Safety Programme. As of May 2012, 107 countries had joined the WHO Medicines Safety Programme. VigiBase is maintained and developed on behalf of the WHO by the Uppsala Monitoring Centre, situated in Uppsala, Sweden. The database system includes the International Conference on Harmonisation of Technical Requirements for Registration of Pharmaceuticals for Human Use (ICH) E2B compatible ICSR database, the WHO Drug Dictionaries (WHO-DD and WHO-DDE), and the medical terminologies WHO Adverse Reaction Terminology (WHO-ART), International Classification of Diseases (ICD), and the Medical Dictionary for Regulatory Activities (MedDRA). VigiBase is used directly by the national centers and is accessed indirectly by other regulatory bodies, the pharmaceutical industry, and academia through data requests to the Uppsala Monitoring Centre. VigiBase contains more than 8,000,000 ICSRs, mainly from Europe and North America [10,11].

Although VigiBase is primarily intended to be a spontaneous ADRs report system, the database includes cases with a varying degree of suspectedness, both on the level of the initial reporter, and on the causality ascertainment made by the national center. Case reports from studies or special monitoring are also included, when provided to the Uppsala Monitoring Centre. Each ICSR can contain more than one ADR [10,11]. It is worth mentioning that, generally, the spontaneous ADR are recorded at the approved therapeutic doses.

To carry out this study, the following search was requested to Vigibase, with output format 'Summary by Year' and coded using MedDRA terminology: all ADRs for users of single drugs and concomitant administration of tramadol and celecoxib as well as for tramadol and celecoxib co-users. That is to say, we requested a separate search for each of the above mentioned five conditions: a, b, c.1, c.2 and c.3.

In order to avoid bias in the comparisons, we focused on the time window when both drugs were marketed. Though the earliest ADRs for tramadol were reported back in 1983 and for celecoxib in 1999, reports in which both are present in the market do not start until 2000. Consequently, this was the starting point, and all reports from January 2000 up to March 2012 were included in the analysis.

Vigibase facilitated us the requested information in an Excel file in March 2012, which was used for the analysis of this study. The following data were gathered: report ID (Vigibase), year, safety report ID, company, MedDRA SOC, PT and LLT Names.

Medical Dictionary for Regulatory Activities (MedDRA)

MedDRA is an international medical terminology dictionary (and thesaurus) was developed under the auspices of ICH and maintained by maintenance and support services organization. It is an international medical dictionary applicable to all phases of biopharmaceutical and medical product development. Therefore, it is used by regulatory authorities in the pharmaceutical industry during the regulatory process, from pre-marketing to post-marketing activities, and for data entry, retrieval, evaluation, and presentation. In addition, it is the adverse event classification dictionary endorsed by ICH [12].

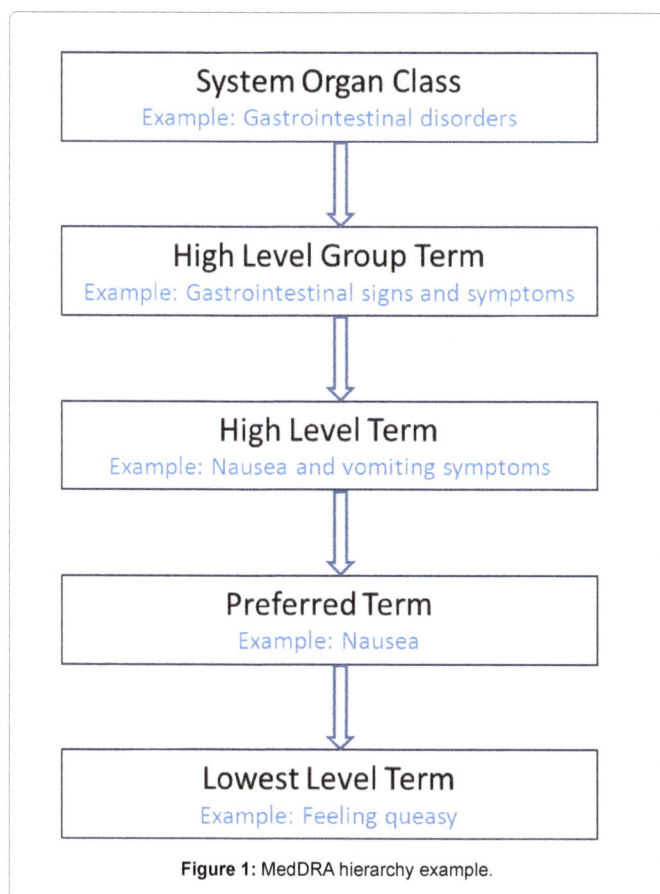

Figure 1: MedDRA hierarchy example.

The MedDRA dictionary is organized in five levels of hierarchy which are, from most specific to most global, as follows: 'Lowest Level Terms' (LLTs) are terms which parallel how information is communicated. These LLTs reflect how an observation might be reported in practice. This level directly supports assigning MedDRA terms within a user database; each member of the next level, 'Preferred Terms' (PTs), is a distinct descriptor (single medical concept) for a symptom, sign, disease diagnosis, therapeutic indication, investigation, surgical or medical procedure, etc. Each LLT is linked to only one PT. Each PT has at least one LLT (itself) as well as synonyms and lexical variants (e.g., abbreviations, different word order). Related PTs are grouped together into 'High Level Terms' (HLTs) based upon anatomy, pathology, physiology, etiology or function. HLTs, related to each other by anatomy, pathology, physiology, etiology or function, are in turn linked to 'High Level Group Terms' (HLGTs). Finally, HLGTs are grouped into 'System Organ Classes' (SOCs) which are groupings by etiology (e.g. Infections and infestations), manifestation site (e.g. Gastrointestinal (GI) disorders) or purpose (e.g. Surgical and medical procedures) [12]. Figure 1 shows the MedDRA hierarchy example.

Standardized MedDRA Queries (SMQs) are used to support signal detection and monitoring. SMQs are validated, standard sets of MedDRA terms that define a search in the database. SMQs include narrow and/or broad terms. Narrow terms are those that are highly likely to represent the condition of interest. For example, the PTs 'pancreatitis acute' and 'pancreatitis haemorrhagic' are narrow terms for the SMQ 'acute pancreatitis' whereas PT 'blood bilirubin' increased is a broad term because not all instances of increased blood bilirubin are indicative of acute pancreatitis [12]. The MedDRA dictionary, version 15.0, was used in this study.

Statistical analysis

The sample size was defined as all ADR contained in the WHO database complying our request specifications in the time period of interest.

Three consecutive types of descriptive analyses were performed for tramadol and celecoxib users in comparison to co-users of tramadol and celecoxib:

First analysis-*Spontaneous ADR by SOC*: ADRs were grouped by primary SOC according to the MedDRA dictionary.

Second analysis: *Spontaneous ADR of 'Special Interest' based on known safety profiles of both drugs. Spontaneous ADR of 'Special Interest'* was defined in agreement with the safety profile included in the summary of product characteristics of both drugs (as given in the ref 8 and 9 in the section 'Special warnings and precautions for use' and the section 'Undesirable effects' very frequent or frequent). The analysis was performed based on SMQ or other *ad hoc* grouping considerations as follows:

a) GI bleeding and GI signs and symptoms, which were reviewed and grouped by PT as follows:

a.1) GI upper bleeding (*ad hoc* grouping): 'GI perforation', 'GI ulceration' and 'GI hemorrhage or bleeding' (PUB).

a.2) GI nonspecific inflammation-dysfunction (SMQ): 'GI nonspecific dysfunction' and 'GI nonspecific inflammation'.

a.3) GI nonspecific symptoms (SMQ): 'GI nonspecific symptoms and therapeutic procedures'.

b) Cardiovascular and Cerebrovascular events, related to 'ischemic and embolic-thrombotic events', were reviewed and grouped by PT as follows:

b.1) Cerebrovascular events (SMQ): 'Ischemic cerebrovascular conditions', 'conditions associated with central nervous system hemorrhages and cerebrovascular accidents'.

b.2) Embolic and thrombotic events (SMQ): 'Embolic and thrombotic arterial events', 'embolic and thrombotic venous events' and 'embolic and thrombotic vessel type unspecified and mixed arterial and venous events'.

b.3) Cardiovascular events (SMQ): 'Myocardial infarction' and 'other ischemic heart disease'.

c) Renal and Renovascular events, including cardiac failure related events, were reviewed and grouped by PT as follows (SMQ): 'Acute renal failure', 'cardiac failure' and 'renovascular disorders'.

d) Central nervous system (CNS) effects: some concrete PTs from the Nervous System Disorders SOC were selected based on the highest reporting frequency in the postmarketing surveillance (*ad hoc* grouping): 'dizziness', 'headache' and 'somnolence'. Another PT, 'fatigue', PT, from the 'General Disorders and Administration Side Conditions' SOC was additionally included.

e) Respiratory depression, and in absence of an appropriate SMQ, the following HLTs were reviewed: 'Breathing abnormalities' and 'respiratory failures' (excluding neonatal).

f) Development of tolerance with repeated administration, including abuse/dependence/withdrawal reported events, were reviewed and grouped by PT as follows (*ad hoc* grouping): 'Drug abuse' and 'drug withdrawal'.

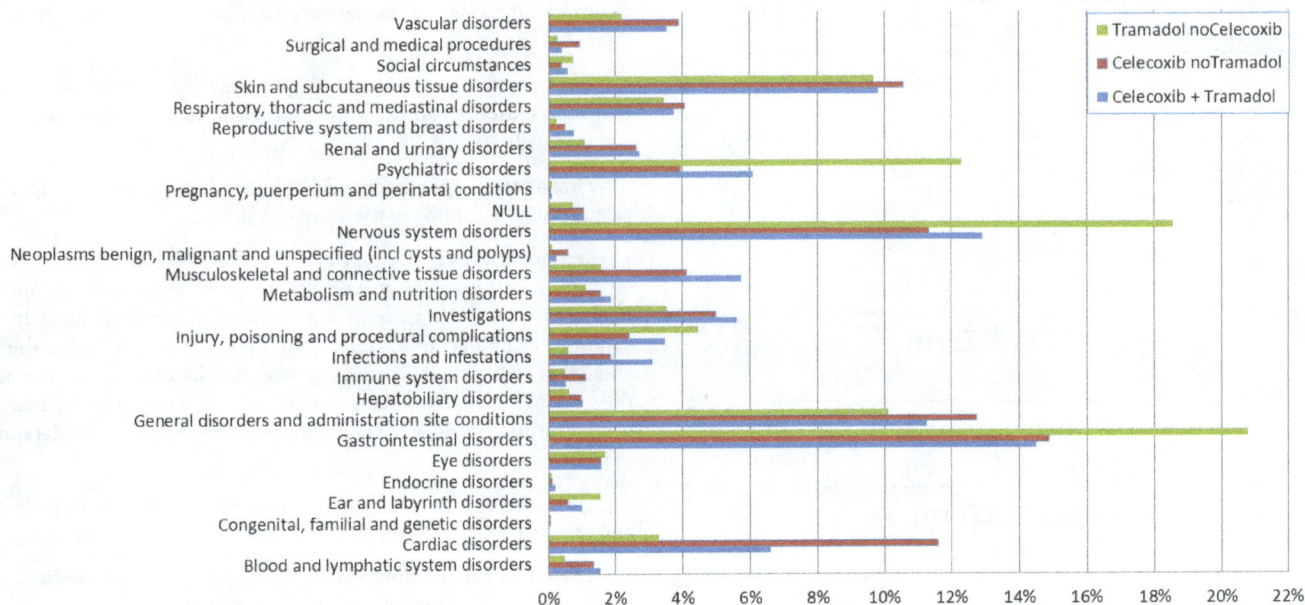

ADR profile by SOC. % over total reported ADRs by drug exposure

NULL: corresponds to ADRs which, for any reason, have not been assigned a MedDRA code in the Vigibase database

Figure 2: Reporting Proportions per 100 Adverse Drug Reactions by System Organ Class and drug-group.

g) Hepatic disorders (drug-related), were reviewed and grouped by PT as Hepatic disorders (drug-related) (*ad hoc* grouping): 'Cholestasis and jaundice of hepatic origin', 'hepatic failure', 'fibrosis' and 'cirrhosis and other liver damage-related conditions' and 'hepatitis, non-infectious'.

h) Skin events, the most clinically relevant Skin events, were reviewed and grouped by PT as follows (SMQ): 'Severe cutaneous adverse reactions'.

i) The most frequent PTs (based on ADRs expected in both SPCs, as given in the references 8 and 9 in the section 'Undesirable effects'), following the specific PTs were analyzed (*ad hoc* grouping): 'Nausea', 'vomiting', 'constipation', 'myocardial infarction' and 'hypertension'.

Third analysis-*Spontaneous ADR of Special Interest but based on observed data*: A data-driven analysis was performed to further evaluate any other potential safety concern different from those detailed above and raised from the free-use of the concomitant administration of tramadol and celecoxib. SOCs showing a higher reporting proportion for 'celecoxib+tramadol' group than for both individual drug-groups were to be explored more in depth, selecting the most reported PTs.

Reporting Proportion (RP): The frequency of reporting of ADRs to Vigibase, among users of the drugs of interest, was described through the calculation of the RP as a summary measure. The RP was defined as the proportion of ADRs (as of PTs) that meet the definition of 'special interest', among all ADRs of a given drug exposure group (drug-group), i.e. 'number of ADRs with the definition of special Interest/total number of reported ADRs'.

For the first analysis, RPs were calculated as the number of ADRs that belong to a given SOC divided by the overall total number of reported ADRs in each drug-group. For the second analysis, RPs were

calculated as the number of ADRs that belong to a given grouping (i.e., SMQ or HLT) divided by the overall total number of reported ADRs in each drug-group. It is important to note that PTs included in more than one SMQ grouping were counted in the calculation of the RP of each of these SMQ groupings. For the third analysis, the RP were calculated as the number of ADRs (single PT) divided by the total number of reported ADRs in the specific SOC for each drug-group. All these analysis focused on the comparison between the RP for the concomitant administration vs. the RP of the 'leading' drug-group primary involved in each particular ADR (marked with an asterisk in tables 1-4).

Results

General characteristics of the spontaneous ADR set

A total of 160,938 ADRs were recorded in the VigiBase database, in which either tramadol or celecoxib administered alone or in a concomitant administration are involved as 'suspected' during the study period. Among them, 2,123 ADRs contained both drugs used concomitantly and reported, at least one of them, as suspected drug; 107,545 contained only 'celecoxib no Tramadol' and 51,270 'Tramadol no Celecoxib'.

Spontaneous ADR findings by System Organ Class

Figure 2 depicts the safety profile of the three defined drug-groups in terms of RPs. These RPs reflect the relative weight of each SOC among all ADRs reported for a given drug-group.

Spontaneous ADR findings of special interest, based on the known safety profiles of both drugs

No detectable safety signals were found. The number of reported ADRs and RPs (per 100 ADRs) concerning GI upper bleeding (PUB),

Drug-group	Total reported	GI upper bleeding (PUB)		GI non-specific inflammation and dysfunction		GI non-specific symptoms	
		(narrow) Count (%)	(broad) Count (%)	(narrow) Count (%)	(broad) Count (%)	(narrow) Count (%)	(broad) Count (%)
Celecoxib+Tramadol	2123	63 (3.0%)	79 (3.7%)	24 (1.1%)	24 (1.1%)	156 (7.4%)	172 (8.1%)
Celecoxib noTramadol	107545	3931 (3.7%)*	5320 (5.0%)*	1719 (1.6%)*	1719 (1.6%)*	6683 (6.2%)	7730 (7.2%)
Tramadol noCelecoxib	51270	122 (0.2%)	220 (0.4%)	148 (0.3%)	148 (0.3%)	9385 (18.3%)*	9691 (18.9%)*
Total	160938	4116 (2.6%)	5619 (3.5%)	1891 (1.2%)	1891 (1.2%)	16224 (10.1%)	17593 (10.9%)

Table 1: Number of reported adverse drug reactions and reporting proportions (per 100 adverse drug reactions) of gastrointestinal bleeding (GI, PUB: Perforation, Ulceration, Bleeding) and GI signs and symptoms (* 'leading' drug-group involved in the ADR).

Drug-group	Total reported	Cardiovascular events		Cerebrovascular events		Embolic-thrombotic events
		(narrow) Count (%)	(broad) Count (%)	(narrow) Count (%)	(broad) Count (%)	Count (%)
Celecoxib+Tramadol	2123	72 (3.4%)	78 (3.7%)	34 (1.6%)	39 (1.8%)	107 (5.0%)
Celecoxib noTramadol	107545	6809 (6.3%)*	6922 (6.4%)*	4715 (4.4%)*	5057 (4.7%)*	12946 (12.0%)*
Tramadol noCelecoxib	51270	136 (0.3%)	200 (0.4%)	83 (0.2%)	244 (0.5%)	259 (0.5%)
Total	160938	7017 (4.4%)	7200 (4.5%)	4832 (3.0%)	5340 (3.3%)	13312 (8.3%)

Table 2: Number of reported adverse drug reactions and reporting proportions (per 100 adverse drug reactions) of cardiovascular and cerebrovascular events (* 'leading' drug-group involved in the ADR).

Drug-group	Total reported	Dizziness Count (%)	Fatigue Count (%)	Headache Count (%)	Somnolence Count (%)
Celecoxib+Tramadol	2123	51 (2.4%)	18 (0.9%)	21 (1.0%)	9 (0.4%)
Celecoxib noTramadol	107545	1294 (1.2%)	761 (0.7%)	1028 (1.0%)	209 (0.2%)
Tramadol noCelecoxib	51270	2252 (4.4%)*	300 (0.6%)*	779 (1.5%)*	757 (1.5%)*
Total	160938	3597 (2.2%)	1079 (0.7%)	1828 (1.1%)	975 (0.6%)

PT from the SOC of General Disorders and Administration Side Condition

Table 3: Number of reported adverse drug reactions and reporting proportions (per 100 adverse drug reactions) concerning central nervous system effects (* 'leading' drug-group involved in the ADR).

Drug-group	Total reported	Constipation Count (%)	Hypertension Count (%)	Myocardial infarction Count (%)	Nausea Count (%)	Vomiting Count (%)
Celecoxib+Tramadol	2123	11 (0.5%)	16 (0.8%)	45 (2.1%)	50 (2.4%)	30 (1.4%)
Celecoxib noTramadol	107545	307 (0.3%)	1144 (1.1%)*	5597 (5.2%)*	1375 (1.3%)	822 (0.8%)
Tramadol noCelecoxib	51270	288 (0.6%)*	211 (0.4%)	54 (0.1%)	4616 (9.0%)*	3698 (7.2%)*
Total	160938	606 (0.4%)	1371 (0.9%)	5696 (3.5%)	6041 (3.8%)	4550 (2.8%)

Table 4: Number of reported Adverse Drug Reactions and Reporting Proportions (per 100 Adverse Drug Reactions) for the most frequent Preferred Terms, by drug-group (* 'leading' drug-group involved in the ADR).

GI non-specific inflammation and dysfunction and GI signs and symptoms are presented in Table 1. Table 2 shows the number of reported ADRs and RPs (per 100 ADRs) concerning Cerebrovascular and Cardiovascular events, related to 'ischemic and embolic/thrombotic events' and 'other embolic/thrombotic events'. The number of reported ADRs and RPs (per 100 ADRs) concerning CNS effects are shown in table 3, and the most frequent PTs ('nausea', 'vomiting', 'constipation', 'myocardial infarction' and 'hypertension') in table 4. Similar results were found in renal and renovascular events, respiratory depression, development of tolerance with repeated administration, hepatic disorders and skin events (data not shown).

Spontaneous ADR of special interest based on observed data

After an in-depth revision of the findings from the above results sections, the following SOCs were also analyzed and evaluated in detail: musculoskeletal and connective tissue disorders, investigations, metabolism and nutrition disorders, infections and infestations as well as blood and lymphatic system disorders. No safety signals from the free concomitant administration of both drugs were detected in these specific spontaneous ADR of special interest (data not shown).

Discussion

To our knowledge, this is the first study that evaluates the safety profile of the concomitant administration use of tramadol and celecoxib, an approach used as multimodal analgesia in clinical practice. No safety signals of this concomitant administration use of tramadol and celecoxib were found. In fact, these findings could be expected. Both active principles, tramadol and celecoxib, have been marketed worldwide for more than 10 years. During this time period, no safety concerns from the concomitant use of both drugs, either in clinical trials data or in post-marketing surveillance data have been raised. Likewise, there is no risk described for the co-administration in any of the labels of the products, neither in the general sections of the summary of product characteristics such as 'Contraindications' and as given in the references 8 and 9 in the section 'Special warnings and special precautions for use' nor in the specific drug-drug interactions as given in the references 8 and 9 in the section 'Interaction with other medicinal products and other forms of interaction' [8,9,13]. Furthermore, the current results are also supported by other lines of knowledge available including as described in the summary of product characteristics of both medicinal products, for instance, that based on the described metabolic routes, no clinically relevant pharmacokinetic drug-drug interactions, that may have safety implications, would be expected with the concomitant use of tramadol and celecoxib at their approved doses.

The observed RPs for the concomitant use of tramadol and

celecoxib were consistent with the safety profile of each individual drug. A consistent safety profile was observed for their concomitant use. RP for global profile (SOC) and for each group of individual ADRs of interest were lower for the concomitant use than for each individual drug, specifically for the main drug (the 'leading': either tramadol or celecoxib) involved in the ADR.

The most frequent reported SOCs for 'tramadol no celecoxib group' were: GI, CNS and psychiatric disorders; and for 'celexoxib no tramadol' group: GI, cardiac and CNS disorders. In all these higher reporting ADRs, the 'celecoxib+tramadol' group presented a lower RPs than the corresponding primary suspected drug for the ADR. Additionally, general disorders and skin and subcutaneous tissue disorders were equally frequent for tramadol, celecoxib and for the concomitant use. The safety profile of the three defined drug groups was also consistent with what is already known referring to the defined safety concerns or to most reported ADRs in each summary of product characteristics [8,9]. For example, it was observed that the RP in the group 'tramadol no celecoxib' were higher for constipation, nausea and vomiting. These results have been previously reported [8,13-15]. In the group 'celecoxib no tramadol' the RPs were higher for PUB, hypertension and myocardial infarction. In fact, these ADRs were also expected [9,16-18]. Based on these results, it can be mentioned that this concomitant administration of two well-known active principles, tramadol and celecoxib, with complementary mechanisms of action, does not present increased or unpredictable safety concerns. Therefore, it could be assumed that nor pharmacokinetic nor deleterious pharmacodynamic clinically relevant drug-drug interactions have been observed. Moreover, it could be hypothesized that, since the most relevant side effects for these drugs are dose-dependent, a lower dose would result in a better benefit/risk profile.

As expected, the number of ADRs reported involving 'celecoxib+tramadol' is substantially lower than for the individual drugs, probably due to a lower number of users of the concomitant administration. Nevertheless, these data provides an idea on the current use of this co-administration. In this line, more than 7,000 patients have been identified to be exposed to the aforementioned concomitant administration in the UK during the same period using the automated health care database Clinical Practice Research Datalink (internal data). Therefore, all these data provide evidence that this co-administration of analgesic medicinal products (tramadol and celecoxib), is administered in clinical practice to the general population.

The main strength of this study is that it is based on a standard ADR register, The WHO Global ICSR Database System, and that it has been used an international medical dictionary, MedDRA. Nevertheless, there are several limitations to this study which should be considered. Limitations related to spontaneous reporting of ADRs and the interpretation of RP as: i) ADRs are under-reported, being estimated between 50-90% (i.e., reporting may be more frequent with severe events and less frequent when the effects are well known) [19,20]; ii) The channeling of a drug to lower or higher risk patients may alter the occurrence of ADRs (i.e. in oncologic pain, patients receiving free concomitant administration of tramadol and celecoxib are in the second step therapy in The WHO Pain Relief Ladder [6,7], pointing to a potentially more severe patient population, which may lead to higher reporting of ADRs [21]; iii) ADRs identification and reporting rates may be higher if there have been recent warnings about a drug (notoriety bias) or early after marketing authorization and other factors (i.e. extent of use, publicity, etc.) which vary over time, from product to product and country to country [10,19]; and iv)

Length of time on the market and familiarity with the drug have been shown to affect reporting rates [10,19]. Another limitation is the lack of information about the number of patients exposed to the product, in addition to uncertainties as to the indication for which an analgesic was prescribed. However, in most cases the spontaneous ADR are recorded on regular clinical practice and thus may correspond to the approved therapeutic doses: for tramadol, 200 mg per day is a usual therapeutic dose and for celecoxib, 200 mg per day is a recommended therapeutic dose. Likewise, the data contained per se in Vigibase and the limited details about each suspected ADR may underestimate the results. The reports, which are submitted to National Centers, come from both regulatory and voluntary sources. Some National Centers accept reports only from medical practitioners; other National Centers accept reports from a wider spectrum of health care professionals. Also, processing time varies from country to country. Therefore, reporting figures obtained from the Collaborating Centre may differ from those obtained directly from National Centers. For the above reasons it is clear that the information is not homogeneous at least with respect to origin or likelihood that the pharmaceutical product caused the adverse reaction. Interpretation of ADRs data, and particularly those based on comparisons between pharmaceutical products, may be overestimating or underestimating the results.

In spite of these limitations, spontaneous reporting of ADRs remains one of the most important methods for monitoring the safety of drugs, and the analyses of adverse events databases have demonstrated to be useful for detecting trends and hypothesis generation. Therefore, the results of this study, based on reporting proportions, allow concluding that no trend to an increased risk for any specific potential safety concern when both drugs, tramadol and celecoxib, are administered concomitantly was observed. These findings should be confirmed with other epidemiological studies or with randomized clinical trials.

The information derived from our analysis does not represent the opinion of The WHO [22].

References

1. IASP® Global Year Against Pain.

2. Buvanendran A, Kroin JS (2009) Multimodal analgesia for controlling acute postoperative pain. Curr Opin Anaesthesiol 22: 588-593.

3. Elvir-Lazo OL, White PF (2010) Postoperative pain management after ambulatory surgery: role of multimodal analgesia. See comment in PubMed Commons below Anesthesiol Clin 28: 217-224.

4. Argoff CE, Albrecht P, Irving G, Rice F (2009) Multimodal analgesia for chronic pain: rationale and future directions. Pain Med: S53-S66.

5. Miranda HF, Silva E, Pinardi G (2004) Synergy between the antinociceptive effects of morphine and NSAIDs. Can J Physiol Pharmacol 82: 331-338.

6. World Health Organization (1996). Cancer pain relief: with a guide to opioid availability. In: Geneva: World Health Organization. (2ndedsn), Geneva, Switzerland.

7. World Health Organization Collaborating Center (2006). Appraising the WHO Analgesic Ladder on its 20th anniversary.Cancer Pain Release.

8. Tramadol. Summary of Product Characteristics of Adolonta 50 mg hard capsules, AEMPS web (Spain). (http://www.aemps.gob.es/cima/ especialidad. do?metodoverFichaWordPdf&codigo=59088&formato=pdf&formulario=FICHA S&file=ficha.pdf)

9. Celebrex 100mg & 200mg Capsules, emc, UK.

10. Lindquist M (2008) VigiBase, the WHO Global ICSR Database System: Basic Facts. Drug Information Journal 42:409-419.

11. http://www.umc-products.com/

12. http://www.meddra.org/

13. Martindale W, Parfitt K (1999) The complete drug reference: Pharmaceutical Press (32ndedn), London UK.

14. Radbruch L, Grond S, Lehmann KA (1996) A risk-benefit assessment of tramadol in the management of pain. Drug Saf 15:8-29.

15. Pergolizzi J, Böger RH, Budd K, Dahan A, Erdine S, et al. (2008) Opioids and the management of chronic severe pain in the elderly: consensus statement of an International Expert Panel with focus on the six clinically most often used World Health Organization Step III opioids (buprenorphine, fentanyl, hydromorphone, methadone, morphine, oxycodone). Pain Pract 8:287-313.

16. Public CHMP Assessment Report for Medicinal products containing Non-Selective Non Steroidal Anti-Inflammatory Drugs (NSAIDS). European Medicines Agency.

17. Kearney PM, Baigent C, Godwin J, Halls H, Emberson JR, et al. (2006) Do selective cyclo-oxygenase-2 inhibitors and traditional non-steroidal anti-inflammatory drugs increase the risk of atherothrombosis? Meta-analysis of randomised trials. BMJ 332: 1302-1308.

18. Castellsague J, Holick CN, Hoffman CC, Gimeno V, Stang MR, et al. (2009) Risk of upper gastrointestinal complications associated with cyclooxygenase-2 selective and nonselective nonsteroidal antiinflammatory drugs. Pharmacotherapy 29: 1397-1407.

19. Strom BL, Kimmel SE, Hennessy S (2012) Pharmacoepidemiology. (5th edsn), John Wiley & Sons, Ltd.

20. Leufkens HG (2000) Pharmacoepidemiology and gastroenterology: a close couple. Scand J Gastroenterol:105-108.

21. de Graaf L, Fabius MA, Diemont WL, van Puijenbroek EP (2003) The Weber-curve pitfall: effects of a forced introduction on reporting rates and reported adverse reaction profiles. Pharm World Sci 25: 260-263.

22. CAVEAT DOCUMENT. Accompanying statement to data released from the Uppsala Monitoring Centre, WHO Collaborating Centre for International Drug Monitoring. Uppsala, Sweden.

33

Buprenorphine Use and Risk of Abuse and Diversion

Michael Soyka[1,2]*

[1]*Department of Psychiatry, Ludwig Maximilian University, Munich, Germany*
[2]*Private Hospital Meiringen, Willigen, CH 3860 Meiringen, Switzerland*

Abstract

Opioid maintenance therapy with methadone or buprenorphine is a well-established first-line treatment for opioid dependence. However, risk of diversion and drug-related mortality are critical issues during maintenance therapy. These issues are discussed controversially in both the scientific and public arenas and are a matter of concern also among medical authorities. In addition to a formulation containing buprenorphine alone, a combination formulation with buprenorphine and naloxone in a 4:1 ratio is available. The combination formulation was developed with the aim to prevent intravenous use or diversion. This critical review summarizes data on the risk of abuse and diversion of buprenorphine.

Keywords: Buprenorphine; Diversion; Abuse; Mortality; Naloxone; Opioids; Opioid dependence

Introduction

Opioid dependence is a chronic relapsing disorder with an excess mortality rate [1-4]. Over than 90% of the estimates relate to heroin, as demonstrated in a global literature review by Degenhardt et al. [5]. Opioid maintenance treatment has proven efficacy in reducing opioid consumption and psychosocial and medical morbidity and in increasing treatment retention rates and social functioning in opioid addicts [6]. Nevertheless, there are persistent and in part increasing concerns about diversion of maintenance drugs, concomitant drug use, and mortality in opioid-maintained patients [1,7,8]. Diversion may be understood differently by clinicians and patients [9]. Usually, it is defined as the unauthorized re-routing or appropriation of a drug. Misuse, on the other hand, is defined as any use of a prescription drug that deviates from medical practice. Risks of diversion and misuse include increased patient morbidity and mortality [10], overdose and fatal respiratory depression [11,12], non-fatal overdose and related emergency admissions [10], blood-borne viruses and infections [13,14], and numerous other complications associated with injection drug use [15,16]. Other considerations include a possible negative impact on the prescribers' practice, threatened reputation of treatment services, and compromised public acceptance for the drug and maintenance treatment [17], as is currently the case in Austria, for example. The economic costs of the non-medical use of prescription opioids are enormous [18].

The misuse of prescription opioids, especially oxycodone but also methadone and others, is very common among street drug users in the USA, UK, and other countries [19-21]. Many patients misuse street methadone to reduce unpleasant addiction-related effects [22]. To diminish the risk of diversion, many countries have implemented regulations on maintenance treatment, which in return restrict access to treatment, among other things [23].

Buprenorphine in Opioid Maintenance Treatment: A Brief Update

Buprenorphine is an established first-line medication for the treatment of opioid dependence (see APA guidelines [24]; WFSBP guidelines [25]; New South Wales clinical guidelines [26]; the British Association for Psychopharmacology guidelines [27]; World Health Organization guidelines [28,29]; for reviews on the risk of buprenorphine diversion and misuse, see Mammen and Bell [30], Orman and Keating [31] and Yokell et al. [32]. In the US, buprenorphine was approved by the FDA in October 2002 for the treatment of addiction.

Buprenorphine is a partial mu-opioid receptor agonist and kappa antagonist with a long half-life of 24-60 hours; it is administered sublingually in opioid replacement therapy [33]. Extensive first-pass liver metabolism results in low bioavailability after oral administration. Dosages of 4 to 16 or 24 mg/day are usually given for maintenance therapy. Two forms of buprenorphine are available: A tablet containing only buprenorphine, and one that combines buprenorphine with the opioid antagonist naloxone in a 4:1 ratio. Naloxone has poor oral bioavailability, which means that after sublingual administration the concentration is too low to cause severe and protracted withdrawal symptoms [34]. However, it has good parenteral bioavailability, with an elimination half-life in plasma of about 30 min [35]. Consequently, if a combination buprenorphine-naloxone tablet is dissolved and administered intravenously, it precipitates an immediate opioid withdrawal syndrome in the majority of patients [36]. This effect is thought to reduce the abuse potential of buprenorphine and improve its safety. The combination tablet has been found to significantly reduce the risk of diversion [24], but it does not eliminate intravenous misuse [30].

Buprenorphine effectively suppresses opioid withdrawal. Clinical studies of the detoxification effects of methadone, primarily in moderate dosages (50-60 mg), and buprenorphine (12-16 mg) have generally demonstrated comparable efficacy for the two drugs [37-39]. For more details on the use of buprenorphine in opioid dependence, see Soyka et al. [25].

*****Corresponding author:** Michael Soyka, MD, Private Hospital Meiringen, P.O. Box 612, CH 3860 Meiringen, Switzerland,
E-mail: Michael.Soyka@privatklinik-meiringen.ch

Aims

This review was performed to evaluate the existing literature concerning the abuse potential and risk of diversion (and illicit use) of buprenorphine and buprenorphine-naloxone (rates of diversion and illicit use and relevance for overdose/mortality in different countries) .

Methods

A systematic literature search was performed in the Medline and Pubmed databases to identify studies on the misuse or diversion of buprenorphine. The search was not limited to certain years or languages. The indexing terms were "buprenorphine AND diversion" (123 citations) and "buprenorphine AND misuse" (132 citations) and "buprenorphine AND diversion" (23 citations). Studies were also identified by examining previous reviews on this issue [32,40,41].

Results

Routes of administration

Buprenorphine is usually misused by the sublingual or intravenous route, but there are also reports of buprenorphine inhalation or intranasal application [42,43]. Intravenous misuse has been recorded since the mid-1980s [44,45]. The consensus seems to be that by far the most common method of abuse is to crush the sublingual tablets and inject the resulting extract [46], which causes morphine-like effects [47].

The abuse potential of buprenorphine, which has been demonstrated in experimental and clinical settings [48-50], is generally considered to be less than that of full opioid agonists [51,52]. Buprenorphine can cause euphoria [53,54], although to a lesser degree than full opioid agonists [31,53-55], and has reinforcing effects, again to a lesser degree than full opioid agonists [56-62]. However, under experimental conditions, buprenorphine was found to be as effective as methadone in producing reinforcing and subjective effects [50,54].

In a randomized, double-blind, placebo-controlled, cross-over study, Middleton et al. [43] evaluated the pharmacokinetic and pharmacodynamic profile and subjective and physiological effects of buprenorphine and buprenorphine/naloxone (crushed tablets) in 10 healthy adults who abused opioids intranasally, but were not physically dependent on them. Subjects reported higher ratings and street values for 8 mg buprenorphine than for the 8 mg buprenorphine/2 mg naloxone combination, but these differences were not statistically different. No significant formulation differences in peak plasma buprenorphine concentration or time course were observed. The authors speculated whether greater bioavailability and faster onset of pharmacodynamic effects compared to sublingual administration might motivate intranasal misuse in non-dependent opioid abusers and concluded that "Significant naloxone absorption from an intranasal buprenorphine/naloxone administration may deter the likelihood of intranasal misuse of buprenorphine/naloxone, but not buprenorphine, in opioid-dependent individuals" [43].

Extent of the problem in the US and non-European countries

Many related studies have been conducted in the US and Australia, but far fewer in Europe and other parts of the world. Data from the US indicate an increasing risk of buprenorphine misuse and diversion [63]. A recent survey indicated that 40% of clinicians believe that the diversion of the buprenorphine-naloxone combination is a dangerous problem [64]. Buprenorphine was introduced to the US market in 2002 and is classified as a Schedule III medication [65]; it is the first-line option for office-based treatment [66,67]. Comparatively low levels of abuse have been found, and buprenorphine and buprenorphine/naloxone rank among the least abused or misused opioids [68-72]. Buprenorphine/naloxone diversion is rather limited, and the drug is used in a "therapeutic," non-medically supervised manner [73-75]. As part of a national post-marketing surveillance program, applicants to substance abuse treatment and physicians certified to prescribe buprenorphine were surveyed about their perceptions of buprenorphine/naloxone diversion and abuse [76]. Measures of diversion and abuse of buprenorphine/naloxone increased from 2005 to 2009. The results from the applicant survey showed that the perceptions of the extent of diversion and abuse were lower than for the positive controls—methadone, oxycodone, and heroin—but higher than for the negative control, amitriptyline. By 2009, 46% of the physicians believed that buprenorphine/naloxone was diverted, 44% believed illegal use was for self-management of withdrawal, and 53% believed the source of the medication was substance-abusing patients. Other measures from national databases showed similar results. When adjusted for millions of tablets sold per year, slopes for measures of diversion and abuse were reduced. The authors concluded that the increases in diversion and abuse measures indicate both the need to take active attempts to curb diversion and abuse and the need for continuous monitoring and surveillance of all buprenorphine products and that "Finding a balance of risk/benefit (i.e. diversion and abuse versus expanded treatment) remains a challenge" [76]. Interestingly, the black market prices for prescription opioids, including buprenorphine, generally follow clinical equianalgesic potency and accurately predict the relative pharmacologic potency of opioid molecules [77].

A recent comprehensive post-marketing postal survey of Australian authorized opioid substitution treatment prescribers [78] found that prescribers perceived that more buprenorphine patients removed supervised doses (7%) and diverted unsupervised doses (20%) than did methadone patients (1% and 4%, respectively) and buprenorphine-naloxone patients (3% and 2%, respectively). In addition, prescribers reported that significantly more buprenorphine and buprenorphine-naloxone patients injected doses (each 5%) than methadone patients did (2%). All in all, the rates reported seem rather low, and the authors discuss that the prescribers may underestimate the levels of diversion.

About one third of injecting drug users in Australia reported injecting buprenorphine in the last 3-6 months [53,79]. Only 10% of injecting drug users (IDUs) reported buprenorphine as the primary drug of abuse [53].

Opioid maintenance drugs are nearly exclusively misused by individuals under substitution treatment who have a history of drug dependence [40] and substance use diagnoses in addition to opioid dependence [80].

An interesting study was performed recently in the US by Lofwall and Havens [81]. The study examined the frequency and source of and risk factors for diverted buprenorphine use over a 6-month period in an Appalachian community sample of prescription opioid abusers. Of the 503 participants at baseline, 471 completed the study. Psychiatric disorders and demographics, drugs use, and social network characteristics were ascertained at baseline and follow-up. Multivariable logistic regression was performed over the 6-month period. Results indicate that lifetime buprenorphine use "to get high" was 70.1%; 46.5% used diverted buprenorphine over the 6-month period; and 9.6% were daily users and 50%-60% sporadic users (1-2 uses over the 6 months). The most common sources were dealers (58.7%) and friends (31.6%). Predictors of increased risk of use of diverted buprenorphine included inability to access buprenorphine treatment (AOR: 7.31), meeting criteria for generalized anxiety disorder, and use in the past 30 days of oxycodone, methamphetamine, and/or alcohol. The authors concluded that these results "suggest that improving, rather than limiting, access to good quality affordable buprenorphine treatment may be an effective public strategy to mitigate buprenorphine abuse. Future work should be an effective public health strategy to mitigate buprenorphine abuse" [81].

Aitken et al. [53] performed a prospective cross-sectional study in 316 injecting drug users in Australia. More than 10% of participants reported buprenorphine as the drug they had most often injected, and 32% had injected buprenorphine at least once in the 3 months before the interview. Sharing a used needle was associated with buprenorphine injection.

Previously, a study reported at the 2006 Australian National Drug Trends Conference showed that of 914 injection drug users asked, 1% cited buprenorphine as their drug of choice, and 6% said that it was the drug they had injected most often in the preceding month [82].

A study examining abuse of buprenorphine with and without naloxone by untreated injection drug users found a strong preference for the formulation without naloxone [54].

Bazazi et al. [74] performed a qualitative epidemiological survey in the US in 51 IDUs and 49 non-injecting opioid users. Seventy-six percent of participants reported having obtained buprenorphine/naloxone illicitly. Diversion was more frequent in IDUs than in non-IDUs (86% vs. 65%). The reasons for use were treatment of withdrawal symptoms (74%), having stopped using other opioids (66%), and not being able to afford drug treatment (64%). The authors concluded that particularly IDUs used diverted buprenorphine for reasons consistent with its therapeutic use, such as alleviating opioid withdrawal symptoms and reducing the use of other opioids.

A US post-marketing surveillance study on methadone and buprenorphine found that between 2003 and 2007, rates of abuse, misuse, and diversion of both compounds increased steadily [83]. Rate ratios (per 100,000 population per quarter) of abuse, misuse, and diversion were consistently higher for methadone than buprenorphine.

A retrospective comparison in Australia of untreated regular IDUs and patients receiving medication-assisted therapy found that buprenorphine/naloxone was injected less frequently than buprenorphine, especially when the rate was corrected for medication availability [84].

An Australian multi-site cross-sectional survey in 508 clients, 442 receiving supervised methadone and 66 buprenorphine, found that the prevalence of recent diversion was more than 10 times higher among those receiving buprenorphine than among those receiving methadone, with 23.8% of buprenorphine-maintained participants reporting diverting their dose in the preceding 12 months [85]. Seventeen percent of methadone clients had injected methadone in the preceding 12 months compared with 9.1% of buprenorphine clients over the same time period. The authors concluded that the higher prevalence of buprenorphine diversion compared to methadone diversion is likely to be due to its sublingual tablet formulation and the difficulty associated with supervising its consumption compared to that of an oral liquid. The authors further discussed that "methadone diversion is also less prevalent likely due to the high levels of methadone take-away provision, which also helps to explain the higher levels of recent methadone injecting compared to buprenorphine injecting. A

clearer understanding of the motivations for diversion and injection of opioid pharmacotherapies, and the relationship between them is required" [85].

Gwin Mitchell et al. [86] conducted a qualitative epidemiological survey in 515 opioid-dependent individuals reporting diversion. The study included self-report data on diversion and semi-structured qualitative interviews. Of the total sample, 84 (16%) reported using diverted (street) methadone 2-3 times/week for six months or more. A subsample (n=22) indicated that street methadone was more widely used than street buprenorphine and that both drugs were largely used as self-medication for detoxification and withdrawal symptoms.

In Singapore, Ho et al. [16] conducted a retrospective data analysis and found that pulmonary hypertension may be a potential comorbidity among intravenous buprenorphine users, among many others.

The question of whether the buprenorphine/naloxone combination lowers the risk of diversion and intravenous use was addressed in Australia in a cross-sectional survey by Larance et al. [87]. Results showed that levels of injection among regular IDUs were lower for buprenorphine/naloxone than for buprenorphine, but comparable to those for methadone. Among patients, fewer buprenorphine/naloxone-treated patients (13%) reported recent injection of their medication than buprenorphine-treated (28%) and methadone-treated patients (23%). Overall, buprenorphine/naloxone was less commonly and less frequently injected than buprenorphine, but both were more frequently diverted than methadone.

Another Australian study [88] in 448 opioid-dependent individuals found that about one fourth of patients had ever injected buprenorphine. The rates of diversion in the 12 preceding months were higher among participants receiving buprenorphine (15.3%) than among those receiving methadone (4.3%).

A US/Canadian cross-sectional survey by Monte et al. [75] in 51 treatment-seeking opioid-individuals tried to characterize buprenorphine/naloxone diversion practices in a region with a high prescribing prevalence. One hundred per cent of patients had diverted buprenorphine/naloxone to modulate withdrawal symptoms arising from attempted "self-detoxification," insufficient funds to purchase preferred illicit opioids, or inability to find a preferred source of drugs.

In summing up the existing literature, Yokell et al. [32] concluded that buprenorphine is effective in opioid dependence treatment and harm reduction. The combination with naloxone may limit its injection misuse potential.

The issue of diversion and abuse of buprenorphine was addressed in a report by Maxwell [41] to the Substance Abuse and Mental Health Services Administration (SAMSHA) that was based on a literature review of papers published since 2002 (n=347). With respect to abuse potential, Maxwell [41] pointed out that while early reports of findings from animal studies suggested that buprenorphine would have minimal abuse potential, varying levels of diversion and abuse were predicted by early investigations in humans [89,90].

Concerning incidence and prevalence of buprenorphine abuse, on the basis of findings from two established informant networks Cicero and Inciardi [46] reported that the level of buprenorphine abuse remained relatively low through the first quarter of 2005 and appeared to be at a much lower level than seen with methadone or oxycodone. In a second report, this group ranked buprenorphine last among other opioids of abuse [68].

Diversion and abuse of buprenorphine in the US is not only restricted to opioid-dependent users: Chronic pain patients may also be affected, because of an increasing amount of nonmedical use of prescription opioids [91]. There are dramatic data concerning emergency department visits due to buprenorphine or other opioids in the US [92,93]. The relative benefit from buprenorphine was discussed by Mendelson et al. [92] in light of the epidemic misuse of prescription opioids. The authors stressed minimal problems with diversion or adverse clinical events, referring to a 2006 SAMSHA/CSAT Evaluation of the Buprenorphine Waiver program.

In their overview of the National Drug Abuse Treatment Clinical Trials Network by the National Institute on Drug Abuse (NIDA), Ling et al. [94] concluded that with the advent of a sublingual tablet containing both buprenorphine and naloxone to mitigate abuse and diversion, buprenorphine appeared poised to be the first-line treatment for opioid addiction.

Findings from a small sample (N=41) in Malaysia suggest that the introduction of the buprenorphine/naloxone combination did not decrease injection-related risk behaviors and was associated with increased benzodiazepine use [95]. A more systematic study in Malaysia, a two-wave survey of buprenorphine IDUs, found that both buprenorphine and buprenorphine/naloxone intravenous misuse occurred in heroin IDUs [60]. Focus group participants reported that buprenorphine/naloxone was not as desirable as buprenorphine, but widespread misuse nevertheless continued. The authors concluded that "the introduction of buprenorphine/naloxone and withdrawal of buprenorphine may have helped to reduce, but did not eliminate the problems with diversion and abuse" [60]. Buprenorphine misuse has been reported also in India [96-98].

Other studies found that switching patients from buprenorphine to buprenorphine/naloxone is an effective measure to reduce diversion and misuse. Amato [99] studied 78 patients for one year after they had switched from buprenorphine to buprenorphine/naloxone and found that the switch had a positive impact on diversion/misuse. Patients were satisfied with treatment and reported improved psychosocial functioning.

Winstock and Lea [88] conducted a survey in 448 clients receiving opioid maintenance treatment. Not surprisingly, the buprenorphine diversion rate in the preceding 12 months was over three times higher among those receiving supervised buprenorphine (15.3%) than among those receiving supervised methadone (4.3%). While 26.5% of participants currently prescribed buprenorphine reported ever injecting buprenorphine, 65.9% of those prescribed methadone reported ever injecting methadone.

Recently, Genberg et al. [100] conducted one of the few systematic assessments of street-obtained buprenorphine use in a community-based sample. Of the 602 respondents, only 9% reported street-obtained buprenorphine use, and only 2% reported getting high. Among active opioid users, 3% reported recent use of diverted buprenorphine. Most patients took street-obtained buprenorphine to avoid withdrawal symptoms.

European Studies

There are reports of buprenorphine misuse/diversion from many European countries, including France, Germany, Spain, the UK, Ireland, and the Scandinavian countries [101-106]. The misuse/ diversion of opioid analgesics in the European community was addressed in a recent systematic review of the literature by Casati et

al. [40]. Methadone and buprenorphine were considered as medicines used for opioid substitution treatment. The authors stated that both drugs have high rates of misuse, including doctor shopping, i.e. seeing multiple treatment providers to procure prescription medications illicitly; illicit intravenous application; snorting; and buying or selling on the black market [107-110].

Buprenorphine is widely used in France, and one study reported that up to 20% of buprenorphine patients misuse the drug intravenously [111]. Another study in France found that 27% of IDUs were exclusively buprenorphine injectors, while another 37% reported polydrug use [112]. Some of these IDUs purchased their buprenorphine from individuals with a prescription [113], while others obtained it by altering or forging prescriptions [51,114,115]. Similar results were provided by Obadia et al. [116]. Intravenous misuse is by far the dominant method in France, but there are also cases of buprenorphine sniffing [117,118].

Guichard et al. [119] reported data of a cross-sectional study on illicit drug use and injection practices among drug users receiving methadone (N=197) and buprenorphine (N=142) treatment in France. Injection was more common among buprenorphine-maintained individuals than among those treated with methadone (40.1% vs. 15.2%, p>0.01). Multivariate analyses indicated that the type of substitution drug was not associated with illicit drug use. Rather surprisingly, the risk of injection increased with dosage in the buprenorphine group but not in the methadone group.

In many cases, methadone and buprenorphine misuse begins even before a subject enters an opioid maintenance treatment program. Cazorla et al. [120] reported that 84000 opioid users have undergone maintenance treatment in France since 2001. Among these patients, 88% were being treated with buprenorphine, and 35% reported having used buprenorphine for the first time without having a prescription for it. An Irish study [109] found even higher rates of methadone misuse before treatment entry among patients in maintenance therapy: 73% of participants reported methadone misuse before starting treatment, while 55% reported methadone misuse during treatment. The main reasons for misuse were management of withdrawal symptoms and hedonistic effects.

German data from patients admitted for detoxification showed that 53.5% misused medical opioids, especially methadone [110], mainly because of difficulty in acquiring heroin.

A recent Italian study by Moratti et al. [107] on heroin-dependent patients in maintenance therapy reported intravenous misuse of buprenorphine by 23.1% of patients. Not surprisingly, patients receiving buprenorphine maintenance therapy were significantly more likely to inject buprenorphine intravenously than those receiving methadone (35.5% vs. 17.8%, respectively). About half (50.7%) of the patients reported injecting buprenorphine to treat their withdrawal symptoms, while only 12.7% of patients reported doing so to experience pleasure or euphoria. In addition, participants were asked to assess the number of patients receiving buprenorphine who had attempted to take it intravenously: 45.9% of participants thought that at least 50% of patients on buprenorphine replacement therapy had injected buprenorphine intravenously, suggesting that the initial results may have underestimated the problem. The authors concluded that misuse was most common among patients currently receiving buprenorphine treatment and among younger patients. "For the majority of patients, the reason for intravenous misuse was to treat their dependence. We believe that the prevalence for buprenorphine misuse could be reduced by adopting appropriate clinical practices and treating patients with the buprenorphine/naloxone combination rather than buprenorphine alone" [107].

A group in Sweden [101] studied buprenorphine misuse among patients in a syringe exchange program and found that 43% of heroin and amphetamine users reported intravenous misuse of buprenorphine and 29% snorting. In addition, 11% of heroin users reported buprenorphine use to induce euphoria compared to 62% of amphetamine users. A Finnish study on the abuse liability of buprenorphine-naloxone tablets among untreated intravenous drug users found that buprenorphine is the most misused intravenous opioid in Finland and that misuse increased sharply in 2001 as heroin availability coincidentally decreased [54]. In order to curb buprenorphine misuse, many treatment centers crush tablets before administering them to patients. Simojoki et al. [121] found that this practice does not significantly alter the clinical effect of the drug, indicating that it is an appropriate method to reduce misuse.

Doctor shopping is a means of acquiring more maintenance drugs than required and is a widespread problem. Some countries, e.g. Germany, have introduced central patient registers to prevent patients obtaining multiple treatments. On the basis of data from the General Health Insurance System in one area of Southern France, Pauly et al. [108] found that 13.2% of the reimbursed high-dose buprenorphine was dispensed with prescriptions obtained from doctor shopping. In addition, results revealed that the more deviant a patient's behavior, the higher the risk for doctor shopping. Another French study on buprenorphine maintenance treatment [122] found that practitioners' attitudes influence the likelihood of doctor shopping, not the other way around: Doctor shopping was lower among general practitioners who induced buprenorphine maintenance treatment with 8 mg/day or more of buprenorphine, as compared with those who prescribed a lower initial dosage; also, doctor shopping was more common among general practitioners with more stringent, "conservative" attitudes towards patients.

An online questionnaire revealed that 72% of 300 opioid-prescribing practitioners in Germany, Italy, France, and the UK believed that buprenorphine or methadone misuse was a huge or significant problem [123]. The results also suggest that often subtherapeutic doses of maintenance drugs were used.

France has quite "liberal" prescribing regulations for buprenorphine, the predominant maintenance medication, which may account for buprenorphine's diversion into the black market [124]. Prescription-monitoring programs may reduce the risk for doctor shopping [125]. The risk of buprenorphine misuse (and benzodiazepine misuse and rates of depression) is underestimated by physicians, as shown in a cross-sectional study by Lavie et al. [126]. Data from France from 2006 show that up to 25% of French buprenorphine doses were diverted into the black market (Narcotics Control Board 2006).

In Germany in 2008, 80%-85% of injecting drug users reported finding it easy to access methadone or buprenorphine on the black market [127].

In a cross-sectional survey in Udine/Italy, Moratti et al. [107] studied opioid-dependent patients treated with methadone (n=214) or buprenorphine (n=93). Significantly more buprenorphine patients (35.5%) than methadone-maintained patients (17.8%) admitted intravenous misuse; the main reason given was self-treatment. Also in Italy, a cross-sectional survey by Montesano et al. [128] studied the effect in 43 opioid-dependent patients of 24 weeks' treatment

with buprenorphine/naloxone after the patients had switched from buprenorphine alone. Only 2% of patients attempted to misuse buprenorphine/naloxone intravenously, and none of them experienced any gratifying effects.

Interestingly, a survey in Finnish intravenous opioid users showed that buprenorphine was the drug most frequently used intravenously (73% of the respondents) [54]. More than 75% used intravenous buprenorphine to self-treat addiction or withdrawal. Most individuals (68%) had tried the buprenorphine/naloxone combination, but 80% reported having a "bad" experience with it. Also interestingly, the street price of buprenorphine/naloxone was less than half that of buprenorphine alone. The authors concluded that buprenorphine/naloxone appears to be a feasible tool for decreasing intravenous abuse of buprenorphine.

A recent Swedish study based on surveys and structured interviews of adolescents and young adults indicated that illicit use of methadone and buprenorphine is rare, only 0.1% of the cohorts sampled had tried these substances, and misuse and diversion of both was not seen as a serious problem by professionals [129].

Risk factors of abuse, which may not be specific for buprenorphine, are younger age, intravenous use of opioids, poor social conditions such as unemployment and withdrawal symptoms, among others [93,130]. Buprenorphine is also cheaper than heroin in many areas [53].

Role of Take-home Doses

Take-home doses of buprenorphine can be prescribed in most countries. In some cases, patients are given take-home doses after they are stabilized, and in others a less than daily dosage of buprenorphine is possible for patient convenience [26]. Advantages of at-home use include saving time for travel, facilitating social integration, emphasizing and promoting patient responsibility for treatment, reinforcing compliance, improving a trusting relationship between staff and patients, engaging in normal day activities, and reducing workload for the dispenser. Some of the apparent risks are the risk of diversion to another person and injection of the oral medication. Patients who should not be candidates for take-home doses include those with repeated intoxication on presentation for dosing at the clinic, concerns about child welfare and safety, current chaotic and unpredictable behavior, risk of self-harm, and hazardous use of opioids [26].

Curcio et al. [131] reported data from a large sample (N=3812) in Italian outpatient centers, 81.5% of whom were treated with methadone and 18.5% with buprenorphine. Patients on buprenorphine treatment were switched to buprenorphine/naloxone, and all patients were followed for about 1 year. The number of patients still in treatment was similar in both groups, but the buprenorphine/naloxone patients reported a significantly greater improvement than the methadone patients in social life status, educational level, and especially toxicological conditions.

In the UK, the number of deaths related to methadone dose clearly declined after the introduction of supervised methadone dosing [132].

Recently, a Finnish study investigated whether electronic medicine dispensers may reduce the risk of diversion of take-home buprenorphine-naloxone, but the authors concluded that further research on this topic is required [133].

Genetics

Recently, the role of genetic variants for treatment response and risk of diversion in buprenorphine maintenance therapy was examined by Gerra et al. [134]. While there was no evidence that genetic variants of the kappa receptor are relevant, a distinct variant of the dopamine transporter gene (DAT 1 allele 10) was more frequent in buprenorphine non-responders. These results must be seen as very preliminary and need confirming.

Risk of Fatal Poisoning/Mortality

A fairly recent scholarly review of 58 prospective studies reporting mortality rates from opioid-dependent samples [135] revealed remarkable mortality rates (all-cause mortality of 2.09 per 100 person years, PY), but confirmed that overall maintenance treatment significantly reduces mortality rates as compared to untreated heroin dependence (1%-3% per year, <50% attributable to heroin overdose). The reasons for death varied, depending on the methodology, but most patients died from overdose; the risk was highest for male patients and during out-of-treatment periods. Although this finding confirms previous reports, core issues remain unresolved, such as mortality risk by type of substitution medication, the degree to which the substitution drug is involved, and mortality during and after dropping out of maintenance. Additional data from Australia also suggest that the majority of deaths in opioid-dependent people are drug related [136].

The general consensus is that overdoses caused by buprenorphine alone are rare [8,137,138]. In an epidemiological review, Okie [139] concluded that deaths from unintentional drug overdoses in the US have risen sharply since the early 1990s and are the second leading cause of accidental death (27,658 in 2007). The increase has been propelled by a rising number of overdoses of opioids, which in 2007 alone caused more deaths than heroin and cocaine combined. Other data show that most of the drug-related unintentional deaths in the US are related to methadone (31%), hydrocodone (19%), alprazolam (15%), and oxycodone (15%) [140]. In general, deaths due to unintentional overdoses of methadone or other opioid analgesics are associated with poverty, unemployment, and prescription opioid drug rates [93].

Very few corresponding data are available from European studies. From 1991 to 2007, the numbers of drug–related deaths due to methadone poisoning increased in Nordic countries [141]. Buprenorphine was the most frequent cause of death among drug-dependent subjects in Finland (25% of all fatal intoxications in 2007), while methadone was the most frequent cause of death in Denmark (51%). Multidrug use was very common in drug-related deaths.

A large German naturalistic follow-up study (N=2694) on one-year outcome in opioid-dependent maintenance patients found an annual mortality rate of 1.04% for methadone- and buprenorphine-treated patients [142]. The study was a nationally representative, prospective, longitudinal naturalistic study program with three waves (baseline, 1 year, 5-7 years) and was based on a nationwide representative sample of physicians and their opioid-dependent patients [143]. During the six-year follow-up phase, n=131 patients died. Mortality rates were 1.2% (n=28/2284) after one year and 5.7% (n=131/2284) after 6 years. The mean crude annual mortality rate was 1.0%, or 1.2 per 100 PY. Mortality rates did not differ significantly between men and women [144]. The most frequent causes of mortality were somatic disorders (n=57, 36.6%), e.g. HIV/Aids (14 cases), cancer (6 cases), cardiovascular disease (6 cases: 5 [0.3%] in the methadone group and 1 [0.2%] in the buprenorphine group, difference not significant); drug overdose (n=37, 28.3%), e.g. heroin, cocaine, benzodiazepine, 6 cases with more than one drug, including the substitution drug; and suicide (16%). Fatal overdose of substitution drugs was almost never

the exclusive reason (n=2, 1.5%), and interactions of the substitution drug with other concomitant drugs were relatively rare as well (n=6, 6.1%). The majority of deceased patients were not in maintenance treatment (n=73, 55.7%) in the weeks before death, either because the treating physician had decided to discontinue maintenance or because the patient had stopped attending appointments. Consistent with this finding, rates of overdose appeared to be elevated for those who died outside treatment. Of the 58 (44.3%) patients who died during maintenance treatment, 52 of a total of 1,690 treated with methadone at baseline were on methadone medication, and 6 out of 578 treated with buprenorphine at baseline were on buprenorphine medication. In this study, buprenorphine patients had a significantly lower mortality risk (OR: 0.27, p=.005) than methadone patients. These results indicated a comparably low mean crude annual mortality rate of 1.0% and a standardized mortality rate of 1.2 per 100 PY. This rate is lower than the annual mortality rate for opioid users indicated by a recent and very comprehensive meta-analysis by Degenhardt et al. [135], possibly reflecting the beneficial effect of the particular characteristics of German maintenance treatment.

In contrast to the meta-analytic findings, the most frequent reason for death in this study was somatic morbidity, followed by fatal overdose/intoxication of multiple substances. The substitution drug itself was rarely (1.5%) involved in premature mortality. Suicide (16%) was another major contributor. Accidents or other violent causes of death were rare (4.6%). Interestingly, the annual mortality rate decreased only moderately over time and not as much as one might have expected and was highest in the first year of the study. Other long-term studies also indicate persistently high mortality among opioid-dependent patients [1] that appears to change over time.

Just over half of the patients (55.7%) were no longer in maintenance treatment at the time of death. In line with previous studies [4], discontinuation for any reason and being out of treatment were the major predictors for death. Also in line with previous studies that addressed shorter follow-up periods [8,135], well-known predictors such as unemployment, higher age, longer opioid use, and comorbid mental or somatic disorders were confirmed in this study.

The substantially lower rate of premature mortality among buprenorphine-treated patients at the 6-year follow-up was remarkable [144]; buprenorphine was found to be a significant predictor for survival. These data are consistent with other findings, especially French and German forensic autopsy data that indicate a low mortality risk with buprenorphine [145,146]. Bell et al. [7] reported that buprenorphine may be safer in the induction phase. In a recent study on risk of death in a large cohort of patients, Cornish et al. [147] found a crude mortality rate of 0.7 per 100 PY among patients in treatment and 1.3 per 100 PY among patients out of treatment. Unlike the mortality risk in the German study, mortality risk was twice as high in men and also higher in the first two weeks of treatment. Variations in outcome and mortality may have been explained also by differences in the clinical samples and by an allocation of severely affected patients to the methadone group, as possibly indicated by a higher rate of baseline comorbid psychiatric diagnosis [148].

Laberke and Bartsch [11] reported that most methadone-associated deaths in Switzerland (N=176) occurred during substitution treatment or illicit intake of methadone. The majority of cases (76%) were related to polydrug intoxication.

Degenhardt et al. [135] estimated the overall reduction in mortality produced by substitution programs to be 29%.

Especially in the US, buprenorphine poisoning and unintentional exposure in children and toddlers has been recognized as a major health problem, because of the increasing number of reports of emergency visits. In nearly all cases, intoxications are nonfatal (4 of 4879 in children under 6, for recent review see [149]). Similar data were published by Lavonas et al. [150], who reported 4 deaths among 2380 cases of unintentional exposures to buprenorphine in children up to 6 years old.

Discussion and Conclusions

Substance use and risk of diversion are central problems in opioid maintenance therapy. All drugs with opioid agonist effects have an abuse potential. Like other "illegal" behaviors, the issue of abuse/diversion is difficult to study. Relevant outcome data do not come from clinical studies, but from surveys of physicians and their clients or poison control centers, among others. With respect to countries, data about opioid misuse, especially prescription opioids, are available predominantly from the US and Australia, and much fewer data are available from Europe. There are significant differences in rates of reported illicit buprenorphine use and diversion between countries. Concerns persist about the increasing misuse and diversion of prescription opioids, especially methadone, oxycodone and others, but to a lesser extent also of buprenorphine, as indicated by a dramatic increase in emergency room visits linked to opioid overdose. To date, this issue is a matter of great public concern in the US, but not in Europe. Rates of diversion depend also on different legal regulations, the "drug market" availability of different drugs, and other factors. One of the apparent advantages of buprenorphine is the very low risk of fatal (mono-) intoxications, at least compared to other opioids. In France, where buprenorphine is by far the most frequently prescribed drug in opioid maintenance therapy, data from 2006 indicate that up to 25% of French buprenorphine doses were diverted into the black market.

Buprenorphine and buprenorphine/naloxone are administered sublingually. A novel buprenorphine film has been developed, but so far it is available only in the US and Australia [151]. Buprenorphine tablets are usually crushed and misused intravenously, and are smoked or inhaled only rarely. The combination buprenor-phine/naloxone was developed to diminish the risk for intravenous use. Naloxone is inactive when taken orally, but immediately precipitates opioid withdrawal when injected, so the combination aims to reduce the risk of abuse/diversion; some data support the effectiveness of the combination in fulfilling this aim. The buprenorphine/naloxone combination is less liked by intravenous opioid users. It may not have eliminated the problem of buprenorphine abuse, but it has clearly decreased it. Fatal intoxications are extremely rare with the combination form and are mostly due to polyintoxications with other CNS depressants. Risk factors for buprenorphine abuse/diversion are younger age, intravenous use of opioids, poor social conditions, and withdrawal symptoms, i.e. all-in-all the typical picture of a polydrug user. Insufficient control of withdrawal symptoms has consistently been reported by buprenorphine abusers as a reason for use. In some cases, a higher dose of buprenorphine and adequate dosing may be helpful to control withdrawal and diminish the risk for buprenorphine misuse.

Careful assessment and supervision of patients given take-home doses of buprenorphine is important for clinical success. If take-home dosing is permitted and the patient is an appropriate candidate, treatment should be initiated with supervised administration and should progress to unsupervised administration when the patient's clinical stability permits. During treatment induction, closer supervision of dosing is

recommended to ensure proper sublingual placement of the dose and to observe the patient's response to treatment as a guide to effective dose titration. As the patient becomes stabilized on treatment, longer intervals between patient assessment may be appropriate, depending on patient compliance, effectiveness of the treatment plan, and overall patient progress. It is also recommended that when determining the prescription quantity for unsupervised administration, the frequency of patient visits and the patient's ability to manage supplies of take-home medication are taken into consideration.

In some cases, crushing the tablets before giving them to patients may be a simple approach to reduce risk of misuse, as shown in Scandinavian studies. In general, one must consider that a reduced risk of buprenorphine/naloxone misuse can be balanced and outweighed by the risk of abusing other drugs, e.g. other opioids, alcohol, or benzodiazepines, which may have an even higher risk for fatal intoxications. A very "conservative" attitude of the treating physician and too low dosages of buprenorphine may encourage doctor shopping and related behaviors, as shown in French studies. On the other hand, too "liberal" regulations may also enhance risk of diversion.

From a scientific point of view, in particular more European studies on the risk of diversion and toxicological studies on safety issues are warranted.

References

1. Bjornaas MA, Bekken AS, Ojlert A, Haldorsen T, Jacobsen D, et al. (2008) A 20-year prospective study of mortality and causes of death among hospitalized opioid addicts in Oslo. BMC Psychiatry 8: 8.

2. Degenhardt L, Randall D, Hall W, Law M, Butler T, et al. (2009) Mortality among clients of a state-wide opioid pharmacotherapy program over 20 years: risk factors and lives saved. Drug Alcohol Depend 105: 9-15.

3. Hser YI, Anglin D, Powers K (1993) A 24-year follow-up of California narcotics addicts. Arch Gen Psychiatry 50: 577-584.

4. Peles E, Schreiber S, Adelson M (2010) 15-Year survival and retention of patients in a general hospital-affiliated methadone maintenance treatment (MMT) center in Israel. Drug Alcohol Depend 107: 141-148.

5. Degenhardt L, Bucello C, Calabria B, Nelson P, Roberts A, et al. (2011) What data are available on the extent of illicit drug use and dependence globally? Results of four systematic reviews. Drug Alcohol Depend 117: 85-101.

6. Mattick RP, Breen C, Kimber J, Davoli M (2009) Methadone maintenance therapy versus no opioid replacement therapy for opioid dependence. Cochrane Database Syst Rev: CD002209.

7. Bell J, Trinh L, Butler B, Randall D, Rubin G (2009) Comparing retention in treatment and mortality in people after initial entry to methadone and buprenorphine treatment. Addiction 104: 1193-1200.

8. Bell JR, Butler B, Lawrance A, Batey R, Salmelainen P (2009) Comparing overdose mortality associated with methadone and buprenorphine treatment. Drug Alcohol Depend 104: 73-77.

9. Winstock AR, Lea T, Sheridan J (2009) What is diversion of supervised buprenorphine and how common is it? J Addict Dis 28: 269-278.

10. Centers for Disease Control and Prevention (CDC) (2010) Emergency department visits involving nonmedical use of selected prescription drugs - United States, 2004-2008. MMWR Morb Mortal Wkly Rep 59: 705-709.

11. Laberke PJ, Bartsch C (2010) Trends in methadone-related deaths in Zurich. Int J Legal Med 124: 381-385.

12. Perret G, Déglon JJ, Kreek MJ, Ho A, La Harpe R (2000) Lethal methadone

intoxications in Geneva, Switzerland, from 1994 to 1998. Addiction 95: 1647-1653.

13. Berson A, Gervais A, Cazals D, Boyer N, Durand F, et al. (2001) Hepatitis after intravenous buprenorphine misuse in heroin addicts. J Hepatol 34: 346-350.

14. Centers for Disease Control and Prevention (2013) HIV/AIDS: DHAP Strategic Plan.

15. Ho RC, Ho EC, Mak A (2009) Cutaneous complications among i.v. buprenorphine users. J Dermatol 36: 22-29.

16. Ho RC, Ho EC, Tan CH, Mak A (2009) Pulmonary hypertension in first episode infective endocarditis among intravenous buprenorphine users: case report. Am J Drug Alcohol Abuse 35: 199-202.

17. Noroozi A, Mianji F (2008) Singapore's experience with buprenorphine (Subutex). Iran J Psychiatry 2: 54-59.

18. Hansen RN, Oster G, Edelsberg J, Woody GE, Sullivan SD (2011) Economic costs of nonmedical use of prescription opioids. Clin J Pain 27: 194-202.

19. Davis WR, Johnson BD (2008) Prescription opioid use, misuse, and diversion among street drug users in New York City. Drug Alcohol Depend 92: 267-276.

20. Duffy P, Baldwin H (2012) The nature of methadone diversion in England: a Merseyside case study. Harm Reduct J 9: 3.

21. Strang J, Sheridan J, Hunt C, Kerr B, Gerada C, et al. (2005) The prescribing of methadone and other opioids to addicts: national survey of GPs in England and Wales. Br J Gen Pract 55: 444-451.

22. Maremmani I, Pacini M, Pani PP, Popovic D, Romano A, et al. (2009) Use of street methadone in italian heroin addicts presenting for opioid agonist treatment. J Addict Dis 28: 382-388.

23. Bell J (2010) The global diversion of pharmaceutical drugs: opiate treatment and the diversion of pharmaceutical opiates: a clinician's perspective. Addiction 105: 1531-1537.

24. Kleber HD, Weiss RD, Anton RF, George TP, Greenfield SF, et al. (2007) Treatment of patients with substance use disorders, second edition. American Psychiatric Association. Am J Psychiatry 164: 5-123.

25. Soyka M, Kranzler HR, van den Brink W, Krystal J, Moller HJ, et al. (2011) The World Federation of Societies of Biological Psychiatry (WFSBP) guidelines for the biological treatment of substance use and related disorders. Part 2: Opioid dependence. World J Biol Psychiatry 12: 160-187.

26. New South Wales Department of Health (2011) Opioid treatment program: Clinical guidelines for methadone and buprenorphine treatment. NSW Government, Sydney.

27. Lingford-Hughes AR, Welch S, Peters L, Nutt DJ; British Association for Psychopharmacology, Expert Reviewers Group (2012) BAP updated guidelines: evidence-based guidelines for the pharmacological management of substance abuse, harmful use, addiction and comorbidity: recommendations from BAP. J Psychopharmacol 26: 899-952.

28. World Health Organization (2009) Guidelines for the psychosocially assisted pharmacological treatment of opioid dependence. World Health Organization, Geneva.

29. Meili D, Broers B, Beck T, Bruggmann P, Hämmig R, et al. (2013) Medical recommendations for maintenance therapy in opioid dependence [in German]. Suchtmed 15: 51-102.

30. Mammen K, Bell J (2009) The clinical efficacy and abuse potential of combination buprenorphine-naloxone in the treatment of opioid dependence. Expert Opin Pharmacother 10: 2537-2544.

31. Orman JS, Keating GM (2009) Spotlight on buprenorphine/naloxone in the treatment of opioid dependence. CNS Drugs 23: 899-902.

32. Yokell MA, Zaller ND, Green TC, Rich JD (2011) Buprenorphine and buprenorphine/naloxone diversion, misuse, and illicit use: an international review. Curr Drug Abuse Rev 4: 28-41.

33. Walsh SL, Preston KL, Stitzer ML, Cone EJ, Bigelow GE (1994) Clinical pharmacology of buprenorphine: ceiling effects at high doses. Clin Pharmacol Ther 55: 569-580.

34. van Dorp E, Yassen A, Dahan A (2007) Naloxone treatment in opioid addiction: the risks and benefits. Expert Opin Drug Saf 6: 125-132.

35. Preston KL, Bigelow GE, Liebson IA (1990) Effects of sublingually given

naloxone in opioid-dependent human volunteers. Drug Alcohol Depend 25: 27-34.

36. Stoller KB, Bigelow GE, Walsh SL, Strain EC (2001) Effects of buprenorphine/naloxone in opioid-dependent humans. Psychopharmacology (Berl) 154: 230-242.

37. Kakko J, Gronbladh L, Svanborg KD, von Wachenfeldt J, Ruck C, et al. (2007) A stepped care strategy using buprenorphine and methadone versus conventional methadone maintenance in heroin dependence: a randomized controlled trial. Am J Psychiatry 164: 797-803.

38. Schottenfeld RS, Pakes JR, Oliveto A, Ziedonis D, Kosten TR (1997) Buprenorphine vs methadone maintenance treatment for concurrent opioid dependence and cocaine abuse. Arch Gen Psychiatry 54: 713-720.

39. Soyka M, Zingg C, Koller G, Kuefner H (2008) Retention rate and substance use in methadone and buprenorphine maintenance therapy and predictors of outcome: results from a randomized study. Int J Neuropsychopharmacol 11: 641-653.

40. Casati A, Sedefov R, Pfeiffer-Gerschel T (2012) Misuse of medicines in the European Union: a systematic review of the literature. Eur Addict Res 18: 228-245.

41. Maxwell JC (2006) Diversion and Abuse of Buprenorphine: A Brief Assessment of Emerging Indicators. Final report. Submitted to the Substance Abuse and Mental Health Services Administration Center for Substance Abuse Treatment. Submitted by JBS International, Inc.

42. Horyniak D, Dietze P, Larance B, Winstock A, Degenhardt L (2011) The prevalence and correlates of buprenorphine inhalation amongst opioid substitution treatment (OST) clients in Australia. Int J Drug Policy 22: 167-171.

43. Middleton LS, Nuzzo PA, Lofwall MR, Moody DE, Walsh SL (2011) The pharmacodynamic and pharmacokinetic profile of intranasal crushed buprenorphine and buprenorphine/naloxone tablets in opioid abusers. Addiction 106: 1460-1473.

44. Harper I (1983) Temgesic abuse. N Z Med J 96: 777.

45. Strang J (1985) Abuse of buprenorphine. Lancet 2: 725.

46. Cicero TJ, Inciardi JA (2005) Potential for abuse of buprenorphine in office-based treatment of opioid dependence. N Engl J Med 353: 1863-1865.

47. Sporer KA (2004) Buprenorphine: a primer for emergency physicians. Ann Emerg Med 43: 580-584.

48. Comer SD, Collins ED (2002) Self-administration of intravenous buprenorphine and the buprenorphine/naloxone combination by recently detoxified heroin abusers. J Pharmacol Exp Ther 303: 695-703.

49. Comer SD, Collins ED, Fischman MW (2002) Intravenous buprenorphine self-administration by detoxified heroin abusers. J Pharmacol Exp Ther 301: 266-276.

50. Comer SD, Sullivan MA, Walker EA (2005) Comparison of intravenous buprenorphine and methadone self-administration by recently detoxified heroin-dependent individuals. J Pharmacol Exp Ther 315: 1320-1330.

51. Baumevieille M, Haramburu F, Begaud B (1997) Abuse of prescription medicines in southwestern France. Ann Pharmacother 31: 847-850.

52. Sigmon SC, Moody DE, Nuwayser ES, Bigelow GE (2006) An injection depot formulation of buprenorphine: extended bio-delivery and effects. Addiction 101: 420-432.

53. Aitken CK, Higgs PG, Hellard ME (2008) Buprenorphine injection in Melbourne, Australia--an update. Drug Alcohol Rev 27: 197-199.

54. Alho H, Sinclair D, Vuori E, Holopainen A (2007) Abuse liability of buprenorphine-naloxone tablets in untreated IV drug users. Drug Alcohol Depend 88: 75-78.

55. Johnson RE, Strain EC, Amass L (2003) Buprenorphine: how to use it right. Drug Alcohol Depend 70: S59-77.

56. Bickel WK, Stitzer ML, Bigelow GE, Liebson IA, Jasinski DR, et al. (1988) Buprenorphine: dose-related blockade of opioid challenge effects in opioid dependent humans. J Pharmacol Exp Ther 247: 47-53.

57. Collins GB, McAllister MS (2007) Buprenorphine maintenance: a new treatment for opioid dependence. Cleve Clin J Med 74: 514-520.

58. Comer SD, Sullivan MA, Whittington RA, Vosburg SK, Kowalczyk WJ (2008)

Abuse liability of prescription opioids compared to heroin in morphine-maintained heroin abusers. Neuropsychopharmacology 33: 1179-1191.

59. Strain EC, Walsh SL, Preston KL, Liebson IA, Bigelow GE (1997) The effects of buprenorphine in buprenorphine-maintained volunteers. Psychopharmacology (Berl) 129: 329-338.

60. Vicknasingam B, Mazlan M, Schottenfeld RS, Chawarski MC (2010) Injection of buprenorphine and buprenorphine/naloxone tablets in Malaysia. Drug Alcohol Depend 111: 44-49.

61. Wesson DR, Smith DE (2010) Buprenorphine in the treatment of opiate dependence. J Psychoactive Drugs 42: 161-175.

62. Who Expert Committee on Drug Dependence (2003) WHO Expert Committee on Drug Dependence: thirty-third report.

63. Wish ED, Artigiani E, Billing A, Hauser W, Hemberg J, et al. (2012) The emerging buprenorphine epidemic in the United States. J Addict Dis 31: 3-7.

64. Schuman-Olivier Z, Connery H, Griffin ML, Wyatt SA, Wartenberg AA, et al. (2013) Clinician beliefs and attitudes about buprenorphine/naloxone diversion. Am J Addict 22: 574-580.

65. U.S. Department of Justice-Drug Enforcement Administration (2013) Drug Fact Sheets.

66. Center for Substance Abuse Treatment (2004) Clinical Guidelines for the Use of Buprenorphine in the Treatment of Opioid Addiction. Treatment Improvement Protocol (TIP) Series 40. DHHS Publication No. (SMA) 04-3939. Substance Abuse and Mental Health Services Administration, Rockville, MD.

67. Fudala PJ, Bridge TP, Herbert S, Williford WO, Chiang CN, et al. (2003) Office-based treatment of opiate addiction with a sublingual-tablet formulation of buprenorphine and naloxone. N Engl J Med 349: 949-958.

68. Cicero TJ, Inciardi JA, Muñoz A (2005) Trends in abuse of Oxycontin and other opioid analgesics in the United States: 2002-2004. J Pain 6: 662-672.

69. Rosenblum A, Parrino M, Schnoll SH, Fong C, Maxwell C, et al. (2007) Prescription opioid abuse among enrollees into methadone maintenance treatment. Drug Alcohol Depend 90: 64-71.

70. Schneider MF, Bailey JE, Cicero TJ, Dart RC, Inciardi JA, et al. (2009) Integrating nine prescription opioid analgesics and/or four signal detection systems to summarize statewide prescription drug abuse in the United States in 2007. Pharmacoepidemiol Drug Saf 18: 778-790.

71. Smith MY, Bailey JE, Woody GE, Kleber HD (2007) Abuse of buprenorphine in the United States: 2003-2005. J Addict Dis 26: 107-111.

72. Hughes AA, Bogdan GM, Dart RC (2007) Active surveillance of abused and misused prescription opioids using poison center data: a pilot study and descriptive comparison. Clin Toxicol (Phila) 45: 144-151.

73. Schuman-Olivier Z, Albanese M, Nelson SE, Roland L, Puopolo F, et al. (2010) Self-treatment: illicit buprenorphine use by opioid-dependent treatment seekers. J Subst Abuse Treat 39: 41-50.

74. Bazazi AR, Yokell M, Fu JJ, Rich JD, Zaller ND (2011) Illicit use of buprenorphine/naloxone among injecting and noninjecting opioid users. J Addict Med 5: 175-180.

75. Monte AA, Mandell T, Wilford BB, Tennyson J, Boyer EW (2009) Diversion of buprenorphine/naloxone coformulated tablets in a region with high prescribing prevalence. J Addict Dis 28: 226-231.

76. Johanson CE, Arfken CL, di Menza S, Schuster CR (2012) Diversion and abuse of buprenorphine: findings from national surveys of treatment patients and physicians. Drug Alcohol Depend 120: 190-195.

77. Dasgupta N, Freifeld C, Brownstein JS, Menone CM, Surratt HL, et al. (2013) Crowdsourcing black market prices for prescription opioids. J Med Internet Res 15: e178.

78. Larance B, Degenhardt L, O'Brien S, Lintzeris N, Winstock A, et al. (2011) Prescribers' perceptions of the diversion and injection of medication by opioid substitution treatment patients. Drug Alcohol Rev 30: 613-620.

79. Jenkinson RA, Clark NC, Fry CL, Dobbin M (2005) Buprenorphine diversion and injection in Melbourne, Australia: an emerging issue? Addiction 100: 197-205.

80. Astals M, Domingo-Salvany A, Buenaventura CC, Tato J, Vazquez JM, et al. (2008) Impact of substance dependence and dual diagnosis on the quality of life of heroin users seeking treatment. Subst Use Misuse 43: 612-632.

81. Lofwall MR, Havens JR (2012) Inability to access buprenorphine treatment as a risk factor for using diverted buprenorphine. Drug Alcohol Depend 126: 379-383.

82. Maxwell JC (2006) Report on the Australian National Drug Trends Conference and the annual meeting of the Australasian Professional Society on Alcohol and Other Drugs. Personal Communication.

83. Dasgupta N, Bailey EJ, Cicero T, Inciardi J, Parrino M, et al. (2010) Post-marketing surveillance of methadone and buprenorphine in the United States. Pain Med 11: 1078-1091.

84. Degenhardt L, Larance BK, Bell JR, Winstock AR, Lintzeris N, et al. (2009) Injection of medications used in opioid substitution treatment in Australia after the introduction of a mixed partial agonist-antagonist formulation. Med J Aust 191: 161-165.

85. Winstock AR, Lea T, Sheridan J (2008) Prevalence of diversion and injection of methadone and buprenorphine among clients receiving opioid treatment at community pharmacies in New South Wales, Australia. Int J Drug Policy 19: 450-458.

86. Gwin Mitchell S, Kelly SM, Brown BS, Schacht Reisinger H, Peterson JA, et al. (2009) Uses of diverted methadone and buprenorphine by opioid-addicted individuals in Baltimore, Maryland. Am J Addict 18: 346-355.

87. Larance B, Degenhardt L, Lintzeris N, Bell J, Winstock A, et al. (2011) Post-marketing surveillance of buprenorphine-naloxone in Australia: diversion, injection and adherence with supervised dosing. Drug Alcohol Depend 118: 265-273.

88. Winstock AR, Lea T (2010) Diversion and injection of methadone and buprenorphine among clients in public opioid treatment clinics in New South Wales, Australia. Subst Use Misuse 45: 240-252.

89. Jaffe JH, O'Keeffe C (2003) From morphine clinics to buprenorphine: regulating opioid agonist treatment of addiction in the United States. Drug Alcohol Depend 70: S3-S11.

90. Robinson GM, Dukes PD, Robinson BJ, Cooke RR, Mahoney GN (1993) The misuse of buprenorphine and a buprenorphine-naloxone combination in Wellington, New Zealand. Drug Alcohol Depend 33: 81-86.

91. Zacny J, Bigelow G, Compton P, Foley K, Iguchi M, et al. (2003) College on Problems of Drug Dependence taskforce on prescription opioid non-medical use and abuse: position statement. Drug Alcohol Depend 69: 215-232.

92. Mendelson J, Flower K, Pletcher MJ, Galloway GP (2008) Addiction to prescription opioids: characteristics of the emerging epidemic and treatment with buprenorphine. Exp Clin Psychopharmacol 16: 435-441.

93. Spiller H, Lorenz DJ, Bailey EJ, Dart RC (2009) Epidemiological trends in abuse and misuse of prescription opioids. J Addict Dis 28: 130-136.

94. Ling W, Jacobs P, Hillhouse M, Hasson A, Thomas C, et al. (2010) From research to the real world: buprenorphine in the decade of the Clinical Trials Network. J Subst Abuse Treat 38 Suppl 1: S53-60.

95. Bruce RD, Govindasamy S, Sylla L, Kamarulzaman A, Altice FL (2009) Lack of reduction in buprenorphine injection after introduction of co-formulated buprenorphine/naloxone to the Malaysian market. Am J Drug Alcohol Abuse 35: 68-72.

96. Chowdhury AN, Chowdhury S (1990) Buprenorphine abuse: report from India. Br J Addict 85: 1349-1350.

97. Panda S, Kumar MS, Lokabiraman S, Jayashree K, Satagopan MC, et al. (2005) Risk factors for HIV infection in injection drug users and evidence for onward transmission of HIV to their sexual partners in Chennai, India. J Acquir Immune Defic Syndr 39: 9-15.

98. Solomon SS, Desai M, Srikrishnan AK, Thamburaj E, Vasudevan CK, et al. (2010) The profile of injection drug users in Chennai, India: identification of risk behaviours and implications for interventions. Subst Use Misuse 45: 354-367.

99. Amato P (2010) Clinical experience with fortnightly buprenorphine/naloxone versus buprenorphine in Italy: preliminary observational data in an office-based setting. Clin Drug Investig 30 Suppl 1: 33-39.

100. Genberg BL, Gillespie M, Schuster CR, Johanson CE, Astemborski J, et al. (2013) Prevalence and correlates of street-obtained buprenorphine use among current and former injectors in Baltimore, Maryland. Addict Behav 38: 2868-2873.

101. Hakansson A, Medvedeo A, Andersson M, Berglund M (2007) Buprenorphine

misuse among heroin and amphetamine users in Malmo, Sweden: purpose of misuse and route of administration. Eur Addict Res 13: 207-215.

102. Lavelle TL, Hammersley R, Forsyth A (1991) The use of buprenorphine and temazepam by drug injectors. J Addict Dis 10: 5-14.

103. Mounteney J, Haugland S (2009) Earlier warning: a multi-indicator approach to monitoring trends in the illicit use of medicines. Int J Drug Policy 20: 161-169.

104. O'Connor JJ, Moloney E, Travers R, Campbell A (1988) Buprenorphine abuse among opiate addicts. Br J Addict 83: 1085-1087.

105. Sakol MS, Stark C, Sykes R (1989) Buprenorphine and temazepam abuse by drug takers in Glasgow--an increase. Br J Addict 84: 439-441.

106. San L, Torrens M, Castillo C, Porta M, de la Torre R (1993) Consumption of buprenorphine and other drugs among heroin addicts under ambulatory treatment: results from cross-sectional studies in 1988 and 1990. Addiction 88: 1341-1349.

107. Moratti E, Kashanpour H, Lombardelli T, Maisto M (2010) Intravenous misuse of buprenorphine: characteristics and extent among patients undergoing drug maintenance therapy. Clin Drug Investig 30 Suppl 1: 3-11.

108. Pauly V, Frauger E, Pradel V, Rouby F, Berbis J, et al. (2011) Which indicators can public health authorities use to monitor prescription drug abuse and evaluate the impact of regulatory measures? Controlling High Dosage Buprenorphine abuse. Drug Alcohol Depend 113: 29-36.

109. Roche A, McCabe S, Smyth BP (2008) Illicit methadone use and abuse in young people accessing treatment for opiate dependence. Eur Addict Res 14: 219-225.

110. Scherbaum N, Kluwig J, Meiering C, Gastpar M (2005) Use of illegally acquired medical opioids by opiate-dependent patients in detoxification treatment. Eur Addict Res 11: 193-196.

111. Auriacombe M, Fatseas M, Dubernet J, Daulouede JP, Tignol J (2004) French field experience with buprenorphine. Am J Addict 13 Suppl 1: S17-28.

112. Moatti JP, Vlahov D, Feroni I, Perrin V, Obadia Y (2001) Multiple access to sterile syringes for injection drug users: vending machines, needle exchange programs and legal pharmacy sales in Marseille, France. Eur Addict Res 7: 40-45.

113. Bouchez J, Vignau J (1998) The French experience--the pharmacist, general practitioner and patient perspective. Eur Addict Res 4 Suppl 1: 19-23.

114. Boeuf O, Lapeyre-Mestre M; French Network of Centers for Evaluation and Information Pharmacodependence (CEIP) (2007) Survey of forged prescriptions to investigate risk of psychoactive medications abuse in France: results of OSIAP survey. Drug Saf 30: 265-276.

115. Lapeyre-Mestre M, Damase-Michel C, Adams P, Michaud P, Montastruc JL (1997) Falsified or forged medical prescriptions as an indicator of pharmacodependence: a pilot study. Community pharmacists of the Midi-Pyrénées. Eur J Clin Pharmacol 52: 37-39.

116. Obadia Y, Perrin V, Feroni I, Vlahov D, Moatti JP (2001) Injecting misuse of buprenorphine among French drug users. Addiction 96: 267-272.

117. Roux P, Villes V, Bry D, Spire B, Feroni I, et al. (2008) Buprenorphine sniffing as a response to inadequate care in substituted patients: results from the Subazur survey in south-eastern France. Addict Behav 33: 1625-1629.

118. Strang J (1991) Abuse of buprenorphine (Temgesic) by snorting. BMJ 302: 969.

119. Guichard A, Lert F, Calderon C, Gaigi H, Maguet O, et al. (2003) Illicit drug use and injection practices among drug users on methadone and buprenorphine maintenance treatment in France. Addiction 98: 1585-1597.

120. Cazorla C, Grenier de Cardenal D, Schuhmacher H, Thomas L, Wack A, et al. (2005) [Infectious complications and misuse of high-dose buprenorphine]. Presse Med 34: 719-724.

121. Simojoki K, Lillsunde P, Lintzeris N, Alho H (2010) Bioavailability of buprenorphine from crushed and whole buprenorphine (subutex) tablets. Eur Addict Res 16: 85-90.

122. Feroni I, Peretti-Watel P, Paraponaris A, Masut A, Ronfle E, et al. (2005) French general practitioners' attitudes and prescription patterns toward buprenorphine maintenance treatment: does doctor shopping reflect buprenorphine misuse? J Addict Dis 24: 7-22.

123. Bacha J, Reast S, Pearlstone A (2010) Treatment practices and perceived challenges for European physicians treating opioid dependence. Heroin Addict Relat Clin Probl 12: 9-19.

124. Fatseas M, Auriacombe M (2007) Why buprenorphine is so successful in treating opiate addiction in France. Curr Psychiatry Rep 9: 358-364.

125. Pradel V, Frauger E, Thirion X, Ronfle E, Lapierre V, et al. (2009) Impact of a prescription monitoring program on doctor-shopping for high dosage buprenorphine. Pharmacoepidemiol Drug Saf 18: 36-43.

126. Lavie E, Fatséas M, Daulouède JP, Denis C, Dubernet J, et al. (2008) Comparison of prescriber evaluations and patient-directed self-reports in office-based practice for buprenorphine treatment of opiate-dependent individuals in France, 2002. Patient Prefer Adherence 2: 369-378.

127. Wickert C, Thane K, Reimer J (2009) Misuse of substitution medication from the users' perspective – motivation, prevalence and consequences. Suchtmedizin 11: 182.

128. Montesano F, Zaccone D, Battaglia E, Genco F, Mellace V (2010) Therapeutic switch to buprenorphine/naloxone from buprenorphine alone: clinical experience in an Italian addiction centre. Clin Drug Investig 30 Suppl 1: 13-19.

129. Richert T, Johnson B (2013) Illicit use of methadone and buprenorphine among adolescents and young adults in Sweden. Harm Reduct J 10: 27.

130. Bouley M, Viriot E, Barache D (2000) Practical reflections on the diversion of drugs. Therapie 55: 295-301.

131. Curcio F, Franco T, Topa M, Baldassarre C; Gruppo Responsabili UO Sert T (2011) Buprenorphine/naloxone versus methadone in opioid dependence: a longitudinal survey. Eur Rev Med Pharmacol Sci 15: 871-874.

132. Strang J, Hall W, Hickman M, Bird SM (2010) Impact of supervision of methadone consumption on deaths related to methadone overdose (1993-2008): analyses using OD4 index in England and Scotland. BMJ 341: c4851.

133. Uosukainen H, Pentikäinen H, Tacke U (2013) The effect of an electronic medicine dispenser on diversion of buprenorphine-naloxone-experience from a medium-sized Finnish city. J Subst Abuse Treat 45: 143-147.

134. Gerra G, Somaini L, Leonardi C, Cortese E, Maremmani I, et al. (2013) Association between gene variants and response to buprenorphine maintenance treatment. Psychiatry Res.

135. Degenhardt L, Bucello C, Mathers B, Briegleb C, Ali H, et al. (2011) Mortality among regular or dependent users of heroin and other opioids: a systematic review and meta-analysis of cohort studies. Addiction 106: 32-51.

136. Degenhardt L, Larney S, Randall D, Burns L, Hall W (2013) Causes of death in a cohort treated for opioid dependence between 1985 and 2005. Addiction.

137. Auriacombe M, Franques P, Tignol J (2001) Deaths attributable to methadone vs buprenorphine in France. JAMA 285: 45.

138. Kintz P (2001) Deaths involving buprenorphine: a compendium of French cases. Forensic Sci Int 121: 65-69.

139. Okie S (2010) A flood of opioids, a rising tide of deaths. N Engl J Med 363: 1981-1985.

140. Piercefield E, Archer P, Kemp P, Mallonee S (2010) Increase in unintentional medication overdose deaths: Oklahoma, 1994-2006. Am J Prev Med 39: 357-363.

141. Simonsen KW, Normann PT, Ceder G, Vuori E, Thordardottir S, et al. (2011) Fatal poisoning in drug addicts in the Nordic countries in 2007. Forensic Sci Int 207: 170-176.

142. Soyka M, Apelt SM, Lieb M, Wittchen HU (2006) One-year mortality rates of patients receiving methadone and buprenorphine maintenance therapy: a nationally representative cohort study in 2694 patients. J Clin Psychopharmacol 26: 657-660.

143. Wittchen HU, Apelt SM, Soyka M, Gastpar M, Backmund M, et al. (2008) Feasibility and outcome of substitution treatment of heroin-dependent patients in specialized substitution centers and primary care facilities in Germany: a naturalistic study in 2694 patients. Drug Alcohol Depend 95: 245-257.

144. Soyka M, Träder A, Klotsche J, Backmund M, Buhringer G, et al. (2011) Six-year mortality rates of patients in methadone and buprenorphine maintenance therapy: results from a nationally representative cohort study. J Clin Psychopharmacol 31: 678-680.

145. Pirnay S, Borron SW, Giudicelli CP, Tourneau J, Baud FJ, et al. (2004) A critical review of the causes of death among post-mortem toxicological investigations: analysis of 34 buprenorphine-associated and 35 methadone-associated deaths. Addiction 99: 978-988.

146. Soyka M, Penning R, Wittchen U (2006) Fatal poisoning in methadone and buprenorphine treated patients--are there differences? Pharmacopsychiatry 39: 85-87.

147. Cornish R, Macleod J, Strang J, Vickerman P, Hickman M (2010) Risk of death during and after opiate substitution treatment in primary care: prospective observational study in UK General Practice Research Database. BMJ 341: c5475.

148. Lieb M, Wittchen HU, Palm U, Apelt SM, Siegert J, et al. (2010) Psychiatric comorbidity in substitution treatment of opioid-dependent patients in primary care: Prevalence and impact on clinical features. Heroin Addict Relat Clin Probl 12: 5-16.

149. Soyka M (2013) Buprenorphine and buprenorphine/naloxone intoxication in children-how strong is the risk? Curr Drug Abuse Rev 6: 63-70.

150. Lavonas EJ, Banner W, Bradt P, Bucher-Bartelson B, Brown KR, et al. (2013) Root causes, clinical effects, and outcomes of unintentional exposures to buprenorphine by young children. J Pediatr 163: 1377-1383.

151. Soyka M (2012) Buprenorphine and buprenorphine/naloxone soluble-film for treatment of opioid dependence. Expert Opin Drug Deliv 9: 1409-1417.

34

Cardiovascular Medicine Safety Profile Evaluation among Urban Private Hospitals

Fredy IC[1], Palatty PL[2]*, Iqbal PT[3], Manikandan TV[3] and Srinivasan R[4]

[1]Pharm D, PES College of Pharmacy, Bangalore, India
[2]Department of Pharmacology Father Muller Medical College, Mangalore, India
[3]Cardiologist, Daya General Hospital & Speciality Centre, Thrissur, India Cardiologist, Elite Mission Hospital, Thrissur, India
[4]Department of Pharmacy Practice, PES College of Pharmacy, Bangalore, India

Abstract

The pharmacovigilance is on-going, mandatory process among medical college hospitals. The private hospitals organization is prioritized and structured differently. Regular efficacy and safety evaluations are not conducted as academic research but occur by default in teaching hospitals. This study investigated and collected adverse drug reactions in this site and contrasted with literature from existing studies to draw comparisons and appropriate interventions.

This was a cross sectional observational study design using conventional ADR form from Central Drugs Standard Control Organization and checklist of cardiovascular medicine specific adverse reactions which was administered for data collection after necessary formalities for patient recruitment. There were statistically significant differences in total number of cardiovascular medications prescribed, the common cardiovascular medicines used, common concomitant medicine prescribed. The ADR profile showed commonly mild and moderate severity with low incidence of severe adverse event.

The adverse reaction profile did have large number of reactions but in the milder range. The cautious prescribing of large number of medicines with low intensity ADRs indicates the discharge of cautious responsibility due to direct liability and awareness. Peer misdemeanors among small circle of professionals would have severe repercussions on their clientele.

Keywords: Cardiovascular drugs; Pharmacovigilance; Drug safety; Adverse drug reactions; ADR reporting in private sector

Introduction

Adverse Drug Reactions (ADRs) are one of the major factors that undermine the therapy. ADRs are unwanted medication effects that have a dramatic impact on economic and clinical perspective often leading to hospital admissions, prolongation of hospital stay and emergency department visits. Premarketing surveillances are conducted to detect and quantify ADRs. Randomized controlled trials have limited sample size and heterogeneity, ADRs occurs in real world during clinical practice rather than clinical trials. Thus post marketing medication safety monitoring including spontaneous reporting, observational studies helps in providing means of ADR detection, quantification and prevention [1].

Cardiovascular diseases are the most common cause of death globally. Every 36 seconds 1 person dies from cardiovascular diseases, and each day about 2500 in US are struck by Cardiovascular Disease (CVD) death overwhelms the death due to cancer, lung diseases, accidents and diabetes combined [2].

Most common cardiovascular diseases includes   coronary heart diseases, stroke, hypertension, congestive cardiac failure, myocardial infarction etc, generally treated with cardiovascular medications falling into classes of diuretics, anti-hyperlipidemics, beta-blockers, calcium channel blockers, ACE inhibitors, nitrates and anti-thrombotics.

Common ADRs for cardiovascular medicines includes hypotension, electrolyte imbalances, dry cough, pedal edema for anti-hypertensives and rhabdomyolysis for statins. The ADRs increases the economic and clinical burden of the treatment [3,4].

This study aims to detect frequency rate, severity, and prevention of ADRs induced by cardiovascular medicines during the course of treatment.

Methodology

The design utilized in this study was of cross sectional-observational study, which was set up in two urban tertiary care hospitals with a sample size of 68.

Patients irrespective of their gender, age group between 30-90 years having history of clinical diagnosis of ischemic heart diseases, myocardial infarction, hypertension, angina pectoris, congestive heart failure were included and those with co-morbid condition of AIDS, severe infection and patients in I.C.U and I.C.C.U were excluded from the study .

Steps:

1.   Data collection forms were filled, from referring patient case file and patient interview.

2.   Observed ADRs were notified in ADR notification form.

*Corresponding author: Palatty PL, Department of Pharmacology Father Muller Medical College, Mangalore, India,
E-mail: drprincylouispalatty @gmail.com

3. Causality of the observed ADRs were assessed and documented.

4. Results were analyzed by using Microsoft excel.

The information collected included, patient general data (initials, age, gender, height, weight), suspected ADR (brief description of the reaction, onset date v/s stop date of occurrence of events, outcome of events, treatment received), suspected medication (name, indication, start date, stop date, dose, frequency, route of administration), medical history (past and present), concomitant medications, and any other relevant history, including the pre-existing medical conditions.

Results

Total of 68 patients of mean age 64yrs were involved in the study and out of which male to female ratio were 1:1.

Commonest diagnosis were hypertension (80.8%), diabetes mellitus (54.4%), AWMI (10.2%), IHD (8%), followed by LVD (7.3%) (Figure 1).The commonest cardiovascular medicines prescribed includes antihyperlipidemics (64.7%) and Anti-anginal (54.4%) (Figure 2).The commonest ADR noted was anorexia (45.5%) and nausea (41.17%) (Figures 3-5). The correlation between number of cardiac medications and number of ADRs were found to 1, which is perfect correlation, positive linear relationship (Figure 6).

Discussion

In this study we explored the ADR profile occurring in cardiac patients among two urban private hospitals. The observations are noteworthy.

The study showed that the gender ratio was almost equal (1:1). The previous articles documented prevalence of ADRs during treatment with cardiovascular medications were common in women compared to men [5].

In a study of ADRs associated with anti-hypertensives by Khurshid et al. among the 192-hypertensive patients, 87 were males and 105 were females. A total of 21 ADRs were observed in 13 out of 192 hypertensive patients. Among the 13 patients reported with ADRs 8 patients were female and 5 were male. Females experienced more ADRs than males [6].

In study conducted by Hussain et al. in medicine OP department by questionnaire based patent interview a total of 34 adverse drug reactions were observed in 250 hypertensive patients during the four month study. A high percentage of adverse drug reactions occurred in middle aged and female patients and frequencies of ADRs were common in poly pharmacy than monotherapy [7].

In our study we have not used the Naranjo's scale for evaluating the ADRs which is the definite limitation of the study but this research was done to answer to the query of ADR occurrence in private sector hospitals.

The mean age of subjects in our study is (64.46 ± 13.05).In the study by Rende et al. claims that most vulnerable age group for ADRs was > 61 yrs who have also been receiving multiple therapies .This high percentage is probably underestimated, because in older adults it may be difficult to recognize an ADR, as it can mimic some features of their age-related disease, Therefore, in elderly patients multiple therapies need to be discouraged, as these enhance the probability of ADRs, due to drug-drug interactions [3].

Diagnosis	%
Diabetes mellitus type 2	54.4
Hypertension	80.8
Left ventricular dysfunction	7.35
Ischaemic heart disease	8.82
AWMI	10.29
COPD	5.8
LRTI	2.9
Hyperlipidemia	4.4
CKD	5.8
Stroke	1.4
Hypothyroidism	5.8
Hypercholestrolemia	4.4
PTCA	2.9
CAD	11.7

*AWMI: Anterior Wall Myocardial Infraction; COPD: Chronic Obstructive Pulmonary Disease;LRTI:Lower Respiratory Tract Infection;CKD:Chronic Kidney Disease;PTCA : Percutaneous Transluminal Coronary Angioplasty; CAD: Coronary artery Disease
Figure 1: Clinical diagnosis

Class of medication prescribed	%
Antihyperlipidemics	64.7
Beta Blockers	13.2
Ca^{2+} channel Blockers	29.4
ACE inhibitors	8.8
Diuretics	26.40
cardiac glycosides	5.80
drugs affecting blood	36.7
antianginal	54.4

Figure 2: Class of medication prescribed

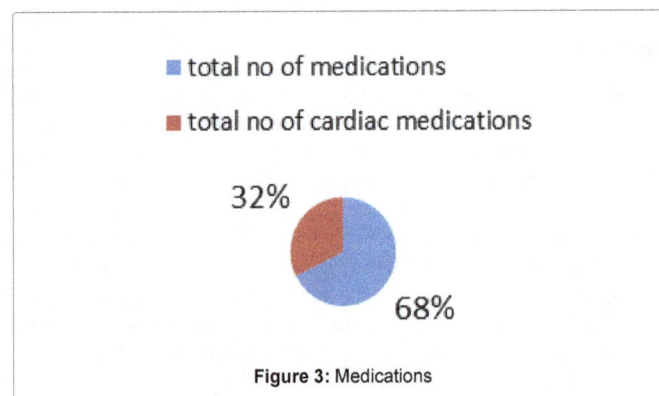

- total no of medications
- total no of cardiac medications

32%

68%

Figure 3: Medications

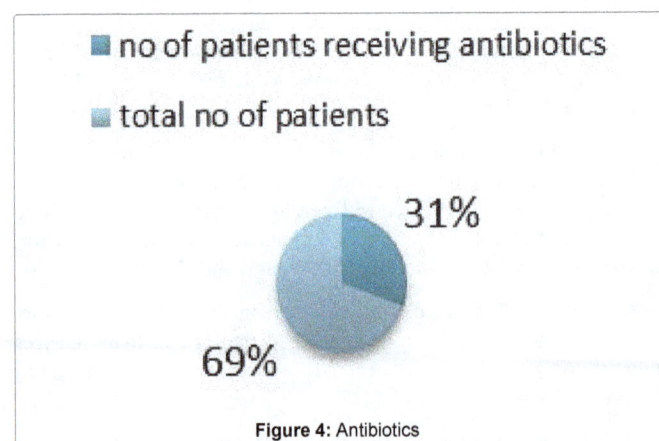

- no of patients receiving antibiotics
- total no of patients

31%

69%

Figure 4: Antibiotics

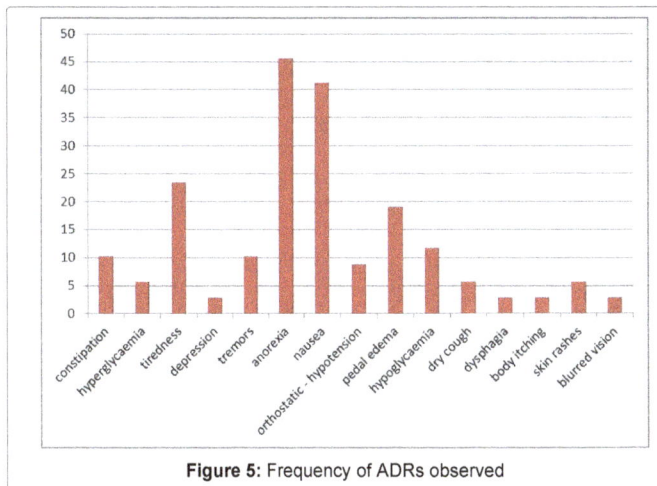

Figure 5: Frequency of ADRs observed

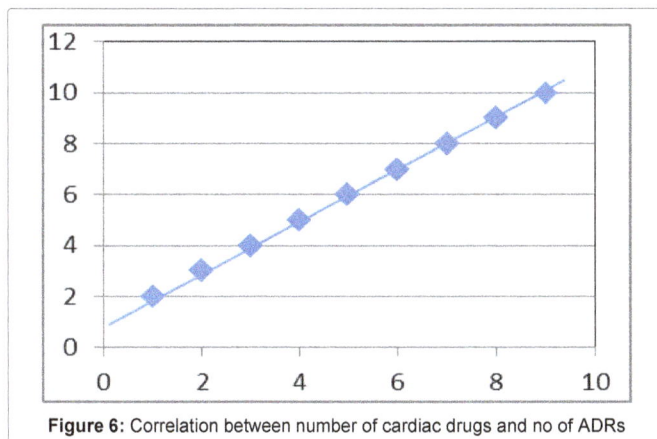

Figure 6: Correlation between number of cardiac drugs and no of ADRs

Study by Venturini et al. on gender differences, polypharmacy, and potential pharmacological interactions in the elderly, out of the 438 elderly patients in the data base, 376 (85.8%) used pharmacotherapy, 274 were female, and 90.4% of females used medications. Women younger than 80 years old used more medications than men in the same age group whereas men older than 80 years increased their use of medications in relation to other age groups [8].

In study by Sriram et al. in private tertiary care hospital, total of 57 documented ADRs were identified in 3117 General Medicine ward admissions during 12 months study period. The results of the age categorization revealed that the patients of 60 years and above age group experienced maximum ADRs which were about, followed by in age group between 30-59 years and 18-29 years age group [9].

Our study shows total number of medicines prescribed for a cardiovascular case is about 5.48, among which the cardiac medications are 2.6, on an average. Study by Venturini et al. The average number of medications used by each individual younger than 80 years was 3.2 ± 2.6 [8].

In our study Most common class of cardiovascular medicines received by the patient was anti-hyperlipidemics (54.4%), antianginal (45.5%), drugs affecting blood (36.6%), CCBs (29.4%), diuretics (26.4%).

In our study general ADRs observed during the treatment were anorexia (45.6%), nausea (41.17%), tiredness (23.52%), pedal edema (19.11%), hypoglycaemia (11.12 %), constipation (10.29%), tremors

(10.29%), orthostatic hypotension (8.8%), dry cough (5.8%). In study by Khurshid et al. calcium channel blockers (CCBs) was found to be the commonest therapeutic class associated with ADRs , followed by diuretics , β-blockers , ARBs and ACE inhibitors. CCBs associated with abdominal pain, ankle edema, sedation, pedal edema, and back pain. Diuretics with fatigue, visual impairment and dizziness. Dry cough was observed with ACE inhibitors [6].

In a study conducted on 19000 admissions in two National Health Services (NHS) units in UK 6.5% were due to ADRs [17].

In a study conducted on in-patients most frequent medications resulting in ADRs were opioid analgesics, antibiotics, diuretics, corticosteroids [18].

Study by Torpet et al. reported the occurrence of oral ADRs due to cardiovascular medications affecting oral mucous membrane, saliva production, and taste [19].

Study by Jimmy et al. shows that evaluation of patient characterization and reaction shows pattern of type A reactions were more common in elderly patients compared with other age groups and type B vice versa [20].

Study by Gallelli et al. on ADRs, NSAIDS was found responsible for 55.2% of ADR. Diclofenac and aspirin (acetylsalicylic acid) were the medications most frequently involved in the development of ADRs, while the skin was the body system most susceptible to NSAID-induced ADRs [10].

Study by Stern et al. suggests that calcium channel blockers are the cause for wide spectrum of cutaneous reactions like toxic epidermal necrolysis with diltiazem, Stevens-Johnson syndrome and erythema multiforme [12].

Study by Diaconu et al. shows that elderly patients prescribed with Diuretics are more likely to develop hypokalaemia and hyponatremia. Female patients had a higher frequency [13].

Study by Zafar et al. found that dry cough occurs with treatment by ACE inhibitors [15].

Study by Arumalni et al. found that the most common medications causing the ADRs were antibiotics associated with about one third of all the ADRs reported (55, 33.5%). Ampicillin produced the highest number of reactions followed by ciprofloxacin and nifedipine. Rashes were the most common ADR reported followed by edema, itching and diarrhoea. Skin was found to be the most commonly affected organ system followed by the central nervous and gastrointestinal systems [11].

Correlation analysis were done and value was found to be +1, which indicates that strong correlation exists between number of ADRs and number of cardiovascular medications in our study. The results of the study were limited by small sample size and geographical region.

Hospital admissions due to ADRs are significant health care problem in these days. As most of these reactions are predictable and preventable an awareness among health care professionals regarding detection, recording and reporting of ADRs following pharmacotherapy will prove to be very valuable for safer and rational drug utilization [14,16].

Conclusion

The present study is a part of Pharmacovigilance program conducted at two urban private hospitals, during this study safety profile of commonly prescribed cardiovascular medications were evaluated and we observed the adverse reaction profile did have large number of reactions but in the milder range, it may be helpful in selection of appropriate treatments enhancing patient adherence, thus reducing unnecessary economic burden to the patients due to unwanted effects of the therapy. Also this study clearly indicates the number of adverse reactions reported with leading questions is definitely more than those by spontaneous reporting. We conclude that quizzing of the patient for various ADRs has a better reflection of ADR reporting than spontaneous.

References

1. Sultana J, Cutroneo P, Trifirò G (2013) Clinical and economic burden of adverse drug reactions. J Pharmacol Pharmacother 4: S73–S77.

2. Myerburg RJ, Kessler KM, Castellanos A (1993) Sudden Cardiac Death: Epidemiology, Transient Risk, and Intervention Assessment. Ann Intern Med 119: 1187-1197.

3. Rende P, Paletta L, Gallelli G, Raffaele G, Natale V (2013) Retrospective evaluation of adverse drug reactions induced by antihypertensive treatment. J Pharmacol Pharmacother 4: S47–S50.

4. Bruckert E, Hayem G, Dejager S, Yau C, Bégaud B (2005) Mild to Moderate Muscular Symptoms with High-Dosage Statin Therapy in Hyperlipidemic Patients-The PRIMO Study. Cardiovasc Drugs Ther 19: 403-414.

5. Mohebbi N, Shalviri G, Salarifar M, Salamzadeh J, Gholami K (2010) Adverse drug reactions induced by cardiovascular medications in cardiovascular care unit patients. Pharmacoepidemiol Drug Saf 19: 889-894.

6. Khurshid F, Aqil M, Alam MS, Kapur P, Pillai KK (2012) Monitoring of adverse drug reactions associated with antihypertensive medicines at a university teaching hospital in New Delhi. Daru 20: 34.

7. Hussain A, Aqil M, Alam MS, Khan MR, Kapur P et al. (2009) A pharmacovigilance study of antihypertensive medicines at a South Delhi hospital. Indian J Pharm Sci.71: 338-341.

8. Venturini CD, Engroff P, Ely LS, Zago LF, Schroeter G (2011) Gender differences, polypharmacy, and potential pharmacological interactions in the elderly. Clinics 66: 1867-1872.

9. Sriram S, Ghasemi A, Ramasamy R, Devi M, Balasubramanian R (2011) Prevalence of adverse drug reactions at a private tertiary care hospital in south India. J Res Med Sci. 16: 16-25.

10. Gallelli L, Colosimo M, Pirritano D, Ferraro M, De Fazio S et al. (2007) Retrospective evaluation of adverse drug reactions induced by nonsteroidal anti-inflammatory drugs. Clin Drug Investig 27: 115-122.

11. Arulmani R, Rajendran SD, Suresh B (2008) Adverse drug reaction monitoring in a secondary care hospital in South India. Br J Clin Pharmacol 65: 210-216.

12. Stern R, Khalsa JH (1989) Cutaneous adverse reactions associated with calcium channel blockers. Arch Intern Med 149: 829-832.

13. Diaconu CC, Balaceanu A, Bartos D (2014) Diuretics, first-line antihypertensive agents: are they always safe in the elderly? Rom J Intern Med 52: 87-90.

14. Subramanian M, Nadig P (2013) Adverse Drug Reactions in rural field pratice area of a teritiary teaching hospital. Int J Pharmacol Therapeut 3: 2-7

15. Israili ZH, Hall WD (1992) Cough and Angioneurotic Edema Associated with Angiotensin-Converting Enzyme Inhibitor Therapy: A Review of the Literature and Pathophysiology. Ann Intern Med 117: 234-242.

16. Palanisamy S, Kumaran K, Rajasekaran A (2011) A study on assessment, monitoring and reporting adverse drug reactions in an indian hospital. Asian J Pharm Clin Res 4: 112-116.

17. Pirmohamed M, James S, Meakin S, Green C, Scott AK et al. (2004) Adverse drug reactions as cause of admission to hospital:prospective analysis of 18 820 patients. BMJ 329: 15.

18. Davies EC, Green CF, Taylor S, Williamson PR, Mottram DR et al. (2009) Adverse drug reactions in hospital in-patients:a prospective analysis of 3695 patient episodes. PLoS ONE 4: e4439.

19. Torpet LA, Kragelund C, Reibel J, Nauntoft B (2004) Oral adverse drug reactions of cardiovascular drugs. Crit Rev Oral Biol Med 15: 28-46.

20. Jose J, Rao PG (2006) Pattern of adverse drug reactions notified by spontaneous reporting in an Indian tertiary care teaching hospital. Pharmacol Res 54: 226-233.

35

A Pharmacovigilance Study Using Tracer Techniques

Yerramilli A[1]*, Veerla S[2], Chintala E[2], Guduguntla M[2], Velivelli P[2], Sharma S[3] and Paul R[4]

[1]Associate Professor, Sri Venkateshwara College of Pharmacy, Hyderabad, India
[2]Pharm. D Interns, Sri Venkateshwara College of Pharmacy, Department of Pharmacy Practice, Osmania University, Hyderabad, India
[3]Clinical Pharmacologist, Apollo Hospitals, Jubilee Hills, Hyderabad, India
[4]General Medicine, Apollo Hospitals, Jubilee Hills, Hyderabad, India

Abstract

Objective: To identify adverse drug reactions by using a comprehensive trigger tool method. To categorize the identified adverse drug reactions based upon their Probability, Severity, Harm and Preventability by using different scales.

Methods: A single-center, Cross-sectional, observational study based on medication and laboratory trigger tool methodology was conducted over a period of six months. The World Health Organization definition of adverse drug reactions was adopted. A list of 17 triggers were used to trace the adverse drug reactions which were then analyzed to assess the causality by using Naranjo's scale, severity by Hartwig and Siegel scale, and harm by the National Coordinating Council for Medication Error Reporting and Preventing Index and preventability by Modified Schumock and Thornton scale.

Results: A total of 100 suspected ADRs were collected and analyzed. The drug classes most commonly implicated with ADRs were cephalosporins (25%) followed by anti-diabetic agents (19%). According to Naranjo's scale, the reactions were categorized as probable (80%), possible (10%) and definite (5%). According to the modified Schumock and Thornton preventability scale, 20 cases (20%) were possibly preventable while 80 cases (80%) were not preventable. In 85 cases (85%) the suspected drug was withdrawn while in 10 cases (10%) no change in dose was made and in 5 cases (5%) the dose was altered.

Conclusion: Pharmacovigilance using tracer techniques significantly increases the identification and reporting of ADRs. The tracer technique is relatively simple, sensitive, less expensive and largely effective compared to traditional methods. The Trigger tool provides an additional instrument in improving patient safety. This technique leads to an increase in awareness and reporting of ADRs and provide opportunities for the health care system to review drug selection and prescribing practices affecting patient outcomes.

Keywords: Adverse drug reactions; Tracer techniques; Triggers; Naranjo's scale; Pharmacovigilance

Introduction

The advent of newer medicines has changed the way in which diseases are managed. Despite their benefits, mounting evidence suggests that drug related Adverse Drug Reactions (ADRs) are common, yet often preventable, cause of illness, disability, death and add to the overall healthcare cost [1]. Early detection, evaluation and monitoring of ADRs are essential to reduce harm to patients and thereby improving public health [2].

The detection of ADRs has become increasingly significant because of the introduction of a large number of newer medicines in the last two or three decades. World Health Organization (WHO) has intervened seriously in this regard and established an international ADR monitoring center at Uppsala, Sweden, which is collaborating with National monitoring centers in around 70 countries [3]. Adverse events occur in nearly one in ten hospitalizations with drug-related adverse events accounting for 15% of these [4].

Assessing the actual safety of drug use has been historically difficult, mainly because traditional methods such as chart audits and voluntary reporting of data which have been shown to be expensive, time consuming, insensitive, and largely ineffective for detecting drug related ADRs. Computerized methods for detecting ADRs, employing "tracer drugs or triggers" in a patient's medical record, are effective and relatively inexpensive [5]. A trigger tool is a simple checklist pro-forma containing a selected number of clinical 'triggers' which a reviewer looks to identify while screening electronic medical records. "Triggers or Tracer drugs" are defined as easily identifiable flags, occurrences or prompts in patient records that alert reviewers to potential adverse events which were previously undetected. The trigger tool methodology is a prospective and retrospective review of a random sample of patient records using triggers to identify possible adverse events associated with patient care. Trigger tools provide clues that an ADR has occurred. It focuses on detecting, quantifying and tracking adverse outcomes over time. The methodology is related to actual clinical injury. It can be used in all clinical environments to detect multiple types of Adverse Drug Event (ADE) [6].

Medication-related harm can be detected using a trigger tool methodology towards an adverse drug event. Medication-related triggers include the sudden withdrawal of a medication, a prescription for an antidote, or an abnormal laboratory test value [5]. Detecting

*Corresponding author: Yerramilli A, Head of Department, Sri Venkateshwara College of Pharmacy, 86, Hitech City Road, Madhapur, Hyderabad, Andhra Pradesh, India, E-mail: svcppharmd.hod@gmail.com

ADEs using 'triggers' from a patient's medical record was first described in the 1970s, and has been shown to be a practical and less labour-intensive approach for identifying ADEs than the traditional extensive retrospective case note review [7,8].

Classen et al. described the use of electronic ADE monitoring using computer database developed in hospital information systems in the early 1990s. While this methodology highlighted a faster method of screening for ADEs in a way that could be used to prevent patient harm rather than voluntary reporting of medical records review, it was deemed to require expensive investment and expertise in such technology [9,10]. The Institute of Healthcare Improvement (IHI) simplified the manual medical record review process and developed the Global Trigger Tool (GTT) consisting of 19 triggers in order to monitor adverse events rates in a way that was easy to replicate in hospitals, with or without computerized records [11]. The methodology cannot capture every adverse event, as it uses the periodic review of small, randomly selected samples of case notes and therefore is more of a surveillance tool. This regular review of notes is meant to take place alongside focused safety and quality improvement activities, with serial measurements of adverse event rates as a guide to their effectiveness.

The objectives of the study include to utilize the tracer methodologies in identifying the ADRs and to categorize the detected ADRs based on probability, severity, Harm and Preventability by using different scales.

There are quite a few studies conducted in India regarding the incidence, monitoring and reporting of ADRs in different departments and settings. But there are no published data regarding the use of triggers to identify ADRs. This is a first of its kind at our institution and will help us to provide insight into the prevalence of ADRs. This will also highlight the tool which could be used by the pharmacists to improve the identification of ADRs and thus their reporting.

Methods

A single-center, cross-sectional and observational drug safety study was conducted for a period of six months between March to August 2013 at a 630 bed tertiary care hospital. The study was initiated after the approval of the study protocol by the Institutional Ethics Committee (IEC) (Protocol No: SVCP/05/2013).

The study involved an active surveillance medication and laboratory module trigger tool methodology adapted from the IHI Global trigger tools and tools used by Rozich et al. [5]. A list of 17 triggers (Appendix-A), were used to trace the ADRs. Some triggers were removed from IHI list as they were either not used or available in our setting. Four new lab triggers were added in our study, which were identified as a potentially valuable trigger.

Data were collected in a questionnaire designed to include all relevant data for the study. Data on patient demographics, medical history, suspected drugs, ADRs, laboratory data were collected from the medical charts, nursing notes and medical records department. Inpatients of both sexes and all age groups who developed an ADR were included in the study; and patients treated on an outpatient basis or cancer patients or who developed an ADR to due to poisoning or administration of fresh blood/blood products were excluded from the study.

During the six month period, all the patient medical charts were reviewed for the presence of triggers. About 300 patient records were found to have the required triggers out of which 200 cases had to be excluded because no ADRs observed in those cases and the triggers

were used for various other indications. If a suspected ADR was reported and met the inclusion and exclusion criteria, data on that particular suspected drug and reaction was collected and documented.

All the investigators were trained to detect ADRs using the trigger tool methodology. The charts were reviewed daily. Each suspected ADR was assessed by all the investigators and approved by the Clinical Pharmacologist. The severity of the ADEs was evaluated using Hartwig and Siegel's scale. Harm was assessed by the National Coordinating Council for Medication Error Reporting and Prevention (NCC MERP) Index, which categorizes harm into E-I that correlates with the actual occurrence of harm to patients. The investigators also determined if hospital acquired ADEs could be preventable or not preventable using Modified Schumock and Thornton preventability scale.

Data was made anonymous and extracted into Excel' for analysis. Descriptive statistics were used to report the results. The Positive Predictive Value (PPV) for each trigger was calculated as the no. of ADRs identified with the Trigger/no. of Triggers found was generated.

Results

In this study, 100 triggers were identified and were found to be associated with ADRs. A total of 15,500 patients were admitted to the hospital during the study period. So the prevalence of ADRs in the institution over a period of six months is 0.64%. About 66% of the patients affected with ADRs were males and 54% were adults. The majority of the patients who developed an ADR were receiving anywhere between 6-10 medications. The demographic characteristics of patients are summarized in the Table 1.

Out of the 17 selected trigger tools, only 7 were identified during our study. The rest were not traced and hence no ADRs reported. The system most commonly affected by an ADR was the dermatology (56%) followed by the endocrine (19%). The PPV of the 7 triggers ranged from 0.17 to 0.65. Three triggers had PPVs at 0.33 or higher (Antihistamines, C difficile positive stool and INR>6). The trigger, PPV, suspected reactions and the systems involved are shown in the Table 2.

The drug class most commonly implicated with ADRs was antibiotics (56%) followed by insulin's (19%). The drug class least implicated were analgesics (1%).

The drugs most commonly implicated with ADRs were cephalosporins (25%) followed by insulins (19%) and penicillins (15%). The results of the drugs implicating ADRs were summarized in Table 3.

The majority of the reactions were type A (80%) followed by type B (10%). The results are summarized in the Figure 1.

Based upon the Naranjo's causality assessment scale, the ADRs were categorized as probable (85%), possible (10%) and definite (5%). According to the modified Hartwig and Siegel's severity assessment scale, the majority of the reactions were moderate (95%) followed

Demographics	No. Of Cases n=100
1. Age	
Paediatrics (<18 years)	6
Adults (18-60 years)	54
Geriatrics (>60 years)	40
2. Sex	
Male	66
Female	34

Table 1: Demographic characteristics.

Trigger Tools	Suspected reaction	Organ systems affected	No. of Triggers found on charts	No. of ADRs (n=100)	PPV
Antihistamines	Drug rashes	Dermatology	86	56	0.65
25% dextrose	Hypoglycemia	Endocrine	108	19	0.17
Calcium Gluconate, Insulin+ 25% dextrose Sodium polystyrene	Hyperkalemia	Systemic	47	12	0.25
Steroids	Hypersensitivity	Immune system	30	6	0.2
Vitamin K INR>6	Warfarin overdose, bleeding	Haematology	20 3	4 1	0.2 0.33
Clostridium difficile positive stool	Antibiotic induced diarrhea	Gastrointestinal	6	2	0.33

PPV=No. of ADRs identified with the Trigger/No. of Trigger found

Table 2: Trigger tools.

Drug class	Medicines	No. of ADR Reports n=100, (%)
1. Antibiotics: Cephalosporins	Cefoperazone Cefuroxime Ceftriaxone Cefotaxime	**25 (25%)**
Penicillins	Amoxicillin Ampicillin Piperacillin Ticarcillin	15 (15%)
Fluoro-quinolones	Ciprofloxacin Levofloxacin Ofloxacin	9 (9%)
Amino-glycosides	Amikacin	4 (4%)
Anti-Fungal	Ketoconazole Fluconazole	4 (4%)
Tetracyclines	Doxycycline	3 (3%)
Carbapenems	Meropenem Ertapenem	2 (2%)
Miscellaneous Antibiotics	Vancomycin	2 (2%)
Sulfonamides	Co-trimaxozole	1 (1%)
Anti-Amoebic	Metronidazole	1 (1%)
2. Insulins		19 (19%)
3. Anticoagulants	Warfarin Acenocoumarin	5 (5%)
4. Anti-Hypertensives	Telmisartan Lisinopril Losartan	3 (3%)
5. Skeletal Muscle Relaxants	Succinylcholine	3 (3%)
6. Immuno-suppressants	Cyclosporine Tacrolimus	2 (2%)
7. Analgesics	Diclofenac + Paracetamol	1 (1%)
8. Hormones and Contraceptives	Medoxyprogestrone	1 (1%)

Table 3: Medications Implicated in ADRs.

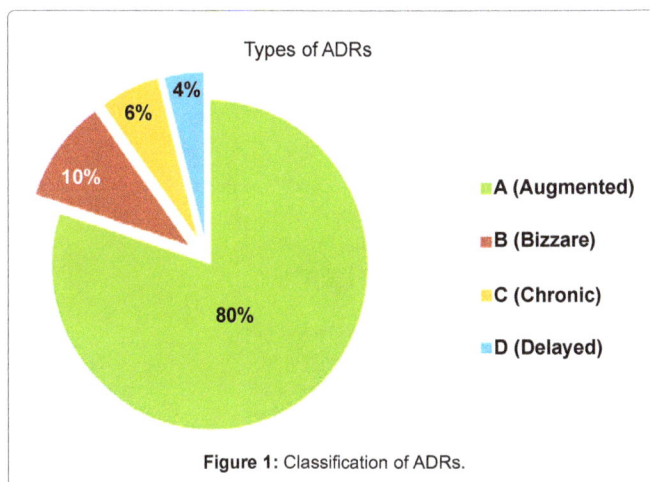

Figure 1: Classification of ADRs.

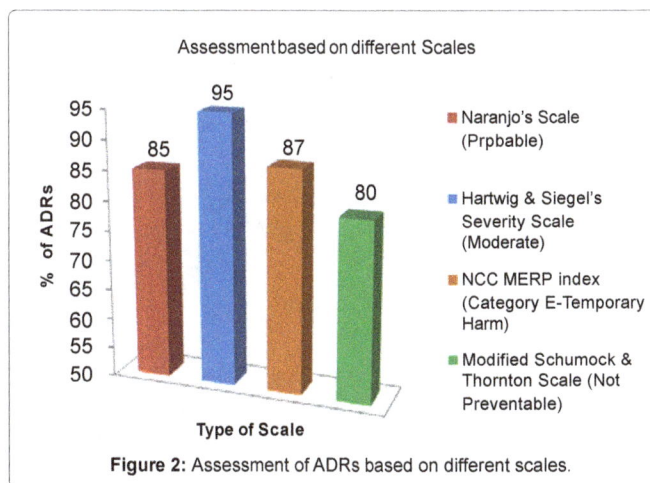

Figure 2: Assessment of ADRs based on different scales.

by severe (5%). Although some of the reactions were mild, patients received antidotes for the reactions as a routine practice in the hospital. According to the National Coordinating Council for Medication Error Reporting and Preventing (NCC MERP) index harm, 87% of the reactions fall under E category i.e., only temporary harm occurred to the patient and required intervention. According to the modified Schumock and Thornton preventability scale, 80% of the ADRs were not preventable. The management of the reported ADRs varied greatly. This study showed that most of the offending antibiotic class of drugs was withdrawn. As an outcome of the management, all the patients are recovered. The results are summarized in the Table 4.

While comparing with different ADR scales, we found that Naranjo's probability scale showing 85% of the reactions were probable, Hartwig and Siegel severity scale showing 95% of the

ADRs were moderate, NCC MERP index harm category showing 87% of the reactions as a category E (temporary harm which requires intervention), and Modified Schumock and Thornton preventability scale showing 80% of the ADRs were not preventable. The results are summarized in Figure 2.

Discussion

Numerous studies reported that approximately 5% to 15% of all hospital admissions are caused by ADRs and as many as 28% of the hospitalized patients experienced an ADR during their hospital stay. Under-reporting by doctors is a well known fact, even in countries with well established ADR reporting and monitoring programs. In India, the

Causality		
Score	**Naranjo's scale**	**No. of ADR Reports n=100, (%)**
≥ 9	Definite	5 (5%)
5-8	Probable	85 (85%)
1-4	Possible	10 (10%)
<1	Doubtful	0 (0%)
Severity		
Level	**Hartwig and Siegel's scale**	**No. of ADR Reports n=100, (%)**
1, 2	Mild	0 (0%)
3, 4, 5	Moderate	95 (95%)
6, 7	Severe	5 (5%)
NCC MERP Index		
Harm	**Category**	**No. of ADR Reports n=100, (%)**
E	Temporary harm and requires intervention	87 (87%)
F	Temporary harm and requires hospitalization	13 (13%)
G	Permanent harm	0 (0%)
H	Intervention required to sustain life	0 (0%)
I	Patient death	0 (0%)
Preventability		
Modified Schumock and Thornton Scale	**No. of Cases n=100, (%)**	
Definitely Preventable	0 (0%)	
Probably Preventable	20 (20%)	
Not Preventable	80 (80%)	
Management		
Management of ADR	**No. of cases n=100, (%)**	
Drug withdrawn	85 (85%)	
No change in dose	10 (10%)	
Dose altered	5 (5%)	
Outcomes		
Category	**No. of ADR Reports n=100, (%)**	
Fatal	0 (0%)	
Continuing	0 (0%)	
Recovering	0 (0%)	
Recovered	100 (100%)	
Unknown	0 (0%)	

Table 4: Assessment of ADRs.

major problem is a lack of a proper system of Pharmacovigilance which has led to a lack of decreased awareness of ADRs and their importance in early detection and prevention.

The reason for an increase in the detection of ADRs was due to the use of a trigger tool reporting system.

Literature surveys have shown that ADRs were common in geriatric and paediatric populations. But in our small study population adults were more prone to ADRs compared to other age groups. This may be due to the fact that most patients who were admitted to the hospital were adults. Another possible reason could be within the adult age group, most reported cases were from the patients who were ≥ 45 years old that those who were aged ≤ 44 years. Higher number of ADRs in the adult and geriatric population are due to the risk factors like co-morbid conditions, polypharmacy, drug interactions, impaired renal and hepatic function and altered physiological effect of the drugs have attributed to this variation.

Out of the 17 selected trigger tools, only 7 were identified ADRs in our study and the majority were antihistamines and the least commonly found were INR>6. Among other identified trigger tools were 25% dextrose, sodium polystyrene, steroids, vitamin K. Naessens et al. showed anti-emetic trigger tool has the maximum probability followed by diphenhydramine and vitamin K [12]. Ganachari et al. reported

abrupt medication stoppage as the maximum probability followed by hypotension [6]. The difference in above mentioned findings may be due to the variability in trigger tool usage.

The maximum number of suspected reactions was allergic rash due to antibiotics and least were diarrhoea induced by antibiotics. These findings were consistent with the study carried out by Palanisamy et al. which reported skin rash was the most commonly identified ADR followed by nausea and vomiting [13].

Antibiotics were found to be the most common class of drugs for ADRs. Among antibiotics, ADRs were maximum with cephalosporins followed by penicillins, fluoroquinolones and aminoglycosides. Our findings are consistent with the study carried out by Krishna et al. However, they reported fluoroquinolones followed by cephalosporins and aminoglycosides as common offenders [14] .This difference may be due to the higher number of cephalosporin prescriptions compared to fluoroquinolones in our study site.

PPVs of the triggers were highly variable. Many PPVs were in the lower range.

According to the type of reactions occurred, the majority were type A followed by type B. This result is consistent with the study carried out by Mandavi et al. [15]. There are no published reports showing prevalence of type C and D reactions.

Based on the Naranjo's causality assessment scale the ADRs were maximum in the category of probable followed by possible and definite. No ADRs were found in doubtful class.

As per the modified Hartwig and Siegel's scale maximum number of ADRs of moderate category was observed in our study. These findings were consistent with the literature reported by Ganachari et al. and Singh et al. [6,16].

As per the NCC MERP index harm category, the majority of the reactions were under the E category i.e., Temporary harm to the patient and requires intervention followed by F category i.e., Temporary harm to the patient and requires hospitalization. As per the Modified Schumock and Thornton preventability scale, maximum number of ADR were in not preventable category followed by probably preventable.

For better patient outcomes ADRs were managed with appropriate interventions and patients recovered. In our study, we found offending drug was withdrawn in the majority of cases followed by no change in dose and alteration of drug dose.

Limitations

In this study, the prevalence of ADRs was less when compared to other healthcare centers which could be due to its relative short duration and also since the hospital selected for our study is known for its highly developed patient safety programs. Thus, the findings cannot be generalized to other centers. As this was a pilot study evaluation of the performance of the trigger tool was not done. An improvement in the patient outcomes before and after the implementation of the trigger tool was not examined.

Conclusion

Adverse drug reactions are inevitable risk factors associated with the use of medicines. The present work is the maiden Pharmacovigilance study using tracer drugs conducted in the institution. It has provided baseline information about the prevalence of ADRs and their distribution among different age groups, genders, organ systems affected, therapeutic classes of medicines, and usage of trigger tools list. As the reporting of ADRs are very poor in the country and in the institution as well these trigger tools will help the clinical pharmacists to improve the identification and thus reporting the ADRs which will improve patient safety. The present study highlights the role of clinical pharmacists in Pharmacovigilance program.

Acknowledgement

We are immensely thankful to Apollo Hospitals, Osmania University, Management and Principal Dr. Prathima Srinivas of Sri Venkateshwara College of Pharmacy, for their constant encouragement and support provided during the study.

References

1. Ramesh M, Pandit J, Parthasaradhi G (2003) Adverse drug reactions in a south Indian hospital-their study and cost involved. Pharmacoepidemiol Drug Saf 12: 687-692.

2. Beijer HJ, de Blaey CJ (2002) Hospitalizations caused by adverse drug reactions: a metaanalysis of observational studies. Pharma World Sci 24: 46-54.

3. WHO (1972) International Drug Monitoring: The Role of National Centers.

4. de Vries EN, Ramrattan MA, Smorenburg SM, Gouma DJ, Boermeester MA (2008) The incidence and nature of in-hospital adverse events: a systematic review. Qual Saf Health Care 17: 216-223.

5. Rozich J, Haraden C, Resar R (2003) Adverse drug event trigger tool: a practical methodology for measuring medication related harm. Qual Saf Health Care 12: 194-200.

6. Ganachari MS, Wadhwa T, Walli S, Disha AK, Aggarwal A (2013) Trigger tools for monitoring and reporting of adverse drug reactions: A Scientific tool for efficient reporting. Open access scientific reports 2: 1-5.

7. Slone D, Jick H, Lewis GP, Shapiro S, Miettinen OS (1969) Intravenously given ethacrynic acid and gastrointestinal bleeding. A finding resulting from comprehensive drug surveillance. JAMA 209: 1668-1671.

8. Resar RK, Rozich JD, Simmonds T, Haraden CR (2006) A trigger tool to identify adverse events in the intensive care unit. Jt Comm J Qual Patient Saf 32: 585-590.

9. Classen DC, Pestotnik SL, Evans RS, Burke JP (1992) Description of a computerized adverse drug event monitor using a hospital information system. Hosp Pharm 27: 774, 776-779, 783.

10. Bates DW, Evans RS, Murff H, Stetson PD, Pizziferri L, Hripcsak G (2003) Detecting adverse events using information technology. J Am Med Inform Assoc 10: 115-128

11. Griffin FA, Resar RK (2009) IHI Global Trigger Tool for Measuring Adverse Events. (2nd edsn),IHI Innovation Series white paper. Cambridge, Massachusetts.

12. Naessens JM, O'Byrne TJ, Johnson MG, Vansuch MB, McGlone CM, et al. (2010) Measuring hospital adverse events: assessing inter-rater reliability and trigger performance of the Global Trigger Tool. Int J Qual Health Care 22: 266-274.

13. Palanisamy S, Kumaran KS, Rajasekaran A (2011) A Study on Assessment, Monitoring, Reporting of Adverse Drug Reactions in Indian Hospital. Asian J Pharm Clin Res 4: 112-116.

14. Krishna KD (2008) An analysis of Adverse Drug Reactions Reported in JIMPER. Drug Alert Regional Pharmacovigilance Centre (South) 4: 1-4.

15. Mandavi, Cruz SD, Sachdev A, Tiwari P (2012) Adverse drug reactions and their risk factors among Indian ambulatory elderly patients. Indian J Med Res. 136: 404-410.

16. Singh H, Kumar BN, Sinha T, Dulhani N (2011) The incidence and nature of drug-related hospital admission: A 6-month observational study in a tertiary health care hospital. J Pharmacol Pharmacother 2: 17-20.

Permissions

All chapters in this book were first published in APDS, by OMICS International; hereby published with permission under the Creative Commons Attribution License or equivalent. Every chapter published in this book has been scrutinized by our experts. Their significance has been extensively debated. The topics covered herein carry significant findings which will fuel the growth of the discipline. They may even be implemented as practical applications or may be referred to as a beginning point for another development.

The contributors of this book come from diverse backgrounds, making this book a truly international effort. This book will bring forth new frontiers with its revolutionizing research information and detailed analysis of the nascent developments around the world.

We would like to thank all the contributing authors for lending their expertise to make the book truly unique. They have played a crucial role in the development of this book. Without their invaluable contributions this book wouldn't have been possible. They have made vital efforts to compile up to date information on the varied aspects of this subject to make this book a valuable addition to the collection of many professionals and students.

This book was conceptualized with the vision of imparting up-to-date information and advanced data in this field. To ensure the same, a matchless editorial board was set up. Every individual on the board went through rigorous rounds of assessment to prove their worth. After which they invested a large part of their time researching and compiling the most relevant data for our readers.

The editorial board has been involved in producing this book since its inception. They have spent rigorous hours researching and exploring the diverse topics which have resulted in the successful publishing of this book. They have passed on their knowledge of decades through this book. To expedite this challenging task, the publisher supported the team at every step. A small team of assistant editors was also appointed to further simplify the editing procedure and attain best results for the readers.

Apart from the editorial board, the designing team has also invested a significant amount of their time in understanding the subject and creating the most relevant covers. They scrutinized every image to scout for the most suitable representation of the subject and create an appropriate cover for the book.

The publishing team has been an ardent support to the editorial, designing and production team. Their endless efforts to recruit the best for this project, has resulted in the accomplishment of this book. They are a veteran in the field of academics and their pool of knowledge is as vast as their experience in printing. Their expertise and guidance has proved useful at every step. Their uncompromising quality standards have made this book an exceptional effort. Their encouragement from time to time has been an inspiration for everyone.

The publisher and the editorial board hope that this book will prove to be a valuable piece of knowledge for researchers, students, practitioners and scholars across the globe.

List of Contributors

Shawaqfeh MS, Bhinder MT, Halum AS, Harrington C, Muflih S and Do T
Nova Southeastern University, Palm Beach Gardens, Florida, United States

Chi-Chen Hong
Department of Cancer Prevention and Control, Roswell Park Cancer Institute, Buffalo NY, USA

Anand B Shah, Caitlin M Jackowiak, Hsin-Wei Fu, George K Nimako, Dimitra Bitikofer and Alice C Ceacareanu
Department of Pharmacy Practice, School of Pharmacy and Pharmacy and Pharmaceutical Sciences, State University of New York at Buffalo, Buffalo NY, USA

Ellen Kossoff
Department of Pharmacy, Roswell Park Cancer Institute, Buffalo NY, USA

Stephen B Edge
Department of Surgical Oncology, Roswell Park Cancer Institute, Buffalo NY, USA

Guo Y, Li Y and Jia Y
Scientific Research Building, Fuwai Hospital, No 167 Beilishi Road, West District, Beijing, People's Republic of China

Gadzhanova S and Roughead E
Division of Health Sciences, School of Pharmacy and Medical Sciences, University of South Australia, City East Campus-R3-17B, Australia

Vitale G, Simonetti G, Conti F, Cursaro C, Scuteri A, Brodosi L, Vukotic R, Loggi E, Gamal N, Pirillo L, Cicero AF and Andreone P
Department of Medical and Surgical Sciences, University of Bologna, Bologna, Italy

Taruschio G and Boncompagni G
Servizio Psichiatrico di Diagnosi e Cura, Azienda USL, Bologna, Italy

Datar P
Sinhgad Institute of Pharmacy, Narhe, Pune, Maharashtra, India

Chedi BAZ
Department of Pharmacology, Bayero University Kano, Nigeria

Abdu-Aguye I and Kwanashie HO
Department of Pharmacology and Therapeutics, Ahmadu Bello University, Zaria, Nigeria

Leblond J
Department of Pharmacy, Centre hospitalier universitaire de Sherbrooke, Sherbrooke, Canada

Beauchesne MF
Department of Pharmacy, Centre hospitalier universitaire de Sherbrooke, Sherbrooke, Canada
Research Center, Hôpital du Sacré-Coeur de Montréal, Montréal, Canada

B Cossette B
Department of Pharmacy, Centre hospitalier universitaire de Sherbrooke, Sherbrooke, Canada
Faculty of Medicine and Health Sciences, Université de Sherbrooke, Sherbrooke, Canada

Blais L
Faculty of Pharmacy, Université de Montréal, Montréal, Canada
Research Center, Hôpital du Sacré-Coeur de Montréal, Montréal, Canada

Garant MP
CR-CHUS, Centre hospitalier universitaire de Sherbrooke, Sherbrooke, Canada

Bernier F
CR-CHUS, Centre hospitalier universitaire de Sherbrooke, Sherbrooke, Canada
Department of Medicine, Centre hospitalier universitaire de Sherbrooke, Sherbrooke, Canada
Faculty of Medicine and Health Sciences, Université de Sherbrooke, Sherbrooke, Canada

Lanthier L
Department of Medicine, Centre hospitalier universitaire de Sherbrooke, Sherbrooke, Canada
Faculty of Medicine and Health Sciences, Université de Sherbrooke, Sherbrooke, Canada

Frédéric Grondin RN
Department of Nursing, Centre hospitalier universitaire de Sherbrooke, Sherbrooke, Canada

Wieslaw A Jedrychowski, Elżbieta Flak, Elzbieta Mroz and Agata Sowa
Chair of Epidemiology and Preventive Medicine, Jagiellonian University Medical College in Krakow, Poland

Maria Butscher
Polish-American Institute of Pediatrics, Jagiellonian University Medical College in Krakow, Poland

Addisu Alemayehu Gube
Department of Nursing, College of Medicine and Health Sciences, Arbaminch University, Arbaminch, Ethiopia

Rufael Gonfa and Tarekegn Tadesse
Department of Pharmacy, College of Medicine and Health Sciences, Ambo University, Ambo, Ethiopia

Badraddin Mohammed Al-Hadiya
Departments of Pharmaceutical Chemistry, College of Pharmacy, King Saud University, Riyadh, Saudi Arabia

Mohamed Fahad AlAjmi
Departments of Pharmacognosy, College of Pharmacy, King Saud University, Riyadh, Saudi Arabia

Kamal Eldin Hussein El Tahir
Departments of Pharmacology, College of Pharmacy, King Saud University, Riyadh, Saudi Arabia

Alomi YA
National Clinical Pharmacy and Pharmacy Practice Programs, Pharmacy R&D Administration, Riyadh, Saudi Arabia

AL- Mudaiheem H
National Drug Information Center, General Administration of Pharmaceutical Care Department, Ministry of Health, Saudi Arabia

Alsharfa A
Drug Information Center, Pharmaceutical Care Department, Ras Tanoura Hospital, East Province, Ministry of Health, Saudi Arabia

Albassri H
Drug Information Center, Pharmaceutical Care Department, Saud Bin Jalawi Hospital, Alahasa, Ministry of Health, Saudi Arabia

Alonizi K
Regional Drug Information Center, Pharmaceutical Care Administration, Tabouk, Ministry of Health, Saudi Arabia

Alothaian M
Drug Information Center, Pharmaceutical Care Department, King Fahad Hospital, Alahasa, Ministry of Health Saudi Arabia

Alreshidi M
Pharmaceutical Care Administration, Hail, Ministry of Health, Saudi Arabia

Alzahrani T
Training and Education Administration, Almadina Amonaoura, Ministry of Health, Saudi Arabia

Gelaw BK, Mohammed A, Tegegne GT, Defersha AD, Fromsa M, Tadesse E, Thrumurgan G and Ahmed M
Department of Pharmacy, College of Medicine and Health Science, Ambo University, Oromia, Ethiopia

Teoh BC and Tew MM
Kuala Muda District Health Office, Kedah, Malaysia

Alrasheedy AA
Pharmacy Practice Department, College of Pharmacy, Qassim University, Saudi Arabia

Hassali MA
School of Pharmaceutical Sciences, Universiti Sains Malaysia, Penang, Malaysia

Samsudin MA
School of Educational Studies, Universitis Sains Malaysia, Penang, Malaysia

Sarah Mahmoud and El Samia Mohamed
Pharmacist, Alexandria Main University Hospital, Egypt

Zahira Metwaly Gad
Professor of Epidemiology, Epidemiology Department, High Institute of Public Health, Alexandria University, Egypt

Nessrin Ahmed El-Nimr
Lecturer of Epidemiology, Epidemiology Department, High Institute of Public Health, Alexandria University, Egypt

Ahmed Abdel Hady Abdel Razek
Lecturer of Critical Medicine, Faculty of Medicine, Alexandria University, Egypt

Yamaguchi H, Satoh M, Iida Y, Matsuura M, Sato M, and Mano N
Department of Pharmaceutical Sciences, Tohoku University Hospital, Sendai, Japan

Obara T
Department of Pharmaceutical Sciences, Tohoku University Hospital, Sendai, Japan
Department of Preventive Medicine and Epidemiology, Tohoku Medical Megabank Organization, Tohoku University, Sendai, Japan

Murai Y
Department of Pharmaceutical Sciences, Tohoku University Hospital, Sendai, Japan

Pharmacy Education and Research Center, Tohoku University Graduate School of Pharmaceutical Sciences, Sendai, Japan

Sakai T
Pharmaceutical Information Center, Faculty of Pharmacy, Meijo University, Nagoya, Japan

Aoki Y
National Institute of Health Sciences, Tokyo, Japan

Ohkubo T
Department of Hygiene and Public Health, Teikyo University School of Medicine, Tokyo, Japan

Iseki K
Department of Pharmacy, Hokkaido University Hospital, Sapporo, Japan

Anne-Marie J W Scheepers-Hoeks and Rene J E Grouls
Department of Clinical Pharmacy, Catharina Hospital, Eindhoven, The Netherlands

Cees Neef
Department of Clinical Pharmacy and Toxicology, Maastricht University Medical Centre, CAPHRI, Maastricht, The Netherlands

Anne-Marie J Doppen
Department of Pharmacy, Rivas Zorggroep, Gorinchem, The Netherlands

Erik H M Korsten
Department of Signal Processing Systems, Faculty of Electronic Engineering, Eindhoven University of Technology, Eindhoven, The Netherlands
Department of Anaesthesiology, Catharina Hospital, Eindhoven, The Netherlands

Almass A Abuzaid
Department of Public Health, University of Medical Sciences and Technology, Khartoum, Sudan

Mohamed A Osman
Kirkwood Regional Center, University of Iowa, Coralville, IA, USA

Abdalla O Elkhawad
Department of Pharmacology, University of Medical Sciences and Technology, Khartoum, Sudan

Kothari DJ and Tabor A
Griffin Memorial Hospital, Norman, Oklahoma, US

Izyan A Wahab, Nicole L Pratt, Lisa M Kalisch and Elizabeth E Roughead
School of Pharmacy and Medical Sciences, Quality Use of Medicines and Pharmacy Research Centre, Sansom Institute, University of South Australia, Adelaide, South Australia, Australia

Shimoyama S
Gastrointestinal Unit, Settlement Clinic, Towa, Adachi-ku, Tokyo, Japan

Vader CI
Epilepsy Center Kempenhaeghe, Heeze, The Netherlands

IJff DM and Majoie MHJM
Epilepsy Center Kempenhaeghe, Heeze, The Netherlands
MHENS School of Mental Health & Neuroscience, Maastricht University, Maastricht, The Netherlands

Kinderen RJ
Epilepsy Center Kempenhaeghe, Heeze, The Netherlands
CAPHRI School for Public Health and Primary Care, Maastricht University, Maastricht, The Netherlands

Aldenkamp AP
Epilepsy Center Kempenhaeghe, Heeze, The Netherlands
MHENS School of Mental Health & Neuroscience, Maastricht University, Maastricht, The Netherlands
Department of Neurology, Maastricht University Medical Center, Maastricht, The Netherlands
Faculty of Electrical Engineering, University of Technology, Eindhoven, The Netherlands

Khaldoon AL-Rahawi
Department of Medicinal chemistry, Faculty of Pharmacy, Sana'a University, Sana'a, 14288, Yemen

Ali AL-Kaf, Shada Yassin and Napila AL-Shoba
Department of Medicinal chemistry, Faculty of Pharmacy, Sana'a University, Yemen

Sameh EL-Nabtity
Department of Pharmacology, Faculty of Veterinary Medicine, Zagazig University, Egypt

Kotb EL-Sayed
Department of Biochemistry and Molecular Biology, Faculty of Pharmacy, Helwan University, Egypt

Caffrey AR
Infectious Diseases Research Program, Veterans Affairs Medical Center, Providence, Rhode Island, USA

Noh E and Morrill HJ
Department of Pharmacy Practice, College of Pharmacy, University of Rhode Island, Kingston, Rhode Island, USA

LaPlante KL
Division of Infectious Diseases,Warren Alpert Medical School of Brown University, Providence, Rhode Island, USA

Mohanad A Al-Bayati and Marawan A Ahmad
University of Baghdad, Collage of Veterinary Medicine, Department of Physiology and Pharmacology, Iraq

Wael Khamas
Western University of Health Science, College of Veterinary Medicine, Pomona, CA, USA

Hua WJ and Hua WX
Department of Pharmacy, The First Affiliated Hospital of Nanchang University, Nanchang, China

Amgad M. Rabie
Pharmaceutical Organic Chemistry Department, Faculty of Pharmacy, Mansoura University, Mansoura, Dakahlia Governorate, Egypt

Nguyen D, Banerjee N and Abdelaziz D and Lewis JH
Division of Gastroenterology, Hepatology Section, Department of Medicine, Georgetown University Medical Center, Washington, USA

Marcos Cardoso Rios, Evelyne de Andrade Mota, Layana Tyara Sandes Fraga, Saulo Makerran Loureiro, Tereza Virgínia Silva Bezerra Nascimento, Ângelo Roberto Antoniolli, Divaldo Pereira de Lyra-Junior and Alex Franca
Universidade Federal de Sergipe, São Cristovão, Sergipe, Brazil

Cáceres MC, Moyano P, Fariñas H, Pijierro A, Dorado P and LLerena A
CICAB Clinical Research Centre, Extremadura University Hospital and Medical School, Badajoz, Spain

Cobaleda J
CICAB Clinical Research Centre, Extremadura University Hospital and Medical School, Badajoz, Spain
Ciudad Jardin Primary Health Care Center.SES Servicio Extremeño de Salud, Badajoz, Spain

Oliveira L and Santos Z
Department of Psychiatry, Psycho-Oncology Unit, Coimbra University Hospital Centre, Coimbra, Portugal

Vaqué A
Drug Safety and Pharmacovigilance. Laboratorios del Dr. Esteve, Barcelona, Spain

Sust M
Clinical Investigation, Laboratorios del Dr. Esteve, Barcelona, Spain

Gascón N
Drug Safety and Pharmacovigilance. Laboratorios del Dr. Esteve, Barcelona, Spain

Puyada A
Clinical Investigation, Laboratorios del Dr. Esteve, Barcelona, Spain

Videla S
Clinical Investigation, Laboratorios del Dr. Esteve, Barcelona, Spain

Michael Soyka
Department of Psychiatry, Ludwig Maximilian University, Munich, Germany
Private Hospital Meiringen, Willigen, CH 3860 Meiringen, Switzerland

Fredy IC
Pharm D, PES College of Pharmacy, Bangalore, India

Palatty PL
Department of Pharmacology Father Muller Medical College, Mangalore, India

Iqbal PT and Manikandan TV
Cardiologist, Daya General Hospital & Speciality Centre, Thrissur, India Cardiologist, Elite Mission Hospital, Thrissur, India

Srinivasan R
Department of Pharmacy Practice, PES College of Pharmacy, Bangalore, India

Yerramilli A
Associate Professor, Sri Venkateshwara College of Pharmacy, Hyderabad, India

Veerla S, Chintala E, Guduguntla M and Velivelli P
Pharm. D Interns, Sri Venkateshwara College of Pharmacy, Department of Pharmacy Practice, Osmania University, Hyderabad, India

Sharma S
Clinical Pharmacologist, Apollo Hospitals, Jubilee Hills, Hyderabad, India

Paul R
General Medicine, Apollo Hospitals, Jubilee Hills, Hyderabad, India

Index

www.ingramcontent.com/pod-product-compliance
Lightning Source LLC
Chambersburg PA
CBHW080641200326
41458CB00013B/4701

9 781632 425782